Worldmark Global Health and Medicine Issues

Worldmark Global Health and Medicine Issues

VOLUME 2

N–Z

Brenda Wilmoth Lerner & K. Lee Lerner, Editors

GALE
CENGAGE Learning

Farmington Hills, Mich • San Francisco • New York • Waterville, Maine
Meriden, Conn • Mason, Ohio • Chicago

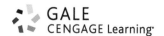

Worldmark Global Health and Medicine Issues

K. Lee Lerner and Brenda Wilmoth Lerner, Editors

Project Editor: Elizabeth P. Manar

Acquisition Editor: Michele P. LaMeau

Editorial: Kathleen J. Edgar, Jacqueline Longe, Rebecca Parks

Rights Acquisition and Management: Moriam Aigoro, Ashley M. Maynard

Imaging: John L. Watkins

Product Design: Kristine A. Julien

Composition: Evi Abou-El-Seoud

Manufacturing: Wendy Blurton

New Products Manager: Douglas A. Dentino

Cover photographs: Image of pollution © Kairos69/Shutterstock.com; Image of world map © PHOTOCREO Michal Bednarek/Shutterstock.com; Image of hand washing © africa924/Shutterstock.com; and Image of scientist in laboratory © A and N photography/Shutterstock.com.

Inside art: Image of DNA strands © vitstudio/Shutterstock.com

While every effort has been made to ensure the reliability of the information presented in this publication, Gale, a part of Cengage Learning, does not guarantee the accuracy of the data contained herein. Gale accepts no payment for listing; and inclusion in the publication of any organization, agency, institution, publication, service, or individual does not imply endorsement of the editors or publisher. Errors brought to the attention of the publisher and verified to the satisfaction of the publisher will be corrected in future editions.

LIBRARY OF CONGRESS CATALOGING-IN-PUBLICATION DATA

Worldmark global health and medicine issues / K. Lee Lerner & Brenda Wilmoth Lerner, editors.
     p. ; cm.
   Includes bibliographical references and index.
   ISBN 978-1-4103-1752-0 (set : alk. paper) — ISBN 978-1-4103-1753-7 (v. 1 : alk. paper) — ISBN 978-1-4103-1754-4 (v. 2 : alk. paper) — ISBN 978-1-4103-1755-1 (e-book)
   I. Lerner, K. Lee, editor.   II. Lerner, Brenda Wilmoth, editor.
   [DNLM: 1. Global Health—Encyclopedias—English.   2. Disease—Encyclopedias—English.   3. International Agencies—Encyclopedias—English.   WB 13]
   RC81.A2
   616.003—dc23
                                                                  2015010922

Gale
27500 Drake Rd.
Farmington Hills, MI 48331-3535

978-1-4103-1752-0 (set)
978-1-4103-1753-7 (vol. 1)
978-1-4103-1754-4 (vol. 2)

This title is also available as an e-book.
ISBN-13: 978-1-4103-1755-1
Contact your Gale sales representative for ordering information.

Printed in China
1 2 3 4 5 6 7 19 18 17 16 15

Table of Contents

VOLUME 2: N-Z

Introduction

Many of the great successes in public health and medicine also serve as important social milestones for humanity, especially with regard to the prevention and treatment of disease. While civic sanitation, water purification, immunization, and antibiotics have dramatically reduced the overall morbidity and the mortality of disease in advanced nations, much of the world is still ravaged by disease and epidemics, and new threats—including lifestyle diseases—constantly appear to challenge the most advanced medical and public health systems.

A collection of 90 entries on topics covering current global health issues, *Worldmark Global Health and Medicine Issues* is devoted to helping students and general readers quickly grasp the essence and complexities of often quickly-evolving global health issues.

At its core, *Worldmark Global Health and Medicine Issues* contains accessible explanations of many recent scientific advances in public health, as well as advances in medicine, molecular biology, genetics, epidemiology, and related fields.

Another key and distinguishing feature of *Worldmark Global Health and Medicine Issues* is an attempt to articulate links between science and social facets of global health issues. Health and medicine issues cannot be distantly cast from their intimate influence over daily life, economic impacts, and social context. Accordingly, a focus of *Worldmark Global Health and Medicine Issues* is the identification of the social determinants of health.

Global health issues can also arouse passionate debate as to effective and appropriate solutions. By illuminating global health issues as a nexus of science, ethics, economics, and policy, *Worldmark Global Health and Medicine Issues* serves both scientists and non-scientists searching to formulate rational opinions on an array of issues. In turn, issues that were once purely social or ethical issues (such as sexuality or alcoholism) are explained as aspects of human behavior and personality determined or influenced by genetics.

Worldmark Global Health and Medicine Issues also attempts to capture the increasing influence of wellness and preventative health measures in responding to public health issues.

The pace of change in facets of global health issues dealing with emerging diseases is daunting, and it is inevitable that as soon as this book went to press, some new threat emerged or some exiting threat reasserted its peril. For this reason, *Worldmark Global Health and Medicine Issues* attempts to lay a broader foundation supporting an understanding of how scientists detect novel diseases and how policy makers have responded to such challenges in the past.

Social and political issues can still arise out of even the most effective and seemingly well-intended of medical advances. For example, although childhood diseases such as measles, mumps, whooping cough, and diphtheria have been effectively controlled by childhood vaccinations, some parents resist or reject vaccinating their own children because they feel that the small personal risk is not mitigated by the larger social benefit of disease control. By opting out of the system (by relying on the immunizations of others to reduce the risk of disease), they simultaneously leave their own children vulnerable while lowering protection for some of most immunologically vulnerable members of their community (infants and immunocompromised individuals).

The interplay of complex ethical and social considerations is also evident when considering the general rise of infectious diseases that sometimes occurs as an unintended side effect of the otherwise beneficial use of medications. Nearly half the world's population, for example, is infected with the bacterium that causes tuberculosis, or TB (although for most people the infection is inactive), yet the organism causing some new cases of TB is evolving toward a greater resistance to the antibiotics that were once effective in treating TB. Such statistics take on added social dimension when considering that TB disproportionately impacts certain social groups, such as the elderly, minority groups, and people infected with HIV.

In an age of globalization, our common biology and biochemistry unite us across culture and geography, but also make us susceptible to contracting and transmitting infectious disease. Increased contact between societies raises new biomedical concerns about the potential spread of disease and sparks social debate regarding the nature and extent of medical cooperation across a varied political landscape. A shrinking global village, beneficial in many cultural and economic aspects, also increases the possibility that the terrible loss of life associated with the plagues of the Middle Ages or with the pandemic influenza outbreak of 1918–1919 might once again threaten humanity on a worldwide scale. Often ominous social and political implications of global health issues cannot be ignored when death continues to cast a disproportionately longer shadow over the poorest nations.

Although specific diseases may be statistically associated with particular regions or other demographics, disease does not recognize social class or political boundary. In our intimately connected world, an outbreak of disease in a remote area may quickly transform into a global threat. Given the opportunity, the agents of disease may spread at the speed of modern travel, and also leap from animals to humans.

Contributors to *Worldmark Global Health and Medicine Issues* include an array of experienced scientists and journalists with expertise in global health issues and a real-world appreciation for the proper context in which issues must be framed.

Brenda Wilmoth Lerner & K. Lee Lerner, Editors
Cambridge, Massachusetts
2015

Organization

All entries in *Worldmark Global Health and Medicine Issues* share a common structure, providing consistent coverage of topics and a simple way of comparing basic elements of one topic with another. Each entry has six parts: introduction, historical background, impacts and issues, future implications, bibliography, and a sidebar, which discusses a related topic, such as an important organization or concept. Some entries also contain an excerpt from a relevant historical text or contemporary article illustrating the topic. The entries are organized A to Z.

Worldmark Global Health and Medicine Issues contains other elements to help guide students studying these topics. It includes a chronology of important historical events; a general bibliography on health and medicine resources; a glossary of important terms in the field; a list of organizations and advocacy groups; about 80 line art images, such as tables and charts, that illustrate various aspects of health and medicine issues; and more than 200 full-color photographs related to the entry topics. Coverage of specific health and medicine subjects can be located in the general index.

Suggestions Welcome

Comments on *Worldmark Global Health and Medicine Issues* are cordially invited. Please write:

The Editors

Worldmark Global Health and Medicine Issues

Gale

27500 Drake Rd.

Farmington Hills, Michigan 48331-3535

Gale, a part of Cengage Learning, does not endorse any of the organizations, products, or methods mentioned in this title.

The websites appearing in *Worldmark Global Health and Medicine Issues* have been reviewed by Gale to provide additional information. Gale is not responsible for the content or operations policies of these websites. Further, Gale is not responsible for the conduct of website providers who offer electronic texts that may infringe on the legal right of copyright holders.

Using Primary Sources

Many of the entries in *Worldmark Global Health and Medicine Issues* contain documents written by or transcribed from (in the case of interviews and speeches) key players in the field covered in the entry. These documents, formally known as *primary sources*, provide insight into the historical setting during which they were produced and offer direct, firsthand witness to the events of their day or thoughts of important people in a particular activity or field. Primary sources come from a wide spectrum of resources, and the definition of what constitutes a primary source depends a great deal on the course of study or the institution of higher learning offering the definition. For the purposes of *Worldmark Global Health and Medicine Issues*, categories of primary sources include:

- Documents containing firsthand accounts of historic events by witnesses and participants. This category includes diaries, journal entries, and blogs; letters and e-mails; newspaper articles; interviews and oral histories; memoirs and autobiographies; and testimony in legal proceedings.

- Documents or works representing the official views of both government leaders and leaders of other organizations. These include policy statements, speeches, interviews, press releases, government reports, and legislation.

- Works of art, including (but not limited to) photographs, poems, and songs, as well as advertisements and reviews of those works that help establish an understanding of the cultural environment with regard to attitudes and perceptions of events.

- Secondary and tertiary sources. In some cases, secondary or tertiary sources may be considered primary sources. For example, a work written many years after an event or to summarize the event that includes quotes, recollections, or retrospectives by participants in the earlier event.

Analysis of Primary Sources

The primary material in *Worldmark Global Health and Medicine Issues* is intended to generate interest and lay a foundation for further inquiry and study.

In order to analyze a primary source properly, readers should remain skeptical and develop probing questions about the source. Using historical documents requires that readers analyze them carefully and extract specific information. However, readers must also read "beyond the text" to garner larger clues about the social impact of the primary source.

In addition to providing information about the topics, primary sources may also supply a wealth of insight into their creator's viewpoint. For example, when reading a news article about an event, consider whether the reporter's words also indicate something about his or her origin, bias, prejudices, or intended audience.

It is important to view the primary source within the historical and social context existing at its creation. Readers should remember that primary sources may contain information later proven to be false or viewpoints and terms unacceptable to future generations. If, for example, a newspaper article is written within hours or days of an event, later developments may reveal some assertions in the original article as false or misleading.

Test Conclusions and Ideas

It is critical to test whatever opinion or working hypothesis you, the reader, form from reading the primary source(s) against other facts and sources related to the incident. For example, it might be wrong to conclude that factual mistakes are deliberate unless evidence can be produced of a pattern and practice of such mistakes with an intent to promote a false idea.

Despite the fact that some primary sources can contain false information or lead readers to false conclusions based on the facts presented, they remain an invaluable resource regarding past events. Primary sources allow readers and researchers to come as close as possible to understanding the perceptions and context of events and thus to more fully appreciate how and why misconceptions occur.

Glossary of Terms

A

ACQUIRED (ADAPTIVE) IMMUNITY: Immunity is the ability to resist infection and is subdivided into innate immunity, with which an individual is born, and acquired, or adaptive, immunity, which develops according to circumstances and is targeted to a specific pathogen. There are two types of acquired immunity, known as active and passive. Active immunity is either humoral, involving production of antibody molecules against a bacterium or virus, or cell-mediated, in which T-cells are mobilized against infected cells. Infection and immunization can both induce acquired immunity. Passive immunity is induced by injection of the serum of a person who is already immune to a particular infection.

ACQUIRED IMMUNE DEFICIENCY SYNDROME (AIDS): A disease of the immune system caused by the human immunodeficiency virus (HIV). It is characterized by the destruction of a particular type of white blood cell and increased susceptibility to infection and other diseases.

ACTIVE INFECTION: An active infection is one that is currently producing symptoms or in which the infective agent is multiplying rapidly. In contrast, a latent infection is one in which the infective agent is present but not causing symptoms or damage to the body nor reproducing at a significant rate.

ADAPTIVE IMMUNITY: Adaptive immunity is another term for acquired immunity, referring to the resistance to infection that develops through life and is targeted to a specific pathogen. There are two types of adaptive immunity, known as active and passive. Active immunity is either humoral, involving production of antibody molecules against a bacterium or virus, or cell-mediated, in which T-cells are mobilized against infected cells. Infection and immunization can

both induce acquired immunity. Passive immunity is induced by the transfer of antibodies from one person to another, and occurs when antibodies in blood products from a person who is immune to a particular disease are injected into a susceptible person.

AIDS (ACQUIRED IMMUNE DEFICIENCY SYNDROME): A disease of the immune system caused by the human immunodeficiency virus (HIV). It is characterized by the destruction of a particular type of white blood cell and increased susceptibility to infection and other diseases.

AIRBORNE PRECAUTIONS: Airborne precautions are procedures that are designed to reduce the chance that certain disease-causing (pathogenic) microorganisms will be transmitted through the air.

AIRBORNE TRANSMISSION: Airborne transmission refers to the ability of a disease-causing (pathogenic) microorganism to be spread through the air by droplets expelled during sneezing or coughing.

ALLELE: Any of two or more alternative forms of a gene that occupy the same location on a chromosome.

ALLERGIES: An allergy is an excessive or hypersensitive response of the immune system to substances (allergens) in the environment. Instead of fighting off a disease-causing foreign substance, the immune system launches a complex series of actions against the particular irritating allergen. The immune response may be accompanied by a number of stressful symptoms, ranging from mild to life threatening. In rare cases, an allergic reaction leads to anaphylactic shock—a condition characterized by a sudden drop in blood pressure, difficulty in breathing, skin irritation, collapse, and possible death.

AMEBIC DYSENTERY: Amebic (or amoebic) dysentery, which is also referred to as amebiasis or amoebiasis, is an inflammation of the intestine caused by the parasite *Entamoeba histolytica*. The severe form of the malady is characterized by the formation of localized lesions (ulcers) in the intestine, especially in the colon; abscesses in the liver and the brain; vomiting; severe diarrhea with fluid loss leading to dehydration; and abdominal pain.

ANAEROBIC BACTERIA: Bacteria that grow without oxygen, also called anaerobic bacteria or anaerobes. Anaerobic bacteria can infect deep wounds, deep tissues, and internal organs where there is little oxygen. These infections are characterized by abscess formation, foul-smelling pus, and tissue destruction.

ANTHRAX: Anthrax refers to a disease that is caused by the bacterium *Bacillus anthracis*. The bacterium can enter the body via a wound in the skin (cutaneous anthrax), via contaminated food or liquid (gastrointestinal anthrax), or can be inhaled (inhalation anthrax).

ANTIBACTERIAL: A substance that reduces the number of or kills germs (bacteria and other microorganisms but not viruses). Also often a term used to describe a drug used to treat bacterial infections.

ANTIBIOTIC: A drug, such as penicillin, used to fight infections caused by bacteria. Antibiotics act only on bacteria and are not effective against viruses.

ANTIBIOTIC RESISTANCE: The ability of bacteria to resist the actions of antibiotic drugs.

ANTIBIOTIC SENSITIVITY: Antibiotic sensitivity refers to the susceptibility of a bacterium to an antibiotic. Each type of bacteria can be killed by some types of antibiotics and not be affected by other types. Different types of bacteria exhibit different patterns of antibiotic sensitivity.

ANTIBODIES: Antibodies, or Y-shaped immunoglobulins, are proteins found in the blood that help to fight against foreign substances called antigens. Antigens, which are usually proteins or polysaccharides, stimulate the immune system to produce antibodies. The antibodies inactivate the antigen and help to remove it from the body. While antigens can be the source of infections from pathogenic bacteria and viruses, organic molecules detrimental to the body from internal or environmental sources also act as antigens. Genetic engineering and the use of various mutational mechanisms allow the construction of a vast array of antibodies (each with a unique genetic sequence).

ANTIGEN: Antigens, which are usually proteins or polysaccharides, stimulate the immune system to produce antibodies. The antibodies inactivate the antigen and help to remove it from the body. While antigens can be the source of infections from pathogenic bacteria and viruses, organic molecules detrimental to the body from internal or environmental sources also act as antigens. Genetic engineering and the use of various mutational mechanisms allow the construction of a vast array of antibodies (each with a unique genetic sequence).

ANTIHELMINTHIC: Antihelminthic drugs are medicines that rid the body of helminths (parasitic worms).

ANTIMICROBIAL: An antimicrobial material slows the growth of bacteria or is able to kill bacteria. Antimicrobial materials include antibiotics (which can be used inside the body) and disinfectants (which can only be used outside the body).

ANTIRETROVIRAL THERAPY (ART): Antiretroviral treatment (ART) with antiretroviral (ARV) drugs prevents the reproduction of a type of virus called a retrovirus. The human immunodeficiency virus (HIV), which causes acquired immune deficiency syndrome (AIDS, also known as acquired immunodeficiency syndrome), is a retrovirus. ARV drugs are therefore used to treat HIV infections. These medicines cannot prevent or cure HIV infection, but they help to keep the virus in check.

ANTISEPTIC: A substance that prevents or stops the growth and multiplication of microorganisms in or on living tissue.

ANTITOXIN: An antidote to a toxin that neutralizes its poisonous effects.

ANTIVIRAL DRUGS: Antiviral drugs are compounds that are used to prevent or treat viral infections, via the disruption of an infectious mechanism used by the virus, or to treat the symptoms of an infection.

ARBOVIRUS: An arbovirus is a virus that is typically spread by blood-sucking insects, most commonly mosquitoes. Over 100 types of arboviruses cause disease in humans. Yellow fever and dengue fever are two examples.

ARENAVIRUS: An arenavirus is a virus that belongs in a viral family known as *Arenaviridae*. The name arenavirus derives from the appearance of the spherical virus particles when cut into thin sections and viewed using a transmission electron microscope. The interior of the particles is grainy or sandy in appearance, due to the presence of ribosomes that have been acquired from the host cell. The Latin designation *arena* means "sandy."

ARTHROPOD-BORNE VIRUS: A virus caused by one of a phylum of organisms characterized by exoskeletons and segmented bodies, such as insects.

ASEPSIS: Asepsis means without germs, more specifically without microorganisms.

ASYMPTOMATIC: A state in which an individual does not exhibit or experience symptoms of a disease.

ATROPHY: Decreasing in size or wasting away of a body part or tissue.

ATTENUATED: An attenuated bacterium or virus has been weakened and is often used as the basis of a vaccine against the specific disease caused by the bacterium or virus.

ATTENUATED STRAIN: A specific strain of bacteria that has been killed or weakened, often used as the basis of a vaccine against the specific disease caused by the bacterium.

AUTOIMMUNE DISEASE: A disease in which the body's defense system attacks its own tissues and organs.

AUTOINFECTION: Autoinfection is the reinfection of the body by a disease organism already in the body, such as eggs left by a parasitic worm.

B

BACTERIA: Single-celled microorganisms that live in soil, water, plants, and animals. Their activities range from the development of disease to fermentation. They play a key role in the decay of organic matter and the cycling of nutrients. Bacteria exist in various shapes, including spherical, rod-shaped, and spiral. Some bacteria are agents of disease. Different types of bacteria cause many sexually transmitted diseases, including syphilis, gonorrhea, and chlamydia. Bacteria also cause diseases such as typhoid, dysentery, and tetanus. Bacterium is the singular form of bacteria.

BACTERIOCIDAL: Bacteriocidal is a term that refers to the treatment of a bacterium such that the organism is killed. A bacteriocidal treatment is always lethal and is also referred to as sterilization.

BACTERIOLOGICAL STRAIN: A bacterial subclass of a particular tribe and genus.

BED NETS: A type of netting that provides protection from diseases caused by insects such as flies and mosquitoes. It is often used when sleeping to allow air to flow through its mesh structure while preventing insects from biting.

BIOINFORMATICS: Bioinformatics, or computational biology, refers to the development of new database methods to store genomic information (information related to genes and the genetic sequence), computational software programs, and methods to extract, process, and evaluate this information. Bioinformatics also refers to the refinement of existing techniques to acquire the genomic data. Finding genes and determining their function, predicting the structure of proteins and sequence of ribonucleic acid (RNA) from the available sequence of deoxyribonucleic acid (DNA), and determining the evolutionary relationship of proteins and DNA sequences are aspects of bioinformatics.

BIOLOGICAL WEAPON: A weapon that contains or disperses a biological toxin, disease-causing microorganism, or other biological agent intended to harm or kill plants, animals, or humans.

BIOSAFETY LEVEL 4 FACILITY: A specialized biosafety laboratory that deals with dangerous or exotic infectious agents or biohazards that are considered high risks for spreading life-threatening diseases, either because the disease is spread through aerosols or because there is no therapy or vaccine to counter the disease.

BIOTECHNOLOGY: Use of biological organisms, systems, or processes to make or modify products.

BLOOD-BORNE PATHOGENS: Disease-causing agents carried or transported in the blood. Blood-borne infections are those in which the infectious agent is transmitted from one person to another via contaminated blood.

BLOOD-BORNE ROUTE: Via the blood. For example, blood-borne pathogens are pathogens (disease-causing agents) carried or transported in the blood. Bloodborne infections are those in which the infectious agent is transmitted from one person to another via contaminated blood. Infections of the blood can occur as a result of the spread of an ongoing infection caused by bacteria such as *Yersinia pestis, Haemophilus influenzae,* or *Staphylococcus aureus.*

BOTULINUM TOXIN: Botulinum toxin is among the most poisonous substances known. The toxin, which can be ingested or inhaled, and which disrupts transmission of nerve impulses to muscles, is naturally produced by the bacterium *Clostridium botulinum.* Certain strains of *C. baratii* and *C. butyricum* can also be capable of producing the toxin.

BOTULISM: Botulism is an illness generally produced by a toxin that is released by the soil bacterium *Clostridium botulinum.* Some strains of *C. baratii* and *C. butyricum* produce the toxin, as well. The toxins affect nerves and can produce paralysis. The paralysis can affect the functioning of organs and tissues that are vital to life.

BROAD-SPECTRUM ANTIBIOTICS: Broad-spectrum antibiotics are drugs that kill a wide range of bacteria rather than just those from a specific family. For example, amoxicillin is a broad-spectrum antibiotic that is used against many common illnesses such as ear infections, pneumonia, and urinary tract infections.

C

CAMPYLOBACTERIOSIS: Campylobacteriosis is a bacterial infection of the intestinal tract of humans. The infection, which typically results in diarrhea, is caused by members of the genus *Campylobacter*. Worldwide, approximately 5 to 14 percent of all diarrhea may be the result of campylobacteriosis.

CARBOLIC ACID: An acidic compound that, when diluted with water, is used as an antiseptic and disinfectant.

CARCINOGEN: A carcinogen is any biological, chemical, or physical substance or agent that can cause cancer. There are over 100 different types of cancer, which can be distinguished by the type of cell or organ that is affected, the treatment plan employed, and the cause of the cancer. Most of the carcinogens that are commonly discussed come from chemical sources artificially produced by humans. Some of the better-known carcinogens are the pesticide DDT (dichlorodiphenyltrichloroethane), asbestos, and the carcinogens produced when tobacco is smoked.

CASE FATALITY RATE: The rate of patients suffering disease or injury that die as a result of that disease or injury during a specific period of time.

CASE FATALITY RATIO: A ratio indicating the amount of persons who die as a result of a particular disease, usually expressed as a percentage or as the number of deaths per 1,000 cases.

CATALYST: Substance that speeds up a chemical process without actually changing the products of reaction.

CD4 T CELLS: CD4 cells are a type of T cell found in the immune system that are characterized by the presence of a CD4 antigen protein on their surface. These are the cells most often destroyed as a result of HIV infection.

CENTERS FOR DISEASE CONTROL AND PREVENTION (CDC): The Centers for Disease Control and Prevention (CDC) is one of the primary public health institutions in the world. The CDC is headquartered in Atlanta, Georgia, with facilities at nine other sites in the United States. The centers are the focus of U.S. government efforts to develop and implement prevention and control strategies for diseases, including those of microbiological origin.

CESTODE: A class of worms characterized by flat, segmented bodies, commonly known as tapeworms.

CHAGAS DISEASE: Chagas disease is a human infection that is caused by a microorganism that establishes a parasitic relationship with a human host as part of its life cycle. The disease is named for the Brazilian physician Carlos Chagas, who in 1909 described the involvement of the flagellated protozoan known as *Trypanosoma cruzi* in a prevalent disease in South America.

CHAIN OF TRANSMISSION: Chain of transmission refers to the route by which an infection is spread from its source to a susceptible host. An example of a chain of transmission is the spread of malaria from an infected animal to humans via mosquitoes.

CHILDBED FEVER: Childbed fever, also known as puerperal infection or postpartum infection, is a bacterial infection occurring in women following childbirth, causing fever and in some cases blood poisoning and possible death.

CHRONIC INFECTION: A chronic infection persists for a prolonged period of time—months or even years—in the host. This lengthy persistence is due to a number of factors, which can include masking of the disease-causing agent (e.g., bacteria) from the immune system, invasion of host cells, and the establishment of an infection that is resistant to antibacterial agents.

CIRRHOSIS: Cirrhosis is a chronic, degenerative, irreversible liver disease in which normal liver cells are damaged and are then replaced by scar tissue. Cirrhosis changes the structure of the liver and the blood vessels that nourish it. The disease reduces the liver's ability to manufacture proteins and process hormones, nutrients, medications, and poisons.

CLINICAL TRIALS: According to the U.S. National Institutes of Health, a clinical trial is "a research study to answer specific questions about vaccines or new therapies or new ways of using known treatments." These studies allow researchers to determine whether new drugs or treatments are safe and effective. When conducted carefully, clinical trials can provide fast and safe answers to these questions.

CLUSTER: In epidemiology, cluster refers to a grouping of individuals contracting an infectious disease or food-borne illness very close in time or place.

COHORT: A cohort is a group of people (or any species) sharing a common characteristic. Cohorts are identified and grouped in cohort studies to determine the frequency of diseases or the kinds of disease outcomes over time.

COHORTING: Cohorting is the practice of grouping persons with similar infections or symptoms together, sometimes in order to reduce transmission of infection to others.

COMMUNITY-ACQUIRED INFECTION: Community-acquired infection is an infection that develops outside of a hospital, in the general community. It differs from hospital-acquired infections in that those who are infected are typically in better health than hospitalized people.

CONTACT PRECAUTIONS: Contact precautions are actions developed to minimize the transfer of microorganisms directly by physical contact and indirectly by touching a contaminated surface.

CONTAGIOUS: A disease that is easily spread among a population, usually by casual person-to-person contact.

CONTAMINATED: The unwanted presence of a microorganism or compound in a particular environment. That environment can be in the laboratory setting, for example, in a medium being used for the growth of a species of bacteria during an experiment. Another environment can be the human body, where contamination by bacteria can produce an infection. Contamination by bacteria and viruses can occur on several levels, and their presence can adversely influence the results of experiments. Outside the laboratory, bacteria and viruses can contaminate drinking water supplies, foodstuffs, and other products, thus causing illness.

CREUTZFELDT-JAKOB DISEASE (CJD): Creutzfeldt-Jakob disease (CJD) is a transmissible, rapidly progressing, fatal neurodegenerative disorder related to bovine spongiform encephalopathy (BSE), commonly called mad cow disease.

CULL: A cull is the selection, often for destruction, of a part of an animal population. Often done just to reduce numbers, a widespread cull was carried out during the epidemic of bovine spongiform encephalopathy (BSE or mad cow disease) in the United Kingdom during the 1980s and has also been carried out in bird populations during outbreaks of avian influenza.

CULTURE: A culture is a single species of microorganism that is isolated and grown under controlled conditions. The German bacteriologist Robert Koch first developed culturing techniques in the late 1870s. Following Koch's initial use of cultures, medical scientists quickly sought to identify other pathogens using such techniques. Today bacterial cultures are used as basic tools in microbiology and medicine.

CULTURE AND SENSITIVITY: Culture and sensitivity refer to laboratory tests that are used to identify the type of microorganism causing an infection and the compounds to which the identified organism is sensitive and resistant. In the case of bacteria, this approach permits the selection of antibiotics that will be most effective in dealing with the infection.

CUTANEOUS: Pertaining to the skin.

CYST: Refers to either a closed cavity or sac or the stage of life during which some parasites live inside an enclosed area. In a protozoan's life, it is a stage when it is covered by a tough outer shell and has become dormant.

CYTOKINE: Cytokines are a family of small proteins that mediate an organism's response to injury or infection. Cytokines operate by transmitting signals between cells in an organism. Minute quantities of cytokines are secreted, each by a single cell type, and regulate functions in other cells by binding with specific receptors. Their interactions with the receptors produce secondary signals that inhibit or enhance the action of certain genes within the cell. Unlike endocrine hormones, which can act throughout the body, most cytokines act locally near the cells that produced them.

D

DEFINITIVE HOST: The organism in which a parasite reaches reproductive maturity.

DEHYDRATION: Dehydration is the loss of water and salts essential for normal bodily function. It occurs when the body loses more fluid than it takes in. Water is very important to the human body because it makes up about 70 percent of the muscles, around 75 percent of the brain, and approximately 92 percent of the blood. A person who weighs about 150 pounds (68 kilograms) will contain about 80 quarts (just over 75 liters) of water. About two cups of water are lost each day just from regular breathing. If the body sweats more and breathes more heavily than normal, the human body loses even more water. Dehydration occurs when that lost water is not replenished.

DEMENTIA: Dementia, which is from the Latin word *dement* meaning "away mind," is a progressive deterioration and eventual loss of mental ability that is severe enough to interfere with normal activities of daily living; lasts more than six months; has not been present since birth; and is not associated with a loss or alteration of consciousness. Dementia is a group of symptoms caused by gradual death of brain cells.

Dementia is usually caused by degeneration in the cerebral cortex, the part of the brain responsible for thoughts, memories, actions, and personality. Death of brain cells in this region leads to the cognitive impairment that characterizes dementia.

DEMOGRAPHICS: The characteristics of human populations or specific parts of human populations, most often reported through statistics.

DEOXYRIBONUCLEIC ACID (DNA): Deoxyribonucleic acid (DNA) is a double-stranded, helical molecule that forms the molecular basis for heredity in most organisms.

DIAGNOSIS: Identification of a disease or disorder.

DIARRHEA: To most individuals, diarrhea means an increased frequency or decreased consistency of bowel movements; however, the medical definition is more exact than this explanation. In many developed countries, the average number of bowel movements is three per day. However, researchers have found that diarrhea, which is not a specific disease, best correlates with an increase in stool weight; a stool weight above 10.5 ounces (300 grams) per day generally indicates diarrhea. This is mainly due to excess water, which normally makes up 60 to 85 percent of fecal matter. In this way, true diarrhea is distinguished from diseases that cause only an increase in the number of bowel movements (hyperdefecation) or incontinence (involuntary loss of bowel contents). Diarrhea is also classified by physicians into acute, which lasts one to two weeks, and chronic, which continues for longer than four weeks. Viral and bacterial infections are the most common causes of acute diarrhea.

DIPHTHERIA: Diphtheria is a potentially fatal, contagious bacterial disease that usually involves the nose, throat, and air passages, but may also infect the skin. Its most striking feature is the formation of a grayish membrane covering the tonsils and upper part of the throat.

DISINFECTANT: Disinfection and the use of chemical disinfectants is one key strategy of infection control. Disinfectants reduce the number of living microorganisms, usually to a level that is considered to be safe for the particular environment. Typically, this entails the destruction of those microbes that are capable of causing disease.

DISSEMINATION: The spreading of a disease in a population, or of disease organisms in the body, is dissemination. A disease that occurs over a large geographic area.

DNA: Deoxyribonucleic acid, a double-stranded, helical molecule that is found in almost all living cells and that determines the characteristics of each organism.

DNA FINGERPRINTING: DNA fingerprinting is the term applied to a range of techniques that are used to show similarities and dissimilarities between the DNA present in different individuals (or organisms).

DROPLET: A droplet is a small airborne drop or particle—less than 5 microns (a millionth of a meter) in diameter—of fluid, such as may be expelled by sneezing or coughing.

DROPLET TRANSMISSION: Droplet transmission is the spread of microorganisms from one space to another (including from person to person) via droplets that are less than 5 microns in diameter. Droplets are typically expelled into the air by coughing and sneezing.

DRUG RESISTANCE: Drug resistance develops when an infective agent, such as a bacterium, fungus, or virus, develops a lack of sensitivity to a drug that would normally be able to control or even kill it. This tends to occur with overuse of anti-infective agents, which selects out populations of microbes most able to resist them, while killing off those organisms that are most sensitive. The next time the anti-infective agent is used, it will be less effective, leading to the eventual development of resistance.

DYSENTERY: Dysentery is the inflammation of the intestines and resulting bloody diarrhea due to infection with the bacteria *Shigella* or the amoeba *Entamoeba histolytica*. Both bacterial and amoebic dysentery are infectious and are still a major problem in developing countries with primitive sanitary facilities.

E

ELECTROLYTES: Compounds that ionize in a solution; electrolytes dissolved in the blood play an important role in maintaining the proper functioning of the body.

EMERGING DISEASE: New infectious diseases such as SARS and West Nile virus, as well as previously known diseases such as malaria, tuberculosis, and bacterial pneumonias that are appearing in forms resistant to drug treatments, are termed emerging infectious diseases.

ENDEMIC: Present in a particular area or among a particular group of people.

ENTERIC: Involving the intestinal tract or relating to the intestines.

ENTEROBACTERIAL INFECTIONS: Enterobacterial infections are caused by a group of bacteria that dwell in the intestinal tract of humans and other warm-blooded animals. The bacteria are all gram-negative and rod-shaped. As a group they are termed Enterobacteriaceae. A prominent member of this group is *Escherichia coli.*

ENTEROVIRUS: Enteroviruses are a group of viruses that contain ribonucleic acid (RNA) as their genetic material. They are members of the picornavirus family. The various types of enteroviruses that infect humans are referred to as serotypes, in recognition of their different antigenic patterns. The different immune response is important, as infection with one type of enterovirus does not necessarily confer protection to infection by a different type of enterovirus. The serotypes include polio viruses, coxsackie A and B viruses, echoviruses, and a large number of what are referred to as non-polio enteroviruses.

ENZYME: Enzymes are molecules that act as critical catalysts in biological systems. Catalysts are substances that increase the rate of chemical reactions without being consumed in the reaction. Without enzymes, many reactions would require higher levels of energy and higher temperatures than exist in biological systems. Enzymes are proteins that possess specific binding sites for other molecules (substrates). A series of weak binding interactions allows enzymes to accelerate reaction rates. Enzyme kinetics is the study of enzymatic reactions and mechanisms. Enzyme inhibitor studies have allowed researchers to develop therapies for the treatment of diseases, including AIDS.

EPIDEMIC: The word *epidemic* comes from the Greek word meaning prevalent among the people and is most commonly used to describe an outbreak of an illness or disease in which the number of individual cases significantly exceeds the usual or expected number of cases in any given population.

EPIDEMIOLOGY: Epidemiology is the study of the various factors that influence the occurrence, distribution, prevention, and control of disease, injury, and other health-related events in a defined human population. By the application of various analytical techniques, including mathematical analysis of the data, the probable cause of an infectious outbreak can be pinpointed.

EPSTEIN-BARR VIRUS (EBV): Epstein-Barr virus (EBV) is part of the family of human herpes viruses. Infectious mononucleosis (IM) is the most common disease manifestation of this virus, which, once established in the host, can never be completely eradicated. Very little can be done to treat EBV; most methods can only alleviate resultant symptoms.

ERADICATE: To get rid of; the permanent reduction to zero of global incidence of a particular infection.

ETIOLOGY: The study of the cause or origin of a disease or disorder.

EXECUTIVE ORDER: Presidential orders that implement or interpret a federal statute, administrative policy, or treaty.

EXOTOXIN: A toxic protein produced during bacterial growth and metabolism and released into the environment.

F

FECAL-ORAL TRANSMISSION: The spread of disease through the transmission of minute particles of fecal material from one organism to the mouth of another organism. This can occur by drinking contaminated water, eating food that was exposed to animal or human feces (perhaps by watering plants with unclean water), or by the poor hygiene practices of those preparing food.

FILOVIRUS: A filovirus is any RNA virus that belongs to the family *Filoviridae.* Filoviruses infect primates. Marburg virus and Ebola virus are filoviruses.

FLEA: A flea is any parasitic insect of the order *Siphonaptera.* Fleas can infest many mammals, including humans, and can act as carriers (vectors) of disease.

FLORA: In microbiology, flora refers to the collective microorganisms that normally inhabit an organism or system. Human intestines, for example, contain bacteria that aid in digestion and are considered normal flora.

FOCUS: In medicine, a focus is a primary center of some disease process (for example, a cluster of abnormal cells). Foci is plural for focus (more than one focus).

FOMITE: A fomite is an object or a surface to which infectious microorganisms such as bacteria or viruses can adhere and be transmitted. Papers, clothing, dishes, and other objects can all act as fomites. Transmission is often by touch.

FOOD PRESERVATION: The term food preservation refers to any one of a number of techniques used to prevent food from spoiling. It includes methods such as canning, pickling, drying and freeze-drying, irradiation, pasteurization, smoking, and the addition of chemical additives. Food preservation has become an increasingly important component of the food industry as fewer people eat foods produced on their own lands, and as consumers expect to be able to purchase and consume foods that are out of season.

FULMINANT: A fulminant infection is an infection that appears suddenly and the symptoms of which are immediately severe.

G

GAMETOCYTE: A germ cell with the ability to divide for the purpose of producing gametes, either male gametes called spermatocytes or female gametes called oocytes.

GAMMA GLOBULIN: Gamma globulin is a term referring to a group of soluble proteins in the blood, most of which are antibodies that can mount a direct attack upon pathogens and can be used to treat various infections.

GANGRENE: Gangrene is the destruction of body tissue by a bacteria called *Clostridium perfringens* or a combination of streptococci and staphylococci bacteria. *C. perfringens* is widespread; it is found in soil and the intestinal tracts of humans and animals. It becomes dangerous only when its spores germinate, producing toxins and destructive enzymes, and germination occurs only in an anaerobic environment (one almost totally devoid of oxygen). While gangrene can develop in any part of the body, it is most common in fingers, toes, hands, feet, arms, and legs, the parts of the body most susceptible to restricted blood flow. Even a slight injury in such an area is at high risk of causing gangrene. Early treatment with antibiotics, such as penicillin, and surgery to remove the dead tissue will often reduce the need for amputation. If left untreated, gangrene results in amputation or death.

GASTROENTERITIS: Gastroenteritis is an inflammation of the stomach and the intestines. More commonly, gastroenteritis is called the stomach flu.

GENE: A gene is the fundamental physical and functional unit of heredity. Whether in a microorganism or in a human cell, a gene is an individual element of an organism's genome and determines a trait or characteristic by regulating biochemical structure or metabolic process.

GENE THERAPY: Gene therapy is the name applied to the treatment of inherited diseases by corrective genetic engineering of the dysfunctional genes. It is part of a broader field called genetic medicine, which involves the screening, diagnosis, prevention, and treatment of hereditary conditions in humans. The results of genetic screening can pinpoint a potential problem to which gene therapy can sometimes offer a solution. Genetic defects are significant in the total field of medicine, with up to 15 out of every 100 newborn infants having a hereditary disorder of greater or lesser severity. More than 2,000 genetically distinct inherited defects have been classified so far, including diabetes, cystic fibrosis, hemophilia, sickle-cell anemia, phenylketonuria, and cancer.

GENETIC ENGINEERING: Genetic engineering is the altering of the genetic material of living cells in order to make them capable of producing new substances or performing new functions. When the genetic material within the living cells (i.e., genes) is working properly, the body can develop and function smoothly. However, should a single gene—even a tiny segment of a gene go awry—the effect can be dramatic: deformities, disease, and even death are possible.

GENOME: All of the genetic information for a cell or organism. The complete sequence of genes within a cell or virus.

GENOTYPE: The genetic information that a living thing inherits from its parents that affects its makeup, appearance, and function.

GEOGRAPHIC FOCALITY: The physical location of a disease pattern, epidemic, or outbreak; the characteristics of a location created by interconnections with other places.

GEOGRAPHIC INFORMATION SYSTEM (GIS): A system for archiving, retrieving, and manipulating data that has been stored and indexed according to the geographic coordinates of its elements. The system generally can utilize a variety of data types, such as imagery, maps, tables, etc.

GEOGRAPHIC MEDICINE: Geographic medicine, also called geomedicine, is the study of how human health is affected by climate and environment.

GERM THEORY OF DISEASE: The germ theory is a fundamental tenet of medicine that states that microorganisms, which are too small to be seen without the aid of a microscope, can invade the body and cause disease.

GLOBAL OUTBREAK ALERT AND RESPONSE NETWORK (GOARN): A collaboration of resources for the rapid identification, confirmation, and response to outbreaks of international importance.

GLOBALIZATION: The integration of national and local systems into a global economy through increased trade, manufacturing, communications, and migration.

H

HARM-REDUCTION STRATEGY: In public health, a harm-reduction strategy is a public-policy scheme for reducing the amount of harm caused by a substance such as alcohol or tobacco. The phrase may refer to any medical strategy directed at reducing the harm caused by a disease, substance, or toxic medication.

HELMINTHIC DISEASE: Helminths are parasitic worms such as hookworms or flatworms. Helminthic disease by such worms is infectious. A synonym for helminthic is verminous.

HELSINKI DECLARATION: A set of ethical principles governing medical and scientific experimentation on human subjects; it was drafted by the World Medical Association and originally adopted in 1964.

HEMOLYSIS: The destruction of blood cells, an abnormal rate of which may lead to lowered levels of these cells. For example, hemolytic anemia is caused by destruction of red blood cells at a rate faster than they can be produced.

HEMORRHAGE: Very severe, massive bleeding that is difficult to control.

HEMORRHAGIC FEVER: A hemorrhagic fever is caused by viral infection and features a high fever and copious (high volume of) bleeding. The bleeding is caused by the formation of tiny blood clots throughout the bloodstream. These blood clots—also called microthrombi—deplete platelets and fibrinogen in the bloodstream. When bleeding begins, the factors needed for the clotting of the blood are scarce. Thus, uncontrolled bleeding (hemorrhage) ensues.

HEPA FILTER: A HEPA (high efficiency particulate air) filter is a filter that is designed to nearly totally remove airborne particles that are 0.3 microns (millionth of a meter) in diameter or larger. Such small particles can penetrate deeply into the lungs if inhaled.

HEPADNAVIRUSES: *Hepadnaviridae* is a family of hepadnaviruses comprised by two genera, *Avihepadnavirus* and *Orthohepadnavirus.* Hepadnaviruses have partially double-stranded DNA, and they replicate their genome in the host cells using an enzyme called reverse transcriptase. Because of this, they are also termed retroviruses. The viruses invade liver cells (hepatocytes) of vertebrates. When hepadna retroviruses invade a cell, a complete viral double-stranded (ds) DNA is made before it randomly inserts into one of the hosta's chromosomes. Once part of the chromosomal DNA, the viral DNA is then transcribed into an intermediate messenger RNA (mRNA) in the host's nucleus. The viral mRNA then leaves the nucleus and undergoes reverse transcription, which is mediated by the viral reverse transcriptase.

HEPATITIS: Hepatitis is an inflammation of the liver, a potentially life-threatening disease most frequently caused by viral infections but which may also result from liver damage caused by toxic substances such as alcohol and certain drugs. There are five major types of viruses that cause hepatitis: hepatitis A (HAV), hepatitis B (HBV), hepatitis C (HCV), hepatitis D (HDV), and hepatitis E (HEV). Hepatitis G (HGV, also known as GB virus C) is also a potential cause.

HERD IMMUNITY: Herd immunity is a resistance to disease that occurs in a population when a large proportion of the population has been immunized against it. The theory is that it is less likely that an infectious disease will spread in a group in which many individuals are unlikely to contract it.

HERPESVIRUS: Herpesvirus is a family of viruses, many of which cause disease in humans. The herpes simplex type 1 and herpes simplex type 2 viruses cause infection in the mouth or on the genitals. Other common types of herpesvirus include chicken pox, Epstein-Barr virus, and cytomegalovirus. Herpesvirus is notable for its ability to remain latent, or inactive, in nerve cells near the area of infection, and to reactivate long after the initial infection. Herpes simplex types 1 and 2, along with chicken pox, cause skin sores. Epstein-Barr virus causes mononucleosis. Cytomegalovirus is also a herpesvirus infection. It usually does not cause symptoms, however it can be dangerous to the developing fetuses of pregnant women, the elderly, infants, and those with weakened immune systems.

HIGHLY ACTIVE ANTIRETROVIRAL THERAPY (HAART): Highly active antiretroviral therapy (HAART) is the name given to the combination of drugs used to treat people with human immunodeficiency virus (HIV) infection to slow or stop the progression of their condition to AIDS (acquired human immune deficiency syndrome). HIV is a retrovirus, and the various components of HAART block its replication by different mechanisms.

HISTOCOMPATIBILITY: The histocompatibility molecules (proteins) on the cell surfaces of one individual of a species are unique. Thus, if a cell from one person is transplanted into another person, the cell will be recognized by the immune system as being foreign. The histocompatibility molecules act as antigens in the recipient and so can also be called histocompatibility antigens or transplantation antigens. This is the basis of the rejection of transplanted material.

HISTOPATHOLOGY: Histopathology is the study of diseased tissues. A synonym for histopathology is pathologic histology.

HIV (HUMAN IMMUNODEFICIENCY VIRUS): The virus that causes AIDS (acquired immune deficiency syndrome).

HOMOZYGOUS: A condition in which two alleles for a given gene are the same.

HORIZONTAL GENE TRANSFER: Horizontal gene transfer is a major mechanism by which antibiotic resistance genes get passed between bacteria. It accounts for many hospital-acquired infections.

HORIZONTAL TRANSMISSION: Horizontal transmission refers to the transmission of a disease-causing microorganism from one person to another, unrelated person by direct or indirect contact.

HOST: An organism that serves as the habitat for a parasite or possibly for a symbiont. A host may provide nutrition to the parasite or symbiont, or it may simply provide a place in which to live.

HUMAN IMMUNODEFICIENCY VIRUS (HIV): The human immunodeficiency virus (HIV) belongs to a class of viruses known as the retroviruses. These viruses are known as RNA viruses because they have RNA (ribonucleic acid) as their basic genetic material instead of DNA (deoxyribonucleic acid).

HUMAN T-CELL LEUKEMIA VIRUS: Two types of human T-cell leukemia virus (HTLV) are known. They are also known as human T-cell lymphotrophic viruses. HTLV-I often is carried by a person with no obvious symptoms. However, HTLV-I is capable of causing a number of maladies. These include abnormalities of the T cells and B cells, a chronic infection of the myelin covering of nerves that causes a degeneration of the nervous system, sores on the skin, and an inflammation of the inside of the eye. HTLV-II infection usually does not produce any symptoms. However, in some people a cancer of the blood known as hairy cell leukemia can develop.

HYGIENE: Hygiene refers to the health practices that minimize the spread of infectious microorganisms between people or between other living things and people. Inanimate objects and surfaces such as contaminated cutlery or a cutting board may be a secondary part of this process.

HYPERENDEMIC: A disease that is endemic (commonly present) in all age groups of a population is hyperendemic. A related term is holoendemic, meaning a disease that is present more in children than in adults.

I

IMMIGRATION: The relocation of people to a different region or country from their native lands; also refers to the movement of organisms into an area in which they were previously absent.

IMMUNE RESPONSE: The body's production of antibodies or some types of white blood cells in response to foreign substances.

IMMUNE SYSTEM: The body's natural defense system that guards against foreign invaders and that includes lymphocytes and antibodies.

IMMUNOCOMPROMISED: A reduction of the ability of the immune system to recognize and respond to the presence of foreign material.

IMMUNODEFICIENCY: In immunodeficiency disorders, part of the body's immune system is missing or defective, thus impairing the body's ability to fight infections. As a result, the person with an immunodeficiency disorder will have frequent infections that are generally more severe and last longer than usual.

IMMUNOLOGY: Immunology is the study of how the body responds to foreign substances and fights off infection and other disease. Immunologists study the molecules, cells, and organs of the human body that participate in this response.

IMMUNOSUPPRESSION: A reduction of the ability of the immune system to recognize and respond to the presence of foreign material.

IMPORTED CASES OF DISEASE: Imported cases of disease happen when an infected person who is not yet showing symptoms travels from his home country to another country and develops symptoms of his disease there.

IN SITU: A Latin term meaning "in place" or in the body or natural system.

INACTIVATED VACCINE: An inactivated vaccine is a vaccine that is made from disease-causing microorganisms that have been killed or made incapable of causing the infection. The immune system can still respond to the presence of the microorganisms.

INACTIVATED VIRUS: An inactivated virus is incapable of causing disease but still stimulates the immune system to respond by forming antibodies.

INCIDENCE: The number of new cases of a disease or injury that occur in a population during a specified period of time.

INCUBATION PERIOD: Incubation period refers to the time between exposure to a disease-causing virus or bacteria and the appearance of symptoms of the infection. Depending on the microorganism, the incubation time can range from a few hours (for example, food poisoning due to *Salmonella*) to a decade or more (for example, acquired immune deficiency syndrome, or AIDS).

INFECTION CONTROL: Infection control refers to policies and procedures used to minimize the risk of spreading infections, especially in hospitals and health care facilities.

INFORMED CONSENT: An ethical and informational process in which a person learns about a procedure or clinical trial, including potential risks or benefits, before deciding to voluntarily participate in a study or undergo a particular procedure.

INNATE IMMUNITY: Innate immunity is the resistance against disease that an individual is born with, as distinct from acquired immunity, which develops with exposure to infectious agents.

INPATIENT: A patient who is admitted to a hospital or clinic for treatment, typically requiring the patient to stay overnight.

INSECT-BORNE VIRUS: A virus carried and transmitted by an insect, such as a mosquito.

INSECTICIDE: A chemical substance used to kill insects.

INTERMEDIATE HOST: An organism infected by a parasite while the parasite is in a developmental form, not sexually mature.

INTERNATIONAL HEALTH REGULATIONS (IHR): International regulations introduced by the World Health Organization (WHO) that aim to control, monitor, prevent, protect against, and respond to the spread of disease across national borders while avoiding unnecessary interference with international movement and trade.

INTRAVENOUS: In the vein. For example, the insertion of a hypodermic needle into a vein to instill a fluid, withdraw or transfuse blood, or start an intravenous feeding.

IONIZING RADIATION: Any electromagnetic or particulate radiation capable of direct or indirect ion production in its passage through matter. In general use: Radiation that can cause tissue damage or death.

IRRADIATION: A method of preservation that treats food with low doses of radiation to deactivate enzymes and to kill microorganisms and insects.

ISOLATION: Within the health community, isolation refers to the precautions that are taken in a hospital to prevent the spread of an infectious agent from an infected or colonized patient to susceptible persons. Isolation practices are designed to minimize the transmission of infection.

ISOLATION AND QUARANTINE: Public health authorities rely on isolation and quarantine as two important tools among the many they use to fight disease outbreaks. Isolation is the practice of keeping a disease victim away from other people, sometimes by treating them in their homes or by the use of elaborate isolation systems in hospitals. Quarantine separates people who have been exposed to a disease but have not yet developed symptoms from the general population. Both isolation and quarantine can be entered voluntarily by patients when public health authorities request it, or it can be compelled by state or national governments or government agencies, such as the U.S. Centers for Disease Control and Prevention.

J

JAUNDICE: Jaundice is a condition in which a person's skin and the whites of the eyes are discolored a shade of yellow due to an increased level of bile pigments in the blood as a result of liver disease. Jaundice is sometimes called icterus, from a Greek word for the condition.

K

KOCH'S POSTULATES: Koch's postulates are a series of conditions that must be met for a microorganism to be considered the cause of a disease. German microbiologist Robert Koch (1843–1910) proposed the postulates in 1890.

L

LATENT: A condition that is potential or dormant, not yet manifest or active, is latent.

LESION: The tissue disruption or the loss of function caused by a particular disease process.

LIVE VACCINE: A live vaccine uses a virus or bacteria that has been weakened (attenuated) to cause an immune response in the body without causing disease. Live vaccines are preferred to killed vaccines, which use a dead virus or bacteria, because they cause a stronger and longer-lasting immune response.

LYMPHATIC SYSTEM: The lymphatic system is the body's network of organs, ducts, and tissues that filters harmful substances out of the fluid that surrounds body tissues. Lymphatic organs include the bone marrow, thymus, spleen, appendix, tonsils, adenoids, lymph nodes, and Peyer's patches (in the small intestine). The thymus and bone marrow are called primary lymphatic organs, because lymphocytes are produced in them. The other lymphatic organs are called secondary lymphatic organs. The lymphatic system also includes thin vessels, capillaries, valves, ducts, nodes, and organs that run throughout the body, helping protect and maintain the internal fluids system of the entire body by both producing and filtering lymph and by producing various blood cells. The three main purposes of the lymphatic system are to drain fluid back into the bloodstream from the tissues, to filter lymph, and to fight infections.

LYMPHOCYTE: A type of white blood cell; includes B and T lymphocytes. These white blood cells function as part of the lymphatic and immune systems by stimulating antibody formation to attack specific invading substances.

M

MAJOR HISTOCOMPATIBILITY COMPLEX (MHC): The proteins that protrude from the surface of a cell that identify the cell as "self." In humans, the proteins coded by the genes of the major histocompatibility complex (MHC) include human leukocyte antigens (HLA), as well as other proteins. HLA proteins are present on the surface of most of the body's cells and are important in helping the immune system distinguish "self" from "non-self" molecules, cells, and other objects.

MALAISE: Malaise is a general or nonspecific feeling of unease or discomfort, often the first sign of disease infection.

MALIGNANT: A general term for cancer cells that can dislodge from the original tumor, then invade and destroy other tissues and organs.

MEASLES: Measles is an infectious disease caused by a virus of the paramyxovirus group. It infects only humans, and the infection results in life-long immunity to the disease. It is one of several exanthematous (rash-producing) diseases of childhood, the others being rubella (German measles), chicken pox, and the now rare scarlet fever. The disease is particularly common in both preschool and young school children.

MENINGITIS: Meningitis is an inflammation of the meninges—the three layers of protective membranes that line the spinal cord and the brain. Meningitis can occur when there is an infection near the brain or spinal cord, such as a respiratory infection in the sinuses, the mastoids, or the cavities around the ear. Disease organisms can also travel to the meninges through the bloodstream. The first signs may be a severe headache and neck stiffness followed by fever, vomiting, a rash, and then convulsions leading to loss of consciousness and potentially death. Meningitis generally involves two types: non-bacterial meningitis, which is often called aseptic meningitis, and bacterial meningitis, which is referred to as purulent meningitis.

MESSENGER RIBONUCLEIC ACID (MRNA): A molecule of RNA that carries the genetic information for producing one or more proteins; mRNA is produced by copying one strand of DNA, but in eukaryotes it is able to move from the nucleus to the cytoplasm (where protein synthesis takes place).

METHICILLIN-RESISTANT *STAPHYLOCOCCUS AUREUS* (MRSA): Methicillin-resistant *Staphylococcus aureus* (MRSA) are bacteria resistant to most penicillin-type antibiotics, including methicillin.

MICROBICIDE: A microbicide is a compound that kills microorganisms such as bacteria, fungi, and protozoa.

MICROFILIAE: Live offspring produced by adult nematodes within the host's body.

MICROORGANISM: Microorganisms are minute organisms. With only a single currently known exception (i.e., *Epulopiscium fishelsonia*, a bacterium that is billions of times larger than the bacteria in the human intestine and is large enough to view without a microscope), microorganisms are minute organisms that require microscopic magnification to view. To be seen, they must be magnified by an optical or electron microscope. The most common types of microorganisms are viruses, bacteria, blue-green bacteria, some algae, some fungi, yeasts, and protozoans.

MIGRATION: In medicine, migration is the movement of a disease symptom from one part of the body to another, apparently without cause.

MMR VACCINE: The MMR (measles, mumps, and rubella) vaccine is a vaccine that is given to protect someone from measles, mumps, and rubella. The vaccine is made up of viruses that cause the three diseases. The viruses are incapable of causing the diseases but can still stimulate the immune system.

MONO SPOT TEST: The mononucleosis (mono) spot test is a blood test used to check for infection with the Epstein-Barr virus, which causes mononucleosis.

MONOCLONAL ANTIBODIES: Antibodies produced from a single cell line that are used in medical testing and, increasingly, in the treatment of some cancers.

MONOVALENT VACCINE: A monovalent vaccine is one that is active against just one strain of a virus, such as the one that is in common use against the poliovirus.

MORBIDITY: The term "morbidity" comes from the Latin word *morbus,* which means sick. In medicine it refers not just to the state of being ill, but also to the severity of the illness. A serious disease is said to have a high morbidity.

MORPHOLOGY: The study of form and structure of animals and plants. The outward physical form possessed by an organism.

MORTALITY: Mortality is the condition of being susceptible to death. The term mortality comes from the Latin word *mors,* which means death. Mortality can also refer to the rate of deaths caused by an illness or injury, i.e., rabies has a high mortality rate.

MOSQUITO COILS: Mosquito coils are spirals of flammable paste that, when burned, steadily release insect repellent into the air. They are often used in Asia, where many coils release octachlorodipropyl ether, which can cause lung cancer.

MOSQUITO NETTING: Fine meshes or nets hung around occupied spaces, especially beds, to keep out disease-carrying mosquitoes. Mosquito netting is a cost-effective way of preventing malaria.

MRSA: MRSA is an abbreviation for methicillin-resistant *Staphylococcus aureus,* which are bacteria resistant to most penicillin-type antibiotics, including methicillin.

MULTI-DRUG RESISTANCE: Multi-drug resistance is a phenomenon that occurs when an infective agent loses its sensitivity against two or more of the drugs that are used against it.

MULTI-DRUG THERAPY: Multi-drug therapy is the use of a combination of drugs against infection, each of which attacks the infective agent in a different way. This strategy can help overcome resistance to anti-infective drugs.

MUTABLE VIRUS: A mutable virus is one whose DNA changes rapidly so that drugs and vaccines against it may not be effective.

MUTATION: A mutation is a change in an organism's DNA that occurs over time and may render it less sensitive to the drugs that are used against it.

MYCOBACTERIA: *Mycobacteria* is a genus of bacteria that includes the bacteria causing leprosy and tuberculosis. The bacteria have unusual cell walls that are harder to dissolve than the cell walls of other bacteria.

MYCOTIC: Mycotic means having to do with or caused by a fungus. Any medical condition caused by a fungus is a mycotic condition, also called a mycosis.

N

NECROPSY: A necropsy is a medical examination of a dead body; also called an autopsy.

NECROTIC: Necrotic tissue is dead tissue in an otherwise living body. Tissue death is called necrosis.

NEEDLESTICK INJURY: Any accidental breakage or puncture of the skin by an unsterilized medical needle (syringe) is a needlestick injury. Health-care providers are at particular risk for needlestick injuries (which may transmit disease) because of the large number of needles they handle.

NEGLECTED TROPICAL DISEASE: Many tropical diseases are considered to be neglected because, despite their prevalence in less-developed areas, new vaccines and treatments are not being developed for them. Malaria was once considered to be a neglected tropical disease, but a great deal of research and money have been devoted to its prevention, treatment, and cure in the twenty-first century.

NEMATODES: Also known as roundworms; a type of helminth characterized by long, cylindrical bodies.

NODULE: A nodule is a small, roundish lump on the surface of the skin or of an internal organ.

NONGOVERNMENTAL ORGANIZATION (NGO): A voluntary organization that is not part of any government; often organized to address a specific issue or perform a humanitarian function.

NORMAL FLORA: The bacteria that normally inhabit some part of the body, such as the mouth or intestines, are normal flora. Normal flora are essential to health.

NOROVIRUS: Norovirus is a type of virus that contains ribonucleic acid as the genetic material and causes an intestinal infection known as gastroenteritis. A well-known example is Norwalk virus.

NOSOCOMIAL INFECTION: A nosocomial infection is an infection that is acquired in a hospital. More precisely, the U.S. Centers for Disease Control in Atlanta, Georgia, defines a nosocomial infection as a localized infection or an infection that is widely spread throughout the body that results from an adverse reaction to an infectious microorganism or toxin that was not present at the time of admission to the hospital.

NOTIFIABLE DISEASES: Diseases that the law requires must be reported to health officials when diagnosed, including active tuberculosis and several sexually transmitted diseases; also called reportable diseases.

NUCLEOTIDE: The basic unit of a nucleic acid. It consists of a simple sugar, a phosphate group, and a nitrogen–containing base.

NUCLEUS, CELL: Membrane-enclosed structure within a cell that contains the cell's genetic material and controls its growth and reproduction. The plural of nucleus is nuclei.

NUTRITIONAL SUPPLEMENTS: Nutritional supplements are substances necessary to health, such as calcium or protein, that are taken in concentrated form to compensate for dietary insufficiency, poor absorption, unusually high demand for a specific nutrient, or other reasons.

O

ONCOGENIC VIRUS: An oncogenic virus is a virus that is capable of changing the cells it infects so that the cells begin to grow and divide uncontrollably.

OPPORTUNISTIC INFECTION: An opportunistic infection is so named because it occurs in people whose immune systems are diminished or are not functioning normally; such infections are opportunistic insofar as the infectious agents take advantage of their hosts' compromised immune systems and invade to cause disease.

ORAL REHYDRATION THERAPY: Patients who have lost excessive water from their tissues are said to be dehydrated. Restoring body water levels by giving the patient fluids through the mouth (orally) is oral rehydration therapy. Often, a special mixture of water, glucose, and electrolytes called oral rehydration solution is given.

OUTBREAK: The appearance of new cases of a disease in numbers greater than the established incidence rate or the appearance of even one case of an emergent or rare disease in an area.

OUTPATIENT: A person who receives health care services without being admitted to a hospital or clinic for an overnight stay.

P

PANDEMIC: Pandemic, which means all the people, describes an epidemic that occurs in more than one country or population simultaneously.

PARAMYXOVIRUS: Paramyxovirus is a type of virus that contains ribonucleic acid as the genetic material and has proteins on its surface that clump red blood cells and assist in the release of newly made viruses from the infected cells. Measles virus and mumps virus are two types of paramyxoviruses.

PARASITE: An organism that lives in or on a host organism and that gets its nourishment from that host. The parasite usually gains all the benefits of this relationship, while the host may suffer from various diseases and discomforts, or show no signs of the infection. The life cycle of a typical parasite usually includes several developmental stages and morphological changes as the parasite lives and moves through the environment and one or more hosts. Parasites that remain on a host's body surface to feed are called ectoparasites, while those that live inside a host's body are called endoparasites. Parasitism is a highly successful biological adaptation. There are more known parasitic species than nonparasitic ones, and parasites affect just about every form of life, including most all animals, plants, and even bacteria.

PASTEURIZATION: Pasteurization is a process in which fluids such as wine and milk are heated for a predetermined time at a temperature that is below the boiling point of the liquid. The treatment kills any microorganisms that are in the fluid but does not alter the taste, appearance, or nutritive value of the fluid.

PATHOGEN: A disease-causing agent or microorganism, such as a bacteria, virus, fungus, etc., that can cause or is capable of causing disease.

PATHOGENIC: Something causing or capable of causing disease.

PAUCIBACILLARY: Paucibacillary refers to an infectious condition, such as a certain form of leprosy, characterized by few, rather than many, bacilli, which are a rod-shaped type of bacterium.

PCR (POLYMERASE CHAIN REACTION): The polymerase chain reaction, or PCR, refers to a widely used technique in molecular biology involving the amplification of specific sequences of genomic DNA.

PERSISTENCE: Persistence is the length of time a disease remains in a patient. Disease persistence can vary from a few days to life-long.

PESTICIDE: Substances used to reduce the abundance of pests, any living thing that causes injury or disease to people, animals, or crops.

PHENOTYPE: The visible characteristics or physical shape produced by an organism's genotype.

PNEUMONIA: Pneumonia is inflammation of the lung accompanied by filling of some air sacs with fluid (consolidation). It can be caused by a number of infectious agents, including bacteria, viruses, and fungi.

POTABLE: Water that is clean enough to drink safely is potable water.

PREVALENCE: The actual number of cases of disease (or injury) that exist in a population.

PRIMARY HOST: The primary host is an organism that provides food and shelter for a parasite while allowing it to become sexually mature, while a secondary host is one occupied by a parasite during the larval or asexual stages of its life cycle.

PRIONS: Prions are proteins that are infectious. The name prion is derived from "proteinaceous infectious particles." The discovery of prions and confirmation of their infectious nature overturned a central dogma that infections were caused only by intact organisms, particularly microorganisms such as bacteria, fungi, parasites, or viruses. Because prions lack genetic material, the prevailing attitude was that a protein could not cause disease.

PROPHYLAXIS: Pre-exposure treatment (e.g., immunization) that prevents or reduces severity of disease or symptoms upon exposure to the causative agent.

PROSTRATION: A condition marked by nausea, disorientation, dizziness, and weakness caused by dehydration and prolonged exposure to high temperatures; also called heat exhaustion or hyperthermia.

PROTOZOA: Single-celled animal-like microscopic organisms that live by taking in food rather than making it by photosynthesis and must live in the presence of water. (Singular: protozoan.) Protozoa are a diverse group of single-celled organisms, with more than 50,000 different types represented. The vast majority are microscopic, many measuring less than 0.0002 inches (0.005 millimeters), but, such as the freshwater *Spirostomun*, may reach 0.17 inches (3 millimeters) in length, large enough to enable them to be seen with the naked eye.

PUERPERAL: An interval of time around childbirth, from the onset of labor through the immediate recovery period after delivery.

PUERPERAL FEVER: Puerperal fever is a bacterial infection present in the blood (septicemia) that follows childbirth. The Latin word *puer* meaning boy or child, is the root of this term. Puerperal fever was much more common before the advent of modern aseptic practices, but infections still occur. Louis Pasteur showed that puerperal fever is most often caused by *Streptococcus* bacteria, which is now treated with antibiotics.

PULMONARY: Having to do with the lungs or respiratory system. The pulmonary circulatory system delivers deoxygenated blood from the right ventricle of the heart to the lungs and returns oxygenated blood from the lungs to the left atrium of the heart. At its most minute level, the alveolar capillary bed, the pulmonary circulatory system is the principle point of gas exchange between blood and air that moves in and out of the lungs during respiration.

Q

QUANTITATED: An act of determining the quantity of something, such as the number or concentration of bacteria in an infectious disease.

QUARANTINE: Quarantine is the practice of separating people who have been exposed to an infectious agent but have not yet developed symptoms from the general population. This can be done voluntarily or involuntarily. In the United States, it can be enacted by the authority of states and the U.S. Centers for Disease Control and Prevention (CDC).

R

RECEPTOR: Protein molecules on a cell's surface that acts as a "signal receiver" and allow communication between cells.

RECOMBINANT DNA: DNA that is cut using specific enzymes so that a gene or DNA sequence can be inserted.

RECOMBINATION: Recombination is a process during which genetic material is shuffled during reproduction to form new combinations. This mixing is important from an evolutionary standpoint because it allows the expression of different traits between generations. The process involves a physical exchange of nucleotides between duplicate strands of deoxyribonucleic acid (DNA).

RED TIDE: Red tides are a marine phenomenon in which water is stained a red, brown, or yellowish color because of the temporary abundance of a particular species of pigmented dinoflagellate (these events are known as "blooms"). Also called phytoplankton, or planktonic algae, these single-celled organisms of the class Dinophyceae move using a tail-like structure called a flagellum. They also photosynthesize, and it is their photosynthetic pigments that can tint the water during blooms. Dinoflagellates are common and widespread. Under appropriate environmental conditions, various species can grow very rapidly, causing red tides. Red tides occur in all marine regions within temperate or warmer climates.

RE-EMERGING INFECTIOUS DISEASE: Re-emerging infectious diseases are illnesses such as malaria, diphtheria, and tuberculosis that were once nearly absent from the world but are starting to cause greater numbers of infections once again. These illnesses are reappearing for many reasons. Malaria and other mosquito-borne illnesses increase when mosquito-control measures decrease or they spread to new areas. Other diseases are spreading because people have stopped being vaccinated, as happened with diphtheria after the collapse of the Soviet Union. A few diseases are re-emerging because drugs to treat them have become less available or drug-resistant strains have developed.

REHYDRATION: Dehydration is excessive loss of water from the body; rehydration is the restoration of water after dehydration.

REPLICATE: To replicate is to duplicate something or make a copy of it. All reproduction of living things depends on the replication of DNA molecules or, in a few cases, RNA molecules. Replication may be used to refer to the reproduction of entire viruses and other microorganisms.

REPLICATION: A process of reproducing, duplicating, copying, or repeating something, such as the duplication of DNA or the recreation of characteristics of an infectious disease in a laboratory setting.

REPORTABLE DISEASE: By law, occurrences of some diseases must be reported to government authorities when observed by health-care professionals. Such diseases are called reportable diseases or notifiable diseases. Cholera and yellow fever are examples of reportable diseases.

RESERVOIR: The animal or organism in which a specific virus or parasite normally resides.

RESISTANCE: Immunity developed within a species (especially bacteria) to an antibiotic or other drug via evolution. For example, in bacteria, the acquisition of genetic mutations that render the bacteria invulnerable to the action of antibiotics.

RESISTANT BACTERIA: Resistant bacteria are microbes that have lost their sensitivity to one or more antibiotic drugs through mutation.

RESISTANT ORGANISM: An organism that has developed the ability to counter something trying to harm it. With infectious diseases, the causative organism, such as a bacterium, has developed a resistance to drugs, such as antibiotics, normally used to fight the disease.

RESPIRATOR: A respirator is any device that assists a patient in breathing or takes over breathing entirely for them.

RESTRICTION ENZYME: A special type of protein that can recognize and cut DNA at certain sequences of bases to help scientists separate out a specific gene. Restriction enzymes recognize certain sequences of DNA and cleave the DNA at those sites. The enzymes are used to generate fragments of DNA that can be subsequently joined together to create new stretches of DNA.

RETROVIRUS: Retroviruses are viruses in which the genetic material consists of ribonucleic acid (RNA) instead of the usual deoxyribonucleic acid (DNA). Retroviruses produce an enzyme known as reverse transcriptase that can transform RNA into DNA, which can then be permanently integrated into the DNA of the infected host cells.

REVERSE TRANSCRIPTASE: An enzyme that makes it possible for a retrovirus to produce DNA (deoxyribonucleic acid) from RNA (ribonucleic acid).

RHINITIS: An inflammation of the mucous lining of the nose. A nonspecific term that covers infections, allergies, and other disorders whose common feature is the location of their symptoms. These symptoms include infected or irritated mucous membranes, production of a discharge, nasal congestion, and swelling of the tissues of the nasal passages. The most widespread form of infectious rhinitis is the common cold.

RIBONUCLEIC ACID (RNA): Any of a group of nucleic acids that carry out several important tasks in the synthesis of proteins. Unlike DNA (deoxyribonucleic acid), RNA has only a single strand. Nucleic acids are complex molecules that contain a cell's genetic information and the instructions for carrying out cellular processes. In eukaryotic cells, the two nucleic acids, ribonucleic acid (RNA) and deoxyribonucleic acid (DNA), work together to direct protein synthesis. Although it is DNA that contains the instructions for directing the synthesis of specific structural and enzymatic proteins, several types of RNA actually carry out the processes required to produce these proteins. These include messenger RNA (mRNA), ribosomal RNA (rRNA), and transfer RNA (tRNA). Further processing of the various RNAs is carried out by another type of RNA called small nuclear RNA (snRNA). The structure of RNA is very similar to that of DNA, however, instead of the base thymine, RNA contains the base uracil in its place.

RING VACCINATION: Ring vaccination is the vaccination of all susceptible people in an area surrounding a case of an infectious disease. Since vaccination makes people immune to the disease, the hope is that the disease will not spread from the known case to other people. Ring vaccination was used in eliminating the smallpox virus.

RNA VIRUS: An RNA virus is one whose genetic material consists of either single- or double-stranded ribonucleic acid (RNA) rather than deoxyribonucleic acid (DNA).

ROUNDWORM: Also known as nematodes; a type of helminth characterized by long, cylindrical bodies. Roundworm infections are diseases of the digestive tract and other organ systems that are caused by roundworms. Roundworm infections are widespread throughout the world, and humans acquire most types of roundworm infection from contaminated food or by touching the mouth with unwashed hands that have come into contact with the parasite larva. The severity of infection varies considerably from person to person. Children are more likely to have heavy infestations and are also more likely to suffer from malabsorption and malnutrition than adults.

ROUS SARCOMA VIRUS: Rous sarcoma virus, named after American doctor Francis Peyton Rous (1879–1970), is a virus that can cause cancer in some birds, including chickens. It was the first virus known to be able to cause cancer.

RUMINANTS: Cud-chewing animals with four-chambered stomachs and even-toed hooves, including cows.

S

SANITATION: Sanitation is the use of hygienic recycling and disposal measures that prevent disease and promote health through sewage disposal, solid waste disposal, waste material recycling, and food processing and preparation.

SCHISTOSOMES: Blood flukes that infect an estimated 200 million people.

SEIZURE: A seizure is a sudden disruption of the brain's normal electrical activity accompanied by altered consciousness and/or other neurological and behavioral abnormalities. Epilepsy is a condition characterized by recurrent seizures that may include repetitive muscle jerking called convulsions. Seizures are traditionally divided into two major categories: generalized seizures and focal seizures. Within each major category, however, there are many different types of seizures. Generalized seizures come about due to abnormal neuronal activity on both sides of the brain,

while focal seizures, also named partial seizures, occur in only one part of the brain.

SELECTION: Process that favors one feature of organisms in a population over another feature found in the population. This occurs through differential reproduction—those with the favored feature produce more offspring than those with the other feature, such that they become a greater percentage of the population in the next generation.

SELECTION PRESSURE: Selection pressure (or selective pressure) refers to factors that influence the evolution of an organism and the tendency of an organism that has a certain characteristic to be eliminated from an environment or to increase in numbers. An example is the overuse of antibiotics, which provides a selection pressure for the development of antibiotic resistance in bacteria and an increased prevalence of bacteria that are resistant to multiple kinds of antibiotics.

SENTINEL: A sentinel is a guard or watcher; in medicine, a sentinel node is a lymph node near the breast in which cancer cells from a breast tumor are likely to be found at an early stage of the cancer's spreading (metastasization).

SENTINEL SURVEILLANCE: Sentinel surveillance is a method in epidemiology where a subset of the population is surveyed for the presence of communicable diseases. Also, a sentinel is an animal used to indicate the presence of disease within an area.

SEPSIS: Sepsis refers to a bacterial infection in the bloodstream or body tissues. This is a very broad term covering the presence of many types of microscopic disease-causing organisms. Sepsis is also called bacteremia. Closely related terms include septicemia and septic syndrome.

SEPTIC: The term "septic" refers to the state of being infected with bacteria, particularly in the bloodstream.

SEPTICEMIA: Prolonged fever, chills, anorexia, and anemia in conjunction with tissue lesions.

SEQUENCING: Finding the order of chemical bases in a section of DNA.

SEROTYPES: Serotypes or serovars are classes of microorganisms based on the types of molecules (antigens) that they present on their surfaces. Even a single species may have thousands of serotypes, which may have medically quite distinct behaviors.

SEXUALLY TRANSMITTED DISEASE (STD): Sexually transmitted diseases (STDs) vary in their susceptibility to treatment, their signs and symptoms, and the consequences if they are left untreated. Some are caused by bacteria. These usually can be treated and cured. Others are caused by viruses and can typically be treated but not cured.

SHED: To shed is to cast off or release. In medicine, the release of eggs or live organisms from an individual infected with parasites is often referred to as shedding.

SHOCK: Shock is a medical emergency in which the organs and tissues of the body are not receiving an adequate flow of blood. This condition deprives the organs and tissues of oxygen (carried in the blood) and allows the buildup of waste products. Shock can result in serious damage or even death.

SOCIOECONOMIC: Concerning both social and economic factors.

SPECIAL PATHOGENS BRANCH: A group within the U.S. Centers for Disease Control and Prevention (CDC) whose goal is to study highly infectious viruses that produce diseases within humans.

SPIROCHETE: A bacterium shaped like a spiral. Spiral-shaped bacteria live in contaminated water, sewage, soil, and decaying organic matter, as well as inside humans and animals.

STANDARD PRECAUTIONS: Standard precautions are the safety measures taken to prevent the transmission of disease-causing bacteria. These include proper hand washing; wearing gloves, goggles, and other protective clothing; proper handling of needles; and sterilization of equipment.

STRAIN: A subclass or a specific genetic variation of an organism.

STREPTOCOCCUS: A genus of bacteria that includes species such as *Streptococci pyogenes*, a species of bacteria that causes strep throat.

SUPERINFECTION: When a new infection occurs in a patient who already has some other infection, it is called a superinfection. For example, a bacterial infection appearing in a person who already had viral pneumonia would be a superinfection.

SURVEILLANCE: The systematic analysis, collection, evaluation, interpretation, and dissemination of data. In public health, it assists in the identification of health threats and the planning, implementation, and evaluation of responses to those threats.

SYSTEMIC: Any medical condition that affects the whole body (i.e., the whole system) is systemic.

T

T CELL: Immune-system white blood cells that enable antibody production, suppress antibody production,

or kill other cells. When a vertebrate encounters substances that are capable of causing it harm, a protective system known as the immune system comes into play. This system is a network of many different organs that work together to recognize foreign substances and destroy them. The immune system can respond to the presence of a disease-causing agent (pathogen) in two ways. In cell-mediated immunity, T cells produce special chemicals that can specifically isolate the pathogen and destroy it. The other branch of immunity is called humoral immunity, in which immune cells called B cells can produce soluble proteins (antibodies) that can accurately target and kill the pathogen.

T-CELL VACCINE: A T-cell vaccine is one that relies on eliciting cellular immunity, rather than humoral antibody-based immunity, against infection. T cell vaccines are being developed against the human immunodeficiency virus (HIV) and hepatitis C.

TAPEWORM: Tapeworms are parasitic flatworms of class *Cestoidea*, phylum *Platyhelminthes*, that live inside the intestine. Tapeworms have no digestive system, but absorb predigested nutrients directly from their surroundings.

TICK: A tick is any blood-sucking parasitic insect of suborder *Ixodides*, superfamily *Ixodoidea*. Ticks can transmit a number of diseases, including Lyme disease and Rocky Mountain spotted fever.

TOPICAL: Any medication that is applied directly to a particular part of the body's surface is termed topical; for example, a topical ointment.

TOXIC: Something that is poisonous and that can cause illness or death.

TRANSFUSION-TRANSMISSIBLE INFECTIONS: Any infection that can be transmitted to a person by a blood transfusion (addition of stored whole blood or blood fractions to a person's own blood) is a transfusion-transmissible infection. Some diseases that can be transmitted in this way are AIDS, hepatitis B, hepatitis C, syphilis, malaria, and Chagas disease.

TRANSMISSION: Microorganisms that cause disease in humans and other species are known as pathogens. The transmission of pathogens to a human or other host can occur in a number of ways, depending upon the microorganism.

TREMATODES: Trematodes, also called flukes, are a type of parasitic flatworm. In humans, flukes can infest the liver, lung, and other tissues.

TYPHUS: A disease caused by various species of *Rickettsia*, characterized by fever, rash, and delirium. Insects such as lice and chiggers transmit typhus. Two forms of typhus, epidemic typhus and scrub typhus, are fatal if untreated.

U

UNIVERSAL PRECAUTION: Universal precaution refers to an infection control strategy in which all human blood and other material is assumed to be potentially infectious, specifically with organisms such as human immunodeficiency virus (HIV) and hepatitis B virus. The precautions are aimed at preventing contact with blood or the other materials.

V

VACCINATION: Vaccination is the inoculation, or use of vaccines, to prevent specific diseases within humans and animals by producing immunity to such diseases. It is the introduction of weakened or dead viruses or microorganisms into the body to create immunity by the production of specific antibodies.

VACCINE: A substance that is introduced to stimulate antibody production and thus provide immunity to a particular disease.

VACCINIA VIRUS: The vaccinia virus is a usually harmless virus that is closely related to the virus that causes smallpox, a dangerous disease. Infection with the vaccinia virus confers immunity against smallpox, so vaccinia virus has been used as a vaccine against smallpox.

VARICELLA ZOSTER IMMUNE GLOBULIN (VZIG): Varicella zoster immune globulin is a preparation that can give people temporary protection against chicken pox after exposure to the Varicella virus. It is used for children and adults who are at risk of complications of the disease or who are susceptible to infection because they have weakened immunity.

VARICELLA ZOSTER VIRUS (VZV): Varicella zoster virus is a member of the alpha herpes virus group and is the cause of both chicken pox (also known as varicella) and shingles (herpes zoster).

VARIOLA VIRUS: Variola virus (or variola major virus) is the virus that causes smallpox. The virus is one of the members of the poxvirus group (Family Poxviridae). The virus particle is brick shaped and contains a double strand of deoxyribonucleic acid. The variola virus is among the most dangerous of all the potential biological weapons.

VARIOLATION: Variolation was the pre-modern practice of deliberately infecting a person with smallpox in order to make them immune to a more serious form of the disease. It was dangerous, but did confer immunity on survivors.

VECTOR: Any agent that carries and transmits parasites and diseases. Also, an organism or chemical used to transport a gene into a new host cell.

VECTOR-BORNE DISEASE: A vector-borne disease is one in which the pathogenic microorganism is transmitted from an infected individual to another individual by an arthropod or other agent, sometimes with other animals serving as intermediary hosts. The transmission depends upon the attributes and requirements of at least three different living organisms: the pathologic agent, either a virus, protozoa, bacteria, or helminth (worm); the vector, commonly arthropods such as ticks or mosquitoes; and the human host.

VENEREAL DISEASE: Venereal diseases are diseases that are transmitted by sexual contact. They are named after Venus, the Roman goddess of female sexuality. They are now more commonly called sexually transmitted diseases.

VESICLE: A membrane-bound sphere that contains a variety of substances in cells.

VIRAL SHEDDING: Viral shedding refers the period of time in which a person with a virus is contagious, allowing the movement of a virus from one person to another. For example, when the herpes virus moves from the nerves to the surface of the skin. During shedding, the herpes virus can be passed on through skin-to-skin contact.

VIRION: A virion is a mature virus particle, consisting of a core of ribonucleic acid (RNA) or deoxyribonucleic acid (DNA) surrounded by a protein coat. This is the form in which a virus exists outside of its host cell.

VIRULENCE: Virulence is the ability of a disease organism to cause disease: a more virulent organism is more infective and liable to produce more serious disease.

VIRUS: A virus is a small, infectious agent that consists of a core of genetic material—either deoxyribonucleic acid (DNA) or ribonucleic acid (RNA)—surrounded by a shell of protein. Viruses are essentially nonliving repositories of nucleic acid that require the presence of a living prokaryotic or eukaryotic cell for the replication of the nucleic acid. Very simple microorganisms, viruses are much smaller than bacteria that enter and multiply within cells. There are a number of different viruses that challenge the human immune system and that may produce disease in humans. Viruses often exchange or transfer their genetic material (DNA or RNA) to cells and can cause diseases such as chicken pox, hepatitis, measles, and mumps.

VISCERAL: Visceral means pertaining to the viscera. The viscera are the large organs contained in the main cavities of the body, especially the thorax and abdomen, for example, the lungs, stomach, intestines, kidneys, and liver.

W

WATERBORNE DISEASE: Waterborne disease refers to diseases that are caused by exposure to contaminated water. The exposure can occur by drinking the water or having the water come in contact with the body. Examples of waterborne diseases are cholera and typhoid fever.

WEAPONIZATION: The use of any bacterium, virus, or other disease-causing organism as a weapon of war. Among other terms, it is also called germ warfare, biological weaponry, and biological warfare.

WILD VIRUS: Wild- or wild-type virus is a genetic description referring to the original form of a virus, first observed in nature. It may remain the most common form in existence but mutated forms develop over time and sometimes become the new wild type virus.

Z

ZOONOTIC: A zoonotic disease is a disease that can be transmitted between animals and humans. Examples of zoonotic diseases are anthrax, plague, and Q-fever.

Chronology of Events

Nineteenth Century

1854 English physician John Snow traces the source of a cholera epidemic to a public water pump in Soho, London. This discovery is generally considered to be the foundation of modern epidemiology.

1857 Louis Pasteur demonstrates that lactic acid fermentation is caused by a living organism. Between 1857 and 1880, he performs a series of experiments that refute the doctrine of spontaneous generation. He also introduces vaccines for fowl cholera, anthrax, and rabies, based on attenuated strains of viruses and bacteria.

1858 Rudolf Virchow publishes his landmark paper "Cellular Pathology" and establishes the field of cellular pathology. Virchow asserts that all cells arise from preexisting cells (*Omnis cellula e cellula*). He argues that the cell is the ultimate locus of all disease.

1859 Charles Darwin publishes his landmark book *On the Origin of Species by Means of Natural Selection*.

1860 Ernst Heinrich Haeckel describes the essential elements of modern zoological classification.

1860 Max Johann Sigismund Schultze describes the nature of protoplasm and shows that it is fundamentally the same for all life forms.

1865 An epidemic of rinderpest kills 500,000 cattle in Great Britain. Government inquiries into the outbreak pave the way for the development of contemporary theories of epidemiology and the germ theory of disease.

1865 French physiologist Claude Bernard publishes *Introduction to the Study of Human Experimentation* that advocates "Never perform an experiment which might be harmful to the patient even if advantageous to science."

1866 The Austrian botanist and monk Johann Gregor Mendel discovers the laws of heredity and writes the first of a series of papers on heredity (1866–1869). The papers formulate the laws of hybridization. Mendel's work is disregarded until 1900, when Hugo de Vries rediscovers it. Unbeknownst to both Darwin and Mendel, Mendelian laws provide the scientific framework for the concepts of gradual evolution and continuous variation.

1870 Lambert Adolphe Jacques Quetelet shows the importance of statistical analysis for biologists and provides the foundations of biometry.

1871 Ferdinand Cohn coins the term bacterium.

1875 Ferdinand Cohn publishes a classification of bacteria in which the genus name Bacillus is used for the first time.

1867 Robert Koch publishes a paper on anthrax that establishes the role of bacteria in causing anthrax, providing the final piece of evidence in support of the germ theory of disease. Koch later formulates postulates that established steps for determining the cause, such as a specific bacteria or virus, of a particular infectious disease.

1877 Paul Erlich recognizes the existence of the mast cells of the immune system.

1877 Robert Koch describes new techniques for fixing, staining, and photographing bacteria.

1878 Joseph Lister publishes a paper describing the role of a bacterium he names *Bacterium lactis* in the souring of milk.

1878 Thomas Burrill demonstrates for the first time that a plant disease (pear blight) is caused by a bacterium (*Micrococcus amylophorous*).

1879 Albert Nisser identifies *Neiserria gonorrhoeoe* as the cause of gonorrhea.

1880 C. L. Alphonse Laveran isolates malarial parasites in erythrocytes of infected people and demonstrates that the organism can replicate in the cells. He is awarded the 1907 Nobel Prize in Medicine or Physiology for this work.

1880 The passage of a nationwide food and drug law is first attempted in the U.S. Congress. Although defeated in Congress, the U.S. Department of Agriculture's findings of widespread food adulteration spur continued interest in food and drug legislation.

1882 The German bacteriologist Robert Koch discovers the tubercle bacillus, the cause of tuberculosis.

1883 Edward Theodore Klebs and Frederich Loeffler independently discover *Corynebacterium* diphtheriae, the bacterium that causes diphtheria.

1884 Elie Metchnikoff discovers the antibacterial activity of white blood cells, which he calls "phagocytes," and formulates the theory of phagocytosis. He also develops the cellular theory of vaccination.

1884 Hans Christian J. Gram develops the Gram stain.

1884 Robert Koch enunciates "Koch's postulates," four steps for determining the source of an infection or disease.

1884 Louis Pasteur and coworkers publish *A New Communication on Rabies*. Pasteur proves that the causal agent of rabies can be attenuated, and the weakened virus can be used as a vaccine to prevent the disease. This work serves as the basis of future work on virus attenuation, vaccine development, and the concept that variation is an inherent characteristic of viruses.

1885 Francis Galton devises a new statistical tool, the correlation table.

1885 French chemist Louis Pasteur inoculates a boy, Joseph Meister, against rabies. Meister had been bitten by an infected dog. The treatment saves his life. This is the first time Pasteur uses an attenuated germ on a human being.

1885 Theodor Escherich identifies a bacterium inhabiting the human intestinal tract that he names *Bacterium coli* and shows that the bacterium causes infant diarrhea and gastroenteritis. The bacterium is subsequently named *Escherichia coli*.

1886 Adolf Mayer publishes the landmark article "Concerning the Mosaic Disease of Tobacco." This paper is considered the beginning of modern experimental work on plant viruses. Mayer assumes that the causal agent was a bacterium, although he was unable to isolate it.

1888 Martinus Beijerinck uses a growth medium enriched with certain nutrients to isolate the bacterium *Rhizobium*, demonstrating that nutritionally-tailored growth media are useful in bacterial isolation.

1888 The Institut Pasteur is formed in France as an international research institute to advance science, medicine, and public health.

1891 Charles-Edouard Brown-Sequard suggests the concept of internal secretions (hormones).

1891 Paul Ehrlich proposes that antibodies are responsible for immunity.

1891 The Prussian State dictates that even jailed prisoners must give consent prior to treatment (even for tuberculosis).

1892 Dmitri Ivanowski demonstrates that filterable material causes tobacco mosaic disease. The infectious agent is subsequently showed to be the tobacco mosaic virus. Ivanowski's discovery creates the field of virology.

1892 George M. Sternberg publishes *Practical Results of Bacteriological Researches*. Sternberg's realization that a specific antibody was produced after infection with vaccinia virus and that immune serum could neutralize the virus becomes the basis of virus serology. The neutralization test provides a technique for diagnosing viral infections, measuring the immune response, distinguishing antigenic similarities and differences among viruses, and conducting retrospective epidemiological surveys.

1892   In an experiment to try to prevent syphilis, Albert Neisser injects human subjects with serum from syphilis patients without their consent. Instead of conferring immunity, the subjects subsequently acquire the disease.

1894   Alexandre Yersin isolates *Yersinia (Pasteurella) pestis,* the bacterium responsible for bubonic plague.

1894   Wilhelm Konrad Roentgen discovers x rays.

1895   Heinrich Dreser, working for the Bayer Company in Germany, produces a drug he believes to be as effective an analgesic as morphine, but without its harmful side effects. Bayer begins mass production of diacetylmorphine, and in 1898 markets the new drug as a cough sedative under the brand name heroin.

1898   Friedrich Loeffler and Paul Frosch publish their *Report on Foot-and-Mouth Disease.* They prove that this animal disease is caused by a filterable virus and suggests that similar agents might cause other diseases.

1898   The First International Congress of Genetics is held in London.

1898   Frederick Manson cites British colonization in the tropics as justification for the new discipline of tropical medicine.

1899   A meeting to organize the Society of American Bacteriologists is held at Yale University. The society will later become the American Society for Microbiology.

Twentieth Century

1900   Carl Correns, Hugo de Vries, and Erich von Tschermak independently rediscover Mendel's laws of inheritance. Their publications mark the beginning of modern genetics. Using several plant species, de Vries and Correns perform breeding experiments that parallel Mendel's earlier studies and independently arrive at similar interpretations of their results. Therefore, upon reading Mendel's publication, they immediately recognize its significance. William Bateson describes the importance of Mendel's contribution in an address to the Royal Society of London.

1900   Karl Landsteiner discovers the blood-agglutination phenomenon and the four major blood types in humans.

1900   Paul Erlich proposes the theory concerning the formation of antibodies by the immune system.

1900   Walter Reed demonstrates that yellow fever is caused by a virus transmitted by mosquitoes. This is the first demonstration of a viral cause of a human disease. Reed injects paid Spanish immigrant workers in Cuba with the agent, paying them if they survive and paying them still more should they contract the disease.

1901   Jokichi Takamine, Japanese-American chemist, and T. B. Aldrich first isolate epinephrine from the adrenal gland. Later known by the trade name Adrenalin, it is eventually identified as a neurotransmitter. This is also the first time a pure hormone is isolated.

1902   The Pan American Health Organization (PAHO), one of the earliest international public health agencies, is founded. PAHO works to improve health and quality of life in the Americas, eventually becoming the Regional Office for the Americas of the World Health Organization and a member of the United Nations system.

1902   Carl Neuberg introduces the term biochemistry.

1903   Willem Einthoven invents the electrocardiograph (EKG).

1906   The U.S. Congress passes, and President Theodore Roosevelt signs, the Pure Food and Drug Act.

1906   Viennese physician and immunological researcher Clemens von Pirquet coins the term allergy to describe the immune reaction to certain compounds.

1906   Doctor of tropical medicine (and later Harvard professor) Richard Strong experiments with cholera on prisoners in the Philippines. Some of the prisoners die because the injections they are given are contaminated by plague.

1909 Sigurd Orla-Jensen proposes that the physiological reactions of bacteria are primarily important in their classification.

1911 (Francis) Peyton Rous publishes the landmark paper "Transmission of a Malignant New Growth by Means of a Cell-Free Filtrate." His work provides the first rigorous proof of the experimental transmission of a solid tumor and suggests that a filterable virus is the causal agent.

1912 Casimir Funk, Polish-American biochemist, coins the term vitamine. Since the dietary substances he discovers are in the amine group, he calls all of them vita-amines (using the Latin word for life, *vita*).

1912 Paul Ehrlich discovers a chemical cure for syphilis. This is the first chemotherapeutic agent for a bacterial disease.

1912 The U.S. Public Health Service is established.

1914 Frederick William Twort, English bacteriologist, and Felix Hubert D'Herelle, Canadian-Russian physician, independently discover bacteriophages, viruses that destroy bacteria.

1916 Felix Hubert D'Herelle carries out further studies of the agent that destroys bacterial colonies and gives it the name "bacteriophage" (bacteria eating agent). D'Herelle and others unsuccessfully attempt to use bacteriophages as bactericidal therapeutic agents.

1918 A global influenza pandemic caused by a virulent strain of Spanish influenza kills more people than the number of soldiers who died fighting during World War I (1914–1918). By the end of 1918, approximately 25 million people have died from influenza.

1918 Thomas Hunt Morgan and coworkers publish *The Physical Basis of Heredity,* a survey of the development of the new science of genetics.

1919 James Brown uses blood agar to study the destruction of blood cells by the bacterium *Streptococcus.* He observes three reactions that he designates alpha, beta, and gamma.

1919 The Health Organization of the League of Nations is established for the prevention and control of disease around the world.

1920 Frederick Grant Banting, Canadian physician, Charles Best, Scottish-American physiologist, and James B. Collip, Canadian biochemist, discover insulin. They develop a method of extracting insulin from the human pancreas. The insulin is then injected into the blood of diabetics to lower their blood sugar.

1922 Elmer Verner McCollum, American biochemist, discovers vitamin D.

1922 Herbert McLean Evans, American physician, and colleagues discover vitamin E.

1924 Albert Jan Kluyver publishes *Unity and Diversity in the Metabolism of Microorganisms.* He demonstrates that different microorganisms have common metabolic pathways of oxidation, fermentation, and synthesis of certain compounds. Kluyver also states that life on Earth depends on microbial activity.

1927 Thomas Rivers publishes a paper that differentiates bacteria from viruses, establishing virology as a field of study that is distinct from bacteriology.

1928 Fred Griffith discovers that certain strains of pneumococci could undergo some kind of transmutation of type. After injecting mice with living R type pneumococci and heat-killed S type, Griffith is able to isolate living virulent bacteria from the infected mice. Griffith suggests that some unknown "principle" had transformed the harmless R strain of the pneumococcus to the virulent S strain.

1929 Francis O. Holmes introduces the technique of local lesion as a means of measuring the concentration of tobacco mosaic virus. The method becomes extremely important in virus purification.

1929 Frank M. Burnet and Margot McKie report critical insights into the phenomenon known as lysogeny (the inherited ability of bacteria to produce bacteriophage in the absence of infection). Burnet and McKie postulate that the presence of a lytic unit is a normal hereditary component of lysogenic bacteria. The lytic unit is proposed to be capable of liberating bacteriophage when it is activated by certain conditions. This concept is confirmed in the 1950s.

1929   Scottish biochemist Alexander Fleming discovers penicillin. He observes that the mold *Penicillium notatum* inhibits the growth of some bacteria. This is the first antibacterial agent, and it opens a new era of "wonder drugs" to combat infection and disease.

1930   Max Theiler demonstrates the advantages of using mice as experimental animals for research on animal viruses. Theiler uses mice in his studies of the yellow fever virus.

1930   The U.S. Food, Drug, and Insecticide Administration is renamed the Food and Drug Administration (FDA).

1931   Alice Miles Woodruff and Ernest W. Goodpasture demonstrate the advantages of using the membranes of the chick embryo to study the mechanism of viral infections.

1931   Joseph Needham publishes his landmark work *Chemical Embryology,* which emphasizes the relationship between biochemistry and embryology.

1931   Rules outlined in Germany's "Regulation on New Therapy and Experimentation" call for consent of patients in medical experimentation and for experiments to be tried on animal subjects prior to testing in humans, as well as other ethical standards for medical experimentation.

1931   Ernst Ruska and Max Knoll develop the first electron microscope. Ruska is awarded the Nobel Prize in 1986 for his work on electron microscopy.

1932   Hans Adolf Krebs, German biochemist, describes and names the citric acid cycle.

1932   William J. Elford and Christopher H. Andrewes develop methods of estimating the sizes of viruses by using a series of membranes as filters. Later studies prove that the viral sizes obtained by this method were comparable to those obtained by electron microscopy.

1932   In an experiment based in Tuskegee, Alabama, African-American sharecroppers become unknowing and unwilling subjects of experimentation on the untreated natural course of syphilis. Even after penicillin came into use in the 1940s, the men remained untreated.

1933   The Twenty-first Amendment to the Constitution repeals the Eighteenth Amendment, reversing the prohibition laws that ban the sale and consumption of alcohol in United States.

1934   John Marrack begins a series of studies that lead to the formation of the hypothesis governing the association between an antigen and the corresponding antibody.

1935   Wendall Meredith Stanley, American biochemist, discovers that viruses are partly protein-based. By purifying and crystallizing viruses, he enables scientists to identify the precise molecular structure and propagation modes of several viruses.

1936   George P. Berry and Helen M. Dedrick report that the Shope virus could be "transformed" into myxomatosis/Sanarelli virus. This virological curiosity was variously referred to as "transformation," "recombination," and "multiplicity of reactivation." Subsequent research suggests that it is the first example of genetic interaction between animal viruses, but some scientists warn that the phenomenon might indicate the danger of reactivation of virus particles in vaccines and in cancer research.

1937   The Marijuana Tax Act effectively criminalizes the use and possession of marijuana, even for medical reasons.

1938   Emory L. Ellis and Max Delbrück perform studies on phage replication that mark the beginning of modern phage work. They introduce the one-step growth experiment, which demonstrates that after bacteriophages attack bacteria, replication of the virus occurs within the bacterial host during a latent period, after which viral progeny are released in a burst.

1938   The Federal Food, Drug, and Cosmetics Act gives regulatory powers over such products to the Food and Drug Administration.

1938   Japanese scientists conduct experiments on Chinese prisoners.

1939   Ernest Chain and H. W. Florey refine the purification of penicillin, allowing the mass production of the antibiotic.

1939   Richard E. Shope reports that the swine influenza virus survived between epidemics in an intermediate host. This discovery is an important step in revealing the role of intermediate hosts in perpetuating specific diseases.

1940   Helmuth Ruska, brother of Ernst Ruska, the inventor of the electron microscope, obtains the first electron microscopic image of a virus.

1941   Nazi scientists perform experiments exposing Buchenwald and Natzweiler concentration camp prisoners to typhus and, in separate experiments, phosphorus burns.

1942   Jules Freund and Katherine McDermott identify adjuvants (e.g., paraffin oil) that act to boost antibody production.

1942   Salvador Luria and Max Delbrück demonstrate statistically that inheritance of genetic characteristics in bacteria follows the principles of genetic inheritance proposed by Charles Darwin. For their work, the two (along with Alfred Day Hershey) are awarded the 1969 Nobel Prize in Medicine or Physiology.

1942   Selman Waksman suggests the word antibiotics be used to identify antimicrobial compounds that are made by bacteria.

1942   Nazi scientists perform experiments subjecting Dachau concentration camp prisoners to high altitude conditions (freezing and low pressure) and, in other experiments, diseases such as malaria.

1944   Salvador E. Luria and Alfred Day Hershey prove that mutations occur in bacterial viruses, and develop methods to distinguish the mutations from other alterations.

1944   A Manhattan Project subprogram experiments with the effects of radioactive implants on U.S. soldiers at Oak Ridge, Tennessee.

1944   U.S. Public Health Service Act passed.

1944   University of Chicago Medical School professor Dr. Alf Alving conducts malaria experiments on more than 400 Illinois prisoners.

1945   Joshua Lederberg and Edward L. Tatum demonstrate genetic recombination in bacteria.

1946   The Communicable Disease Center is organized in Atlanta, Georgia, as part of the U.S. Public Health Service. Its first mission is to prevent the spread of malaria. The agency eventually becomes the Centers for Disease Control and Prevention, a division of the U.S. Department of Health and Human Services.

1946   Felix Bloch and Edward Mills Purcell develop nuclear magnetic resonance (NMR) as a viable tool for observation and analysis.

1946   Max Delbrück and W. T. Bailey, Jr. publish a paper titled *Induced Mutations in Bacterial Viruses*. Despite some confusion about the nature of the phenomenon in question, this paper establishes the fact that genetic recombinations occur during mixed infections with bacterial viruses. Alfred Hershey and R. Rotman make the discovery of genetic recombination in bacteriophage simultaneously and independently. Hershey and his colleagues prove that this phenomenon can be used for genetic analyses. They construct a genetic map of phage particles and show that phage genes can be arranged in a linear fashion.

1948   James V. Neel reports evidence that sickle-cell disease is caused by a Mendelian autosomal recessive trait.

1948   The World Health Organization's Constitution comes into force, as proposed by diplomats at the formation of the United Nations in 1945.

1948   Alfred Kinsey publishes *Sexual Behavior in the Human Male*.

1949   Atomic Energy Commission's "Green Run" study takes place, using intentional release of radioactive iodine and xenon 133 over Hanford, Washington.

1949   John F. Ender, Thomas H. Weller, and Frederick C. Robbins publish "Cultivation of Polio Viruses in Cultures of Human Embryonic Tissues." The report by Enders and coworkers is a landmark in establishing techniques for the cultivation of poliovirus in cultures on non-neural tissue and for further virus research. The technique leads to the polio vaccine and other advances in virology.

1949   Macfarlane Burnet and his colleagues begin studies that lead to the immunological tolerance hypothesis and the clonal selection theory. Burnet receives the 1960 Nobel

Prize in Physiology or Medicine for this research.

1949 The role of mitochondria is revealed. These slender filaments within the cell, which participate in protein synthesis and lipid metabolism, are the cell's source of energy.

1950 British physician Douglas Bevis demonstrates that amniocentesis can be used to test fetuses for Rh-factor incompatibility.

1950 Robert Hungate develops the roll-tube culture technique, which is the first technique that allows anaerobic bacteria to be grown in culture.

1950 Dr. Joseph Stokes of the University of Pennsylvania infects 200 women prisoners with viral hepatitis.

1951 Esther M. Lederberg discovers a lysogenic strain of *Escherichia coli*, K12, and isolates a new bacteriophage, called lambda.

1952 Alfred Hershey and Martha Chase publish their landmark paper "Independent Functions of Viral Protein and Nucleic Acid in Growth of Bacteriophage." The famous "blender experiment" suggests that DNA is the genetic material. When bacteria are infected by a virus, at least 80 percent of the viral DNA enter the cell and at least 80 percent of the viral protein remain outside.

1952 James T. Park and Jack L. Strominger demonstrate that penicillin blocks the synthesis of the peptidoglycan of bacteria. This represents the first demonstration of the action of a natural antibiotic.

1952 Karl Maramorosch demonstrates that some viruses could multiply in both plants and insects. This work leads to new questions about the origins of viruses.

1952 Esther and Joshua Lederberg develop the replica plating method that allows for the rapid screening of large numbers of genetic markers. They use the technique to demonstrate that resistance to antibacterial agents such as antibiotics and viruses is not induced by the presence of the antibacterial agent.

1952 Renato Dulbecco develops a practical method for studying animal viruses in cell cultures. His so-called plaque method is comparable to that used in studies of bacterial viruses, and the method proves to

be important in genetic studies of viruses. These methods are described in his paper *Production of Plaques in Monolayer Tissue Cultures by Single Particles of an Animal Virus.*

1952 William Hayes isolates a strain of *Escherichia coli* that produces recombinants thousands of times more frequently than previously observed. The new strain of K12 is named Hfr (high-frequency recombination) Hayes.

1953 Jonas Salk begins testing a polio vaccine comprised of a mixture of killed viruses.

1954 Seymour Benzer deduces the fine structure of the rII region of the bacteriophage T4 of *Escherichia coli*, and coins the terms cistron, recon, and muton.

1955 Fred L. Schaffer and Carlton E. Schwerdt report on their successful crystallization of the polio virus. Their achievement is the first successful crystallization of an animal virus.

1955 Heinz Fraenkel-Conrat and Robley C. Williams prove that tobacco mosaic virus can be reconstituted from its nucleic acid and protein subunits. The reconstituted particles exhibit normal morphology and infectivity.

1956 Alfred Gierer and Gerhard Schramm demonstrate that naked RNA from tobacco mosaic virus is infectious. Subsequently, infectious RNA preparations are obtained for certain animal viruses.

1956 The American Medical Association defines alcoholism as a disease.

1957 Alick Isaacs and Jean Lindemann discover interferon, a protein made by the immune system that responds to pathogens such as viruses.

1957 The World Health Organization advances the oral polio vaccine developed by Albert Sabin as a safer alternative to the Salk vaccine.

1959 English biochemist Rodney Porter begins studies that lead to the discovery of the structure of antibodies. Porter receives the 1972 Nobel Prize in Physiology or Medicine for this research.

1959 Sydney Brenner and Robert W. Horne publish a paper titled "A Negative Staining

Method for High Resolution Electron Microscopy of Viruses." The two researchers develop a method for studying the architecture of viruses at the molecular level using the electron microscope.

1961   French pathologist Jacques Miller discovers the role of the thymus in cellular immunity.

1961   Noel Warner establishes the physiological distinction between the cellular and humoral immune responses.

1961   Rachel Carson publishes *Silent Spring,* exposing harmful effects of pollutants, including DDT, a commonly used insecticide.

1962   After thousands of birth deformities are blamed on the drug, Thalidomide is withdrawn from the market.

1962   The U.S. Food and Drug Administration requires multiphase human clinical trials before drugs can be released to market.

1964   The first Surgeon General's Report on Smoking and Health is released, and the U.S. government first acknowledges and publicizes that cigarette smoking is a leading cause of cancer, bronchitis, and emphysema.

1964   The World Medical Association adopts the Helsinki Declaration, a set of ethical principles governing the use of human subjects in medical experimentation.

1965   At the height of tobacco use in America, surveys show 52 percent of adult men and 32 percent of adult women use tobacco products.

1966   Bruce Ames develops a test to screen for compounds that cause mutations, including those that are cancer causing. The so-called Ames test utilizes the bacterium *Salmonella typhimurium.*

1966   The U.S. Food and Drug Administration and National Academy of Sciences begin investigation of the effectiveness of 4,000 drugs previously approved because they were safe, though they had not been proven effective.

1966   The United States passes the Fair Packaging and Labeling Act.

1966   The U.S. National Institutes of Health Office for Protection of Research Subjects (OPRR) is created.

1967   Dr. Christiaan Barnard performs the first successful transplant of a human heart. The recipient, Louis Washkansky, survives for 18 days.

1967   British physician M. H. Pappworth publishes "Human Guinea Pigs," advising "No doctor has the right to choose martyrs for science or for the general good."

1968   The U.S. Food and Drug Administration administratively moves to the U.S. Public Health Service.

1968   Werner Arber discovers that bacteria defend themselves against viruses by producing DNA-cutting enzymes. These enzymes quickly become important tools for molecular biologists.

1969   Julius Adler discovers protein receptors in bacteria that function in the detection of chemical attractants and repellents. The so-called chemoreceptors are critical for the directed movement of bacteria that comes to be known as chemotaxis.

1969   Max Delbrück, Alfred D. Hershey, and Salvador E. Luria are awarded the Nobel Prize in Medicine or Physiology for their discoveries concerning the replication mechanism and the genetic structure of viruses.

1970   The Controlled Substance Act (CSA) puts strict controls on the production, import, and prescription of amphetamines. Many amphetamine forms, particularly diet pills, are removed from the over-the-counter market.

1970   The U.S. Food and Drug Administration requires a patient information package insert in oral contraceptives. The insert must contain information regarding specific risks and benefits.

1970   The U.S. Congress passes the Controlled Substance Act (CSA).

1971   Médecins Sans Frontières (MSF) is founded by a group of young French doctors to aid victims of conflict and disaster. Known in English as Doctors Without Borders, MSF is awarded the Nobel Peace Prize in 1999 "in recognition of the organization's pioneering humanitarian work on several continents."

1972   Recombinant technology emerges as one of the most powerful techniques of molecular biology. Scientists are able to splice together pieces of DNA to form recombinant genes. As the potential uses, therapeutic and industrial, became increasingly clear, scientists and venture capitalists establish biotechnology companies.

1973   Herbert Wayne Boyer and Stanley H. Cohen create recombinant genes by cutting DNA molecules with restriction enzymes. These experiments mark the beginning of genetic engineering.

1974   Peter Doherty and Rolf Zinkernagl discover the basis of immune determination of self and non-self.

1975   César Milstein and George Kohler create monoclonal antibodies.

1975   David Baltimore, Renato Dulbecco, and Howard Temin share the Nobel Prize in Medicine or Physiology for their discoveries concerning the interaction between tumor viruses and the genetic material of the cell and the discovery of reverse transcriptase.

1975   John R. Hughes, Scottish physiologist, and others discover enkephalin. This first known opioid peptide, popularly called brain morphine, occurs naturally in the brain, indicating that the brain's chemicals block the transmission of pain signals.

1975   Scientists at an international meeting in Asilomar, California, call for the adoption of guidelines regulating recombinant DNA experimentation.

1975   E. O. Wilson publishes *Sociobiology,* proposing the interrelation of biology, human behavior, and culture.

1976   The U.S. Federal Bureau of Investigation (FBI) warns "crack" cocaine use and cocaine addiction are on the rise in the United States.

1976   The first outbreak of Ebola virus is observed in Zaire, Africa. There are more than 300 cases with a 90 percent death rate.

1976   Michael J. Bishop, Harold Elliot Varmus, and coworkers establish definitive evidence of the oncogene hypothesis. They discover that normal genes can malfunction and cause cells to become cancerous.

1976   Swine flu is identified in soldiers stationed in New Jersey. The virus, identified as H1N1, causes concern due to its similarities to H1N1 responsible for Spanish flu pandemic of 1918. President Gerald Ford calls for an emergency vaccination program. More than 20 deaths result from Guillain-Barre syndrome related to the vaccine.

1977   Philip Allen Sharp and Richard John Roberts independently discover that the DNA making up a particular gene could be present in the genome as several separate segments. Although both Roberts and Sharp use a common cold-causing virus, called adenovirus, as their model system, researchers later find split genes in higher organisms, including humans. Sharp and Roberts are subsequently awarded the Nobel Prize in Medicine or Physiology in 1993 for the discovery of split genes.

1977   The first known human fatality from H5N1 avian flu occurs in Hong Kong.

1977   The World Health Organization develops the first list of essential medicines, describing them as "those drugs that satisfy the health care needs of the majority of the population; they should therefore be available at all times in adequate amounts and in appropriate dosage forms, at a price the community can afford."

1977   The last reported smallpox case is recorded. Ultimately, the World Health Organization declares the disease eradicated in 1980.

1978   The Alma Ata Declaration, one of the first declarations to promote health as a basic human right, is adopted at the International Conference on Primary Health Care in Almaty (present day Kazakhstan). The resolution calls for building health care capacity in rural as well as urban areas and encourages partnership with community health workers and traditional healers for extending the reach of health care providers.

1978   Louise Brown, the world's first "test-tube baby," is born.

1981   The U.S. Centers for Disease Control and Prevention recognizes acquired immune deficiency syndrome (AIDS) as an emergent infectious disease.

1981   Karl Illmensee clones baby mice.

1982   The U.S. Food and Drug Administration approves the first genetically engineered drug, a form of human insulin produced by bacteria.

1983   *Escherichia coli* O157:H7 is identified as a human pathogen.

1983   Luc Montainer and Robert Gallo discover the human immunodeficiency virus (HIV) that is believed to cause acquired immune deficiency syndrome (AIDS).

1984   Steen A. Willadsen successfully clones a sheep.

1985   Alec Jeffreys develops genetic fingerprinting, a method of using DNA polymorphisms (unique sequences of DNA) to identify individuals. The method, which has been used in paternity, immigration, and murder cases, is generally referred to as DNA fingerprinting.

1985   American molecular biologist and physician Leroy Hood leads a team that discovers the genes that code for the T cell receptor.

1985   Japanese molecular biologist Susuma Tonegawa discovers the genes that code for immunoglobulins. He receives the 1986 Nobel Prize in Physiology or Medicine for this discovery.

1986   Congress passes the National Childhood Vaccine Injury Act, requiring patient information on vaccines and reporting of adverse events after vaccination.

1986   Robert A. Weinberg and coworkers isolate a gene that inhibits growth and appears to suppress retinoblastoma (a cancer of the retina).

1986   The U.S. Food and Drug Administration approves the first genetically engineered human vaccine for hepatitis B.

1986   A U.S. Surgeon General's report focuses on the hazards of environmental tobacco smoke (secondhand smoke) to nonsmokers.

1987   The U.S. Congress charters a Department of Energy (DOE) advisory committee, the Health and Environmental Research Advisory Committee (HERAC), that recommends a 15-year, multidisciplinary, scientific, and technological undertaking to map and sequence the human genome. DOE designates multidisciplinary human genome centers. National Institute of General Medical Sciences at the National Institutes of Health begins funding genome projects.

1988   Harvard and Dow Chemical patent a genetically engineered mouse with plans to use it in cancer studies.

1988   The Human Genome Organization (HUGO) is established by scientists in order to coordinate international efforts to sequence the human genome.

1989   Cells from one cow embryo are used to produce seven cloned calves.

1990   Michael R. Blaese and French W. Anderson conduct the first gene replacement therapy experiment on a four-year-old girl with adenosine deaminase (ADA) deficiency, an immune-system disorder. T cells from the patient are isolated and exposed to retroviruses containing an RNA copy of a normal ADA gene. The treated cells are returned to her body where they help restore some degree of function to her immune system.

1990   The U.S. National Council on Alcoholism and Drug Dependence, along with the American Society of Addictive Medicine, defines alcoholism as a chronic disease influenced by genetic, psychological, and environmental factors. Alcoholism is described as a loss of control over drinking and a preoccupation with drinking despite negative consequences to one's physical, mental, and emotional makeup as well as one's work and family life.

1990   The U.S. Supreme Court decides in *Employment Division v. Smith* that the religious use of peyote by Native Americans is not protected by the First Amendment.

1990   The U.S. Congress passes the Nutrition Labeling and Education Act, permitting manufacturers to make some health claims for foods, including dietary supplements.

1991   Mary-Claire King concludes, based on her studies of the chromosomes of women in cancer-prone families, that a gene on chromosome 17 causes the inherited form of breast cancer and also increases the risk of ovarian cancer.

1991   The gender of a mouse is changed at the embryo stage.

1991   The Genome Database, a human chromosome mapping data repository, is established.

1992 The United Nations' Earth Summit is held in Rio de Janeiro, Brazil. The United Nations Framework Convention on Climate Change (UNFCCC) is adopted, with the goal of stabilizing "greenhouse gas concentrations in the atmosphere at a level that would prevent dangerous anthropogenic interference with the climate system."

1992 American and British scientists develop a technique for testing embryos *in vitro* for genetic abnormalities such as cystic fibrosis and hemophilia.

1992 U.S. Congress passes the Prescription Drug User Fee Act requiring the U.S. Food and Drug Administration to use product application fees collected from drug manufacturers to hire more reviewers to assess applications.

1992 Craig Venter establishes The Institute for Genomic Research (TIGR) in Rockville, Maryland. TIGR later sequences the genome of *Haemophilus influenzae* and many other bacterial genomes.

1992 The U.S. Army begins collecting blood and tissue samples from all new recruits as part of a "genetic dog tag" program aimed at better identification of soldiers killed in combat.

1993 An international research team led by Daniel Cohen of the Center for the Study of Human Polymorphisms in Paris produces a rough map of all 23 pairs of human chromosomes.

1993 George Washington University researchers clone human embryos and nurture them in a Petri dish for several days. The project provokes protests from ethicists, politicians, and critics of genetic engineering.

1993 Hantavirus emerges in the United States in a 1993 outbreak on a Four Corners area (the juncture of Utah, Colorado, New Mexico, and Arizona) Native American Reservation. The resulting hantavirus pulmonary syndrome (HPS) has a 43 percent mortality rate.

1993 Scientists identify p53, a tumor suppressor gene, as the crucial factor preventing uncontrolled cell growth. In addition, scientists find that p53 performs a variety of functions ensuring cell health.

1994 Geneticists determine that DNA repair enzymes perform several vital functions, including preserving genetic information and protecting the cell from cancer.

1994 The Human Genome Project website is made available to researchers and the public.

1994 The U.S. Congress passes the Dietary Supplement Health and Education Act expressly defining a dietary supplement as a vitamin, a mineral, an herb or other botanical, an amino acid, or any other "dietary substance." This law prohibits claims that herbs can treat diseases or disorders, but it allows more general health claims about the effect of herbs on the "structure or function" of the body or about the "well-being" they induce. Under this law, the Food and Drug Administration bears the burden of having to prove an herbal supplement is unsafe before restricting its use. This law also establishes the Office of Dietary Supplements within the National Institutes of Health to promote and compile research on dietary supplements.

1995 Public awareness of the potential use of chemical or biological weapons by terrorist groups increases following the release of sarin gas in a Tokyo subway by the Japanese cult Aum Shinrikyo. The gas kills a dozen people and sends thousands to hospitals.

1995 Researchers at Duke University Medical Center report that they have transplanted hearts from genetically altered pigs into baboons. All three transgenic pig hearts survive at least a few hours, suggesting that xenotransplants (cross-species organ transplantation) might be possible.

1995 The sequence of *Mycoplasma genitalium* is completed. *Mycoplasma genitalium*, regarded as the smallest known bacterium, is considered a model of the minimum number of genes needed for independent existence.

1996 Chris Paszty and co-workers successfully employ genetic engineering techniques to create mice with sickle-cell anemia, a serious human blood disorder.

1996 H5N1 avian flu virus is identified in Guangdong, China.

1996 Researchers C. Cheng and L. Olson demonstrate that the spinal cord can be regenerated in adult rats. Experimenting on rats with severed spinal cords, Cheng and Olson use peripheral nerves to connect white matter and gray matter.

1996   Researchers find that abuse and violence can alter a child's brain chemistry, placing him or her at risk for various problems including drug abuse, cognitive disabilities, and mental illness later in life.

1996   Scientists discover a link between apoptosis (cellular suicide, a natural process whereby the body eliminates useless cells) gone awry and several neurodegenerative conditions, including Alzheimer's disease.

1996   Dolly, the world's first cloned sheep, is born. Several European Union nations ban human cloning. The U.S. Congress debates a bill to ban human cloning.

1996   Scientists report further evidence that individuals with two mutant copies of the CC-CLR-5 gene are generally resistant to HIV infection.

1996   The South Carolina Supreme Court decides in favor of the Medical University of South Carolina (MUSC) policy to secretly test pregnant patients for cocaine use. The court upholds MUSC's drug testing in an effort to protect the unborn. Cocaine greatly increases the chances of a miscarriage. Low birth weight "crack babies" have 20 times as great a risk of dying in their first month of life as normal weight babies. Those who survive are at increased risk for birth defects. Subsequently, in 2001 the U.S. Supreme Court rules that based on the Fourth Amendment, hospitals cannot test pregnant women for drugs without their consent and then inform the police.

1996   William R. Bishai and coworkers report that SigF, a gene in the tuberculosis bacterium, enables the bacterium to enter a dormant stage.

1997   The Kyoto Protocol, an international treaty on climate change, is adopted by the United Nations. Signatories are legally bound to emission reduction targets.

1997   Donald Wolf and coworkers announce that they have cloned rhesus monkeys from early stage embryos, using nuclear transfer methods.

1997   Researchers identify a gene that plays a crucial role in establishing normal left-right configuration during organ development.

1997   The DNA sequence of *Escherichia coli* is completed.

1997   The United States passes the Food and Drug Administration Modernization Act and reauthorizes the Prescription Drug User Fee Act of 1992. The changes in policy allow for a more rapid review of drugs and delivery devices. The Act also expands U.S. Food and Drug Administration regulatory powers over advertising, especially with regard to health claims.

1997   William Jacobs and Barry Bloom create a biological entity that combines the characteristics of a bacterial virus and a plasmid (a DNA structure that functions and replicates independently of the chromosomes). This entity is capable of triggering mutations in *Mycobacterium tuberculosis*.

1998   Craig Venter forms a company (later named Celera), and predicts that the company will decode the entire human genome within three years. Celera plans to use a "whole genome shotgun" method, which would assemble the genome without using maps.

1998   The U.S. Department of Energy funds bacterial artificial chromosome and sequencing projects.

1998   Dolly, the first cloned sheep, gives birth to a lamb that had been conceived by a natural mating with a Welsh Mountain ram. Researchers say the birth of Bonnie proves that Dolly is a fully normal and healthy animal.

1998   Immunologist Ellen Heber-Katz, researcher at the Wistar Institute in Philadelphia, reports that a strain of laboratory mice can regenerate tissue in their ears, closing holes which scientists had created for identification purposes. This discovery reopens the discussion on possible regeneration in humans.

1998   Scientists find that an adult human's brain can replace cells. This discovery heralds potential breakthroughs in neurology.

1998   Two research teams succeed in growing embryonic stem cells.

1999   Scientists announce the complete sequencing of the DNA making up human chromosome 22. The first complete human chromosome sequence is published in December 1999.

Twenty-First Century

2000 The United Nations, at its Millennium Summit, establishes eight international Millennium Development Goals. They are: (1) eradicate extreme poverty and hunger; (2) achieve universal primary education; (3) promote gender equality and empower women; (4) reduce child mortality; (5) improve maternal health; (6) combat HIV/AIDS, malaria, and other diseases; (7) ensure environmental stability; and (8) create a global partnership for development. These goals are agreed to by all countries of the world.

2000 The first volume of *Annual Review of Genomics and Human Genetics* is published. Genomics is defined as the new science dealing with the identification and characterization of genes and their arrangement in chromosomes and human genetics as the science devoted to understanding the origin and expression of human individual uniqueness.

2000 The National Cancer Institute (NCI) estimates that 3,000 lung cancer deaths, and as many as 40,000 cardiac deaths per year among adult nonsmokers in the United States can be attributed to passive smoke or environmental tobacco smoke (ETS).

2000 The U.S. Congress considers but does not pass the Pain Relief Promotion Act, which would have amended the Controlled Substances Act to say that relieving pain or discomfort—within the context of professional medicine—is a legitimate use of controlled substances. The bill does not pass in the Senate.

2000 The U.S. Congress passes a transportation spending bill that includes the establishment of a national standard for drunk driving for adults at a 0.08 percent blood alcohol level. States are required to adopt this stricter standard by 2004 or face penalties. By 2001, more than half the states adopt this stricter standard. All states adopt it by 2005.

2000 The U.S. Drug Addiction Treatment Act allows opioids to be distributed to physicians for the treatment of opioid dependence.

2001 In February 2001, the complete draft sequence of the human genome is published. The public sequence data is published in the British journal *Nature* and the Celera sequence is published in the American journal *Science*. Increased knowledge of the human genome allows greater specificity in pharmacological research and drug interaction studies.

2001 Scientists from the Whitehead Institute announce test results that show patterns of errors in cloned animals that might explain why such animals die early and exhibit a number of developmental problems. The report stimulates new debate on ethical issues related to cloning. In the journal *New Scientist*, Ian Wilmut, the scientist who headed the research team that cloned the sheep Dolly, argues that the findings demand "a universal moratorium against copying people."

2001 The company Advanced Cell Technology announces that its researchers have created cloned human embryos that grew to the six cell stage.

2001 The United States announces that the National Institutes of Health will fund research on only 64 embryonic stem cell lines created from human embryos.

2001 Research conducted by the U.S. National Institute of Drug Abuse asserts that children exposed to cocaine prior to birth sustain long-lasting brain changes. Eight years after birth, children exposed to cocaine prior to birth had detectable brain chemistry differences from children not exposed to the drug prior to birth.

2001 The U.S. Office of National Drug Control Policy's annual report asserts that about 80 percent of Americans abusing illegal drugs used marijuana.

2001 Study titled "Global Illicit Drug Trends," conducted by the United Nations Office for Drug Control and Crime Prevention, estimates that 14 million people use cocaine worldwide.

2001 The annual Monitoring the Future study, conducted by the University of Michigan and funded by the National Institute on Drug Abuse, finds that 17.1 percent of eighth-graders had abused inhalants at some point in their lives.

2001   The U.S. military endorses the situational temporary usefulness of caffeine, recommending it as a safe and effective stimulant for its soldiers in good health.

2001   The U.S. Supreme Court rules 8 to 0 in *United States vs. Oakland Cannabis Buyers' Cooperative* that the cooperatives permitted under California law to sell marijuana to medical patients who had a physician's approval to use the drug were unconstitutional under federal law.

2001   In August 2001, U.S. President George W. Bush announces the United States will allow and support limited forms of stem cell growth and research.

2001   Terrorists attack the United States on September 11, 2001, and kill thousands by crashing airplanes into the World Trade Center buildings in New York City. Several weeks later, an unknown terrorist sends four mailings, including letters to U.S. government leaders, that contain anthrax. The anthrax ultimately kills five people.

2002   Following the September 11, 2001, terrorist attacks on the United States, the Public Health Security and Bioterrorism Preparedness and Response Act of 2002 is passed in an effort to improve ability to prevent and respond to public health emergencies.

2002   Health Canada, the Canadian health regulatory agency, requests a voluntary recall of products containing both natural and chemical ephedra.

2002   In June 2002 traces of biological and chemical weapon agents are found in Uzbekistan on a military base used by U.S. troops fighting in Afghanistan. Early analysis dates and attributes the source of the contamination to former Soviet Union biological and chemical weapons programs that formerly utilized the base.

2002   The Best Pharmaceuticals for Children Act passes in an effort to improve safety and efficacy of patented and off-patent medicines for children.

2002   The planned destruction of stocks of smallpox causing Variola virus at the two remaining depositories in the United States and Russia is delayed over fears that large scale production of vaccine might be needed in the event of a bioterrorist action.

2003   An unusual pneumonia is reported in Hanoi, Vietnam. It is later identified as SARS.

2003   World Health Organization (WHO) officer Dr. Carlo Urbani identifies sudden acute respiratory syndrome or SARS. Urbani later dies of the disease.

2003   The U.S. Commissioner of Food and Drugs establishes an obesity working group to deal with the U.S. obesity epidemic. In March 2004 the group releases "Calories Count: Report of the Obesity Working Group."

2003   Differences in influenza outbreaks in Hong Kong between 1997 and 2003 cause investigators to conclude that the H5N1 virus has mutated.

2003   The United States invades Iraq and finds chemical, biological, and nuclear weapons programs but no actual weapons.

2003   The U.S. Food and Drug Adminsitration requires food labels to include trans fat content. This is the first major change to the nutrition facts panel on foods since 1993.

2003   SARS is added to the list of quarantinable diseases in the United States.

2003   The World Health Organization Global Influenza Surveillance Network intensifies work on development of a H5N1 vaccine for humans.

2004   Based on results from controlled clinical studies indicating that Cox-2 selective agents may be connected to an elevated risk of serious cardiovascular events, including heart attack and stroke, the U.S. Food and Drug Administration issues a public health advisory urging health professionals to limit the use of these drugs.

2004   The U.S. Food and Drug Administration bans dietary supplements containing ephedrine.

2004   The U.S. Food Allergy Labeling and Consumer Protection Act requires the labeling of foods that contain proteins derived from peanuts, soybeans, cow's milk, eggs, fish, crustacean shellfish, tree nuts, and wheat, which account for a majority of food allergies.

2004   In the United States, the Project BioShield Act of 2004 authorizes U.S. government agencies to expedite procedures related to rapid distribution of treatments as countermeasures to chemical, biological, and nuclear attack.

2004   The most powerful earthquake in more than 40 years occurs underwater off the Indonesian island of Sumatra. The resulting tsunami produces a disaster of unprecedented proportion in the modern era, affecting 14 countries and killing over 230,000 by some estimates. Some experts stated it was one of the costliest, longest, and most difficult recovery periods ever endured as a result of a natural disaster.

2005   H5N1 virus, responsible for avian flu, moves from Asia to Europe. The World Health Organization attempts to coordinate multinational disaster and containment plans. Some nations begin to stockpile antiviral drugs.

2005   Hurricane Katrina slams into the U.S. Gulf Coast, causing levee breaks and massive flooding in New Orleans. Damage is extensive across the coasts of Louisiana, Mississippi, and Alabama. The Federal Emergency Management Agency is widely criticized for lack of coordination in relief efforts. Three other major hurricanes make landfall in the United States within a two-year period, straining relief and medical supply efforts. Long-term health studies begin of populations in devastated areas.

2005   The World Health Assembly adopts International Health Regulations (IHR) 2005, the purpose of which is "to prevent, protect against, control and provide a public health response to the international spread of disease in ways that are commensurate with and restricted to public health risks, and which avoid unnecessary interference with international traffic and trade." The IHR, which would enter into force in 2007, are binding on 194 countries.

2005   The U.S. Food and Drug Administration Drug Safety Board is founded.

2005   A massive 7.6-magnitude earthquake leaves more than three million homeless and without food or basic medical supplies in the Kashmir mountains between India and Pakistan. Approximately 80,000 die.

2006   More than a dozen people are diagnosed with avian flu in Turkey, but United Nations health experts assure the public that human-to-human transmission is still rare and only suspected in a few cases in Asia.

2006   The European Union bans the importation of avian feathers (non-treated feathers) from countries neighboring or close to Turkey.

2006   In an effort to aid vaccine development, the WHO influenza pandemic task force officials ask that all countries share H5N1 (avian flu) virus samples and genetic sequencing results.

2006   Mad cow disease (bovine spongiform encephalopathy) is confirmed in an Alabama cow as the third reported case in the United States.

2007   The Intergovernmental Panel on Climate Change scientists, composed of scientists from 113 countries, issues a consensus report stating that global warming is caused by humans and predicting that warmer temperatures and rises in sea level will continue for centuries, unless humans begin to control their pollution.

2007   Studies announced in 2007 show the ability to create stem cells from cloned monkey embryos and normal adult skin cells rather than from destroyed human embryos. Stem cells are undifferentiated cells that can give rise to diverse types of differentiated (specialized) cells. The results of the studies offer a potential solution to ethical concerns about the origins of stem cells.

2007   Henrik Clausen at the University of Copenhagen in Denmark announces in the journal *Nature Biotechnology* the discovery of enzymes (proteins that help control the rates of reaction) and a method to convert any blood type into the universal Type O, a discovery that could lead to reduction in blood shortages.

2007   The U.S. Food and Drug Administration concludes that food products containing meat or products from cloned animals and their offspring are safe for human consumption.

2007   The environmental group Greenpeace launches an attack on genetically modified corn developed by U.S. biotech company Monsanto, saying that rats fed on one variety developed liver and kidney problems.

2008   Agricultural testing demonstrates that a genetically modified, drought-tolerant wheat developed to boost harvests in water-challenged areas yields up to 20 percent more harvestable wheat than similar non-modified crops used as research controls.

2008   The 1000 Genome Project embarks on its mission to sequence the profiles of a large group of people in order to catalog and better understand variation in humans.

2008   Trials of an HIV vaccine on nonhuman primates show that the vaccine, based on cell-mediated immunity, fails to prevent HIV-1 infection. The vaccine also fails to produce significant reductions in levels of the virus in newly infected specimen. Researchers continue to test whether cell-mediated immune responses might reduce replication of the HIV virus.

2008   Oil and food prices rise sharply on a global scale, increasing dangers of famine and poverty. Critics contend increased prices for petroleum lead to the diversion of food crops to biofuel production.

2009   Pandemic influenza H1N1 is confirmed in over 208 countries and territories, leading to at least 12,220 deaths, according to the World Health Organization.

2009   Yellow fever outbreaks in several African nations lead to large scale emergency vaccination programs.

2009   The U.S. Food and Drug Administration (FDA) approves clinical trials for human embryonic stem cell therapies.

2010   The Patient Protection and Affordable Care Act is signed into law by U.S. President Barack Obama, making quality health care affordable and accessible to all U.S. citizens. The law brings the United States into line with the rest of the developed world of middle- and high-income countries in the provision of universal health coverage.

2010   The *Deepwater Horizon* oil spill in the Gulf of Mexico is effectively stopped when a well cap is successfully placed. Cleanup efforts include use of microorganisms selected, modified, and tested using an array of biotechnology.

2011   The U.S. Department of Agriculture introduces MyPlate, a nutrition guide using a graphic of a plate to illustrate recommended serving proportions from the five food groups. MyPlate is widely praised as simpler and easier to understand than food pyramid diagrams, which it replaces.

2011   An international team of researchers construct the first carbon-nanotube yarns to build artificial muscles.

2012   The first reported cases of Middle East respiratory syndrome (MERS), a new coronavirus, are noted in Saudi Arabia. MERS is linked to countries in or near the Arabian Peninsula.

2014   The World Health Organization (WHO) reports the largest outbreak of Ebola virus disease to date, beginning in Guinea, West Africa. The WHO statement says, "The Ebola epidemic ravaging parts of West Africa is the most severe acute public health emergency seen in modern times. Never before in recorded history has a biosafety level four pathogen infected so many people so quickly, over such a broad geographical area, for so long."

2014   The World Health Organization announces that the spread of polio—a serious vaccine-preventable disease—presents a renewed global public health risk, and requires a coordinated international response.

2015   Measles cases in the United States reach a 20-year high, fueled by an 18-state outbreak traced to unvaccinated children exposing others at California's Disneyland amusement park.

2015   On May 9, Liberia is declared Ebola free following the West African Ebola outbreak that began the previous year. The World Health Organization estimates that by that date, almost 27,000 people had been infected by Ebola and more than 11,000 had died in the outbreak.

Neglected Tropical Diseases

🌐 Introduction

Neglected tropical diseases (NTDs) are a diverse collection of specific diseases that afflict more than 1 billion people and threaten billions more worldwide yet receive only a fraction of the money and media attention directed toward programs that fight such well-known diseases as acquired immune deficiency syndrome (AIDS), malaria, and tuberculosis. In addition to suffering and death, NTDs create devastating economic burdens that often perpetuate poverty for individuals, communities, and nations.

The World Health Organization (WHO) officially classifies a group of 17 diseases as NDTs. In addition to killing tens of thousands of people in tropical and subtropical areas of the developing world each year, NTDs contribute to chronic disability in millions of people. Children under five years of age are often the most vulnerable, both to illness and to the consequences of poverty. Included in the group of NTDs are lymphatic filariasis (elephantiasis), leprosy, and dengue fever.

🌐 Historical Background

The diseases that the WHO officially classifies as NTDs are Buruli ulcer, Chagas disease, cysticercosis, dengue, dracunculiasis (parasitic guinea worm disease), echinococcosis, fascioliasis, human African trypanosomiasis, leishmaniasis, leprosy, lymphatic filariasis, onchocerciasis, rabies, schistosomiasis, soil transmitted helminthiasis, trachoma, and yaws.

The WHO's list of NTDs are caused by a diverse array of causative pathogens. Protozoa cause Chagas disease, human African trypanosomiasis (sleeping sickness), and leishmaniasis. Bacteria cause Buruli ulcer, leprosy (Hansen's disease), trachoma, and yaws. Helminths are responsible for cysticercosis/taeniasis, dracunculiasis (guinea worm disease), echinococcosis, food-borne trematodiases, lymphatic filariasis, onchocerciasis (river blindness), schistosomiasis, and soil-transmitted helminthiases. Viruses cause dengue, chikungunya, and rabies.

Buruli Ulcer

Buruli ulcer, also called Bairnsdale ulcer, is a chronic, infectious disease caused by the bacterium *Mycobacterium ulceranus*. This bacterium is a member of the family Mycobacteriaceae, the same family that includes the bacteria responsible for tuberculosis and leprosy.

Infection from the disease leads to deformation and destruction of blood vessels, nerves, soft skin tissues, and, occasionally, bones. Large ulcers often form on the body, usually on the legs or arms. The name Buruli is often associated with the infection because of its widespread incidence during the 1960s in Buruli County (now Nakasongola District) of Uganda.

Buruli ulcer disease is one of the most ignored tropical diseases. Unfortunately, it is also one of the most treatable tropical diseases. Though the Buruli ulcer bacterium is in a family that causes other serious diseases in mammals, including leprosy and tuberculosis, these diseases have garnered much more attention that Buruli ulcer disease.

Chagas Disease

Chagas disease is caused by infection with the parasite *Trypanosoma cruzi*, which is transmitted from an animal reservoir to a human or other animal host by insects. Chagas disease occurs mostly in Latin America and is endemic (occurs naturally in a region) to rural areas in Mexico, Central America, and South America. However, through migration and other mass movements of people, the disease has been spread all over the world. Since parasites can be transmitted via the bloodstream, another mode of infection is via exposure to infected blood. This is the main mode of infection in non-endemic countries.

Drug treatment for Chagas disease is usually only effective during acute stages of the disease and is aimed at removing the parasite. However, during the chronic stages, treatment targets the effects of the disease, such as damaged organs. Chagas disease is best prevented through avoidance of insects that may be infected with *T. cruzi*, or through preventing infection from contaminated blood.

Cysticercosis

Cysticercosis is a tissue infection caused by the tapeworm *Taenia solium* in its larval cyst stage. Tapeworms are parasitic animals also known as cestodes. The life cycle of the tapeworm involves humans as either a primary or intermediate host. Both of these situations cause infection in humans. Humans become infected with tapeworms when they either ingest meat containing encysted tapeworms or when they ingest tapeworm eggs. In the first case, humans act as primary hosts. In the second case, humans act as intermediate hosts.

While tapeworm infections tend to be asymptomatic, some symptoms may appear, including abdominal pain, nausea, diarrhea, stools containing mucus, and the passing of tapeworm segments, or proglottids. However,

if a human is infected with eggs, more serious complications can arise. The cysts formed by the larvae in tissues can cause damage, including damage to vital organs such as the brain.

Tapeworm infections occur worldwide, but are more prevalent in countries with low hygiene and sanitation conditions or in areas where humans live close to livestock. Tapeworms are passed on predominantly through ingesting meat containing encysted tapeworms or ingesting food and water contaminated with infected human feces. Treatment involves antiparasitic medications, such as praziquantel, and is usually effective.

Dengue Fever

Global public health experts argue that the fastest-spreading NTD, dengue fever, poses an increasingly potent threat to public health on a global scale. Dengue fever, also known as breakbone fever in many developing countries, is regarded by many infectious disease experts as a looming 21st-century pandemic. Dengue is endemic in at least 115 countries and is spreading globally. There is no cure. Of the 30,000 to 50,000 people who die from

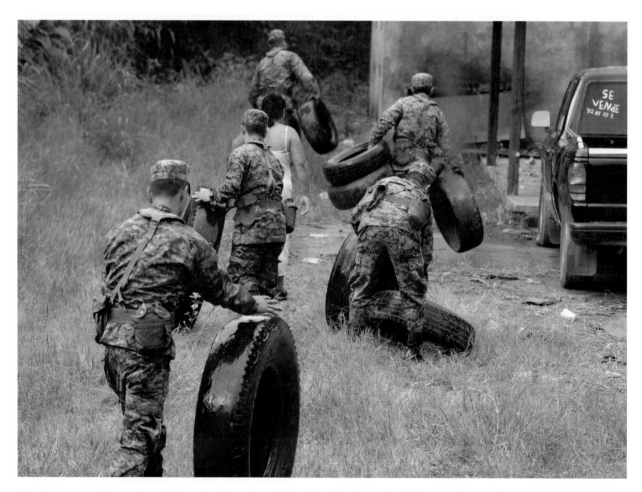

Honduran army soldiers seek to eliminate breeding places of the *Aedes aegypti* mosquito in Tegucigalpa, Honduras. *© Orlando Sierra/AFP/ Getty Images.*

it each year, children under age five are especially vulnerable. Caused by four unique viruses, dengue spreads wherever its carrier, the *Aedes aegypti* mosquito, thrives due to standing water or lack of sanitation. Except for its more deadly form, dengue hemorrhagic fever, dengue fever is usually less lethal than influenza. Breakbone fever earned its name by causing excruciating and incapacitating joint pain that often keeps children from going to school and farmers from working their fields.

More troubling to public health experts, according to the U.S. Centers for Disease Control and Prevention's (CDC) *Morbidity and Mortality Weekly Report* released in July 2011, is that typical precautions exercised by travelers to areas where dengue virus is endemic are not proving effective. The discovery of dengue in travelers returning from Haiti, where the virus is endemic, was not unexpected. The results of additional studies on a group of missionaries, however, provided unexpected surprises for investigators. In cooperation with state-level public health agencies, CDC epidemiologists surveyed all group members in an attempt to study the effectiveness of disease education and mosquito-avoidance practices (including but not limited to the use of repellents and nets). The investigators found that pretravel education and mosquito-avoidance practices did not deter dengue infection in this case.

Dracunculiasis (Guinea Worm Disease)

The guinea worm (*Dracunculus medinensis*) is a parasite that infects humans who drink water infested with "water fleas," which are the carriers of its larvae. Over the course of about a year, the adult female larvae grow into adults that are 2 to 3 feet (60–100 centimeters) long. To escape from the human host, a guinea worm forms a blister on the human's skin and emerges from the wound. When the worm emerges it releases more larvae. The process of the worm escaping from the skin may last several days to weeks and is painful, disabling, and can lead to other

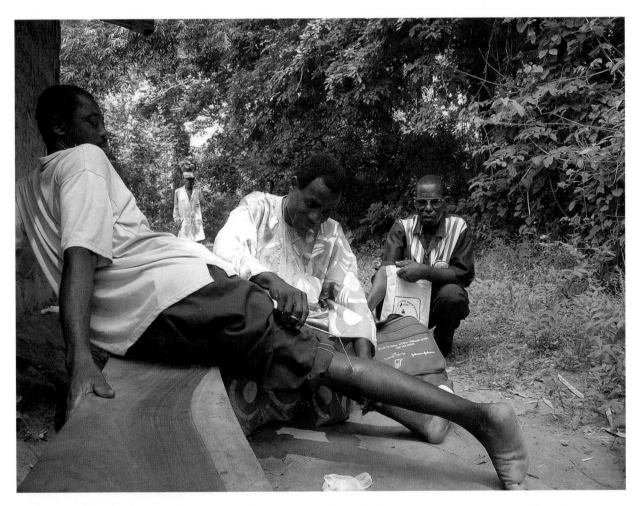

A Nigerian man has a guinea worm, *Dracunculus medinensis*, extracted from his right lower leg, where it has emerged from its subcutaneous burrow. Once the white, spaghetti-like worm emerges from the wound, it is pulled out only a few centimeters each day, and wrapped around a small stick or piece of gauze. Sometimes a worm can be pulled out completely within a few days, but this painful process often takes weeks. *E. Staub/U.S. Centers for Disease Control and Prevention/The Carter Center.*

complications. People may try to alleviate the pain by putting the affected area into water, which begins the cycle again.

Although people rarely die as a direct effect of the parasite, the social and economic burden at both the individual and community level is great. During the weeks that worms are emerging, victims usually are unable to work or carry out family duties. This debilitation often continues for several months after worms are no longer visible. In severe cases, arthritis-like conditions can develop in infected joints, and the person may be permanently crippled.

There is not a specific medication or vaccine for guinea worm. Prevention is the key to stopping the spread of the parasite. Dracunculiasis was targeted for eradication by the world health community in 1986, when there were 3.5 million cases worldwide. The CDC reported in 2015 that the almost 20 years of campaigns to eliminate the disease had decreased the number of cases from millions in the mid-1980s to 148 in 2013 and to 126 in 2014. It is hopeful that the disease will become the second human disease (after smallpox in 1980) and the first human parasite to be eradicated globally.

Echinococcosis

Alveolar echinococcosis is an infection caused by the tapeworm *Echinococcus multilocularis*. The infection is rare in humans, although is serious when it occurs as, if not treated, the infection is nearly always lethal. Tumor-like formations—due to the growth of the larval form of the tapeworm—occur most commonly in the liver, but can also be present in the brain, lungs, and elsewhere in the body.

Fascioliasis and Opisthorchiasis

Liver fluke infections are the result of infestation by parasitic worms known as liver flukes. There are two main types of liver fluke infections, fascioliasis and opisthorchiasis. Although each infection is caused by different species of flukes, they share similarities in characteristics and transmission. Humans become infected when they ingest the cysts containing parasitic forms of the flukes. These cysts open in the digestive system and release the parasites. Humans most often ingest the cysts after drinking contaminated water or eating raw or undercooked food that contains the cysts.

Infection can be asymptomatic or can be either acute or chronic. Mild cases of both fascioliasis and opisthorchiasis result in tiredness, fever, aches, swollen liver, abdominal pain, and rash. Symptoms of chronic forms include exacerbated versions of the acute symptoms with possible diarrhea, nausea, swelling of the face, blockage of the bile ducts, and sometimes complications such as migration of flukes to other regions in the body. Administration of one of a variety of antihelminthic drugs is usually effective, with recovery likely to occur.

Trypanosomiasis

Trypanosomiasis, also known as African sleeping sickness because of the semiconscious stupor and excessive sleep that can occur in someone who is infected, is an infection passed to humans through the bite of the tsetse fly. Thus, it is a vector-borne disease. The fly bite transfers either *Trypanosoma brucei rhodesiense*, which causes a version of the disease called East African trypanosomiasis, or *T. brucei gambiense*, which causes West African trypanosomiasis. If left untreated, trypanosomiasis is ultimately fatal.

Trypanosomiasis is common in Africa. In the 1960s the disease was almost eradicated, but interruptions in the delivery of public health to affected regions due to government indifference and warfare caused a reemergence of the disease, that resulted in tens of thousands of cases reported every year in the 1990s. The WHO estimates that in 2005 there were 50,000–70,000 new cases. This was a drop from higher numbers reported during the 1990s. An ongoing effort involving the WHO, Médecines Sans Frontières (Doctors Without Borders), and several pharmaceutical companies has attempted to bring trypanosomiasis under control. The numbers continued to decrease after 2005 to fewer than 10,000 in 2009 and down to 7,216 in 2012.

Leishmaniasis

Leishmaniasis is a parasitic disease caused by a protozoan of the genus *Leishmania* and spread by the bite of a sand fly. It has three main forms: cutaneous (which causes skin ulcers), mucocutaneous (which affects the mucosal membranes), and visceral (also known as kala-azar, which affects vital organs). The disease is endemic in 88 countries worldwide. (See map.) Specific forms of the disease may be more common in different countries, for example, 90 percent of mucocutaneous leishmaniasis occur in Bolivia, Brazil, and Peru, according to the WHO. About 2 million cases of the various forms occur each year.

Leishmaniasis usually affects people living in tropical and subtropical regions frequently exposed to the sand fly. Signs and symptoms vary depending on the form of infection, but mild cases present with skin sores on the face, arms, and legs that eventually heal with treatment. The more severe cases of visceral leishmaniasis affect organs such as the spleen and liver and may be fatal if untreated.

Leprosy

Leprosy, also known as Hansen's disease, is a chronic (long-term) disease caused by infection with the bacillus *Mycobacterium leprae* (*M. leprae*). The disease was greatly feared for many centuries because of the extreme disfigurement it can cause; it is widely known today from references to *Tzaraath* in the Hebrew Bible, translated as "leprosy," although the translation probably included a wide range of skin diseases. Leprosy is treatable by

New Cases of Visceral Leishmaniasis Reported in 2012

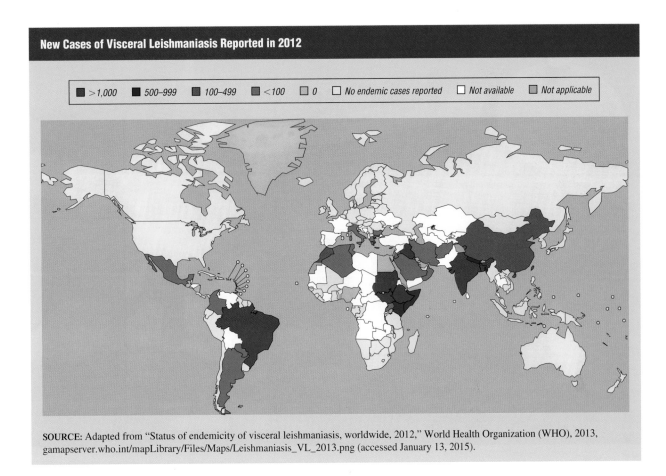

■ >1,000   ■ 500–999   ■ 100–499   ■ <100   □ 0   □ No endemic cases reported   □ Not available   ☐ Not applicable

SOURCE: Adapted from "Status of endemicity of visceral leishmaniasis, worldwide, 2012," World Health Organization (WHO), 2013, gamapserver.who.int/mapLibrary/Files/Maps/Leishmaniasis_VL_2013.png (accessed January 13, 2015).

combination drug therapy, and eradication campaigns are under way in Africa, India, Brazil, and other places where the disease remains common.

Leprosy does not, as commonly assumed, cause fingers, toes, and noses to drop off: this is a side effect of the disease's attack on the peripheral nerves. Loss of sensation makes patients unable to respond to minor injuries and infections in their fingers, toes, and elsewhere, and it is these secondary causes that lead to the characteristic loss of body parts. However, leprosy can also cause puffy, deforming lesions on the face and elsewhere, as well as a number of other symptoms.

Lymphatic Filariasis

Filariasis is a preventable parasitic disease caused by the threadworms *Wuchereria bancrofti*, *Brugia malayi*, and *Brugia timori*. The parasite attacks the lymphatic system, but symptoms may not appear for years. It is endemic in over 80 countries and is considered to be the main cause of permanent disability worldwide.

When symptomatic, patients may present with severe lymphedema (limb swelling caused by excess fluid), commonly referred to as elephantiasis. The disfigurations resulting from elephantiasis may cause stigma among some communities and add to the socioeconomic impacts of this debilitating disease.

Infection is transmitted through mosquito bites, where both the vector (disease carrier) and the human host are necessary in the successful completion of the parasitic life cycle. Antiparasitic treatment is available but is expensive and can take around a year to eliminate the parasites. Filariasis infection has been successfully curtailed in countries such as China, which has given hope for the campaign of global eradication.

Onchocerciasis

Onchocerciasis is caused by a type of parasitic worm called a helminth and occurs mainly in Africa. The worms are spread by the bite of infected black flies, which live mainly near fast-running rivers and streams. Hence, the alternative name—river blindness—for the condition.

Once they have invaded the body, the worms reproduce and millions of microscopic offspring migrate to the eye. When they die, the toxic effects cause severe and chronic inflammation of the cornea and related areas of the eye that lead to loss of vision. The threat of river blindness led to mass migration of people in West Africa away from areas infested with the black fly. This had severe economic consequences, because the people settled in less productive upland areas. Fortunately, the antiparasitic drug ivermectin can be used to treat river

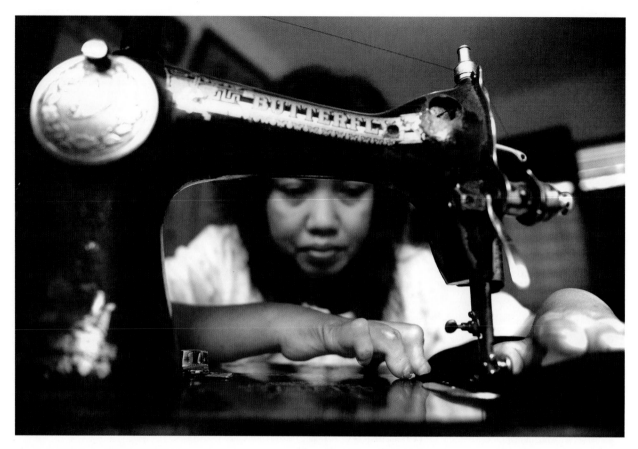

A former leper sews a skirt at Babat Jerawat Leprosy Shelter in Surabaya, Indonesia. Leprosy remains a largely neglected disease, especially in the rural areas of the country where little is known about it, and many suffer from the stigma and lack of knowledge surrounding the disease. Indonesia has around 25,000 leprosy sufferers, 30 percent of them in East Java Province, giving it the third-highest number of cases in the world behind India and Brazil. The number of new leprosy patients worldwide dropped from around 10 million in 1991 to around 230,000 in 2014. The majority of cases (about 60 percent) were in India, according to the World Health Organization. © *Robertus Pudyanto/Getty Images.*

blindness. Mass treatment programs have decreased the burden of river blindness in recent years.

Rabies

Rabies, from the Latin word *rabies* for "mad," has long been one of the most-feared of diseases. It was described by the Greek philosopher Aristotle (384–322 BCE) who realized that humans could contract rabies through being bitten by infected dogs, which is still the most common way the disease is transmitted. Rabies claims the lives of around 55,000 people around the world each year, mainly in rural parts of Africa and Asia.

Rabies is an acute viral illness that affects the brain and nervous system. Left untreated, it is invariably fatal. The symptoms are dramatic, including seizures, hallucinations, foaming at the mouth, and violent throat spasms. Rabies is a zoonosis—a disease of animals which can affect humans. Wild mammals are the reservoir of the rabies virus and they can, in turn, affect domestic animals like cats and dogs. Humans usually become infected through a bite from a wild or domestic animal with

rabies. Fortunately, an effective vaccine against rabies is available and this can be used either before or after exposure to the virus.

Schistosomiasis

Schistosomiasis, also called human blood fluke disease or bilharziasis, is a parasitic disease that is estimated to affect more than 207 million people worldwide. About 700 million people live in areas where it is endemic, mostly in the tropics. Although sometimes fatal, schistosomiasis more commonly results in chronic ill-health and low energy levels.

The disease is caused by small parasitic flatworms of the genus *Schistosoma*. Of the three species that cause disease in humans, two (*S. haematobium* and *S. mansoni*) are found in Africa and the Middle East, the third (*S. japonicum*) in Asia. *S. haematobium* lives in the blood vessels of the urinary bladder and is responsible for over 100 million human cases of the disease a year. *S. mansoni* and *S. japonicum* reside in the intestine; the former species infect 75 million people a year and the latter 25 million.

Schistosomiasis is spread when infected people urinate or defecate into open waterways and introduce parasite eggs that hatch in the water. Each egg liberates a microscopic free-living larva called the miracidium, which bores into the tissues of a water snail of the genus *Biomphalaria*, *Bulinus*, or *Onchomelania*, the intermediate host. Inside the snail, the parasite multiplies in sporocyst sacs to produce masses of larger, mobile, long-tailed larvae known as cercariae. The cercariae emerge from the snail into the water, actively seek out a human host, and bore deep into the skin. More than 700 million people worldwide are at risk of infection with the parasite, as their farming, domestic chores, and recreation put them in contact with infested water.

Soil-Transmitted Helminthiasis (Roundworm, Whipworm, and Hookworm Infections)

Soil-transmitted helminth infections are common worldwide (the CDC estimates that up to 2 billion people are affected), but are mostly prevalent in poor and developing areas where sanitation is inadequate. The main helminth species that infect people are the roundworm *Ascaris lumbricoides*, the whipworm *Trichuris trichiura*, and the hookworms *Necator americanus* and *Ancylostoma duodenale*. Transmission is via eggs shed into in human feces that contaminate soil.

Trachoma

Trachoma, also called granular conjunctivitis and Egyptian ophthalmia, is a contagious bacterial disease of the eye caused by the bacterium *Chlamydia trachomatis*.

Flies become infected when they lay eggs on human feces lying in soil. The infection occurs when a host fly, infected with the bacterium, bites a human. A fly can also become a host and harbor the bacteria when it makes direct contact with eye, nose, or throat secretions from an infected person. The bacterium can also be carried directly to humans from contaminated hands by fomites (objects contaminated with infective material) such as clothing. The disease is reported as one of the leading infectious causes of blindness.

Yaws

Yaws is a chronic infection that primarily affects the skin, bones, and cartilage of its victims. Yaws is nearly unknown in developed countries.

A spiral-shaped bacterium called *Treponema pertenue* causes yaws. These bacteria, called spirochetes, are closely related to the bacteria that cause syphilis. The spirochetes spread from person to person by direct contact of skin with infectious yaws sores. Crowding, poor sanitation, and dirty water all contribute to spreading yaws, and the disease primarily affects the poor in tropical areas of Africa, Asia, and Latin America.

⊕ Impacts and Issues

Tropical infectious diseases have an impact upon many millions of people, particularly in Africa, causing death, disability, loss of economic productivity, and impaired quality of life. There are many approaches to keeping these diseases under control or eliminating them. Where the disease is well understood and a cure or vaccine is available, then surveillance, monitoring, and effective distribution are key to targeting supplies where they are needed. Public-private partnerships—between the WHO and drug companies, for instance—can be very valuable.

In May 2013, the 66th World Health Assembly (WHA) adopted resolution WHA66.12 calling for "intensified, integrated measures and planned investments to improve the health and social well-being of affected populations." Representatives from 32 countries and representatives of nongovernmental organizations (NGOs) participated in debate and discussions before voting to adopt the resolution urging that countries "ensure country ownership of prevention, control, elimination and eradication programmes; expand and implement interventions and advocate for predictable, long-term international financing for activities related to control and capacity strengthening; integrate control programmes into primary health-care services and existing programmes; ensure optimal programme management and implementation; and achieve and maintain universal access to interventions and reach [targeted goals]."

Although a number of NGOs are involved in a grassroots effort to treat and eliminate NTDs, the majority of funding to combat NTDs currently comes from international pharmaceutical companies, the World Bank, and the Bill & Melinda Gates Foundation. In 2012, the Global Network for Neglected Tropical Diseases launched the END7 campaign, targeting seven NTDs, in partnership with the NGO Wunderman UK, the WHO, and the Bill & Melinda Gates Foundation. The UK government, hoping to help finance 1 billion treatments per year worldwide, also made a £245 million (US$381 million) international commitment to fight NTDs in 2012.

Medical researchers are making significant progress in the effort to eradicate some NTDs. Global cases of parasitic guinea worm disease, for example, have dropped dramatically from 3.5 million per year in 1986 to only 126 in 2014 due to international public health efforts. As of 2014, local cases of parasitic guinea worm disease occurred only in South Sudan, Mali, Ethiopia, and Chad. Public health officials continue to combat parasitic disease by instituting programs to improve sanitation and drinking water, provide shoes, and increase access to larvicides.

Although NTD rates are highest in sub-Saharan Africa and Southeast Asia, the poorest inhabitants of the Oceania (Pacific Island nations) region have NTD rates comparable to those locations. Hookworm infections,

SCHOLARS AND HEALTH-CARE WORKERS DISCUSS NTD ISSUES

The first global gathering of neglected tropical disease (NTD) experts specifically dedicated to discussing and articulating issues related to NTDs took place in Cambridge, Massachusetts, in July 2011 at the International Society for Infectious Diseases (ISID)—NTD meeting. The meeting focused on diseases that globally afflict more than 1 billion people, yet receive only a fraction of the money and media attention directed toward acquired immune deficiency syndrome (AIDS), malaria, and tuberculosis programs.

Long-standing tensions among researchers, clinicians, and public health advocates about the best allocation of limited resources created spirited debate. During the plenary session, lectures and exchanges among meeting participants twice became heated and emotional, with open challenges to the validity of scientific data and the effectiveness of various treatment programs. Arguments concerning the best use of funding and ways to spur awareness of NTD impacts found passionate supporters who differed about whether basic science research, vaccine development, nongovernmental organization (NGO) treatment programs, or community-based public health programs should receive future priority.

Daniel Lew, ISID president, said that the NTD meeting was part of ISID's mission to "encourage collaboration in tackling the world's infectious disease problems." Although less deadly in comparison to the "big three" (i.e., AIDS, malaria, and tuberculosis), Lew said that the NTD burden was economically devastating for individuals and communities. "In addition to causing death and suffering, NTDs perpetuate poverty," Lew argued in welcoming remarks. During the opening sessions, Lew and other speakers unanimously agreed that the fastest-spreading NTD, dengue fever, poses an increasingly potent threat to public health on a global scale.

During her plenary session lecture, Mirta Roses Periago, director of the Pan American Health Organization (PAHO) also lamented the comparative lack of media attention and money devoted to NTDs. "Those who suffer from NTDs don't make the headlines," Roses said. "Even physicians have trouble pronouncing some of these diseases." Roses emphatically declared that the elimination of NTDs was a "moral imperative," arguing that, "NTDs combine to rob millions of people, many among the most vulnerable in the world, of the freedom to live long, productive, and healthy lives."

Attracting NTD specialists from every continent, the meeting mixed scientists and clinicians with representatives from international pharmaceutical companies, the World Bank, and the Bill & Melinda Gates Foundation. Meeting participants also included delegates from at least eight other NGOs.

for example, affect more than half the population of Papua New Guinea.

Large-scale population movements have led to an increased risk of diseases in areas where they are not normally endemic. In non-endemic areas, the diseases encounter typically vulnerable populations with little to no exposure history. As humans continue to invade new ecological habits, contact with wild reservoirs of pathogens increases—along with increased chances of transmission between a vector and human.

🌐 Future Implications

According to the WHO, the 17 NTDs prioritized are endemic in 149 countries and affect an estimated 1.4 billion people. Economic costs are difficult to estimate with certainty but, at a minimum, the burden on developing countries is significant, and in some cases debilitating.

Experts fear that the dangerous set of dengue viruses will be tough to stop without an effective vaccine, and dengue fever will require a vaccine that is biologically complex. Several tetravalent vaccines (capable of offering protection against all four serotypes of dengue) were in development as of 2014. Global vaccine experts agree that the world faces an uphill challenge in developing a dengue vaccine, as only six pharmaceutical production facilities, all located in North America or Europe, have the capacity to produce a complex tetravalent vaccine.

Some scientists predict that global climate change may increase the incidence of tropical diseases. Warmer temperatures and increased surface water may increase the habitat of disease vectors such as insects. Some assert that tropical diseases will become more common, more widespread, and increasingly virulent. A study at Bournemouth University, published in *Emerging Microbes and Infections* in 2014, found a strong link between outbreaks of Buruli ulcer in French Guiana and shifting weather and climate patterns. Extreme rainfall events, such as those driven by El Niño, help spread and worsen outbreaks of the waterborne disease.

NTDs bring significant impact to local societies and economies. Since NTDs often strike subsistence cultures, the ability to work and grow food is vitally important to survival. Endemic threat of NTDs such as sleeping sickness has forced many people to flee productive—and sometimes scarce—farm and grazing lands in river valleys. Farming less-productive soils has contributed to food scarcity in some regions. Migration and increased local population density has exacerbated malnutrition and fueled incidence of disease. Some survivors of NTDs experience lifelong pain or physical disability, curtailing their ability to work. Despite the significant social and economic effects of NTDs, less than 1 percent of all new drugs registered between 1975 and 2000 were indicated to treat or prevent tropical diseases. Belen Pedrique and colleagues published an assessment in *The Lancet Global*

Health in 2013 showing that between 2000 and 2011 only 4 percent of new drugs and vaccines were targeted for neglected diseases, however, their definition included malaria, tuberculosis, diarrheal diseases, and 19 other diseases, still reflecting a lack research and development for combating NTDs.

The WHO and other organizations have reenergized international research on tropical diseases. Several NTDs can be treated with drugs that cost as little as two U.S. cents per dose. International health organizations have focused on educating health officials and training community volunteers to administer and distribute therapeutic drugs. Improved sanitation and hygiene programs, increased access to clean drinking water, and use of anti-insect pesticides, traps, and mosquito netting have helped to reduce incidence of NTDs. However, treatments for some NTDs remain expensive, outdated, and toxic or dangerous if administered incorrectly. Development of vaccines and cheaper, more effective, and safer drugs are vital to combating these NTDs.

PRIMARY SOURCE

Sustaining the Drive to Overcome the Global Impact of Neglected Tropical Diseases

SOURCE *"Summary," in* Sustaining the Drive to Overcome the Global Impact of Neglected Tropical Diseases: Second WHO Report on Neglected Tropical Diseases. *Geneva: World Health Organization (WHO), 2013, 2–3, 5–6. http://apps. who.int/iris/bitstream/10665/80245/1/WHO_ HTM_NTD_2013.2_eng.pdf (accessed January 25, 2015).*

INTRODUCTION *This primary source is from a summary of the second World Health Organization report on neglected tropical diseases, published in 2013. It gives an update of progress on global response since publication of the original report.*

BACKGROUND

SUSTAINING THE DRIVE TO OVERCOME THE GLOBAL IMPACT OF NEGLECTED TROPICAL DISEASES builds on the growing sense of optimism generated by the publication in 2012 of the WHO roadmap *Accelerating work to overcome the global impact of neglected tropical diseases....*

The roadmap set targets for the prevention, control and elimination of 17 neglected tropical diseases, including the eradication of dracunculiasis (by 2015) and yaws (by 2020). It marked a major strategic advance since the publication in 2010 of WHO's first report on neglected tropical diseases. The roadmap set a further 6 targets for the elimination of 5 neglected tropical diseases by 2015, and 10 elimination targets for 2020, either globally or in selected geographical areas, for 9 neglected tropical diseases. Targets for the intensified control of dengue, Buruli ulcer, cutaneous Leishmaniasis, selected zoonoses and helminthiases were also set....

SUSTAINABLE PROGRESS

Since 2010, more than 710 million people worldwide have received preventive chemotherapy treatment annually for at least one disease. The number of people treated for schistosomiasis almost tripled between 2005 and 2010, entirely due to expansion of programmes in the African Region. Coverage with treatment of populations at risk for soil-transmitted helminthiases reached 31% between 2005 and 2010....

Impressive progress is also being made in eradicating dracunculiasis. At the end of 2012, transmission was limited to four countries where the disease is endemic. The number of reported cases continued to decrease, with a total of 542 cases in 2012 compared with 1058 confirmed cases in 2011. Heightened community-based surveillance, combined with national integrated disease surveillance and response programmes such as for poliomyelitis, are expected to intensify case detection and further reduce transmission. Despite achievements and successes, operational challenges remain in Chad, Ethiopia, Mali and South Sudan.

Another disease targeted by WHO for eradication by 2020 is yaws. WHO's new Morges strategy uses a new treatment policy designed to replace those developed in the 1950s, which mainly centred on delivering injections of benzathine benzylpenicillin. Published in January 2012, the findings of a study in Papua New Guinea show that a single dose of oral azithromycin is as effective as intramuscular benzathine benzylpenicillin in treating yaws, thus revitalizing prospects for eradication through the delivery of large-scale treatment to infected and at-risk populations in the estimated 14 countries where yaws is endemic. This new strategy of treating the entire community overcomes the limitations of penicillin injections, which require trained healthcare personnel to deliver case-by-case treatment.

Management of diseases such as Buruli ulcer, Chagas disease, human African trypanosomiasis and the Leishmaniases has significantly improved. New cases of human African trypanosomiasis have continued to drop, raising prospects for elimination of the disease. Early diagnosis and treatment of cases, prompt management of complications, systematic screening of patients and adoption of strategies that respond appropriately to different levels of endemicity and health-system capacity have all contributed to reducing infection and morbidity.

SEE ALSO *Climate Change: Health Impacts; Global Health Initiatives; Parasitic Diseases; Waterborne Diseases*

BIBLIOGRAPHY

Books

Adams, Jonathan, Karen Gurney, and David Pendlebury. *Neglected Tropical Diseases.* Leeds, UK: Evidence, 2012.

Bentivoglio, Marina, et al., eds. *Neglected Tropical Diseases and Conditions of the Nervous System.* New York: Springer, 2014.

Biehl, João, and Adriana Petryna, eds. *When People Come First: Critical Studies in Global Health.* Princeton, NJ: Princeton University Press, 2013.

Crisp, Nigel. *Turning the World Upside Down: The Search for Global Health in the Twenty-First Century.* London: Royal Society of Medicine Press, 2010.

Davidson, Ronald J., ed. *Neglected Tropical Diseases: Background, Identification, and Prevention.* New York: Nova Science, 2011.

Elliott, Richard L., ed., et al. *Third World Diseases.* Berlin: Springer, 2011.

Farmer, Paul, Jim Yong Kim, Arthur Kleinman, and Matthew Basilico. *Reimagining Global Health.* Berkeley: University of California Press, 2013.

Hall, Peter A., and Michele Lamont, eds. *Successful Societies: How Institutions and Culture Affect Health.* New York: Cambridge University Press, 2009.

Hotez, Peter J. *Forgotten People, Forgotten Diseases The Neglected Tropical Diseases and Their Impact on Global Health and Development,* 2nd ed. Washington, DC: ASM Press, 2013.

McDowell, Mary Ann, and Sima Rafati, eds. *Neglected Tropical Diseases—Middle East and North Africa.* Vienna: Springer, 2014.

Palmer, Michael J., and Timothy N. C. Wells, eds. *Neglected Diseases and Drug Discovery.* Cambridge, UK: Royal Society of Chemistry, 2011.

Rothe, Camilla. *Clinical Cases in Tropical Medicine.* Philadelphia: Elsevier Saunders, 2015.

Walraven, Gijsbertus Engelinus Laurentius. *Health and Poverty: Global Health Problems and Solutions.* London: Earthscan, 2011.

Periodicals

Feasey, Nick, et al. "Neglected Tropical Diseases." *British Medical Bulletin* 93, no. 1 (2010): 179–200.

Friedrich, M. J. "Neglected Tropical Diseases." *JAMA* 304, no. 19 (2010): 2116.

Hotez, Peter J. "Enlarging the Audacious Goal: Elimination of the World's High Prevalence Neglected Tropical Diseases." *Vaccine* 29 (2011): 104–110.

Hotez, Peter J., and Jurg Utzinger. "The Global Burden of Disease Study 2010: Interpretation and Implications for the Neglected Tropical Diseases." *PLOS Neglected Tropical Diseases* 8, H7 (2014): e28658.

Keiser, Jennifer, Jurg Utzinger, Johannes A. Blum, and Christoph Hatz. "Neglected Tropical Diseases: Diagnosis, Clinical Management, Treatment and Control." *Swiss Medical Weekly* 142 (2012): w13726.

Molyneux, D. "Neglected Tropical Diseases." *Community Eye Health / International Centre for Eye Health* 26, no. 82 (2013): 21–24.

Tomczyk, S., and Jurg Utzinger. "Association between Footwear Use and Neglected Tropical Diseases: A Systematic Review and Meta-Analysis." *PLOS Neglected Tropical Diseases* 8, H.11 (2014): e3285.

Yang, Guo-Jing, Marcel Tanner, and Jurg Utzinger. "China's Sustained Drive to Eliminate Neglected Tropical Diseases." *The Lancet Infectious Diseases* 14 (2014): S881–892.

Websites

"Neglected Tropical Diseases." *PLOS.* http://journals.plos.org/plosntds/ (accessed March 1, 2015).

"Neglected Tropical Diseases." *U.S. Centers for Disease Control and Prevention (CDC).* http://www.cdc.gov/globalhealth/ntd/ (accessed March 1, 2015).

"Neglected Tropical Diseases." *World Health Organization (WHO).* http://www.who.int/neglected_diseases/diseases/en/ (accessed March 1, 2015).

Pedrique, Belen, et al. "The Drug and Vaccine Landscape for Neglected Diseases (2000–11): A Systematic Assessment." *The Lancet Global Health,* October 24, 2013. http://www.thelancet.com/journals/langlo/article/PIIS2214-109X(13)70078-0/abstract (accessed March 19, 2015).

K. Lee Lerner

NGOs and Health Care: Deliverance or Dependence

⊕ Introduction

Nongovernmental organizations (NGOs) play an essential role in the delivery of health services and contribute to health systems and strategies in the developing world. The term NGO refers to different types of entities that do not work within the public sector and do not operate for financial gain. Though NGOs are integral to health care throughout much of the world, they often have been controversial; detractors accuse many NGOs of inefficiency and fostering dependency.

Because many national governments are unable to provide sufficient health care for their citizens, NGOs are considered safe and useful institutions able to supply health care efficiently and cost-effectively. There has been rapid growth of NGOs, and significant public funds are used to pay for their activities in the health field. Smaller NGOs normally do not work alone in the health-care sector and often cooperate with United Nations (UN) agencies, which technically are also NGOs, such as the World Health Organization (WHO), Pan American Health Organization (PAHO), United Nations High Commissioner for Refugees (UNHCR), and the United Nations Children's Fund (UNICEF). These international agencies partner with smaller NGOs to achieve their missions and extend health care capabilities to nations in need.

In addition to providing health care to the poor across the globe, NGOs are crucial elements of a democratic culture, fostering social integration, building civil society, and engaging in public discourse and participatory democracy. However, there is criticism that NGOs often do not meet expectations and that their actions have the potential to exacerbate rather than ameliorate access to and availability of health-care services in developing countries.

The main tasks of NGOs in the health-care arena are to provide health advocacy, policy, and services. Provisions of health services often consist of medical, social, and psychological services, as well as nursing, material support, education, and training. Health advocacy includes actions designed to gain political commitment, policy support, social acceptance, and support for various health goals and objectives. In addition, NGOs are responsible for developing health policies to assist governments to implement effective responses to health needs. NGOs operate in every part and level of the health system, contributing surveillance (monitoring population health and the occurrence of disease), immunizations, community engagement, emergency services, and medical supplies in developing countries.

⊕ Historical Background

The origin of NGO involvement in health care can be traced to the perceived failure of state-led development in the world in the 1970s and 1980s. To complement and improve state functions, NGOs offered dynamic alternatives, using innovative and patient-centered approaches for health service delivery, advocacy, and policy. Specifically, development NGOs sought new and effective approaches to address systemic poverty and challenge social and health inequalities resulting from inadequate and inefficient public services. Often operating at the ground level with local communities, NGOs were able to deliver programs and projects based on community participation to treat and empower poor, vulnerable, and marginalized populations.

Until the late 1970s and early 1980s, NGOs gained little recognition for their implementation of development projects or influence on health policy. However, during the 1970s NGOs became a popular, new component in global development. This coincided with the rise of capitalism and liberalization as the Soviet and socialist models failed to provide for and inspire populations across the globe. As a result, structural adjustments in aid policies were made, largely reducing government services and spending. The market, rather than the state, became the foundation of development strategies, because economic growth was seen as essential to aid development and to help the poor.

By the 1990s, with the emerging good governance agenda, which refocused the use of government service, the state again became central to the effort to alleviate mass poverty through the implementation of state-oriented strategies and interventions. According to Nicola Banks and David Hulme's article "The Role of NGOs and Civil Society in Development and Poverty Reduction" in the *Brooks World Poverty Institute Working Paper*, the emphasis on state-centered responsibility acted to diminish the role of NGOs while the good governance agenda, with its focus on democracy, human rights, and public participation, supported the importance of NGOs in development.

In the 21st century, about one-fifth of international NGOs focus on health care, health advocacy, and health policy development. A new model for development and aid emerged, promoting greater communication between donors and recipients and designating poverty as a state responsibility. With a new emphasis on strengthening civil society, NGOs achieved greater recognition as an integral part of a free, democratic civil society.

As a major contributor to international development, NGOs have adopted diverse and complex relationships with governments, from conciliatory and complementary to critical and oppositional. These relationships, along with prevailing institutional arrangements, have largely supported the growth of NGOs in developing countries, but also ensured that NGOs and their relationships with state governments varied in different regions of the world.

Banks and Hulme note that in south Asia, the relationships between the state, NGOs, and global policies produced a diverse combination of sociopolitical environments, NGO activities, donor presence, and agendas during the 1970s. The decline of public sector institutions and the indifference of dominant political parties helped fuel an explosion of NGOs in India. Similarly, in the Philippines, the failure of political parties to treat and represent a major segment of its population left a political void that NGOs filled. In contrast, NGOs in Indonesia and Vietnam were established to expand public representation in response to state power rather than the weakness of their institutions.

Africa experienced its own NGO boom starting in the 1990s. In Kenya and Tanzania, NGOs multiplied throughout the decade with thousands of NGOs focused on indigenous memberships. In contrast, in Uganda, NGOs were viewed with suspicion, and critics worried that their primary focus was not the public good. In addition, African NGOs have been susceptible to political influence with some participating in patronage networks of political leaders.

Historically, in Latin America NGOs operated in opposition to authoritarian governments; they worked to strengthen civil society. In Mexico NGOs flourished under the leadership of college-educated members of the middle class hoping to treat and mobilize marginalized and underrepresented communities. As countries in the region transitioned to democracy, NGOs fragmented, losing their identity as organizations promoting resistance and social change. Foreign aid also fostered growing government collaboration with NGOs. NGOs continue to expand and operate in Latin America as they refocus on providing health care services to indigenous populations and persons who are disabled.

⊕ Impacts and Issues

Characteristics of NGOs

In the health-care arena, there is significant variety among the types of NGOs, though they can be divided broadly by their scope, according to Maria Piotrowicz and Dorota Cianciara's article "The Role of Non-governmental Organizations in the Social and Health System" in *Przeglad Epidemiologiczny* journal. International NGOs work around the world to facilitate development, deliver humanitarian aid, and address international public health problems. Commonly, international NGOs attempt to create access to basic health care in developing countries; they establish hospitals and clinics, implement vaccination drives, and respond to emergencies.

Usually operating within a single country, national NGOs often focus on specific health problems while addressing the needs and promotion of health service institutions. There has been growth of NGOs that seek to meet the health and social needs of specific groups and minorities while promoting their rights. In addition, there has been an increase in NGOs that attempt to treat and promote the rights of patients and families who suffer from chronic illness or disabilities.

Legally, NGOs can have either an informal or formal structure, which can be registered based on rules of a given country that certify the responsibilities and privileges of the classification. These privileges may include status that exempts the NGO from paying taxes and the ability to apply for and secure grant funding.

Along with the WHO, some of the largest and best-known international NGOs that work in the health-care arena are Médecins Sans Frontières (MSF; also known as Doctors Without Borders); the Bill & Melinda Gates Foundation; World Vision International; Save the Children; the International Federation of Red Cross and Red Crescent Societies (IFRC); the Global Fund to Fight AIDS, Tuberculosis and Malaria; the Joint United Nations Programme on HIV/AIDS (UNAIDS); the Wellcome Trust; and the World Bank.

Main Functions: Health Advocacy

Health advocacy is a combination of social and individual actions intended to achieve popular support for specific purposes, programs, and health initiatives. One form of advocacy is lobbying to make legislative changes through

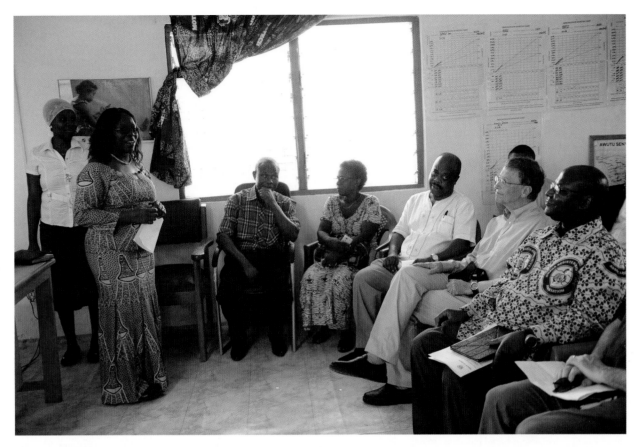

Microsoft's chairman, Bill Gates, one of world's richest men and high-profile aid donors, listens as a health official speaks on immunization coverage plans for the Awutu Senya district, a central region in Ghana. Gates was in Ghana to meet with government and health officials on ways to combat global health problems. The Bill & Melinda Gates Foundation, an NGO, donates at least 5 percent of its assets each year to fight poliomyelitis, HIV/AIDS, tuberculosis, malaria, and other diseases across the globe. © *Pius Utomi Ekpei/AFP/Getty Images.*

participatory and representative political bodies. Advocacy also encompasses persuasion through the use of meetings and forums, coordinating with political coalitions of interested organizations, and using the media to inform and educate the public.

The types and methods of health advocacy vary throughout the world, depending largely on the degree of development, local culture and tradition, the political system, resources, and specific needs. In low- and middle-low income countries, NGOs focus on human rights, service delivery, raising awareness, and prevention campaigns. In countries with middle to high incomes, NGOs often are more specialized; they combat specific diseases or champion specific preventive measures such as smoking cessation or diabetes prevention. In high-income countries patients have expanded opportunities to influence the development of NGO health delivery services and policy.

Main Functions: Health Policy

Another major task of NGOs is participating in the formulation of health policy. NGOs, along with organizations representing medical professionals, insurers, other health-care providers, consumers, commercial groups, and governments, take part in the process of creating and modifying health policies.

NGOs involved in the development of global policy initiatives include:

1. Center for Strategic and International Studies Global Health Policy Center, which links the public health and foreign policy communities and helps to develop strategies for U.S. involvement in basic global health issues such as the provision for food and water and preventing the spread of disease;

2. Global Alliance for Chronic Diseases, which funds and arranges research international collaborations to combat the rise of chronic diseases such as high blood pressure, a risk factor for heart disease, stroke, kidney disease, and other conditions that affect an estimated 1 billion people worldwide;

3. Global Health Council, which advocates for U.S. investment in global health policy and partners with the global health advocacy community to help ensure continuous funding for global health programs;

NGO HEALTH CARE IN PAKISTAN

In many developing countries, weaknesses and gaps in government health services have hampered progress and resulted in poor health outcomes (how patients fare as a result of health-care treatment or lack of treatment). This leaves considerable room for non-state actors, especially NGOs, to operate in an attempt to repair and improve public sector health services. For example, the public sector in Pakistan has long lacked the capacity to satisfy the health needs of its population. Historically, Pakistan has been plagued by public corruption that has resulted in uneven quality and poor management of health services and insufficient planning. State industries have suffered as a result of political instability caused by frequent military coups, and dramatically fewer merit-based promotions in public services have contributed to the health system's inability to address the needs of Pakistan's impoverished population.

According to Iram Ejaz, Babar T. Shaikh, and Narjis Rizvi in their article "NGOs and Government Partnership for Health Systems Strengthening: A Qualitative Study Presenting Viewpoints of Government, NGOs and Donors in Pakistan" in the journal *BMC Health Services Research*, international and national NGOs have been largely successful in filling the gaps in health service delivery, research, and advocacy due to their targeted, population-based programs to better Pakistan's health system. Ejaz and colleagues assert that NGOs have improved health care in the country through enhanced coordination and public private partnerships.

As a result, 206 public-private service organizations and 600 NGOs are engaged in health service delivery, research, and advocacy to fix the country's ailing health. For example, public-private partnerships with NGOs, such as the Leprosy Control Program and the National Action Plan to respond to noncommunicable diseases, have been tremendously successful. These partnerships have implemented new health education, promotion, and advocacy programs. The success of these NGOs is attributed to their ability to hire more staff quickly at acceptable salaries, acquire specialized equipment, and serve populations in specific geographic areas. NGO health services are considered to be more reliable, better managed, and of better quality than services provided by the public sector.

Though NGOs play a major role in Pakistan's health system, difficulties with capacity along with a lack of trust between NGOs and the government persist. Officials fear that partnerships can erode confidence in the public sector and undermine potential improvements in the system. Clear strategies, engagement, and smart regulations have the potential to provide a foundation for the government and NGOs to further coordinate to better Pakistan's beleaguered health-care system. Collaboration between NGOs and the public sector has the potential to help Pakistan achieve its goal of alleviating its health-care deficiencies.

4. Global Health Technologies Coalition, which champions innovation and use of technology to address pressing health problems such as HIV/AIDS, tuberculosis, malaria, and childhood killers such as diarrhea and pneumonia;

5. Kaiser Family Foundation U.S. Global Health Policy, which focuses on the U.S. role in global health policy and regularly surveys Americans to identify their priorities for global health efforts; and

6. Research!America Global Health R&D Advocacy, which advocates for research and development policies and funding to address global public health issues.

As more and more diverse groups participate in health policy formation, the process of planning and implementing policies becomes more complex. Though NGOs have grown increasingly powerful, the government begins, regulates, and governs the process of cooperation. NGOs can, however, exert real pressure during this process because of their alliances and coalitions with government representatives, professional groups, scientists, and media organizations.

Main Functions: Health Services

NGOs operate in every major field of the health-care system, including provision of basic health services, disease prevention, health promotion, and collaboration with state structures and organizations. Health services consist of education and training in addition to various types of support, including medical, social, psychological, nursing, and material, as well as financial assistance. In the global health context, NGOs often are the backbone of support for disease surveillance (monitoring the occurrence and spread of disease), immunizations, community engagement, emergency services, and medical supplies, according to the Center for Disaster and Humanitarian Assistance Medicine.

Before beginning operations, NGOs assess the region and population they plan to serve by analyzing surveillance results and other relevant medical data. Often this means using information provided by state governments and international organizations such as the UN. In addition, NGOs use a variety of surveillance methods and surveys to analyze the overall nutritional status, occurrence of disease and death rates, and health-care coverage in a given region.

A popular method of surveying promoted by John Seaman of Save the Children (United Kingdom) uses the household economy approach, which suggests that rural economic conditions and other pertinent information should be considered to comprehend fully the status of healthcare in a region. Assessing malnutrition and nutritional health levels in a population also may involve using body measurements, such as mid-upper arm circumference and weight-for-height measurements. NGO surveillance also includes monitoring communicable (infectious) diseases by measuring infection rates of specific diseases, which is used to analyze and anticipate potential outbreaks and epidemics. Such surveillance not only helps NGOs better do their jobs but also enables them to detect threats to international public health safety.

NGOs play a crucial role in immunizing populations, often those affected by a recent natural disaster, when circumstances such as a lack of water and sanitation create an ideal climate for the spread of disease. Working with local communities and international agencies, NGOs have spearheaded efforts to immunize against a range of communicable diseases including measles, meningitis, diphtheria, pertussis, tetanus, and polio to help contain and prevent major outbreaks of these diseases.

NGOs engage with local communities, operating programs that aim to enhance health awareness and strengthen local medical training and health-care capacity. To strengthen weak health-care systems, NGO health initiatives often involve training local community health workers, village health aides, and even traditional birth attendants to implement health education and support service programs. Training local health workers to deliver

reproductive health programs that educate about and provide access to birth control and ensuring adequate nutrition during pregnancy and after birth are popular strategies employed by NGOs that emphasize family and community planning.

One key role of NGOs is to respond to emergencies and public health crises. Often on the ground in an emergency or already in the region before a crisis, NGOs are poised to respond quickly, providing essential information to the international community as well as immediate, ground-level implementation of emergency health services.

NGOs are supported technically and financially by international agencies such as the UN and organizations and donors such as the WHO, UNICEF, the United Nations Office for the Coordination of Humanitarian Affairs, the U.S. Agency for International Development, and the Canadian International Development Agency. Coordinating with the international community, NGOs respond rapidly to implement health service priorities so that limited resources can be used to meet urgent needs. According to USAID's Field Operations Guide, NGOs and the international community prioritize specific actions, such as providing clean water and vaccinations and assessing the need for food and shelter as well

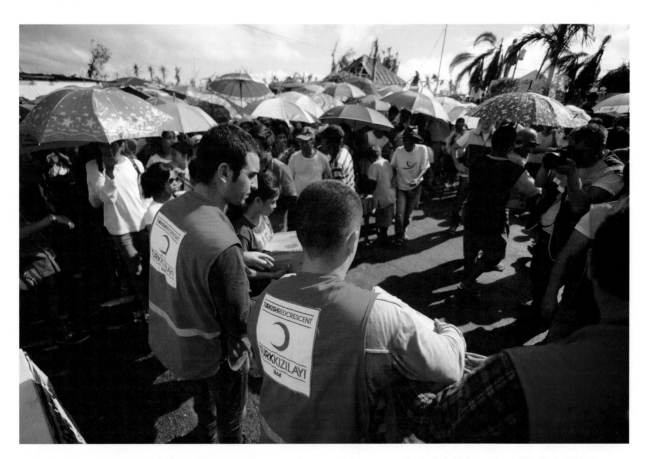

The Turkish Red Crescent arrives in the Philippines, carrying 110 tons (100 metric tons) of relief aid for victims of Typhoon Haiyan (Yolanda) on November 27, 2013, in Tacloban, Philippines.   © *Omer Urer/Anadolu Agency/Getty Images.*

as identifying vulnerable populations such as children and older adults who may require special assistance.

NGOs play a significant role in procuring and delivering pharmaceutical and medical supplies across the globe, especially to regions in crisis. Often, NGOs do more than any other groups to deliver medicines to affected areas during an emergency. Major NGO medical suppliers include Direct Relief International, Americares, MAP (formerly Medical Assistance Programs), and Operation USA. Each maintains ongoing relationships with pharmaceutical and medical supply companies that donate their overstock. These NGOs stockpile medical supplies and ship their inventory via air and ocean freight to local NGOs and agencies to distribute them.

Criticism of NGOs

As NGOs have grown, criticism of them has increased as well. The chief criticism of NGOs is that although they are promoted as decentralized, efficient alternatives to state agencies, they can be as inefficient and bureaucratic as the state agencies themselves. Critics suggest that NGOs are prone to embellish their productivity while actually failing to cater to more than a small percentage of the populations they are intended to serve, according to S. Akbar Zaidi's article "NGO Failure and the Need to Bring Back the State" in the *Journal of International Development*. For example, Zaidi points out that the largest NGOs in Bangladesh reach only 20 percent of the landless population, those most in need of and desperate for care.

Detractors also assert that NGOs' dependence on donors with short-term goals creates inefficiencies in health-care delivery. According to Jessica Maltha's article "NGOs in Primary Health Care: A Benefit or a Threat?" in *Global Medicine Magazine*, NGOs are blamed for carrying out projects to meet donor requirements, instead of using the ideas and acquired knowledge of locals to fulfill their needs. Often NGOs arrive in a foreign country with their own agendas and programs, approved by their donors, which include very specific objectives and targets that must be met to ensure continued funding. As a result, NGOs may neglect to address critical health needs or the overall functioning of the health-care system in favor of their own predetermined assessments and action plans.

In addition to NGOs' dependence on donors, critics argue that NGOs, with state support, foster dependency between the developed and developing nations, which recalls and reenacts a long history of colonialism. According to the Edelstein Center for Social Research, NGOs are an antidemocratic innovation that claim humanitarian goals but ultimately are not accountable to the people they treat and are intended to serve. Maltha also claims that NGOs foster dependence through their hiring and compensation practices. In many cases, international NGOs employ their own Western staff and pay them considerably more than the local health workers are paid. NGOs that do hire local staff pay them more too, which serves to undermine the public health care system by hiring away government workers. When economic incentives motivate local workers to work for NGOs instead of the state, state public health services suffer the loss of their expertise and diminished capacity.

In response to these criticisms and problems with NGO policies and operations, a group of leading service and advocacy organizations adopted the NGO Code of Conduct for Health Systems Strengthening in 2008. The code, which is composed of six articles, outlines how NGOs can strengthen public health care systems while supporting international health. It addresses the roles and responsibilities of international NGOs and offers guidance for NGO hiring and compensation practices, training of local health workers, and describes ways to minimize the management burden for ministries of health that are often created by multiple NGO projects.

⊕ Future Implications

As populations grow in developing countries, NGOs continue to play an important role in international health care, advocacy, and policy. In addition to delivering vital health services, NGOs play a crucial role in the development of civil societies by promoting public health campaigns, responding to public health emergencies, and pursuing basic human rights. NGOs continue to grow and mature, working to enhance local capacity, engage professionals, and balance private-sector interests.

NGOs also have responded to criticism that they frequently foster dependency and undermine local health care delivery systems. In a May 2010 report, Health Alliance International assessed the implementation of the NGO Code of Conduct, concluding that problems remain though progress is being made. Increased donor presence and funding has resulted in a higher demand for and hiring of trained personnel from the public health-care sector. In addition, NGOs continue to fan the flames of the human resource crisis in low-income countries by hiring health workers who would otherwise work for the local ministries of health or in other public employment.

Despite these concerns, Health Alliance International remains optimistic about the future and is confident that NGOs, governments, and donors can and will cooperate and collaborate to strengthen public health systems and provide equitable health care throughout the world, especially for poor and vulnerable populations.

SEE ALSO *Health-Care Worker Safety and Shortages*

BIBLIOGRAPHY

Books

Edwards, Michael, ed. *The Oxford Handbook of Civil Society.* New York: Oxford University Press, 2011.

Fowler, Alan. *The Virtuous Spiral: A Guide to Sustainability for NGOs in International Development.* London: Earthscan, 2000.

Lewis, David, and Nazneen Kanji. *Non-governmental Organizations and Development.* London: Routledge, 2009.

Periodicals

Banks, Nicola, and David Hulme. "The Role of NGOs and Civil Society in Development and Poverty Reduction." *Brooks World Poverty Institute Working Paper* 171 (June 1, 2012). Available online at http://www.slideshare.net/purbitaditecha/bwpi-wp17112 (accessed April 13, 2015).

Cooley, Alexander, and James Ron. "The NGO Scramble: Organizational Insecurity and the Political Economy of Transnational Action." *International Security* 27, no. 1 (Summer 2002): 5–39.

Ejaz, Iram, Babar T. Shaikh, and Narjis Rizvi. "NGOs and Government Partnership for Health Systems Strengthening: A Qualitative Study Presenting Viewpoints of Government, NGOs and Donors in Pakistan." *BMC Health Services Research* 11, no. 1 (May 2011): 122.

Gellert, George A. "Non-governmental Organizations in International Health: Past Successes, Future Challenges." *International Journal of Health Planning Management* 11, no. 1 (January 1996): 19–31.

Maltha, Jessica. "NGOs in Primary Health Care: A Benefit or a Threat?" *Global Medicine Magazine,* 7 (July 2009): 6–9.

Piotrowicz, Maria, and Dorota Cianciara. "The Role of Non-governmental Organizations in the Social and the Health System." *Przeglad Epidemiologiczny* 67, no. 1 (June 2013): 69–74.

Zaidi, S. Akbar. "NGO Failure and the Need to Bring Back the State." *Journal of International Development* 11 (December 1999): 259–271.

Websites

"Can NGOs Help Build the Public-Sector Health Workforce? Successes and Challenges Implementing the NGO Code of Conduct for Health Systems Strengthening." *Health Alliance International.* http://ngocodeofconduct.org/wp-content/uploads/implementing_ngo_code_of_conduct_report_may-2010.pdf (accessed January 29, 2015).

"Civil Societies North-South Relations: NGOs and Dependency." *Edelstein Center for Social Research.* http://www.centroedelstein.org.br/PDF/Working Papers/WP_1_English.pdf (accessed January 29, 2015).

"A Guide to Nongovernmental Organizations for the Military." *Center for Disaster and Humanitarian Assistance Medicine.* http://www.fas.org/irp/doddir/dod/ngo-guide.pdf (accessed January 29, 2015).

"Nongovernmental Organizations (NGOs)." *Nongovernmental Organizations (NGOs) Working in Global Health Research.* http://www.fic.nih.gov/Global/Pages/NGOs.aspx (accessed March 10, 2015).

"Strategic Alliances: The Role of Civil Society in Health." *World Health Organization (WHO).* http://www.who.int/civilsociety/documents/en/alliances_en.pdf (accessed January 29, 2015).

"Understanding Civil Society Issues for WHO." *World Health Organization (WHO).* http://www.who.int/civilsociety/documents/en/understanding_en.pdf?ua=1 (accessed January 29, 2015).

"WHO and Civil Society: Linking for Better Health." *World Health Organization (WHO).* http://www.who.int/civilsociety/documents/en/CSICaseStudyE.pdf?ua=1 (accessed January 29, 2015).

Yahya Zaffir Chaudhry

Noncommunicable Diseases (Lifestyle Diseases)

🌐 Introduction

Noncommunicable diseases are illnesses or conditions that are the result of lifestyle and behavioral characteristics in a population. Unlike infectious diseases that are spread from person to person, these afflictions are the result of lifestyle factors like poor nutrition, physical inactivity, aging, and tobacco use. The World Health Organization (WHO) estimates that noncommunicable diseases killed 38 million people in 2012.

Noncommunicable, or "lifestyle," diseases typically develop and progress slowly over longer periods than infectious diseases. According to the WHO, the most common noncommunicable illnesses include cardiovascular ailments (stroke and coronary heart disease), varying forms of cancer, respiratory conditions (asthma and chronic obstructive pulmonary disease [COPD]), and diabetes.

The majority of deaths from noncommunicable diseases are now occurring in low- and middle-income countries. Most low- and middle-income countries do not have universal health-care coverage, meaning individuals in these developing countries commonly bear the sole cost of these chronic conditions.

In 2012, 42 percent of the 38 million deaths from noncommunicable disease occurred during a time of life that individuals are often considered to be of working ages. This loss of income and reduction in workforce can have significant detrimental impacts on low- and middle-income economies. The cost of treatment for noncommunicable diseases can be overwhelming for developing nations as well. In 2011, the combined financial burden of cancer and COPD was estimated to be $700 billion.

🌐 Historical Background

As societies develop, their population demographics and disease characteristics change. Communicable diseases tend to gradually account for fewer deaths over time. In 1996, a WHO report indicated noncommunicable diseases accounted for 47 percent of annual worldwide deaths in 1990, with the remaining deaths attributable to injuries (11 percent) and communicable diseases (42 percent). The report also projected that by 2020, the rates of noncommunicable diseases would increase by at least 20 percent, causing a subsequent decrease in the rates of communicable diseases.

The "epidemiological transition" described above represents a theory described by the researcher A. R. Omran in 1971. Omran postulated that changes in population demographics (age, mortality rates, fertility, etc.) would shift as a societies moved from agrarian civilizations and became industrialized. The theory operates on the premise that mortality is the principal component of population change. This statement might seem straightforward, considering that birthrates might impact population numbers much like mortality. After all, would not any population stop growing if birthrates dropped to zero, regardless of how low the mortality rate was? Omran pointed out that although birthrates could potentially rise to maximum biological levels, there are no such restraints on mortality.

The second premise in Omran's theory involved distinct changes in the common diseases a population would be exposed to as a society develops. As stated in his original article, "During the transition, a long-term shift occurs in mortality and disease patterns whereby pandemics of infection are gradually displaced by degenerative and man-made diseases as the chief form of morbidity and primary cause of death."

Epidemiological Transition Stages

The epidemiological transition theory consists of three stages that describe changes in population demographics and mortality from disease. The first stage, "the age of pestilence and famine," is characterized by high mortality rates and short life spans. As early human beings became less nomadic and community sizes grew, animals were domesticated and crops were farmed. Unfortunately, this led to an increased exposure to human and animal waste, which spread endemic diseases that could wipe out the

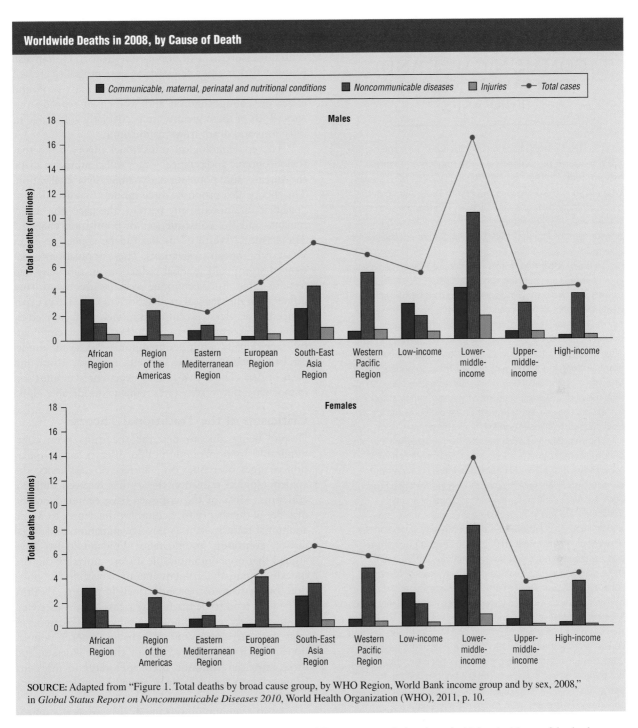

Worldwide Deaths in 2008, by Cause of Death

SOURCE: Adapted from "Figure 1. Total deaths by broad cause group, by WHO Region, World Bank income group and by sex, 2008," in *Global Status Report on Noncommunicable Diseases 2010*, World Health Organization (WHO), 2011, p. 10.

According to the World Health Organization (WHO), lower- to middle-income populations have the highest incidence of deaths due to noncommunicable diseases.

majority of a population. Death from communicable diseases and nutritional deficiencies are common during this stage, and the average life expectancy at birth is between 20 to 40 years.

The second stage, "the age of receding pandemics," is marked by a fewer peaks in mortality rates. This period represents the initial shift from infectious diseases

causing high rates of mortality to noncommunicable, or chronic, diseases generating the majority of deaths in a population. There are many reasons for this transition to occur, for example, improvements in hygiene and sanitation, increases in food supplies, less crowded living environments, etc. Each factor makes varying contributions. Infant mortality rates decline, and parents begin waiting

BLURRED LINES BETWEEN COMMUNICABLE AND NONCOMMUNICABLE DISEASES

"It is time to close the book on infectious diseases, and declare the war against pestilence won." This quote is often mistakenly attributed to U.S. Surgeon General Dr. William H. Stewart, who served in the position from 1965 to 1969. Although this particular statement was never actually uttered, the sentiment was adopted in medical and scientific circles following the development of antibiotics, vaccines, and other advancements against infectious agents.

It is now clear that there is considerable overlap between communicable and noncommunicable diseases. A variety of cancers and cardiovascular diseases are caused by infections, and treatment methods have been developed to combat these conditions. However, it is often difficult to identify the interactions between infectious and lifestyle diseases because they can, and often do, occur within the same person at the same time. For example, patients infected with human immunodeficiency virus often develop chronic tuberculosis. Diabetic patients are also at high risk of developing infections. Many environmental concerns (sanitation, hygiene, air quality, etc.) have profound impacts on both communicable and noncommunicable diseases.

Globalization has also increased the rate at which low- and middle-income countries adopt unhealthy lifestyle behaviors. Tobacco use has dropped in many developed countries, but remains high in less wealthy nations. Sugar-sweetened beverages, a known contributor to childhood obesity and type 2 diabetes, are sold in huge quantities to high-, low-, and middle-income countries. The strategies to reduce tobacco use in developing nations are often used to develop programs to address the high rates of soda consumption. Unfortunately, these products are not analogous. In many areas of the world, soda is a main source of calories and one way for individuals to increase caloric intake. For example, according to Janet M. Wojcicki and Melvin B. Heyman in "Malnutrition and the Role of the Soft Drink Industry in Improving Child Health in Sub-Saharan Africa," in rural areas of South Africa, infants under the age of 2 are consuming soda two to three times per week. Thus, programs must be put in place to combat hunger, undernutrition, and inadequate nutrient consumption, conditions that also lead to increased susceptibility to communicable diseases.

Preventive measures for communicable disease must be implemented concurrently with programs to address noncommunicable disease to reduce the double burden of disease in low- and middle-income countries.

mortality rates decrease until they eventually plateau. It is during this stage that fertility replaces mortality as the central measurement of population growth. Omran also postulated that any safeguards against mortality created during the third stage would have the most profound effect on young children and women of reproductive ages. Both of these groups are particularly vulnerable to infections and death from malnutrition.

The epidemiological transitional theory notes that socioeconomic and political forces will continue to shape the disease and population dynamics in a civilization. The theory also proposes three models that account for "peculiar variations in the pattern, the pace, the determinants and the consequences of population change." The classical "Western" model can be applied to most Western European civilizations. These populations experienced steady and gradual reductions in mortality and fertility rates. Socioeconomic systems are the driving influence in the classical model. Societies like Japan experienced an accelerated transition model, characterized by a relatively shorter time to reach the third epidemiological stage. Finally, a third contemporary "delayed" model can be applied to societies in South America, Africa, and parts of Asia. These civilizations experienced a reduction in mortality, but fertility rates remain considerably high.

Criticisms of the Traditional Theory

Despite being able to describe the shifts from communicable to noncommunicable diseases and population changes over time on a variety of continents, the epidemiological transition theory has received multiple criticisms. Most of the critiques have centered on the inability of the theory to account for the degree to which additional factors, such as poverty, nutrition, and social justice, contribute to mortality. Epidemiologists have argued that noncommunicable disease mortality can rise quickly among the affluent members within a population, but remain low for individuals in poverty. Wealthy individuals tend to be the first to access healthy lifestyles, causing a divergence in noncommunicable disease mortality between socioeconomic groups. Poorer populations often have a delayed rise in chronic illnesses, and these rates can continue even after rates of mortality begin to drop for more prosperous groups in the same population.

Another limitation of Omran's theory is the simplified association of risks that are made between disease and mortality. The risk for dying from any particular cause differs considerably among demographic groups within a population. For example, in 2013, the most common form of death for men in the United Kingdom was cancer, but for women it was circulatory diseases. In 2011, homicide was the most common cause of death in the United States for black men between the ages of 20–24, accounting for 49 percent of the total deaths. The percentage of deaths from homicide for white males in the same age group was 8 percent.

longer to have additional children. The average life expectancy at birth increases to approximately 30 to 50 years.

The third stage in the theory, "the age of degenerative and man-made diseases," consists of continued increases in the average life expectancy at birth, and

Variations in risk and mortality rates within a population are often much more complicated than the traditional theory explains. For example, a rapid drop in the risk for a certain disease can cause the proportional risks of other diseases appear larger, even if the actual risk for these diseases has also declined. It has also been discovered that the separation between communicable and noncommunicable diseases is not so clear cut. Medical science has now shown that chronic conditions like some types of cancer and cardiovascular disease have infectious etiologies.

⊕ Impacts and Issues

Cardiovascular Diseases

Cardiovascular diseases (CVDs) accounted for 17.5 million deaths in 2012, according to the WHO. Nearly half of all the deaths from noncommunicable diseases were from CVDs. Although they are commonly grouped together, CVDs actually make up a collection of several separate disorders that affect the heart and circulatory system. Coronary artery disease often results from a buildup of a fatty substance called plaque, which adheres to the inner walls of the vessels that supply blood to bodily organs. If these vessels become too narrow to allow adequate blood supply to pass through, this can lead to tissue death. For example, coronary heart disease is caused by the occlusion of blood vessels that cause the heart muscles to stop receiving enough sufficient blood supplies.

As time goes on, plaque deposits inside the vessels begin to harden and cause the arteries to lose their elasticity; this can cause several types of CVDs. Cerebrovascular disease is caused by an obstruction in the vessels that supply blood to the brain, resulting in a stroke. Peripheral arterial disease is the result of plaque occluding the arteries in the arms, legs, and other areas distal to the heart. If the large veins that reside in the leg develop a blockage, or clot, the result is referred to as a deep vein thrombosis. An embolism occurs if a piece of plaque breaks free and flows though the bloodstream, blocking blood flow to the brain, heart, or lungs.

Other types of CVDs can occur, as well. Congenital heart diseases are present at birth, and result in dysfunctional blood flow to the heart. These diseases can cause the blood flow to be weakened, blocked, or even reversed. Rheumatic heart disease is a unique form of CVD because it is caused by bacteria, specifically group A streptococcal. If the initial infection is not treated with antibiotics, the bacteria can cause rheumatic fever. This condition stimulates an abnormal generation of fibrous tissue in the heart valves. If the condition is not addressed, the valves that pump blood through the heart become unable to function, resulting in heart failure.

Over 80 percent of deaths from noncommunicable diseases are due to CVD. Recently, this disease has begun to disproportionally affect low- and middle-income countries. The rates of CVDs in these countries are now higher than those in high-income countries. Thirty-one percent of all global deaths are from CVDs, and strokes are the second-leading cause of death for individuals over 60 years of age.

Cancers

Cancer is a broad term that applies to a collection of diseases that are usually the result of irregular and uncontrolled growth of tissue cells. In 2012, the estimated prevalence rate for individuals over 15 years old who had received a cancer diagnosis in the last five years was 32.6 million. That year, cancers killed 8.2 million people worldwide. The WHO expected this number to increase by 70 percent over the next 20 years.

Although all of the causes of cancer remain unknown, environmental agents have been identified that produce cancerous cells. These substances are referred to as carcinogens, and they cause cancer by inducing mutations in human cells. A mutation is an alteration to the genetic information contained within every living cell. Between 60 to 90 percent of all human cancers are thought to be caused by environmental carcinogens. Cigarette smoke, radon gas, and ultraviolet radiation from the sun are all examples of known carcinogens. Some cancers can also be caused by infectious agents such as viruses, bacteria, and parasites. The WHO states that tobacco use is the number one cause of preventable deaths worldwide due to its links to lung cancer and other noncommunicable diseases.

Cancer risks vary for men and women. In 2012, lungs were the most common area for cancer diagnosis among men. Lung cancers were also the most deadly form of the disease, causing a total of 1.6 million deaths. The prostate is the second-leading location for cancer in males. Most prostate cancers involve gland cells that generate reproductive fluids. Despite being common, prostate cancer tends to have a very low mortality rate.

Breast cancer is the leading diagnosis of cancer in women. Unlike prostate cancer, breast cancer has a high mortality rate. There were over half a million deaths from breast cancer in 2012. Colorectal cancers are the second-leading area for diagnosis in women. Colorectal cancers are the fourth-deadliest form of cancer, and the third-most commonly diagnosed cancer for men.

Some types of cancer are caused by viral infections. Liver cancer, the second-most deadly form of cancer worldwide, can result from chronic exposure to the hepatitis B and C viruses. Prolonged infections from hepatitis B or C cause a form of scaring on the liver, referred to as cirrhosis. If left untreated, cirrhosis can lead to liver cancer. The human papillomavirus (HPV) is transmitted during sexual intercourse and can cause cancers in both men and women. The cervix is the fourth-most-common site for cancer diagnosis in women, and its primary cause is exposure to HPV. Exposure to HPV has also been linked to cancers in the penis, anus, mouth, and throat.

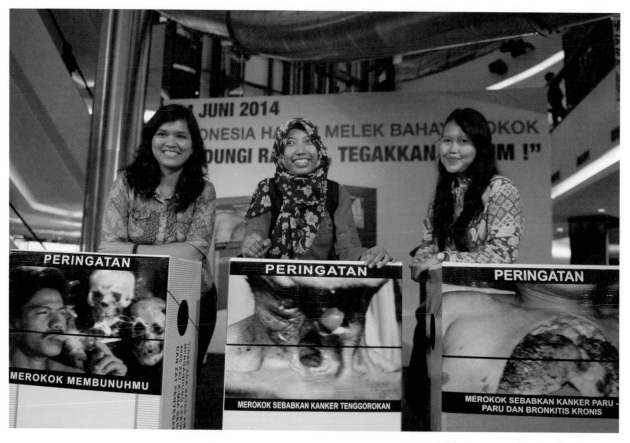

Indonesian youths have their photographs taken next to oversized cigarette pack mockups with graphic images of medical conditions caused by smoking in Jakarta. An Indonesian law requiring manufacturers to display pictorial health warnings on cigarette packs came into force on June 24, 2014, but antismoking campaigners said the rule was widely ignored. The government had given the tobacco industry 18 months to comply with the 2012 regulation on tobacco control, which demands pictures or graphics on packs to warn about the hazards of smoking in addition to written warnings.   *© Adek Berry/AFP/Getty Images.*

Respiratory Diseases

Chronic obstructive pulmonary disease (COPD) is characterized by a reoccurring lack of airflow, resulting in breathlessness and persistent coughing that generate high levels of phlegm. Formerly known as emphysema and chronic bronchitis, these disease is caused by cigarette smoke, air pollution, pulmonary infections, and exposure to hazardous occupational dusts and gases. Inhalation of these substances causes destruction of the small, distended sacs within the lungs referred to as alveoli. As the alveoli are damaged, they lose the ability to expel air upon exhalation. Over time, the remaining excess air increases the size of the chest cavity. COPD also causes the mucosal lining of the airway to thicken, trapping pathogens and causing breathlessness.

Asthma is a combination of chronic inflammation, hypersensitivity, and obstruction of the airway. Asthma symptoms can be caused by muscle spasms in the bronchi, the primary inlet for air to enter the lungs. Sometimes the airway obstructions are caused by an increase in the mucus secreted within the lungs. Individuals with asthma have reactions to lower concentrations of irritants that do not typically affect individuals without asthma. The exact cause of asthma remains unknown, but it is triggered by allergens like pollen, household dust mites, molds, cigarette smoke, exercise, and even certain food preservatives. If untreated, asthma can lead to chronic inflammation and eventually death of lung tissue.

Diabetes

Type 1 diabetes, also known as insulin-dependent diabetes, is characterized by low levels of insulin. Insulin is an important storage hormone that triggers the absorption of glucose from the bloodstream. Glucose, a simple sugar, is the primary energy source for humans. In type 1 diabetes, the immune system spontaneously targets and destroys the cells that produce insulin. Individuals with low levels of insulin have difficulty absorbing glucose, which causes the body to resort to breaking down fat stores for energy. When fat stores are used for energy, the by-products produced can cause the blood to become more acidic, a condition known as ketoacidosis. If not treated, ketoacidosis can be deadly. Breaking down fat stores for energy also increases the amount of fat in the bloodstream, which can lead to blocked vessels and arteries. The unabsorbed glucose also interferes with the lens in the eye, eventually leading to blindness. Type 1 diabetes is more common in individuals of northern European descent. For example, in Finland approximately 1 percent of the population develops type 1 diabetes by age 15.

Type 2 diabetes, or non-insulin-dependent diabetes, is much more common than type 1. Unlike the low insulin level indicative of type 1 diabetes, type 2 diabetics suffer from an excess of insulin in the bloodstream. Insulin is released in response to food intake, and cell receptors identify the hormone and begin absorbing glucose from the bloodstream. If too much insulin is present in the bloodstream, the cell receptors become desensitized and do not respond by absorbing glucose from the bloodstream. Sugar-sweetened beverage intake, low physical activity levels, and tobacco use increase the risk for developing type 2 diabetes. The WHO estimates that type 2 diabetes accounts for 90 percent of the diabetes cases worldwide, and that type 2 diabetes will become the seventh-leading cause of death by 2030.

⊕ Future Implications

Current prevention strategies for addressing noncommunicable diseases include tobacco cessation programs, healthful diet advice, physical activity promotion, and a reduction in alcohol intake. These are all considered to be modifiable risk factors, either at the individual or policy level. In 2013 the WHO published the *Global Action Plan for the Prevention and Control of Noncommunicable Diseases.* This report outlines efforts and strategies member nations can take to reduce the burden from noncommunicable disease.

WHO Goals for 2020

Nine voluntary goals are outlined in the Global Action Plan report, the first being a "25% relative reduction in overall mortality" from the top four noncommunicable diseases. This measurement applies to individuals that die from a common noncommunicable disease between the ages of 30 and 70. Two goals target a 10 percent relative reduction in the amount of alcohol consumed and the prevalence of physical inactivity. Another two goals aim for reduction in the average population salt intake

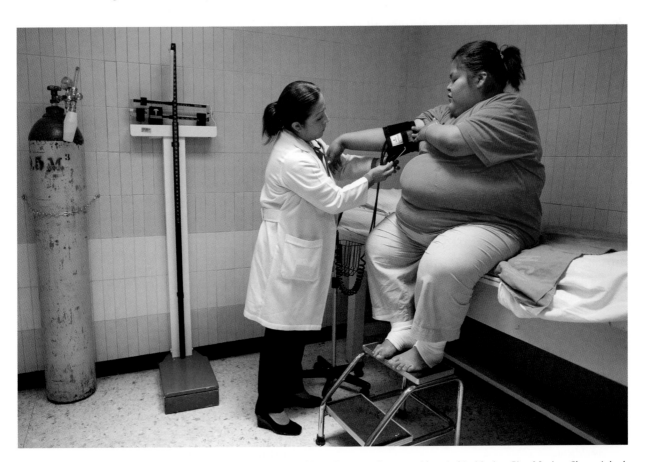

A 17-year-old Mexican girl with severe, morbid obesity is checked by a doctor at the general hospital in Mexico City, Mexico. She weighed in at 315 pounds and was 5 feet and 2 inches (159 centimeters) tall, with a BMI of 56.7. She was diagnosed with diabetes mellitus type 2, arterial hypertension, metabolic syndrome, and deep venous insufficiency. Her mother died as a result of complications from diabetes.
© Benedicte Desrus / Alamy.

and tobacco use by 30 percent, relative to each country's starting point.

High blood pressure, otherwise known as hypertension, is an early indicator for a cluster of noncommunicable diseases, including coronary heart disease, stroke, and type 2 diabetes. High blood pressure can cause damage to the blood vessel walls and induce inflammation, similar to plaque buildup. In countries currently recording population blood pressure statistics, the report advises reducing high blood pressure by 25 percent. For countries not documenting blood pressure statistics, obtaining the current prevalence of high blood pressure is sufficient.

Obesity, a medical condition determined by an individual's body mass index (BMI), increases an individual's risk for CVD, certain forms cancer, and type 2 diabetes. Since the mid-1980s, obesity rates have climbed globally. More importantly, the rates of childhood obesity have increased the prevalence of type 2 diabetes in low- and middle-income countries. The report calls for a halt in the rise of obesity and diabetes rates, regardless of current estimates.

The last two goals are specific to the accessibility of prevention and treatment medicines. The first seeks to ensure that "at least 50% of eligible people receive drug therapy and counseling to prevent heart attacks and strokes." Eligible people are individuals over 40 years old with a 10-year cardiovascular risk greater than 30 percent. These individuals are most at risk for suffering a cardiac event and should be prioritized to reduce the burden from CVD. The final goal is to provide an 80 percent availability of "affordable basic technologies and essential medicines" to treat noncommunicable disease in public and private medical facilities.

PRIMARY SOURCE

Global Action Plan for the Prevention and Control of Noncommunicable Diseases, 2013–2020

SOURCE *"Overview," in* Global Action Plan for the Prevention and Control of Noncommunicable Diseases, 2013–2020. *Geneva: World Health Organization (WHO), 2013, 3–5. http://apps.who.int/iris/bitstream/10665/94384/1/9789241506236_eng.pdf (accessed January 25, 2015).*

INTRODUCTION *This primary source is an excerpt from a World Health Organization publication outlining long-term goals for eradication of noncommunicable diseases, a category of disease that has emerged as a major cause of death worldwide.*

Vision:

A world free of the avoidable burden of noncommunicable diseases.

Goal:

To reduce the preventable and avoidable burden of morbidity, mortality and disability due to noncommunicable diseases by means of multisectoral collaboration and cooperation at national, regional and global levels, so that populations reach the highest attainable standards of health and productivity at every age and those diseases are no longer a barrier to well-being or socioeconomic development.

Overarching Principles

- Life-course approach
- Empowerment of people and communities
- Evidence-based strategies
- Universal health coverage
- Management of real, perceived or potential conflicts of interest
- Human rights approach
- Equity-based approach
- National action and international cooperation and solidarity
- Multisectoral action

Objectives

1. To raise the priority accorded to the prevention and control of noncommunicable diseases in global, regional and national agendas and internationally agreed development goals, through strengthened international cooperation and advocacy.

2. To strengthen national capacity, leadership, governance, multisectoral action and partnerships to accelerate country response for the prevention and control of noncommunicable diseases.

3. To reduce modifiable risk factors for noncommunicable diseases and underlying social determinants through creation of health-promoting environments.

4. To strengthen and orient health systems to address the prevention and control of noncommunicable diseases and the underlying social determinants through people-centred primary health care and universal health coverage.

5. To promote and support national capacity for high-quality research and development for the prevention and control of noncommunicable diseases.

6. To monitor the trends and determinants of noncommunicable diseases and evaluate progress in their prevention and control.

Voluntary Global Targets

- A 25% relative reduction in risk of premature mortality from cardiovascular diseases, cancer, diabetes, or chronic respiratory diseases.

- At least 10% relative reduction in the harmful use of alcohol, as appropriate, within the national context.

- A 10% relative reduction in prevalence of insufficient physical activity.

- A 30% relative reduction in mean population intake of salt/sodium.

- A 30% relative reduction in prevalence of current tobacco use in persons aged 15+ years.

- A 25% relative reduction in the prevalence of raised blood pressure or contain the prevalence of raised blood pressure, according to national circumstances.

- Halt the rise in diabetes and obesity.

- At least 50% of eligible people receive drug therapy and counselling (including glycaemic control) to prevent heart attacks and strokes.

- An 80% availability of the affordable basic technologies and essential medicines, including generics, required to treat major noncommunicable diseases in both public and private facilities.

SEE ALSO *Cancer; Cardiovascular Diseases; Diabetes; High Blood Pressure; Tobacco Use*

BIBLIOGRAPHY

Books

Ben-Shlomo, Yoav, Sara Brookes, and Matthew Hickman. *Epidemiology, Evidence-Based Medicine and Public Health Lecture Notes,* 6th ed. Oxford: Wiley-Blackwell, 2013.

Papadakis, Maxine, Stephen McPhee, and Michael W. Rabow. *2013 Current Medical Diagnosis and Treatment.* New York: McGraw-Hill Medical, 2013.

Somerville, Margaret, K., and Rob Anderson. *Public Health and Epidemiology at a Glance.* Oxford: Wiley-Blackwell, 2012.

Periodicals

Basu, Sanjay, Paula Yoffe, Nancy Hills, and Robert H. Lustig. "The Relationship of Sugar to Population-Level Diabetes Prevalence: An Econometric Analysis of Repeated Cross-Sectional Data." *PLOS ONE* (February 27, 2013). doi: 10.1371/journal. pone.0057873. Available online at http://journals. plos.org/plosone/article?id=10.1371/journal. pone.0057873 (accessed March 25, 2015).

Beaglehole, Robert, et al. "Priority Actions for the Non-communicable Disease Crisis." *The Lancet: Health Policy* 377 (2011): 1438–1447.

Habib, Samira Humaira, and Soma Saha. "Burden of Non-communicable Disease: Global Overview." *Diabetes & Metabolic Syndrome: Clinical Research & Reviews* 4, no. 1 (January–March 2010) 41–47.

Magnusson, Roger S. "Global Health Governance and the Challenge of Chronic, Non-communicable Disease." *Journal of Law, Medicine & Ethics* 38, no. 3 (Fall 2010): 490–507.

McKeown, Robert E. "The Epidemiologic Transition: Changing Patterns of Mortality and Population Dynamics." *American Journal of Lifestyle Medicine* 3, Suppl. 1 (2009): 19S–26S. doi:10.1177/1559827609335350.

Omran, A. R. "The Epidemiologic Transition: A Theory of the Epidemiology of Population Change." *Milbank Quarterly* 83, no. 4 (2005): 731–757.

Spellberg, Brad, and Bonnie Taylor-Blake. "On the Exoneration of Dr. William H. Stewart: Debunking an Urban Legend." *Infectious Diseases of Poverty*, 2, no. 3 (2013). Available online at http://www. ncbi.nlm.nih.gov/pmc/articles/PMC3707092/ (accessed March 25, 2015).

Wojcicki, Janet M., and Melvin B. Heyman. "Malnutrition and the Role of the Soft Drink Industry in Improving Child Health in Sub-Saharan Africa." *Pediatrics* 126, no. 6 (December 2010): e1617–e1621. doi:10.1542/peds.2010-0461. Available online at http://www.ncbi.nlm.nih.gov/pmc/articles/PMC3139541/ (accessed March 25, 2015).

Websites

"Global Action Plan for the Prevention and Control of Noncommunicable Diseases 2013–2020." *World Health Organization (WHO).* http://www.who. int/nmh/events/ncd_action_plan/en/ (accessed March 20, 2015).

"Global Status Report on Noncommunicable Diseases 2014." *World Health Organization (WHO),* 2014. http://www.who.int/nmh/publications/ncd-status-report-2014/en/ (accessed March 20, 2015).

Martin James Frigaard

Nutrition

⊕ Introduction

An analysis of the Global Burden of Disease Study 2010 published in 2012 by S. S. Lim and colleagues in *The Lancet* showed that 10 percent of global disability-adjusted life years (DALYs)—a measure of the number of years lost as a result of disease, disability, or death—in 2010 were accounted for by unhealthful diets and physical inactivity. The key dietary risk factors were low intakes of fruits and vegetables and high intakes of sodium. Lim and colleagues also found that worldwide, childhood nutrition-related risk factors such as underweight, micronutrient deficiencies, and low rates of breast-feeding had fallen in rank between 1990 and 2010 relative to adult nutrition-related risk factors such as hypertension. The shift in disease burden from the traditional global health concerns of infectious, or communicable, diseases and undernutrition to chronic, or noncommunicable, diseases such as obesity, diabetes, and heart disease, is called the epidemiological transition.

Another analysis of the Global Burden of Disease Study 2010 published by R. Lozano and colleagues in the same 2012 issue of *The Lancet* found that in 2010, two-thirds of deaths worldwide were from noncommunicable diseases, and only one-quarter of deaths were from communicable, maternal, neonatal, and nutritional (undernutrition) causes. In that year, the top two causes of death worldwide were ischemic heart disease and stroke; diabetes was the ninth-leading cause of death; and hypertensive heart disease was the 14th-leading cause of death. It is important to note that some noncommunicable diseases, such as diabetes and heart disease, are attributable to, or exacerbated by obesity, which is in part caused by overnutriton and unhealthful diets. Protein-energy malnutrition, considered the dominant cause of undernutrition, was ranked 21st in 2010, compared with 11th in 1990. It is therefore evident that substantial progress on alleviating undernutrition around the world has been made over the past two decades.

However, the analysis by Lozano and colleagues also identified huge health disparities across regions. For example, in sub-Saharan Africa, communicable, maternal, neonatal, and nutritional (undernutrition) causes accounted for 76 percent of years of life lost in 2010. But over the next decade, the greatest increases in nutrition-related noncommunicable diseases such as diabetes are expected to occur in sub-Saharan Africa. According to the sixth edition of the International Diabetes Federation's *Diabetes Atlas*, the number of people with diabetes in Africa will increase by an estimated 109 percent between 2013 and 2035. Thus, addressing the dual burden of under- and overnutrition is one of the biggest issues facing low- and middle-income countries today.

An important issue is how to measure nutrition. Typically, two methods have been used to assess the nutritional status of individuals: (1) micronutrient deficiencies, particularly vitamin A, iodine, iron, and zinc, and (2) anthropometrics, including weight, length for children under two years old, height for children over two years old and adults, and various circumferences (head, arm, waist, and hip). This individual-level information is then used to estimate the proportion of the population that is malnourished, either undernourished or overnourished. In global health, the best methods are those that are feasible across a wide range of settings, are inexpensive, and that can be carried out in a standardized way by study staff after minimal training. Anthropometry is especially field-friendly, thus many international nutrition studies use anthropometric data.

The choice of nutritional status indicator depends on the age group of interest. For example, in adults, body mass index (BMI) is calculated as the individual's weight in weight in pounds divided by his or her height in inches-squared $\times$ 703 (lbs/inches^2 $\times$ 703) or kilograms divided by his or her height in meters-squared [kg/m^2]. The proportion of individuals with a BMI less than 18.5 is then calculated to determine the prevalence of underweight, according to a cut-point recommended by a 2003 World Health Organization (WHO)/Food and Agriculture Organization (FAO) Expert Consultation. Similarly, the proportion of individuals with a BMI of at least 25 is calculated to determine the prevalence of overweight/obesity.

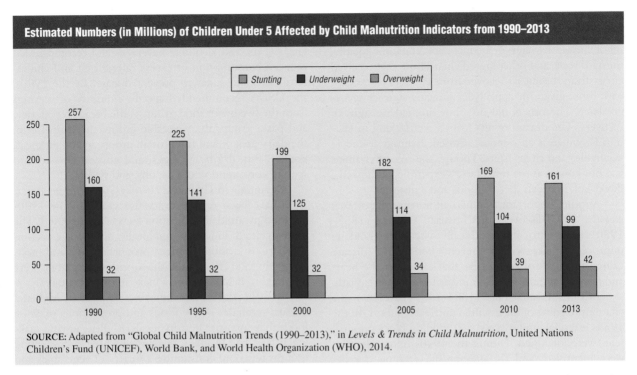

Estimated Numbers (in Millions) of Children Under 5 Affected by Child Malnutrition Indicators from 1990–2013

■ *Stunting* ■ *Underweight* ■ *Overweight*

SOURCE: Adapted from "Global Child Malnutrition Trends (1990–2013)," in *Levels & Trends in Child Malnutrition*, United Nations Children's Fund (UNICEF), World Bank, and World Health Organization (WHO), 2014.

The WHO estimates that stunting impacted about 161 million children in 2013. Lower than in previous years, nutrition in children under five is still a major public health concern. Interventions in early childhood feeding have been shown to reduce stunting and obesity in young children.

In contrast, for infants and children, growth is considered the best overall indicator of nutritional status. To assess population-level infant nutritional status, the proportion of babies that weigh less than about 5.5 pounds (2,500 grams) at birth is calculated to determine the incidence of low birth weight. In low-income countries with a high incidence of low birth weight, it is usually the result of intrauterine growth restriction, such as fetal malnutrition. However, in higher-income countries with lower incidences of low birth weight, it is usually the result of preterm delivery.

In children under five years old, two nutritional status indicators are typically used: (1) wasting, or low weight for height, and (2) stunting, or low height for age. Wasting is usually the result of acute protein-energy malnutrition, whereas stunting is usually the result of chronic protein-energy malnutrition. To determine whether or not a child is suffering from wasting or stunting, his or her height must be compared to child growth standards—that is, the pattern of growth in a large population of healthy, breast-fed children.

The WHO and the U.S. Centers for Disease Control and Prevention (CDC) both have age- and sex-specific growth charts available. In international settings, WHO Child Growth Charts are often used, while in the United States, CDC Growth Charts are used. Given the strong influence of early life nutrition on cognitive development, measures of cognition and school performance may also be used to assess nutritional adequacy in this

age group. Finally, in adolescents, pubertal stage may be used in conjunction with anthropometric indices (such as BMI) to assess nutritional status.

In addition to anthropometrics, micronutrient deficiencies may be measured to assess the nutritional status of a particular population. Anemia, typically the result of iron deficiency, is one of the most commonly used micronutrient deficiency indicators and is assessed by measuring hemoglobin levels in blood. This test is relatively easy and inexpensive to do in the field. The hemoglobin cut-points used to calculate the proportion of individuals with anemia vary according to age, sex, and pregnancy status, and are provided in the WHO's 2008 publication *Worldwide Prevalence of Anemia 1993–2005*.

⊕ Historical Background

The relationship between nutrition and health was recognized in early times. Hippocrates (c. 460– c. 377 BCE) the Greek physician considered the founder of Western medicine said, "Let thy food be thy medicine and thy medicine be thy food." More direct links of specific foods to health were tested by James Lind (1716–1794), a Scottish naval physician, who performed experiments to test a variety of food-related treatments for scurvy (a disease that causes bleeding gums, loss of teeth, sores, anemia, and potentially death), which afflicted many sailors or those at sea for long periods. Lind assigned test subjects with scurvy various treatments. The patients were assigned apple cider; citrus fruits; vinegar; diluted oil of vitriol; seawater; or a concoction containing garlic, mustard seed, and other ingredients. Those that received citrus fruits began to recover from the scurvy quickly, with those given the apple cider showing signs of recovery later. The others did not show immediate signs of recovery. The disease results from a diet lacking in vitamin C, which is an essential nutrient typically found in vegetables and citrus fruits. Though the role of vitamins was not known at the time, Lind's experiments showed a direct link between specific foods and a disorder.

Another important landmark in nutritional research was the 1897 discovery of Christiaan Eijkman (1858–1930) that nutrients—specifically vitamins found in unprocessed rice—could prevent beriberi, a disease caused by a lack of vitamin B1 that can affect the heart and nervous system and if left untreated will cause death.

In 1912, Casimir Funk (1884–1967) gave the name vitamins to some of the essential nutrients in food. In the 1930s essential amino acids, the building blocks of protein, were identified. During the 1940s, more vitamins were identified, and throughout the ensuing decades understanding of the roles of essential nutrients in health and disease has increased.

Evolving Standards of Nutrition

Like other evolving disciplines, nutrition information and recommendations have changed over time. For example, in the United States, the Department of Agriculture (USDA) has been issuing dietary recommendations for more than a century. The first guidance, published in 1894, before vitamins and minerals had been identified, advised a diet consisting of "protein, carbohydrate, fat, and mineral matter (ash)." In 1902, the recommendations emphasized balance and moderation, cautioning that "The evils of overeating may not be felt at once, but sooner or later they are sure to appear—perhaps in an excessive amount of fatty tissue, perhaps in general debility, perhaps in actual disease."

By 1921, USDA guidelines were based on food groups—milk and meat, cereals, vegetables and fruits, fats and fatty foods, and sugars and sugary foods. In 1941, the first set of recommended dietary allowances (RDAs)—specific intakes for calories and nine essential nutrients—protein, iron, calcium, vitamins A and D, thiamin, riboflavin, niacin, and ascorbic acid (vitamin C)—were issued. From 1956 through the early 1970s, recommendations focused on consuming a minimum number of foods from four basic food groups—milk, meat, fruits and vegetables, and grain products.

In 1977 the dietary guidelines warned about overconsumption of fat, saturated fat, cholesterol, and sodium because of their relationship to increased risk of developing chronic diseases such as heart disease and stroke. The guidelines specified targets for protein, carbohydrates, fats, cholesterol, sugar, and sodium consumption. In 1979 the guidance also advised moderation in intake of fats, sweets, and alcoholic beverages and recommended reduced consumption of excess calories, fat and cholesterol, salt, and sugar to prevent disease. By the 1990s, the USDA recommended specific numbers of servings from the five major food groups—the bread, cereal, rice, and pasta group; the vegetable group; the fruit group; the dairy group; and the protein group, including meat, poultry, fish, dry beans, eggs, and nuts. It also advised sparing consumption of fats, oils, and sweets.

Beginning in 1980, the *Dietary Guidelines for Americans* have been revised every five years. In the 1990s the food pyramid and nutrition facts labels debuted. The food pyramid aimed to graphically display key recommendations including variety, proportionality, and moderation in food choices and the nutrition facts labels were intended to help consumers make informed choices.

In 2011, the food pyramid was replaced by MyPlate, a visual reminder of the foods and proportions of those foods that comprise healthy meals. MyPlate advises making at least half of grains consumed whole grains, eating lean protein, and consuming a variety of vegetables and fruit and calcium-rich dairy.

Concepts of Malnutrition

The recommendations adopted in the United States highlight disparities between what may be recommended by various government agencies and what is actually available to many people. Impoverished people in both developed and developing countries may spend large percentages of their incomes on food, yet they are often malnourished because of limited incomes or poor food

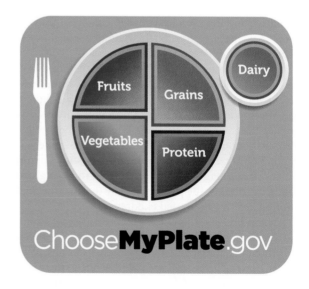

MyPlate, created by the U.S. Department of Agriculture in 2011, serves as a visual representation of the types of food and proportions that healthy meals comprise. *U.S. Department of Agriculture.*

availability. Worldwide organizations such as the United Nations Children's Fund (UNICEF) have focused on reducing levels of malnutrition. The conceptual framework of the underlying causes of malnutrition first developed by UNICEF in 1990 continues to be used by global health researchers and international development organizations. It takes a socio-ecological approach, recognizing the important role that the political, economic, and social situation (including empowerment of women) can have on nutrition, as well as the immediate causes of insufficient access to food (food insecurity) and subsequent food intake. The UNICEF framework also emphasizes the substantial impact insufficient health care and disease can have on nutrition.

A second conceptual framework commonly used in international nutrition was proposed by the United Nations Administrative Committee on Coordination (ACC)/Subcommittee on Nutrition (SCN) in 2000 and emphasizes a life course approach to understanding the direct causes and effects of undernutrition at the individual level. The ACC/SCN 2000 framework identifies critical periods of intervention—pregnancy, infancy, childhood, and adolescence—and recognizes the potential for trans-generational effects of malnutrition.

⊕ Impacts and Issues

The concept of the developmental origins of disease recognizes that nutrition during the first 1,000 days of life can have long-term effects on health. Today, most experts agree that an individual's risk of noncommunicable diseases begins very early in life, likely during fetal development. Evidence is beginning to accumulate suggesting trans-generational effects of these early-life risk factors. Efforts to improve adult nutrition and health must therefore also address early-life nutrition and health.

Pregnancy

Due to the increased nutrient requirements during pregnancy, pregnant women are at increased risk of micronutrient deficiencies, particularly vitamin A, iodine, iron, and zinc. Given that maternal anemia, most often caused by iron deficiency, is associated with adverse pregnancy outcomes including preterm birth and low birth weight, a 2014 WHO policy brief on anemia recommends iron and folic acid supplementation as part of prenatal care and for at least three months following delivery. Micronutrient fortification of foods such as wheat and maize flours, rice, and sugar, and increasing dietary diversity, are also WHO-recommended strategies for addressing micronutrient deficiencies in pregnant women.

Birth weight, an important pregnancy outcome, was one of the first early-life markers of nutritional status and growth to be linked with future risk of adult noncommunicable disease. In a series of papers published in the *British Medical Journal* by C. Osmond and colleagues

in 1993, low birth weight was found to be significantly associated with cardiovascular disease among men and women in England. Subsequent studies have found associations between low birth weight and diabetes in cohorts from low- and middle-income countries. Thus, interventions to improve pregnancy outcomes such as low birth weight will be an important aspect of life course approaches to nutrition-related noncommunicable disease prevention.

Infancy and Early Childhood

Exclusive breast-feeding (i.e., no other fluids or foods, including water) for the first six months of life is the primary focus of nutrition interventions to improve infant health, highlighted in the WHO and UNICEF's *Global Strategy for Infant and Young Child Feeding*, published in 2003. This is because breast milk is an excellent source of energy and nutrients, particularly vitamin A, a key nutrient of concern for infants and young children. From a life course perspective, breast-feeding is also important because it is associated with reduced risk of hypertension and overweight/obesity in adulthood.

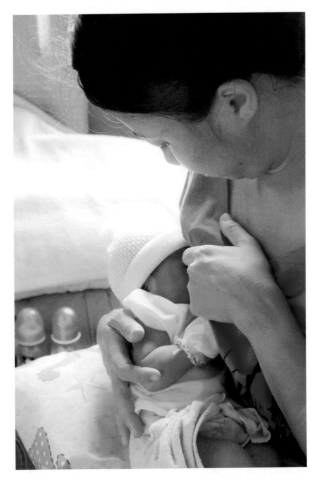

Breast-feeding optimizes health of the infant and the reproductive health of the mother. © *Atthapol Saita/Shutterstock.com*

Beginning at six months of age, safe complementary foods should be introduced because breast milk alone is not sufficient to meet the energy and nutrient needs of infants. Worldwide, complementary foods are often inadequate in energy density, protein, and key micronutrients. Thus, interventions to improve complementary practices such as weaning are an important aspect of improving child nutrition. These interventions may focus on maternal education on feeding infants culturally acceptable, high-protein foods (for example, eggs, fish, chicken livers, or caterpillars), increasing variety in infant diets, and/or providing lipid-based nutritional supplements.

The introduction of nutrient-dense and safe complementary foods is critically important because this period of life (from six months to two years of age) coincides with the peak of nutrient deficiencies, which in turn can lead to stunting. According to a 2004 review by Ian Darnton-Hill, C. Nishida, and W. P. James, published in the journal *Public Health Nutrition*, stunting is associated with several noncommunicable diseases later in life, including stroke, heart disease, and diabetes. Height is the result of genetics but is also strongly associated with socioeconomic and nutritional status, especially total energy and protein intake, during childhood.

Thus, appropriate calories and protein during infancy and early childhood are essential.

Recent evidence of growth trajectories during early life, including a study using data from five longitudinal studies (Brazil, Guatemala, India, the Philippines, and South Africa), suggests that faster growth (height) and weight gain during the first two years of life reduces the risk of adult short stature. However, this "catchup growth" was also associated with an increased risk of overweight and hypertension in adulthood. Thus, life course approaches to preventing adult noncommunicable diseases must consider not only stunting of attained adult stature (height), but also the trajectory of growth over time.

Nutrition and Infectious Disease

The relationship between nutrition and infectious disease is complex and reciprocal. Malnutrition can impair the immune system, thus increasing susceptibility to pathogens (disease-causing microorganisms). Infections that lead to diarrhea and vomiting can result in nutrient losses; fever can increase caloric requirements; infection can increase protein requirements; and a condition called tropical enteropathy (subclinical damage to the intestinal lining) caused by frequent infections can

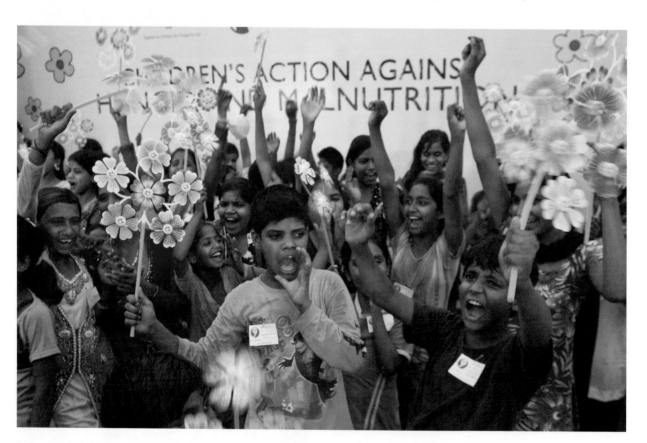

Indian youths hold flower-shaped pinwheels, with each petal representing a child death caused by malnutrition, during a Global Day of Action against Hunger event in New Delhi on June 7, 2013. The event was held ahead of the Hunger Summit in London hosted by the UK and Brazilian governments calling for action on global hunger. © *Prakash Singh/AFP/Getty Images.*

result in impaired nutrient absorption. Moreover, given the strong connection between water, sanitation, and hygiene (often referred to as WASH) and infections, many new interventions targeting nutritional status also consider these relationships.

As discussed in the previous section, breast-feeding is critical to achieving optimal infant nutritional status. This is through both direct effects (breast milk is optimally formulated for human infants) and indirect effects: exclusive breast-feeding is associated with fewer diarrheal infections in infants, and subsequently better nutritional status. However, settings where the prevalence of human immunodeficiency virus/acquired immune deficiency syndrome (HIV/AIDS) is high require special consideration given that without preventive intervention, HIV-infected mothers can pass the virus onto their children through breast milk. Since giving mothers antiretroviral drugs can significantly reduce the risk of transmission of HIV through breast-feeding, it is extremely important that HIV-infected mothers take antiretroviral drugs and continue to exclusively breast-feed for the first six months. Indeed, given the importance of breast-feeding, particularly in settings with limited water, sanitation, and hygiene, the 2010 WHO guidelines still recommend exclusive breastfeeding when antiretroviral drugs are not available.

Finally, as relates to nutrition and infectious disease, evidence from randomized controlled trials suggests that iron supplementation may increase the risk of infection, particularly malaria. However, as noted previously, iron deficiency anemia is associated with numerous adverse health outcomes in pregnant women, infants, and children, and iron supplementation is beneficial in these populations. Given these conflicting data, the WHO 2007 Consultation on the Prevention and Control of Iron Deficiency in Malaria-Endemic Areas recommends that in sub-Saharan Africa and other malaria-endemic areas, children should be screened for iron deficiency before beginning supplementation. Alternatively, iron supplementation should be combined with malaria-prevention interventions such as vector control and provision of insecticide-treated bed nets.

Food Insecurity

Food insecurity exists when there is a chronic lack of access to food, and as a result, dietary intake fails to meet nutrition needs. According to the FAO, at least one in nine people worldwide are chronically undernourished, and the vast majority (98 percent) live in low- and middle-income countries. Food insecurity can exist at individual, household, community, or national levels, and its causes vary widely. The root causes of food insecurity, namely, political and economic instability and social organization, are highlighted in the UNICEF framework.

Food security and nutrition are intricately connected. Food security is not just providing enough calories through foods but also providing nutrient-dense foods. Micronutrient fortification of staple crops is one strategy to address food insecurity. Other approaches include crop and livestock diversification, and nutrition education through school and workplace gardens.

The Nutrition Transition

Industrialization, urbanization, globalization, and economic development have all contributed to improvements in the standard of living around the world. However, they have also contributed to a shift away from traditional, healthful diets to Westernized, unhealthful diets, and from active lifestyles to sedentary lifestyles. This shift is called nutrition transition, and has been reported in all regions of the world, from Latin America to Southeast Asia to sub-Saharan Africa. Specifically, diets shift from plant-based, high-fiber, and complex carbohydrate norms to diets characterized by low fiber and high levels of refined carbohydrates, added sugar, and saturated fat from animal products. Studies suggest that this nutrition transition may be responsible for a transition from diseases caused or worsened by undernutrition to diseases attributable to overnutrition.

An analysis of dietary quality in 187 countries by F. Imamura and colleagues, published in *The Lancet Global Health*, found that from 1990 to 2010, consumption of healthful foods (for example, whole grains, fruits, vegetables, fish, and nuts) worldwide increased, but so did consumption of unhealthful foods (for example, sugar-sweetened beverages and red meats). Importantly, their analysis identified substantial regional and socioeconomic differences in the relative change of healthful foods versus unhealthful foods. For example, in some high-income countries, improvements in both healthful and unhealthful foods were observed, but in some low-income countries, healthful foods decreased in the face of increasing unhealthful foods. Overall, this study highlighted the need for country-specific tailoring of food policy interventions.

Several countries have implemented policies and campaigns targeting dietary intake and physical activity. U.S. First Lady Michelle Obama's anti-obesity campaign, called Let's Move!, has involved multiple stakeholders, including suppliers of school lunches, the food and beverage industry, the American Academy of Pediatrics, and state and local governments. The U.S. Dietary Guidelines and MyPlate, described earlier, have also been an important part of education about healthful food and beverage choices.

A recent systematic review by Carl Lachat and colleagues published in *PLOS Medicine* focused on policies in low- and middle-income countries' efforts to improve dietary quality and physical activity. Researchers found that only 12 percent of countries (14 of 116 countries included) had policies that addressed all four of the leading diet and activity risk factors (salt consumption, fat consumption, fruit and vegetable intake, and physical activity), confirming that there is much progress to be made.

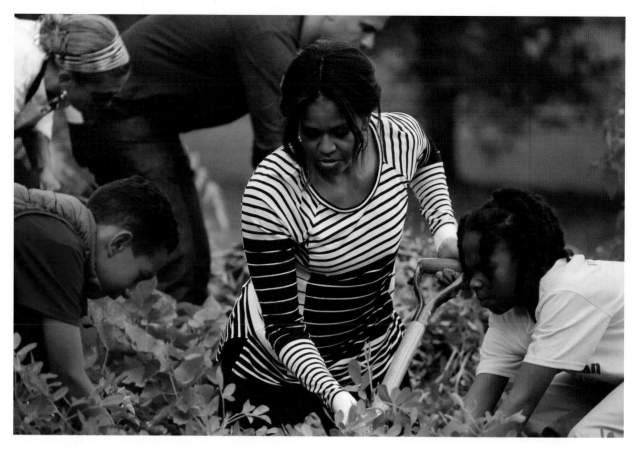

U.S. First Lady Michelle Obama (center) helps schoolchildren harvest fruits and vegetables from the White House kitchen garden during an event on October 14, 2014, in Washington, D.C. During her time as first lady, Mrs. Obama has been promoting greater fresh fruit and vegetable consumption and increased physical activity by children with the Let's Move! campaign.   © *Mark Wilson/Getty Images.*

⊕ Future Implications

Looking ahead to the future of nutrition and global health, the biggest challenge will be addressing both ends of the nutrition spectrum: undernutrition and overnutrition, which can co-occur in individuals (for example, stunted obesity), within households (for example, underweight grandparents and overweight grandchildren), and within countries (for example, significant burdens of food insecurity and obesity). The classical interventions used to address undernutrition, such as nutrient-based supplements and agricultural fortification and intensification, will not completely address overnutrition. Nor will the classical interventions used to address overnutrition, such as individual-level behavioral interventions and reformulations of products by the food industry, completely address undernutrition.

Additional approaches to improving nutritional status, including those that address underlying risk factors such as poverty, should be used to increase the cost-effectiveness, efficiency, and long-term impact of existing efforts to improve nutritional status worldwide. Given the persistence of global hunger and undernutrition, and the rising obesity and noncommunicable disease epidemic,

there is an urgent need for the development and implementation of innovative interventions and policies.

PRIMARY SOURCE

Essential Nutrition Actions

SOURCE Essential Nutrition Actions: Improving Maternal, Newborn, Infant and Young Child Health and Nutrition. *Geneva: World Health Organization (WHO), 2013, 2–5. http://apps.who.int/iris/bitstr eam/10665/84409/1/9789241505550_eng.pdf (accessed January 25, 2015).*

INTRODUCTION *This primary source is a section of a report developed by the World Health Organization (WHO) on maternal, infant, and young child nutrition. It summarizes the updated WHO guidelines on effective nutrition programs under various circumstances, particularly for pregnant women and children in the first years of life.*

Timing of interventions

New analyses, using the WHO Growth Standards, confirm the importance of the first two years of life as a window of opportunity for growth promotion. An important feature of the WHO standards is that they reveal a much greater problem of undernutrition during the first six months of life than previously believed, bringing coherence between the rates of undernutrition observed in young infants and the prevalence of low birth weight and early abandonment of exclusive breastfeeding. These findings highlight the need for prenatal and early-life interventions to prevent the growth failure that primarily happens during the first two years of life, including the promotion of appropriate infant feeding practices. The deficits acquired by this age are difficult to reverse later.

Strategies to improve nutritional status and growth in children should include interventions to improve nutrition of pregnant and lactating women; early initiation of breastfeeding with exclusive breastfeeding for six months; promotion, protection, and support of continued breastfeeding along with appropriate complementary feeding from six months up to two years and beyond; and micronutrient supplementation, targeted fortification and food supplementation, when needed.

Recommended nutrition practices targeting women, infants and young children

In 1999 WHO, in collaboration with UNICEF and BASICS, proposed effective, feasible, available and affordable interventions. These interventions worked best when combined with interventions to reduce infections, such as water, sanitation and hygiene.

Focusing on a package of essential nutrition actions (ENAs), health programmes could reduce infant and child mortality, improve physical and mental growth and development, and improve productivity. These essential actions protect, promote and support priority nutrition outcomes:

- exclusive breastfeeding for six months;

- adequate complementary feeding starting at six months with continued breastfeeding for two years;

- appropriate nutritional care of sick and malnourished children;

- adequate intake of vitamin A for women and children;

- adequate intake of iron for women and children; and

- adequate intake of iodine by all members of the household.

The actions proposed to obtain the priority nutrition outcomes included ones that health workers could implement, such as complementary feeding counselling and active feeding, growth monitoring and promotion, and supplementary feeding or food-based interventions. At the same time, health managers aiming for adequate intake of vitamin A for women and children could encourage daily intake of vitamin A-rich foods and adequate breastfeeding, give high-dose vitamin A supplements to children with infections, train staff to detect and treat clinical VAD, and design a plan for preventive supplementation of vitamin A for children and postpartum women in populations at risk of VAD.

Improving nutrition involves actions at health facility and population levels. At district level, these could include monitoring nutrition, identifying sub-populations at risk of nutrition problems, updating nutrition policies and protocols, and providing resources and tools to implement nutrition activities at health facilities and at community venues.

At health facilities, ENAs should be carried out at all contacts with pregnant and lactating women and their children. Outside facilities in the community, follow-up of mothers and children and support to community workers and groups are key.

SEE ALSO *Child Health; Diabetes; Food Security and Hunger; Malnutrition; Maternal and Infant Health; Noncommunicable Diseases (Lifestyle Diseases); Obesity*

BIBLIOGRAPHY

Books

International Diabetes Federation (IDF). *IDF Diabetes Atlas*, 6th ed. Brussels: International Diabetes Federation, 2013.

Maire, B., and F. Delpeuch. *Nutrition Indicators for Development*. Rome: Food and Agriculture Organization of the United Nations, 2005.

United Nations Administrative Committee on Coordination (ACC)/Sub-committee on Nutrition (SCN). *4th Report on the World Nutrition Situation: Nutrition throughout the Life Cycle*. Washington, DC: International Food Policy Research Institute, 2000.

World Health Organization (WHO). *Global Nutrition Targets 2025: Anaemia Policy Brief*. Geneva: World Health Organization, 2014.

World Health Organization (WHO). *HIV and Infant Feeding: Guidelines on Principles and Recommendations for Infant Feeding in the Context of HIV and a Summary of the Evidence*. Geneva: World Health Organization, 2010.

World Health Organization (WHO). *Worldwide Prevalence of Anaemia 1993–2005*. Geneva: World Health Organization, 2008.

World Health Organization (WHO) and Food and Agriculture Organization (FAO) of the United Nations. *Diet, Nutrition, and the Prevention of Chronic Diseases: Report of a Joint WHO/FAO Expert Consultation*. Geneva: World Health Organization, 2003.

World Health Organization (WHO) and United Nations Children's Fund (UNICEF). *Global Strategy for Infant and Young Child Feeding.* Geneva: World Health Organization, 2003.

Periodicals

Adair, L. S., et al., for the COHORTS group. "Associations of Linear Growth and Relative Weight Gain during Early Life with Adult Health and Human Capital in Countries of Low and Middle Income: Findings from Five Birth Cohort Studies." *The Lancet* 382, no. 9891 (August 2013): 523–534.

Darnton-Hill, Ian, C. Nishida, and W. P. James. "A Life Course Approach to Diet, Nutrition and the Prevention of Chronic Diseases." *Public Health Nutrition* 7, no. 1A (February 2004): 101–121.

Humphrey, J. H. "Child Undernutrition, Tropical Enteropathy, Toilets, and Handwashing." *The Lancet* 374, no. 9694 (September 2009): 1032–1035.

Imamura, F., et al., for the Global Burden of Diseases Nutrition and Chronic Diseases Expert Group (NutriCoDE). "Dietary Quality among Men and Women in 187 Countries in 1990 and 2010: A Systematic Assessment." *The Lancet Global Health* 3, no. 3 (March 2015): e132–e142.

Lachat, Carl, et al. "Diet and Physical Activity for the Prevention of Noncommunicable Diseases in Low- and Middle-Income Countries: A Systematic Policy Review." *PLOS Medicine* 10, no. 6 (2013): e1001465.

Lim, S. S., et al. "A Comparative Risk Assessment of Burden of Disease and Injury Attributable to 67 Risk Factors and Risk Factor Clusters in 21 Regions, 1990–2010: A Systematic Analysis for the Global Burden of Disease Study 2010." *The Lancet* 380, no. 9859 (December 2012): 2224–2260.

Lozano, R., et al. "Global and Regional Mortality from 235 Causes of Death for 20 Age Groups in 1990 and 2010: A Systematic Analysis for the Global Burden of Disease Study 2010." *The Lancet* 380, no. 9859 (December 2012): 2095–2128.

Norris, S. A., et al., for the COHORTS Group. "Size at Birth, Weight Gain in Infancy and Childhood, and Adult Diabetes Risk in Five Low- or Middle-Income Country Birth Cohorts." *Diabetes Care* 35, no. 1 (January 2012): 72–79.

Osmond, C., D. J. Barker, P. D. Winter, C. H. Fall, and S. J. Simmonds. "Early Growth and Death from Cardiovascular Disease in Women." *British Medical Journal* 307, no. 6918 (December 1993): 1519–1524.

Popkin, B. M. "Nutritional Patterns and Transitions." *Population Development and Review* 19, no. 1 (March 1993): 138–157.

World Health Organization (WHO). "Conclusions and Recommendations of the WHO Consultation on Prevention and Control of Iron Deficiency in Infants and Young Children in Malaria-Endemic Areas." *Food and Nutrition Bulletin* 28, suppl. 4 (December 2007): S621–S627.

Websites

"About Us: MyPlate." *U.S. Department of Agriculture (USDA).* http://www.choosemyplate.gov/about.html (accessed March 27, 2015).

Davis, Carole, and Etta Saltos. "Chapter 2 Dietary Recommendations and How They Have Changed Over Time." *U.S. Department of Agriculture (USDA).* http://www.ers.usda.gov/media/91022/aib750b_1_.pdf (accessed March 27, 2015).

"UNICEF Conceptual Framework." *United Nations Children's Fund (UNICEF).* http://www.unicef.org/nutrition/training/2.5/4.html (accessed March 14, 2015).

Lindsay M. Jaacks

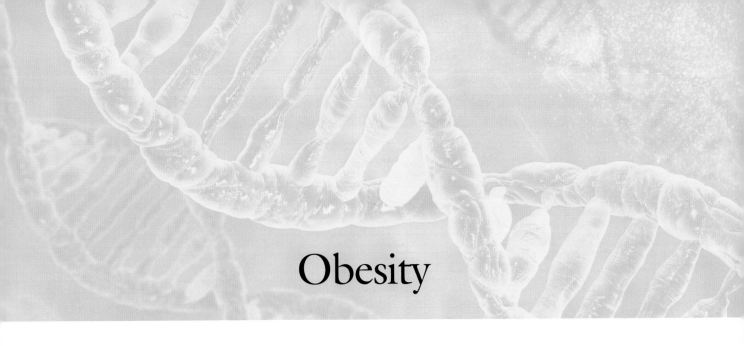

Obesity

Introduction

According to an analysis of the Global Burden of Disease Study 2013 published in *The Lancet* by M. Ng and colleagues in 2014, between 1980 and 2013, the prevalence of overweight/obesity in adult men increased from 28.8 percent to 36.9 percent and in adult women from 29.8 percent to 38 percent. That is, nearly two-fifths of men and women around the world were overweight or obese. And the problem is not restricted to adults. Between 1980 and 2013, the prevalence of overweight/obesity in children increased 47.1 percent. By 2013, 23.8 percent of boys and 22.6 percent of girls in high-income countries, and 12.9 percent of boys and 13.4 percent of girls in low- and middle-income countries were overweight/obese. In summary, worldwide, 2.1 billion people are overweight or obese. This is clearly an unprecedented global health issue.

The most commonly used metric for defining overweight and obesity is body mass index (BMI). BMI is calculated as the individual's weight in pounds divided by height in inches squared × 703 (pounds/inches² × 703) or the individual's weight in kilograms divided by his or her height in meters-squared (kg/m²). In adults (over 18 years old), the proportion of individuals with a BMI of at least 25 is calculated to determine the prevalence of overweight and obesity combined, which is in accordance with a 2003 World Health Organization (WHO)/Food and Agriculture Organization (FAO) Expert Consultation. However, as the rate of obesity increases, the prevalence of overweight and obesity separately are more often calculated. In this case, overweight is defined as a BMI of at least 25 but less than 30, and obesity is defined as a BMI of 30 or higher.

In children (18 years or younger), overweight and obesity are defined using age- and sex-specific cut-points. These cut-points are derived using growth charts, either from the International Obesity Task Force (for international studies) or from the U.S. Centers for Disease Control and Prevention (for U.S. studies). In addition

to BMI, other markers of adiposity include waist circumference, hip circumference, waist-to-height and waist-to-hip ratios, and skinfolds. More direct assessments of fat composition, such as bioelectrical impedance (BIA) and dual energy x-ray absorptiometry (DXA), can also be used. While BIA can be measured in the field and is relatively inexpensive, DXA—considered the "gold standard" for body fat composition—is expensive and requires special equipment and highly trained staff. Thus, most global health studies rely on anthropometrics (e.g., BMI and waist circumference) and select studies also measure BIA.

The drivers of the obesity epidemic witnessed by all regions of the world since the 1980s are still not fully understood. Increases in energy intake, decreases in physical activity, increases in sedentary time, changes in dietary composition, environmental pollutants, and changes in the gut microbiome are all thought to contribute. Given that a BMI of more than 25 has consistently been associated with increased risk of cardiovascular disease, diabetes, osteoarthritis, some cancers, and chronic kidney disease, interventions to prevent the rising tide of obesity are urgently needed. However, in order to develop effective obesity prevention strategies, a greater understanding of the causes of the global obesity epidemic are needed.

Historical Background

The United States continues to stand out as having a high prevalence of obesity: in 2013, 31.6 percent of U.S. men and 33.9 percent of U.S. women were obese. Mexico also stands out, surpassing the United States as having the highest prevalence of obesity in the world in 2013 according to an FAO report. This is in contrast to China and India, where the prevalence of obesity is increasing but still much lower than that in the United States and Mexico: in China, 3.8 percent of men and 5 percent of women were obese in 2013, and in India,

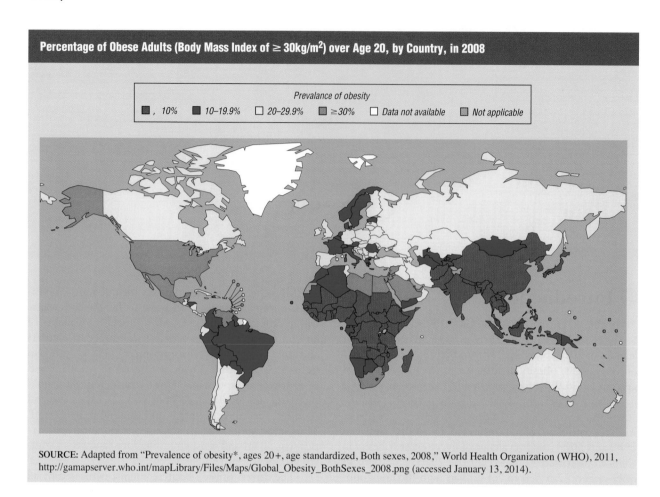

Percentage of Obese Adults (Body Mass Index of ≥ 30kg/m²) over Age 20, by Country, in 2008

Prevalance of obesity

■ , 10% ■ 10–19.9% □ 20–29.9% ■ ≥30% □ Data not available ■ Not applicable

SOURCE: Adapted from "Prevalence of obesity*, ages 20+, age standardized, Both sexes, 2008," World Health Organization (WHO), 2011, http://gamapserver.who.int/mapLibrary/Files/Maps/Global_Obesity_BothSexes_2008.png (accessed January 13, 2014).

these numbers were 3.7 percent and 4.2 percent, respectively. However, given the large populations of China and India, these relatively low prevalence rates translate into very large absolute numbers of people. Half of the 671 million obese (not including overweight) individuals around the world live in just 10 countries: the United States, China, India, Russia, Brazil, Mexico, Egypt, Germany, Pakistan, and Indonesia.

The analysis of the Global Burden of Disease Study by Ng and colleagues did have some positive findings: the rate of increase in overweight/obesity peaked between 1992 and 2002, and has been slowing down in the years since. This decline in the rate of increase (note: this is not the same as a decrease in the rate of obesity, it is just an increase at a slower rate) is especially evident in high-income countries. Nonetheless, the prevalence of obesity remains higher across all ages in high-income compared to low- and middle-income countries. Central America, the Middle East, and island nations in the Pacific and Caribbean are the exceptions and have especially high rates of obesity. Of course, given the large absolute populations of low- and middle-income countries, despite their relatively low prevalence rates, nearly two-thirds of the world's obese population lives in developing countries.

⊕ Impacts and Issues

The comorbidities of obesity lead to significant economic costs. An analysis by Y. C. Wang and colleagues found that between 2008 and 2030, the cost of treating obesity-related diseases in the United States alone will increase by an estimated US$66 billion per year. A study by Ketevan Rtveladze and colleagues published in the journal *Public Health Nutrition* in 2014 predicted that the cost of treating obesity-related diseases in Mexico would increase from $806 million in 2010 to $1.2 billion in 2030. Thus, the heavy economic burden of obesity is carried not only by high-income countries, but also low- and middle-income countries.

An analysis by S. S. Lim and colleagues published in *The Lancet* in 2012 found that high BMI accounted for 3.4 million deaths in 2010 and 3.8 percent of global disability-adjusted life years, a measure of the number of years lost as a result of disease, disability, or death. Most of the deaths associated with obesity are from cardiovascular diseases such as coronary heart disease and stroke. This is because obesity increases the risk of three important cardiovascular disease risk factors: high blood pressure (hypertension), dyslipidemia (high low-density lipoprotein [LDL] cholesterol and triglycerides and low

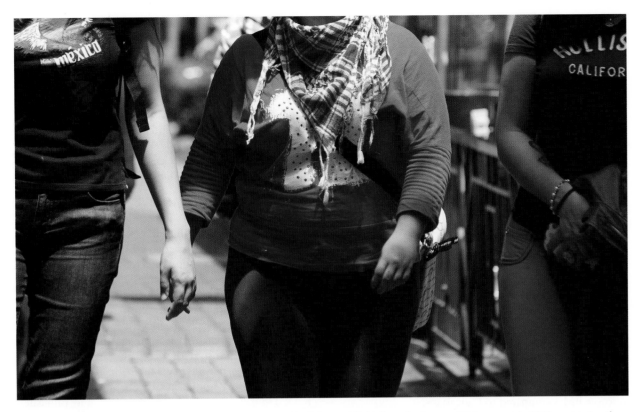

A woman walks down a street in Mexico City, Mexico. Mexico had the world's highest obesity rate, 32.8 percent, in 2013, surpassing the United States' 31.8 percent according to the 2013 report "The State of Food and Agriculture" published by the United Nations Food and Agriculture Organization. *© Susana Gonzalez/Bloomberg via Getty Images.*

high-density lipoprotein [HDL] cholesterol), and high blood glucose (hyperglycemia).

A recent analysis by the Global Burden of Metabolic Risk Factors for Chronic Diseases Collaboration published in *The Lancet* (2014), found that 46 percent of the excess risk from BMI for coronary heart disease and 76 percent of the excess risk from BMI for stroke could be accounted for by these three risk factors. The most important of the three was high blood pressure, which alone accounted for 31 percent and 65 percent of the excess risk for coronary heart disease and stroke, respectively. Importantly, this study showed that treatment of these comorbidities in obese individuals would only eliminate half of the risk from BMI for coronary heart disease. Thus, even with drug therapy, obese individuals are at increased risk of cardiovascular events such as myocardial infarction (heart attack) and stroke. Weight loss is critical to fully reduce risk.

Obesity is also an independent risk factor for diabetes. A meta-analysis published by C. L. Gillies and colleagues in the *British Medical Journal* in 2007 evaluated 17 randomized controlled trials and found that individuals with prediabetes who received a lifestyle intervention focused on weight loss had half the risk of developing diabetes compared to those who received standard advice. As such, the American Diabetes Association recommends

weight loss of 7 percent of initial body weight and increasing physical activity to at least 150 minutes per week for prevention of diabetes.

Metabolically Healthy Obesity

Many studies are beginning to identify a subgroup of obese individuals who are metabolically healthy, with normal blood pressure, lipid levels, and insulin sensitivity. Lack of a precise and uniform definition of metabolically healthy obesity has led to wide variation in the reported prevalence of this condition. A study by R. P. Wildman and colleagues of the National Health and Nutrition Examination Surveys (NHANES), published in the journal *Archives of Internal Medicine* in 2008, found that 51.3 percent of overweight adults in the United States and 31.7 percent of obese adults were metabolically healthy. A more recent systematic review of reported prevalence rates in the literature, conducted by J. P. Rey-Lopez and colleagues and published in *Obesity Reviews* in 2014, found that the prevalence of metabolically healthy obesity reported in 27 identified studies ranged from 6 percent to 75 percent. Studies conducted in the United States, including the previously mentioned Wildman study of NHANES, ranged from 19 percent to 40 percent.

In regard to health outcomes associated with metabolically healthy obesity, a systematic review conducted by L. L. Roberson and colleagues and published in *BMC Public Health* in 2014 found mixed results across studies, with some studies finding a significant association with all-cause mortality, cardiovascular disease–associated mortality, and incident cardiovascular disease, while other studies found no significant associations. Given these results, some experts posit that this condition of metabolically healthy obesity is not without risk, and represents an early, subclinical stage in the transition to a more unhealthy metabolic profile. More research is needed to understand heterogeneity between obese individuals so that personalized treatment strategies can be developed.

Not All Fat Is Created Equal

Related to the concept of heterogeneity in metabolic profile between obese individuals is heterogeneity in disease risk dependent on where fat is stored. It is now well established that visceral adiposity (abdominal fat or central obesity) is more strongly associated with future risk of diseases such as diabetes and coronary heart disease than subcutaneous adiposity (fat found directly below the skin throughout the body, not just abdominally). This distinction in fat storage is thought to be one of the reasons underlying the observation that Asians and particularly South Asians are at increased risk of diabetes at lower BMIs compared to Caucasians.

In addition to differences in future disease risk stemming from differences in where fat is stored, it is also now recognized that not all fat is of the same type. In general, there are two types of adipose tissue with antagonistic functions: white adipose tissue and brown adipose tissue. White adipose tissue is the classic type of fat; it is where excess energy is stored. Brown adipose tissue, on the other hand, uses energy to produce heat. Thus, individuals with greater amounts of white adipose tissue tend to have higher body weights, whereas individuals with greater amounts of brown adipose tissue tend to have lower body weights. These observations have led to a new line of research into potential ways of mimicking the action of brown adipose tissue to treat obesity.

Obesity Interventions

The analysis of the Global Burden of Disease Study by Ng and colleagues did not find a single country (out of 188 countries analyzed) in which the prevalence of obesity is decreasing. To date, most countries have relied on self-regulation by the food and beverage industry, and mass education campaigns that put the burden of change on the individual. Yet most experts agree that government regulation is absolutely necessary to "level the playing field" and provide consumers with healthy, affordable alternatives. In a review by B. A. Swinburn and colleagues published in *The Lancet* in 2011, experts concluded that policies to address environments promoting unhealthful diets and sedentary behavior must be implemented. Interventions at the clinical level focusing on behavior change of individuals will not be sufficient.

An important aspect of any intervention or policy is monitoring and evaluation of effects. Importantly, an analysis by K. D. Hall and colleagues published in *The Lancet* in 2011 found that very small changes in energy intake (10 calories per day) can lead to slight changes in body weight (one pound per year), and that there is a significant lag in realizing these effects—up to three years. Thus, follow-up of intervention participants and populations exposed to policy changes must continue for more than a couple of weeks or months. If follow-up is stopped early, some important effects may be missed.

Individual-Level Treatment   To date, much of the work on individual-level interventions for the treatment of obesity and community-level interventions for the prevention of obesity has focused on improving dietary intake and physical activity. Interventions targeting other potential causes of obesity such as environmental pollutants have not been conducted, but should be a part of comprehensive population prevention strategies.

Achieving clinically meaningful weight loss (5 to 7 percent of body weight) is difficult, and few interventions have demonstrated success in sustaining weight loss over long periods. A systematic review of long-term weight-loss studies in obese adults, conducted by J. D. Douketis and colleagues in 2005 and published in the *International Journal of Obesity*, found that lifestyle interventions result in, on average, fewer than 5 kilograms (11 pounds) of weight loss after two to four years, drug therapy results in 5 to 10 kilograms (11 to 22 pounds) of weight loss after one to two years, and bariatric surgery results in 25 to 75 kilograms (55 to 165 pounds) of weight loss after two to four years. The American College of Cardiology (ACC), the American Heart Association (AHA), and the Obesity Society (TOS) recommend lifestyle intervention as the first and primary treatment for weight loss. In individuals with extreme obesity or with lesser obesity but with comorbidities, other treatments may also be prescribed such as weight-loss drugs or bariatric surgery.

Since the first drug for obesity treatment, methamphetamine, was approved by the U.S. Food and Drug Administration (FDA) in 1947, several other drugs have been approved. Many were subsequently withdrawn from the market due to serious side effects, such as damage to heart valves by the drug Fen-Phen (fenfluramine), which was withdrawn in 1997, and heart attack and stroke for the drug Meridia (sibutramine), withdrawn in 2010. After 13 years without the emergence of any new FDA-approved drugs for weight loss, the FDA approved two new drugs for long-term use—Qsymia (phentermine and topiramate) and Belviq (lorcaserin)—in 2012, and Contrave (extended release form of naltrexone and bupropion) and Saxenda (liraglutide) in 2014. The only other FDA-approved weight-loss drug for long-term use is Xenical (orlistat), which is also sold over the counter in a lower-dose form called Alli.

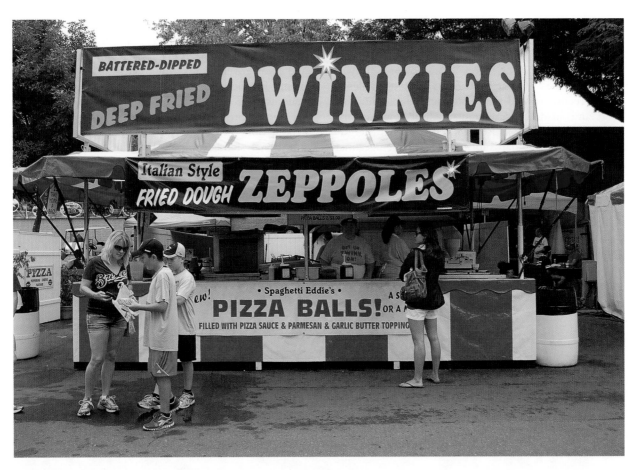

In the United States, many deep fried and unhealthful foods are available, illustrating trends in eating patterns that have become more common across the globe. Food industry interventions and education programs regarding healthful diets at the government level are now being recommended by some experts. © *miker/Shutterstock.com.*

Most FDA-approved drugs for weight loss have adverse side effects, and in all clinical trials of weight-loss drugs, the drugs are used in combination with lifestyle interventions such as healthful diet and physical activity. The dropout rate for many clinical trials of weight-loss drugs is more than 50 percent. Thus, while weight-loss drugs are effective at reducing weight, they are typically not a sustainable option for obese individuals. Furthermore, none is approved for use in children.

Bariatric surgery is effective for weight loss but is expensive, invasive, and not without risk. There are several different types of bariatric surgeries, and the effects of surgery on weight loss, comorbidities, and complications vary according to which procedure is used. The five major types include: laparoscopic adjustable gastric banding, laparoscopic Roux-en-Y gastric bypass, open Roux-en-Y gastric bypass, biliopancreatic diversion with and without duodenal switch, and sleeve gastrectomy.

According to the ACC/AHA/TOS guidelines for management of obesity in adults, mean weight loss 10 years following bariatric surgery is 16 percent of initial weight, and the incidence of diabetes remains significantly lower in those who have surgery compared to those who do not. A systematic review, conducted by V. L. Gloy and colleagues and published in the *British Medical Journal* in 2013, found that the most common complications of bariatric surgery were iron deficiency anemia (because some types of bariatric surgery bypass sections of the intestine, thus reducing absorption of nutrients) and reoperations.

Similar to weight-loss drugs, bariatric surgery is not approved for children, though some types are approved for adolescents. Early results of the Teen Longitudinal Assessment of Bariatric Surgery (Teen-LABS) study, published in the *Journal of the American Medical Association-Pediatrics* by T. H. Inge and colleagues, supported that bariatric surgery is safe for select adolescents: major complications (such as reoperation) were seen in 8 percent of participants and minor complications (such as dehydration) were seen in 15 percent. Nonetheless, lifestyle intervention is still the mainstay of obesity treatment for adolescents and adults.

Community-Level Prevention The U.S. Institute of Medicine (IOM) as of 2012 recommends that governments and the private sector (i.e., food and beverage industry) should work together to decrease access to unhealthful foods such as sugar-sweetened beverages and increase access and affordability of healthful foods such as fresh fruits and vegetables. It is also recommended that restaurants, including fast-food and sit-down restaurants, adopt lower-calorie, more healthful options for children, and that the government adopt standards for foods and beverages marketed directly to children. Other policy interventions include consistent and clear front-of-package nutrition labeling and menu board labeling that encourages healthful food choices.

In regard to physical activity, the IOM recommends that communities and urban planners should rethink community design and enhance the built environment so that it is conducive to safe physical activity that can be integrated into people's daily routines. Concurrent with this, communities and organizations should develop and implement high-visibility media campaigns that promote physical activity. The IOM also recommends that state and local governments adopt physical activity requirements for licensed child-care providers and schools. Schools have long been recognized as an ideal venue for obesity prevention. Requiring physical-activity education, time for physical activity during school, strong nutritional standards for school lunches and vending machines, and nutrition education are key examples of interventions that are recommended for implementation in schools in the United States.

Taking a more international approach, a review by S. L. Gortmaker and colleagues published in *The Lancet* in 2011 found that the top three most cost-effective obesity prevention interventions were: (1) an unhealthful food and beverage tax of 10 percent, (2) front-of-package traffic light nutrition labeling, and (3) reduction of advertising

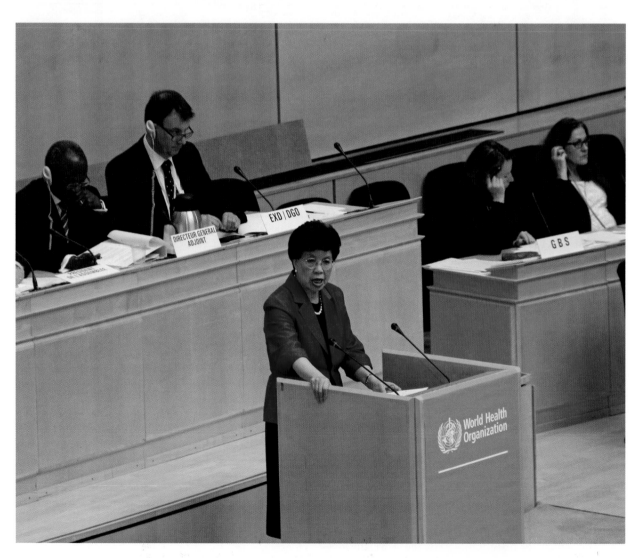

As the 67th Session of World Health Assembly begins in Geneva, Switzerland, on May 19, 2014, World Health Organization Director-General Dr. Margaret Chan speaks about the increase worldwide of childhood obesity during the session.   © *Fatih Erel/Anadolu Agency/Getty Images.*

of junk food and beverages to children. All of these interventions require government action. Other cost-saving interventions identified in that review were school-based, including education programs to reduce screen time and sugar-sweetened beverage consumption. There is no "magic bullet." The causes of obesity are multiple, and the solution will therefore have to be multifaceted.

⊕ Future Implications

Given the substantial health and economic costs of obesity, if action is not taken now to address the obesity epidemic, health systems around the world will be inundated, and gains made in other areas may be lost. Unique to the obesity epidemic (as compared to other global health issues such as human immunodeficiency virus/ acquired immune deficiency syndrome (HIV/AIDS), tuberculosis, and undernutrition), there are no exemplars for prevention or reversal of the trend of increasing overweight/obesity in adults and children. Also unique to obesity, many of the efforts to prevent the problem through improving diet and physical activity will also treat the problem.

Several environmental factors within countries may explain the wide variation in obesity prevalence across countries. The built environment, including, for example, pedestrian-friendly streets and green spaces that encourage physical activity; cuisines; and cultural body-size preferences can all affect national obesity prevalence and are important areas of intervention. Individual behaviors also undoubtedly contribute, and while the genetic underpinnings of obesity have been extensively researched, results have been largely disappointing, with no single abnormality identified as being responsible. Thus, it is up to federal and local governments, industry, community-based organizations, schools, and workplaces to change the environment from one that is conducive to poor diets and sedentariness to one that encourages healthful diets and active lifestyles. Urgent action involving multiple sectors is needed to reverse the rising tide of obesity.

PRIMARY SOURCE

Prevention of Childhood Obesity

SOURCE *"Introduction,"* in Prioritizing Areas for Action in the Field of Population-Based Prevention of Childhood Obesity: A Set of Tools for Member States to Determine and Identify Priority Areas for Action. *Geneva: World Health Organization (WHO), 2012, 11–12. http://www. who.int/dietphysicalactivity/childhood/Childhood_ obesity_Tool.pdf (accessed February 4, 2015).*

INTRODUCTION *This primary source is an excerpt from a publication on childhood obesity prepared by the World Health Organization that recognizes the health consequences of childhood obesity and the challenges of implementing public health policies to prevent it. The document seeks to address tackling the problem of obesity in a manner "that is both systematic and locally relevant" to each member state.*

INTRODUCTION

1.1 Childhood obesity

Over the past three decades the prevalence of overweight and obesity has increased substantially. Globally, an estimated 170 million children (aged < 18 years) are estimated to be overweight, and in some countries the number of overweight children has trebled since 1980. The high prevalence of overweight and obesity has serious health consequences. Raised body mass index (BMI) is a major risk factor for diseases such as cardiovascular disease, type 2 diabetes and many cancers (including, colorectal cancer, kidney cancer and oesophageal cancer). These diseases, often referred to as noncommunicable diseases (NCDs), not only cause premature mortality but also long-term morbidity. In addition, overweight and obesity in children are associated with significant reductions in quality of life and a greater risk of teasing, bullying and social isolation. Due to the rapid increase in obesity prevalence and the serious health consequences, obesity is commonly considered one of the most serious health challenges of the early 21st century.

1.2 The Global Strategy on Diet, Physical Activity and Health

The *Global Strategy on Diet, Physical Activity and Health (DPAS)* was developed by the World Health Organization (WHO) in 2004 to address the increasing prevalence and burden of NCDs. More specifically, the strategy focuses on improving global diet and physical activity patterns, two of the main risk factors for NCDs.
The four main objectives addressed by DPAS are:

1. To encourage the implementation of public health action and preventative intervention to reduce the risk factors which result from unhealthy diet and physical inactivity.

2. To increase recognition of the implications of unhealthy diet and inadequate physical activity levels and knowledge of preventative measures.

3. To promote policies and action plans at all levels to address diet and physical activity behaviours.

4. To encourage monitoring, evaluation and further research.

DPAS calls for priority to be given to the socially, economically and politically disadvantaged, and for the unhealthy diet and physical activity behaviours of, in particular, children and adolescents to be addressed.

1.3 WHO framework for the implementation of DPAS at country level

WHO developed a framework to assist Member States in monitoring and evaluating the implementation of DPAS at country level. The framework proposes that national governments demonstrate leadership and facilitate collaborative action in the implementation of policies and programmes to promote supportive environments for health. These actions are expected, in turn, to facilitate positive changes in diet and physical activity behaviours. The framework indicates that immediate- short- and long-term health, social, environmental, and economic outcomes should be measured regularly to assess changes. Furthermore, monitoring, evaluation and surveillance are core aspects of the implementation framework.

The original schematic model developed by WHO for monitoring the implementation of DPAS has subsequently been modified to focus specifically on areas for obesity prevention action.... The model enables a comprehensive and systematic analysis of potential obesity prevention action areas in multiple sectors and settings and incorporates three public health promotion approaches for tackling the issue: "Upstream" or socio-ecological, "Midstream" or behavioural and "Downstream" for health services.

SEE ALSO *Cardiovascular Diseases; Diabetes; Noncommunicable Diseases (Lifestyle Diseases); Nutrition*

BIBLIOGRAPHY

Books

Food and Agriculture Organization, International Fund for Agricultural Development, and World Food Programme. *The State of Food Security in the World*. Rome: Food and Agriculture Organization, 2013.

Institute of Medicine (IOM). *Accelerating Progress in Obesity Prevention: Solving the Weight of the Nation*. Washington, DC: National Academy of Sciences, 2012.

World Health Organization (WHO) and Food and Agriculture Organization (FAO) of the United Nations. *Diet, Nutrition and the Prevention of Chronic Diseases: Report of a Joint WHO/FAO Expert Consultation*. Geneva: World Health Organization, 2003.

Periodicals

Douketis, J. D., et al. "Systematic Review of Long-Term Weight Loss Studies in Obese Adults: Clinical Significance and Applicability to Clinical Practice." *International Journal of Obesity* 29 (July 2005): 1153–1167.

Gillies, C. L., et al. "Pharmacological and Lifestyle Interventions to Prevent or Delay Type 2 Diabetes in People with Impaired Glucose Tolerance: Systematic Review and Meta-Analysis." *British Medical Journal* 334, no. 7588 (February 10, 2007): 299.

Gloy, V. L., et al. "Bariatric Surgery versus Non-surgical Treatment for Obesity: A Systematic Review and Meta-analysis of Randomised Controlled Trials." *British Medical Journal* 347 (October 2013): f5934.

Gortmaker, S. L., et al. "Changing the Future of Obesity: Science, Policy, and Action." *The Lancet* 378, no. 9793 (August 2011): 838–847.

Hall, K. D., et al. "Quantification of the Effect of Energy Imbalance on Bodyweight." *The Lancet* 378, no. 9793 (August 2011): 826–837.

Inge, T. H., et al., for the Teen-LABS Consortium. "Perioperative Outcomes of Adolescents Undergoing Bariatric Surgery: The Teen-Longitudinal Assessment of Bariatric Surgery (Teen-LABS) Study." *Journal of the American Medical Association-Pediatrics* 168, no. 1 (January 2014): 47–53.

Jensen, M. D., et al. "2013 AHA/ACC/TOS Guideline for the Management of Overweight and Obesity in Adults: A Report of the American College of Cardiology/American Heart Association Task Force on Practice Guidelines and the Obesity Society." *Circulation* 129, suppl. 25 (June 2014): S102–S138.

Lim, S. S., et al. "A Comparative Risk Assessment of Burden of Disease and Injury Attributable to 67 Risk Factors and Risk Factor Clusters in 21 Regions, 1990–2010: A Systematic Analysis for the Global Burden of Disease Study 2010." *The Lancet* 380, no. 9859 (December 2012): 2224–2260.

Ng, M., et al. "Global, Regional, and National Prevalence of Overweight and Obesity in Children and Adults During 1980–2013: A Systematic Analysis for the Global Burden of Disease Study 2013." *The Lancet* 384, no. 9945 (August 2014): 766–781.

Rey-López, J. P., L. F. de Rezende, M. Pastor-Valero, and B. H. Tess. "The Prevalence of Metabolically Healthy Obesity: A Systematic Review and Critical Evaluation of the Definitions Used." *Obesity Reviews* 15, no. 10 (October 2014): 781–790.

Roberson, L. L., et al. "Beyond BMI: The 'Metabolically Healthy Obese' Phenotype and Its Association with Clinical/Subclinical Cardiovascular Disease and All-Cause Mortality: A Systematic Review." *BMC Public Health* 14 (January 2014): 14.

Rtveladze, Ketevan, et al. "Obesity Prevalence in Mexico: Impact on Health and Economic Burden." *Public Health Nutrition* 17, no. 1 (January 2014): 233–239.

Swinburn, B. A., et al. "The Global Obesity Pandemic: Shaped by Global Drivers and Local Environments." *The Lancet* 378, no. 9793 (August 2011): 804–814.

Wang, Y. C., Ketevan. McPherson, T. Marsh, S. L. Gortmaker, and M. Brown. "Health and Economic Burden of the Projected Obesity Trends in the USA and
the UK." *The Lancet* 378, no. 9793 (August 2011):
815–825.

Wildman, R.P., et al. "The Obese without Cardiometabolic Risk Factor Clustering and the Normal Weight
with Cardiometabolic Risk Factor Clustering: Prevalence and Correlates of 2 Phenotypes among the
US Population (NHANES 1999-2004)." *Journal of
Internal Medicine* 168, no. 15 (August 11, 2008):
1617–1624.

Websites

"FDA Approves Weight-Management Drug Saxenda."
U.S. Food and Drug Administration (FDA), December 23, 2014. http://www.fda.gov/NewsEvents/
Newsroom/PressAnnouncements/ucm427913
.htm (accessed March 16, 2015).

"Obesity and Overweight," Fact Sheet No. 311. *World
Health Organization (WHO)*, January 2015.
http://www.who.int/mediacentre/factsheets/
fs311/en/ (accessed March 15, 2015).

Lindsay M. Jaacks

Organ Donation and Transplantation

⊕ Introduction

To people with a disease that is causing an organ to fail, transplant can be a lifesaving miracle. Organ failure is when an organ of the body is so damaged that it starts to fail in its function. Many different conditions, for example congenital defects, and diseases, for example diabetes, liver diseases such as cirrhosis (scarring and hardening of the liver), and various forms of hepatitis (infectious or chemical inflammation), can cause organs to fail. A transplant involves taking an organ from a donor and placing it into the patient whose organ has failed; it often means the recipient will have many more years of life.

Many organs can be used for transplant. Corneas (the clear covering of the eye), kidneys, lungs, hearts, bones, skin (the body's largest organ), livers, and intestines can all be transplanted. Organs can be taken from living donors or cadavers (dead bodies). Living donors are more often used in kidney and liver transplants, because the human body has two kidneys and part of the liver can be removed, leaving the donor with enough organ to survive.

In the United States in 2012, the five-year transplant survival rate after receiving an organ from a cadaver was 83 percent; from living donors the rate was 92 percent, though rates differ depending on the organ. In 2014, 62 percent of living donors were women; of deceased donors, 60 percent were men. Fifty-seven percent of deceased donors were white; 16 percent black; 15 percent Latino; and 6 percent Asian, native Hawaiian, or other islanders. As of January 2015, 42 percent on the waiting list for organ transplant were white; 30 percent black; 19 percent Latino; and almost 9 percent were Asian, native Hawaiian, or other islanders. These statistics are important because donor matches are more likely to be found within ethnic groups.

According to the Global Observatory on Donation and Transplantation (GODT), about 114,690 transplants were performed worldwide in 2012, with the majority of those being kidney transplants (77,818).

Kidney transplants generally have good outcomes around the world, according to the World Health Organization (WHO), though the one-year survival rate depends on several factors, including whether the donor was alive or deceased and the region in which the transplant was performed. Outcomes were generally good worldwide after one year, with those receiving grafts from deceased donors having survival rates ranging from 78 percent to 97 percent and from live donors from 82 to 99 percent.

⊕ Historical Background

The concept of transplanting body parts is as old as civilization, and myths regarding the replacement of organs can be found in all cultures. Christian texts have numerous references to restoring lost limbs, from the time of Jesus to the saints of the Middle Ages (c. 500–c. 1500). The taking of body parts, often from animals, was believed to be the work of gods and healers. Ancient humans often looked to the supernatural to restore body parts lost due to disease, war, or punishment, believing that if bodies were not healed, resurrection was impossible. An ancient Greek myth tells of an island populated by large sea turtles whose blood could glue body parts back on. A traditional Irish tale speaks of a ruler who lost his hand; because he was forbidden to rule if not whole, a physician who had replaced his own eye with the eye of a cat dug up the ruler's hand and reattached it using incantations. A heart transplant features in the Chinese story of a judge who replaced a man's heart with one taken from someone in the netherworld. Ethical aspects of transplants were also noted in ancient literature. In one myth, a goddess switched the heads of a married man and his brother and created a dilemma: which was the husband? A folktale from the brothers Grimm tells of a hand transplanted from a thief that causes the recipient to start stealing.

By 800 BCE, it is believed Indian doctors had begun to treat wounds by replacing damaged skin from one part

AM I A MATCH?

When a person is need of a transplant, whether new bone marrow or a heart, finding the right donor can increase the success of the transplant and reduce complications. In a 2014 *American Journal of Transplantation* article, "Transplantation Genetics: Current Status and Prospects," the authors report that approximately 60 percent of transplant recipients still experience rejection, with 40 percent experiencing the rejection within the first year following transplant.

While there are some variations in match testing and needs depending on the organ, all transplant workups have basic requirements. The simplest and first test is blood type. There are four basic types: O, A, B, and AB. The most common type, O, is considered the universal donor because it may be given to any of the other types. The rarest type is AB; it is the universal recipient, meaning it can receive any of the other types.

Following a blood type match, human leukocyte antigens (HLA) matching is done. While not necessary in all organ transplants, it is important in kidney and bone marrow transplants. HLA are proteins on white blood cells that can cause immune reactions. While not totally eliminating rejection, a good match of the six major proteins can ensure a better chance of survival of the graft (organ) and decrease the complications of the recipient.

Next, antibodies are measured in the recipient: the more antibodies, the higher the risk of rejection. Antibodies can be acquired by previous transfusions, by a previous transplant, or during pregnancy with an incompatible blood type fetus. Just prior to a transplant, crossmatching is done. Cells of the donor and recipient are mixed, and the reaction is observed. If the result is positive, the two are not compatible, and the transplanted organ will experience rejection.

Other factors are also considered, depending on the organ. Time is critical in heart and lung transplants; those organs can only survive for a few hours once removed from the donor. Distance from the donor hospital may affect who gets the organ. The body size of the recipient is also important, as the new organ must fit into the patient. When an organ becomes available, the health of the recipient is considered, as the patient may be too ill to undergo the procedure. Gender and race are not considerations.

Recent advances in genetic testing are leading to new ways of evaluating recipients. It has been shown that there are numerous non-HLA proteins that may affect the rejection process. Polymorphism, the existence of an organism in multiple colors or forms, occurs at a rate of approximately 3.5 million between two unrelated individuals of European descent and at least 10 million in those of African descent. Although race is not a factor in choosing recipients, matching donors and recipients of similar race can have a good effect on organ survival. Efforts are ongoing to enroll minorities in donor programs. A blood test used in Europe for some time but only recently introduced in the United States is able to uncover genetic variation in blood types, helping to prevent mismatches.

of the body with healthy skin from another. These techniques did not reach Europe until the 1200s. In the 16th century, an Italian surgeon named Gasparo Tagliacozzi (1545–1599) reconstructed noses and ears using tissue from the arm of the patient. When Tagliacozzi attempted the procedure using tissue from donors, however, the procedure often failed. Although he did not understand the reason for this result, it is now known as rejection.

In the early 1900s, European doctors attempted to save dying kidney patients with transplanted animal kidneys. The patients all died within days. However, in 1905, Eduard Zirm, an Austrian ophthalmologist, or eye surgeon, transplanted a cornea and restored the sight of a man blinded in an occupational accident. A few years later, in 1912, French surgeon and biologist Alexis Carrel (1873–1944) received the Nobel Prize for his successful kidney transplant procedures between dogs and techniques for suturing blood vessels. He and U.S. aviator Charles Lindbergh (1902–1974) invented a device to keep organs alive outside of the body. This device was the precursor to the artificial heart.

An attempt was made in Russia in 1936 to transplant a cadaver kidney into a patient, but the patient soon died of rejection. The first successful human transplant took place in 1954. Plastic surgeon Dr. Joseph Murray (1919–2012) of Boston, Massachusetts, transplanted a kidney from one identical twin into the other twin. He won a Nobel Prize in 1990 for his work. The twin receiving the new kidney lived for 10 more years, and suffered no rejection because identical twins have the same genetic makeup. In 1967, Dr. Christiaan Barnard (1922–2001) performed the first heart transplant at a hospital in South Africa. The male patient, Louis Washkansky, was dying of heart failure, while the donor was a 25-year-old woman who was killed in a car accident. The recipient lived only 18 days, dying not of the transplant but from pneumonia. Barnard's achievement was based on the work of Dr. Norman Shumway (1923–2006), who pioneered heart transplant procedures and performed the first such surgery in the United States in 1968. Throughout the rest of the 1960s and early 1970s, there were several firsts in transplant surgery, but the pivotal moment was the introduction of the drug cyclosporine. This drug could suppress the body's immune system, thus preventing rejection of an organ.

Side Effects and Risks of Transplants

While transplants can offer a second chance at life for the recipient, survival can be just as challenging after surgery. There are many complications that follow surgery, such as bleeding, infection, and pain. The most feared complication is rejection. Since donor and recipient do not have identical genes, the body's immune system, which is designed to protect the body against invaders, sees the new organ as foreign and will actively work to destroy it. In the 1970s, the development of cyclosporine changed the game. Cyclosporine is a drug that blocks immune response, allowing the recipient's body to accept the new organ. However, by blocking the immune system, the drugs predispose the recipient to potentially life-threatening infections from both bacteria and viruses. Newer and more effective drugs continue to be developed, but patients must remain on these powerful drugs for the rest of their lives or risk rejection. Other problems often develop, such as depression. In many cases, someone had to die in order for the recipient to live, which produces guilt over receiving the organ. Also, antirejection drugs are extremely expensive, often costing US$20,000 to US$30,000 annually, which can cause enormous financial strain.

Living donors also experience repercussions. Some have experienced surgical complications, others have developed chronic pain, and some have progressed to failure in their remaining organ. According to a 2012 CNN report, a healthy 57-year-old donor died of massive blood loss at Lahey Clinic in Massachusetts while donating part of his liver to his brother-in-law. While there are many organizations available to help transplant patients, donors can feel forgotten; often there is no one to help with medical costs or psychological issues.

⊕ Impacts and Issues

While transplants offer hope, there is a great shortage of organs compared to the number of people who need them. In the United States, approximately 79 people receive a transplant each day, but 21 others will die each day waiting for their chance. As of 2012, there were over 200,000 patients on the waiting list in the United States alone, and another 100,000 in Europe. The WHO estimates that only 1 in 10 people who need an organ transplant will ever receive an organ. There are several problematic issues when obtaining organs for this purpose. One early concern was the concept of brain death. Before an accepted definition of brain death existed, organs could only be removed from patients whose hearts had stopped beating. This limited the number of organs available, as lack of oxygen flow to those organs caused them to be unusable. In 1968, a team at Harvard University Medical School developed the first standard definition of brain death. In the United States, all 50 states have now adopted the criteria, which allow a brain dead patient to be kept on a ventilator. All organs are thus supplied with blood flow and oxygen until they can be removed for transplant.

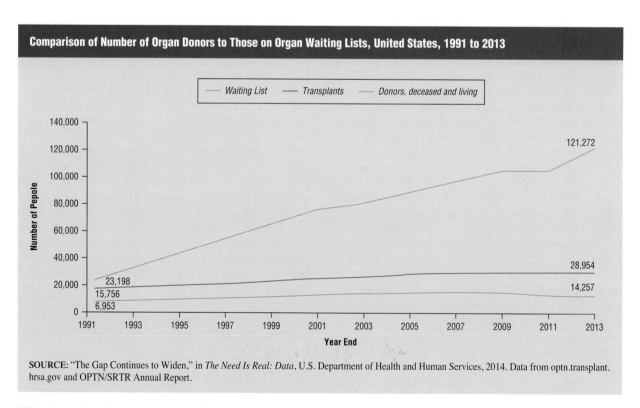

Comparison of Number of Organ Donors to Those on Organ Waiting Lists, United States, 1991 to 2013

Legend: Waiting List — Transplants — Donors, deceased and living

121,272

28,954

14,257

23,198

15,756

6,953

Number of Pepole (y-axis); Year End (x-axis: 1991, 1993, 1995, 1997, 1999, 2001, 2003, 2005, 2007, 2009, 2011, 2013)

SOURCE: "The Gap Continues to Widen," in *The Need Is Real: Data*, U.S. Department of Health and Human Services, 2014. Data from optn.transplant.hrsa.gov and OPTN/SRTR Annual Report.

While the number of organ transplants and the number of donors have remained relatively constant in the United States, the wait list for organs continues to grow at a considerable rate.

Not all cultures have readily accepted the concept of brain death. In Japan, the idea that brain death allows for the continued beating of the heart is inconsistent with the cultural belief in death of the whole person, not just one organ. After the country passed a law in 1997 allowing use of brain dead donors, it took 16 months for the performance of the first transplant under the law. In 2010, Japan revised the Organ Transplant Act, further easing organ donation after brain death and allowing for family consent of organ donation after a patient dies without a signed will stating consent. Yet an estimated 70 percent of transplanted kidneys and 80 percent of transplanted liver segments in Japan are supplied by living donors. This is in contrast to the United States, where in 2014, according to the Organ Procurement and Transplantation Network (OPTN) of the U.S. Department of Health and Human Services, 42 percent of kidneys and less than 4 percent of livers came from live donors. Although Japanese law protects the voluntary nature of the donation as well as family rights, distrust in the system remains. Some of this relates to the controversial history of transplants in Japan. In 1968, Dr. Juro Wada (1922–2011) used a heart from a brain dead donor in the world's second heart transplant. Because of issues surrounding the case, he was subsequently arrested for murder, and it took six years of litigation to clear him. Heart transplant was banned in Japan for 15 years thereafter.

In 2007, China banned living donors, excluding spouses, blood relatives, and adopted/stepfamily members. Then in 2014, due to international criticism over ethics, China ended its use of executed prisoners as a source of organs, further increasing shortages. While they have 300,000 people each year on the waiting list, only 1 in 30 will receive a transplant.

Religious considerations can also hinder availability of organs. No religion specifically outlaws transplants or donations. Religious beliefs, however, can affect the number of organs available. Among Christian religions, there are subtle nuances between various denominations. Protestant, Anglican, and Catholic doctrines support organ donation as an act of selflessness. In 1990, there was a joint declaration of the Catholic and Protestant churches in Germany encouraging donations. The Mormon and Quaker religions consider it an individual decision.

The Jewish faith proscribes unnecessary interference with the bodies of the deceased. Some Jewish scholars use three scriptural prohibitions to discourage donation: desecration of the body, delay of burial, and benefit from death of another. However, preservation of life is also a fundamental tenet of the religion. As viewed by Jewish scholars, the definition of brain death is important. The ultraorthodox believe brain death is not true death. The Halachic organ donor card offers two options: one allows donation after brain death, while the other only permits donation following heart cessation. As of 2010, only 8 percent of Israelis are registered organ donors.

Islamic beliefs on the subject are also complicated. As with Judaism, desecrating the body is forbidden, but altruism is an important principle. In 1988, the Islamic Jurisprudence Assembly Council in Saudi Arabia issued a religious ruling that organ transplant is in keeping with Islam. Other Islamic nations followed suit, including Egypt, Iran, and Pakistan. In 1996, The UK Muslim Law Council allowed Muslims in the United Kingdom to carry donor cards. Live donation is considered an act of merit. Both Jewish and Islamic patients or donors can request directed donations, giving or receiving organs only with those of the same faith.

The integrity of the body is not important in Hinduism, Sikhism, or Buddhism. Sustaining life, continuous rebirth, and the transitory nature of time on Earth are all concepts that allow acceptance of transplantation.

Illegal Organ Trafficking

Because of the shortage in organ donations, the selling and trafficking of organs has emerged as a global problem. The United Nations has stated that organ trafficking occurs in three categories. In the first category, traffickers force or deceive victims into giving up an organ. In the second category, victims willingly give up an organ for payment, but are paid less than was agreed upon; a donor may receive between US$1,000 and $5,000 for a kidney, when the recipient has paid the broker between US$100,000 and $200,000. The third category includes impoverished migrants, or homeless or illiterate people who are treated for an illness that may not exist; the organs are then removed without their knowledge or consent. It is estimated that at least 10,000 black market kidney transplants take place each year. Illegal organ trade generates between $600 million and $1.2 billion annually. Organs often come from impoverished countries in South America, Africa, Asia, and Eastern Europe, while recipients include patients in wealthier nations such as the United States, Canada, United Kingdom, Australia, Japan, and Israel. Patients of these illegal operations have a higher rate of complications from transplant related human immunodeficiency virus (HIV), incompatibility, and poor condition of the organs.

Trafficking, run by organized criminal groups, was first brought to light in 1990. Because these groups operate in at least 50 different countries, tracking and prosecution can be difficult. The WHO has taken the role of trying to document and track illegal organ transactions. Organ Watch is another agency that works to draw attention to this activity. It was founded in 1997 by Berkeley, California, anthropology professor, author, and human rights activist, Nancy Scheper-Hughes (1944–).

Around the world, nations have created laws to deal with this criminal activity. In 1994, India banned the sale of organs. The National Organ Transplant Act was passed by the U.S. Congress in 1984, making it illegal to sell organs in the United States. In June 2012,

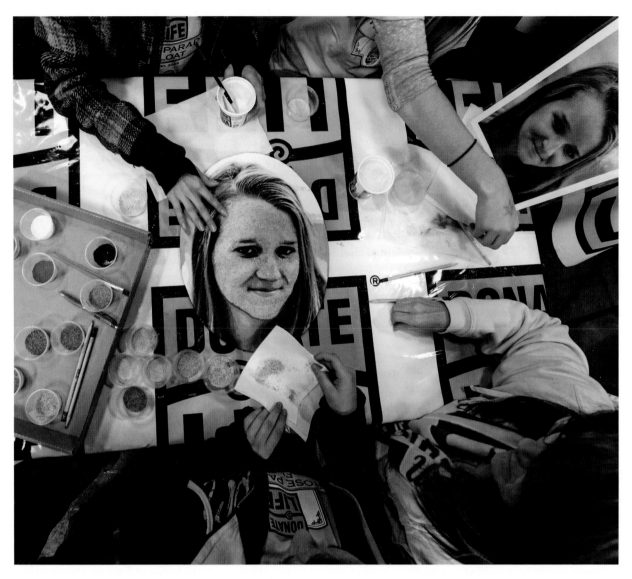

Family members work on the "floragraph" of organ donor Lindsey Denae Woodward for the Donate Life float entry, "Light Up the World," for its appearance in the 125th Rose Parade on January 1, 2014. On June 14, 2011, 14-year-old Lindsey was declared brain dead after an automobile accident; her parents donated her organs, corneas, and tissue. More than 28,000 lives are saved each year in the United States through organ donation, and the Donate Life float calls attention each New Year's Day to the need for people to register in their state to be organ, eye, and tissue donors and to donate blood in their communities. *© Brian Cahn/ZUMAPRESS.com/Alamy.*

representatives of some Central American countries and the Dominican Republic established a minimum penalty for organ trafficking. Prosecutors have been reluctant to go after the purchasers of the organs. As of 2014, Iran had the only legal and regulated kidney-selling program in existence, but limited the trade to donors and recipients within the country. Singapore and Australia allow for limited payments to compensate for a donor's time off of work.

Ethical Issues

Ethical issues, including how and where organs are allocated, arise frequently in transplantation. Due to the scarcity of available organs, transplants must be rationed.

Should the sickest, who may not tolerate surgery, be at the top of the list? Is it wrong to compensate someone for a donation? Should patients be allowed to designate their recipients? Some ethicists propose giving preference for transplants to patients also listed as donors, as mandated in Singapore. In Europe, allocations are based on the national ratio of donors to recipients: countries that have more donors get a higher percentage of the organs available for transplant. In the United States, however, 70 percent of the people receiving organs are not donors themselves.

Directed donations are allowed by U.S. law. An organization founded in 2002, LifeSharers, is a nonprofit network of organ donors. Members pledge their organs, upon death, for use in transplants. In exchange, should the member need a transplant, the LifeSharer member is given priority for organs donated by other LifeSharers. A six-month waiting period is enforced to discourage people from joining because they need an organ. There is no membership fee.

Other issues persist. There are methods to "jump the line"; for example, those with financial means can place themselves on multiple lists, increasing the chance an organ will become available. There is also the issue of those not able to consent to donation, such as the mentally disabled, who need a transplant.

In 2014, 10-year-old Sarah Murnaghan of Pennsylvania was denied a lung transplant because of her age. While on a pediatric list, Sarah was prohibited from being matched against a list of adult donors because of a rule that prevents children under age 12 from being given adult lungs, usually because of the size limitations of transferring an adult organ to a child. Her parents sued, and the judge ruled in their favor. As a result, U.S. Secretary of Health and Human Services Kathleen Sebelius had to reverse a decision not allow the transplant to go ahead, giving a one-time exception to the 12-year-old cut-off rule. In 2014 OPTN ruled that such exceptions could be granted on a case-by-case basis.

Allocation of Organs

In an attempt to ensure that the limited supply of organs is fairly allocated, most countries have developed resources and enacted laws regulating transplants. In the United States, the National Organ Transplant Act (1984) called for the development of the OPTN. It is run by the United Network for Organ Sharing (UNOS), a nonprofit organization under federal contract. UNOS has established an organ-sharing network and collects data pertaining to waiting lists, matching of organs, and transplant operations. U.S. Medicare law was amended in 1978 to allow coverage of renal (kidney) transplant. Other laws have been passed over the years to include coverage of pediatric transplants, Medicaid coverage of transplants, and federal employee leave to serve as a living donor. Since 2006, the Uniform Anatomical Gift Act bars others from revoking the consent of a donor following his or her death.

In the United States, UNOS maintains a centralized computer network that links all procurement organizations and transplant centers. If a patient's physician feels the criteria for a transplant are met, the patient is referred to a center for evaluation. Both physical and mental health are evaluated, as well as the individual's support system. If accepted, the patient is placed into the database. If a donor becomes available, the computer will match the two and rank according to blood type, tissue match, length of time on the waiting list, immune status, and distance between donor and recipient. In cases of heart, lung, and intestinal transplants, medical urgency

is also assessed. In addition to not matching a donor, a person at the top of the list may not get the available organ if surgery is too risky, if immediate transplant is not possible, or if the procedure is otherwise unfeasible.

The European Union has established a number of rules governing transplants. Member states must set up national authorities to monitor, maintain quality, and ensure safety standards for organs intended for transplant. All donations must be voluntary and unpaid, although living donors may receive compensation for expenses and lost wages due to the procedure. Advertising of organs available is prohibited. Within the United Kingdom, requirements differ among different areas. For example, in Bolton, one must actively sign the Donor Register to become a donor, while in Wales, people are automatically donors unless they specifically opt out.

Japan revised its Organ Transplant Law in 2010; anyone can now donate, even children. The original law, passed in 1997, stated that there must be written consent by the donor given prior to death and the consent of the next of kin. Written consent is no longer needed but the consent of the family is still required. Some lawmakers did not support the legislation because of the problematic definition of brain death. There was concern over how that definition would relate to children who have healthy hearts that can beat for many years following brain death.

In 2014, China started a new donor program. One problem already identified is lack of transparency that exists in other countries. Unlike the United States, where the public can log on to the database, China offers no open access to information regarding donors and operations. In its early days, this program showed an increase in transplants from voluntary donors, but the number of organs available since the cessation of using executed prisoners has dropped by 50 percent. The government is stating that hospitals using organs from outside the established network will lose their certifications, although it is not known how this will be enforced.

⊕ Future Implications

Many aspects of transplant procedures continue to be featured in news stories, including issues of organ availability, ethics, and medical research.

In many countries and religions, the definition of death is problematic. A universally accepted definition of death could increase organ availability.

While the option of allowing people to sell their organs has been suggested, the possibility of financial gain raises concern that the poor and desperate could become entrapped in these transactions.

Several changes in priorities on the U.S. waiting list took effect in 2014. Length of time on dialysis is now factored in for potential kidney recipients. Younger patients, in whom the transplanted organ may have a better chance to survive, will be given priority. Almost

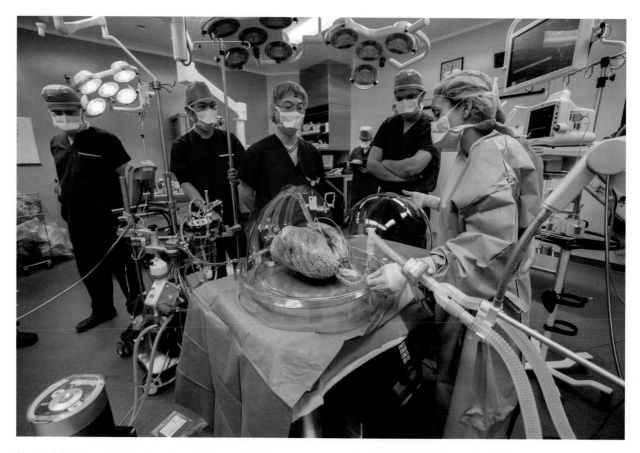

Dr. Virginia Linacre (right), places donor lungs in the XVIVO lung perfusion machine at Toronto General Hospital for a potential double-lung transplant. The air left inside lungs can keep them from the immediate deterioration seen in other organs, and the machine helps preserve the lungs, allowing the transplant team run a series of tests to verify the condition of the donor organ prior to transplant. As medical urgency is one factor in determining who gets a lung due to their fragility, it is hoped the machine may add time to how long the lungs can remain viable. © *Randy Risling/Toronto Star via Getty Images.*

15 percent of those on the waiting list already have undergone a failed transplant. In initiating the changes, it is thought that this will prevent re-transplant rates and free up organs for others. As in some European countries, donors will be advanced up the waiting list if they need a future transplant.

Spain, Italy, Austria, Belgium, and other European countries have presumed consent laws; under this system, only those who choose to sign an opt-out card are excluded. In the United States alone, there are over 2.5 million deaths a year due to lack of organs for transplants. A presumed consent law would create a large supply of available organs. However, presumed consent could be interpreted as a violation of the Fifth Amendment over taking property without due process and compensation.

Research on subjects such as stem cells could open new avenues to replacement or repair of organs. Cloning of organs is also being studied. In 2014, surgeons in Australia successfully performed three "dead heart" transplants, in which the donated hearts had stopped beating for up to 20 minutes. A device developed by Massachusetts-based TransMedics, Inc., revives a non-beating heart by warming it and perfusing it with a preservation solution and oxygenated nutrient-rich blood. Doctors involved believe the technique could save 30 percent more lives.

Organ transplants will continue to present a challenge as long as recipients outnumber donors. Research, new techniques, and changes in attitudes continue to evolve.

PRIMARY SOURCE

2012 National Survey of Organ Donation Attitudes and Behaviors

SOURCE *"Executive Summary," from* 2012 National Survey of Organ Donation Attitudes and Behaviors, *Rockville, MD: U.S. Department of Health and Human Services, September 2013, 1–5. http://www.organdonor.gov/dtcp/national-surveyorgandonation.pdf (accessed January 25, 2015).*

INTRODUCTION *This primary source summarizes the results of a 2012 survey of attitudes and behavior in the United States regarding organ donation. It was published by the U.S. Department of Health and Human Services.*

EXECUTIVE SUMMARY

The 2012 National Survey of Organ Donation Attitudes and Behavior is a nationally representative sample of more than 3,200 U.S. adults. The survey included measures of attitudes and behaviors related to donation of organs for transplantation, discussing donation wishes with family, granting permission to donate, beliefs about the donation process, and opinions on policies related to donation. This study, conducted for the Health Resources and Services Administration (HRSA), built upon two previous studies—one sponsored by HRSA in 2005 and the other by the Partnership for Organ Donation in 1993. All three surveys were conducted under contract by Gallup, Inc. While some items remained the same in all three survey instruments, some were new in 2012, and others were variants of topics examined in the 2005 and 1993 reports.

Support for Organ Donation

There was high and sustained support for the donation of organs for transplant with 94.9 percent of U.S. adults supporting or strongly supporting donation in 2012. Similar to the proportions in 1993 and 2005, adults in the U.S. continued to express a positive sentiment toward organ donation. Although the total support was consistent from 2005 to 2012, the percentage of the adult population that strongly supported the donation of organs for transplant has increased significantly since 2005. In 2012, 48.8 percent of the population strongly supported the donation of organs for transplantation, a significantly greater percentage than the 39.4 percent of the population who strongly supported it in 2005. Strong support for donation was significantly higher among women than men, significantly higher among Whites and Native Americans than in other racial or ethnic groups, significantly lower among those aged 66 and older, and significantly lower among the population with an education level of high school or less.

Granting Permission for Organ Transplant

There was a significant increase from 2005 to 2012 in the percentage of U.S. adults who granted permission for donation on their driver's license. In 2005, 51.3 percent had granted permission on a driver's license compared with the 60.1 percent who said the same in 2012. Although there was also a significant increase between 2005 and 2012 in the percentage of U.S. adults who reported they joined their state donor registry, some portion of the increase may reflect the increase in the number of states that instituted a donor registry during this period. There was no difference in the percentage of the U.S. adult population who reported having a signed donor card during the same time.

The key finding with regard to granting permission for donation pertains to the 66 and older group in 2012. In 2005, 26.3 percent of the 66 and older group granted permission for organ donation on their driver's license; this was the lowest of all age groups. In 2012, 52.2 percent of the 66 and older age group granted permission for organ donation on their driver's license, roughly twice the proportion of the same population in 2005.

Of the population who had not yet granted permission for organ donation, roughly one-third (36.8 percent) said they had reservations about donation, and more than half (59.2 percent) said they were open to considering donation. Among racial groups who had not yet granted permission, Native Americans were most open to donation (32.8 percent *definitely yes*) while African-Americans were least open to considering donation (9.5 percent *definitely yes*).

Donating a Family Member's Organs

In 2012, the likelihood of donating family members' organs upon their death was very high (96.7 percent) when family members' wishes to donate were known. This finding is in line with the number observed in 2005 (95.9 percent). When unsure of their family members' wishes, a majority of U.S. adults were still likely to donate (75.6 percent), but to a lesser extent. A little over half (51.3 percent) of the population reported a family member had informed them about his or her wishes to donate or not donate organs upon death. When comparing across time, those who reported being *very likely* to donate a family member's organs without knowing that family member's preference, there was a significant increase in 2012 (44.3 vs. 30.0 percent in 2005) among the 66 and older group. When the family member's wish to donate was known, the percentage of the population 66 and older that was *very likely* to honor the donation request was still significantly greater in 2012 (87.6 percent) than in 2005 (74.0 percent).

Communicating Intent to Donate

There were distinct age variations regarding sharing donation wishes with family. Discussing donation wishes was less common among the youngest population (67.0 percent) in 2012 compared with the two middle-age groups—the 35- to 54-year-olds (82.0 percent) and 55- to 65-year-olds (78.9 percent). The eldest population in 2012 was significantly less likely to report that a member of their family had told them about their donation wishes. For those aged 66 and older, this proportion was 38.5 percent, compared with more than half of the population for the other age groups.

Living Donation

The proportion of the U.S. adult population who indicated they were *very likely* to donate an organ while alive was closely aligned to the relationship they have with the potential recipient. Overall, most U.S. adults were significantly more likely to be a living donor for a family member (73.3 percent) than for any other relationship, such as an acquaintance. A significantly greater proportion of women (76.3 percent) than men (70.0 percent) reported being *very likely* to be a living donor for a family member. The 35- to 54-year-old group was *very likely* (78.1 percent), which was significantly more than the 18- to 34-year-old group (73.8 percent), the 55- to 65-year-old group (68.3 percent), or the 66 and older group (67.2 percent). There were no differences in willingness to donate to a family member among racial or ethnic groups in 2012. The likelihood of a living donation to a family member was high among 77.5 percent of the some college educational group. This is significantly higher than the high school or less educational group (69.5 percent) in 2012.

In comparing 2012 with 2005, there was a significant increase in the percentage of adults who reported they were *very likely* to be willing to be a living donor for a family member. In 2012, 73.3 percent of U.S. adults were *very likely* (20.2 percent *somewhat likely*) compared with the 61.1 percent of adults who said the same in 2005 (29.0 percent *somewhat likely* in 2005). The trend was the same regarding a close friend. Eighty-five percent (85.4 percent) of the population was at least *somewhat likely* to be a living donor (45.0 percent *very likely* and 40.4 percent *somewhat likely*) for a close friend compared with 74.3 percent in 2005. There was a significant increase from 2005 to 2012 in willingness to be a living donor for a stranger. In 2012, 15.1 percent of adults reported being *very likely* and 39.6 percent of adults reported being *somewhat likely* to be a living donor for someone they don't know. Both of these percentages were significantly higher than in 2005, where only 8.0 percent reported they were *very likely* and 29.5 percent reported being *somewhat likely* to donate to a stranger.

In comparing the 2012 racial groups to their counterparts in 2005, there was a significant difference in the Asian American population. In 2005, 52.1 percent of the Asian population reported being *very likely* to be a living donor for a family member. This increased significantly to 72.8 percent of the Asian population in 2012.

Donating Hands and Face

For the first time, the 2012 survey included questions about the public's attitudes toward donation of hands and face. While the majority of the population supported both hand and face donation, the public was more open to the donation of their hands (80.3 percent) than the donation of their face (58.2 percent).

When considering gender, there were no significant differences between men and women on donating their hands or their face. There were no substantial differences among different age groups when asked about donating hands, but there were several distinctions related to donating a face. One-quarter (25.1 percent) of the youngest group (18- to 34-year-olds) were *very willing* to donate their face. This was significantly lower than the percentage of those who reported being *very willing* to donate their face in the 35- to 54-year-old group (34.3 percent) and in the 55- to 65-year-old group (35.6 percent). There was also a significant difference in the opposite extreme of the scale with 14.0 percent of the 55- to 65-year-old group being *not at all willing* to donate their face, significantly lower than all other age groups where a larger proportion said they were *not at all willing*.

Presumed Consent

Half of the U.S. adult population (51.1 percent) would *support* or *strongly support* a system of presumed consent in the United States. This was significantly more than the 41.9 percent who supported such a system in 2005. Regardless of support for a presumed consent system, there was little question of the utility of presumed consent. Most U.S. adults believed that this policy would increase the number of available organs for transplants. This reflects virtually no difference between 2005 (80.4 percent) and 2012 (80.0 percent). About one-quarter of the population (23.4 percent) said that under a system of presumed consent they would sign up as a non-donor, significantly less than the 29.7 percent reported in 2005.

Strong support for a presumed consent system was double for the 66 and older population in 2012 (19.1 percent) compared with the same population in 2005 (8.1 percent). The youngest age group, 18- to 34-year-olds, was significantly more likely than all other age groups (87.3 percent) to believe that presumed consent will increase the number of available organs for donation. The youngest age group was also least likely to opt out of a presumed consent system.

Financial Incentives

In 2012, one-quarter (25.4 percent) of the population reported that a financial incentive would increase their likelihood to donate their own organs. This represented a significant increase from the 16.7 percent who held this belief in 2005. Although more respondents were supportive of financial incentives, a majority of the population (63.6 percent) continued to report that a financial incentive would have no effect on their decision to donate their organs.

Hispanics (39.2 percent) and Native Americans (35.5 percent) were similar to African-Americans (28.9 percent) but significantly more likely than Asians (24.5

percent) and Whites (23.5 percent) to say that financial incentives would increase their willingness to donate.

The willingness to donate a family member's organs if offered a financial incentive has increased significantly since 1993 and mirrored the data of willingness to donate one's own organs if offered a financial incentive. In 2012, 25.8 percent of respondents indicated that a financial incentive would increase their willingness to donate a family member's organs—a significant increase from the 18.3 percent of respondents who said the same in 2005.

SEE ALSO *Noncommunicable (Lifestyle) Diseases*

BIBLIOGRAPHY

Books

Hakim, Nadey S., ed *Introduction to Organ Transplantation.* 2nd ed, Singapore: World Scientific, 2012.

Hamilton, David. *A History of Organ Transplantation: Ancient Legends to Modern Practice.* Pittsburgh, PA: University of Pittsburgh Press, 2012.

Jensen, Steven J., ed *The Ethics of Organ Transplantation.* Washington, DC: Catholic University of America Press, 2011.

Norris, Lisa. *Transplant Administration.* Chichester, UK: Wiley, 2014.

Weimer, David L. *Medical Governance: Values, Expertise, and Interests in Organ Transplantation.* Washington, DC: Georgetown University Press, 2010.

Periodicals

Almoguera, B., A. Shaked, and B. J. Keating. "Transplantation Genetics: Current Status and Prospectus." *American Journal of Transplantation* 14, Issue 4 (April 2014): 764–778.

Bramstedt, Katrina A. "Is It Ethical to Prioritize Patients for Organ Allocation According to Their Values about Organ Donation?" *Progress in Transplantation* 16, no. 2 (June 2006): 170–174.

Bruzzone, P. "Religious Aspects of Transplantation." *Transplant Proceedings* 40, no. 4 (May 2008): 1064–1067.

Byram-Coers, Susanna, and Michael L. Ault. "Con: The Challenges of Utilizing Expanded-Criteria Donors for Orthotopic Heart Transplant" *Journal of Cardiothoracic and Vascular Anesthesia* 28, no. 6 (December 2014): 1688–1690.

Oliver, Michael, et al. "Organ Donation, Transplantation and Religion." *Nephrology Dialysis Transplantation* 26, no. 2 (2011): 437–444. Available online at http://ndt.oxfordjournals.org/content/26/2/437 (accessed January 25, 2015).

Websites

"A Brief History of Heart Transplantation." *Columbia University Department of Surgery.* http://hearttransplant.com/history.html (accessed January 25, 2015).

Hooper, Rowan. "Japan's Live Organ Donors Enjoy Better Health Than 'Normal' Citizens Do." *Japan Times,* November 11, 2012. http://www.japantimes.co.jp/news/2012/11/11/national/science-health/japans-live-organ-donors-enjoy-better-health-than-normal-citizens-do/#.VSXURJOVRps (accessed April 8, 2015).

"How the Transplant System Works." *United Network for Organ Sharing.* http://www.unos.org/donation/index.php?topic=fact_sheet_1 (accessed January 25, 2015).

Li Hui, and Ben Blanchard. "China to End Use of Prisoners' Organs for Transplants in Mid-2014." *Reuters,* November 2, 2013. http://www.reuters.com/article/2013/11/02/us-china-organs-id USBRE9A011N20131102 (accessed January 25, 2015).

Mayo Clinic Staff. "Organ Donation: Don't Let These Myths Confuse You." *Mayo Clinic.* http://www.mayoclinic.org/healthy-living/consumer-health/in-depth/organ-donation/art-20047529 - 40k (accessed January 25, 2015).

Organ Procurement and Transplantation Network (U.S.) http://optn.transplant.hrsa.gov/ (accessed April 8, 2015).

"Organ Trafficking and Transplantation Pose New Challenges." *World Health Organization (WHO),* September 1, 2004. http://www.who.int/bulletin/volumes/82/9/feature0904/en/ (accessed January 25, 2015).

"Organ Transplantation." *Virtual Mentor* 14, no. 3 (March 2012): 181–295. Available online at http://virtualmentor.ama-assn.org/2012/03/toc-1203.html (accessed January 25, 2015).

"Religious Views on Donation." *Organdonor.gov.* http://www.organdonor.gov/about/religious-views.html (accessed January 25, 2015).

"Timeline of Historical Events Significant Milestones in Organ Donation and Transplantation." *Organdonor.gov.* http://www.organdonor.gov/legislation/timeline.html (accessed January 25, 2015).

Williams, Heidi. "Allocating a Future: Ethics and Organ Transplantation." *Santa Clara University.* http://www.scu.edu/ethics/publications/submitted/allocating_organs.html (accessed January 25, 2015).

Virginia Herbert McDougall

Pan American Health Organization (PAHO)

🌐 Introduction

The Pan American Health Organization (PAHO) is the world's oldest functioning international health agency. Originated in 1902 as the International Sanitary Bureau, dominated by the U.S. Public Health Service, and concerned mainly with quarantine regulations, it has evolved into an important international body. Since an agreement concluded in 1949 under the auspices of the United Nations (UN), PAHO functions as the Regional Office of the World Health Organization (WHO) for the Americas, or AMRO. Following an agreement in 1950 with the Organization of American States (OAS), it is also a specialized agency within the Inter-American system.

PAHO's numerous health, sanitary, environmental, nutritional, and social development programs express its commitment to equitable access to public health and health services as well as equity in the social determinants of health. The mission of the organization, as stated in its constitution, is "to promote and coordinate efforts of the countries of the Western Hemisphere to combat disease, lengthen life, and promote the physical and mental health of the people."

PAHO is a multilateral intergovernmental organization integrating all the countries of the Western Hemisphere as member states, as well as territories under the jurisdiction of the United Kingdom, the Netherlands, and France as participating states. It also includes Spain and Portugal as observer states and Puerto Rico, Aruba, Curaçao, and Saint Martin as associated members.

🌐 Historical Background

The organization's directing bodies, as established in 1947, are the Pan American Sanitary Conference, which meets every five years and is its supreme authority, in which all member and participating states are represented by high-level government officials and elect the director; the Directing Council, which meets annually in the years between the meetings of the Conference; and the Executive Committee of the Directing Council, which meets twice a year. The Directing Council and the Conference also serve as the Regional Committee of WHO for the Americas.

PAHO's secretariat, called Pan American Sanitary Bureau (PASB), is responsible for formulating plans, policies, programs, and budget proposals for consideration by the governing bodies and for the implementation of their decisions as well. The PASB has field offices in every country of Latin America and the Caribbean. Approximately 2,000 health professionals, specialists, and administrative personnel are serving in the PASB, 30 percent at the headquarters and 70 percent in the field offices.

The PASB's Technical Cooperation Programs are organized into seven main areas: communicable diseases and epidemics, noncommunicable diseases and risk factors, sustainable development and health equity, family health and cultural diversity, health systems and services, regional observatory on public health and health situation analysis, and knowledge management and Virtual Health Library. PAHO's activities, as well as its name, have evolved during its history.

Origins and Evolution

In 1901, the second conference of the International Union of the American Republics, precursor of OAS, met in Mexico City, where it proposed to convene representatives of the different republics with the goal of creating agreements and regulations on health, to be followed periodically by further conferences. The First General International Sanitary Convention of the American Republics was held on December 2, 1902, in Washington, D.C. It established the International Sanitary Bureau, which would be renamed the Pan American Sanitary Bureau in 1923 and would finally become Pan American Health Organization in 1958.

During the period before World War I (1914–1918), additional International Sanitary Conventions met in Washington, D.C., including in 1905; in Mexico City, Mexico, in 1907; in San José, Costa Rica, in 1910; and in Santiago, Chile, in 1911. Both of the PASB's successive two directors, Walter Wyman and Rupert Blue, were surgeons general of the U.S. Public Health Service.

The main achievements in the first 10 years were the substantial reforms of the quarantine systems in conformity with new discoveries about the transmission of yellow fever, cholera, and bubonic plague, and the implementation of maritime public health measures, particularly strict sanitation of ports and vessels. An important turning point was the confirmation in 1901 by U.S. Army physician Walter Reed of the hypothesis that had been advanced in 1881 by Cuban physician Carlos J. Finlay, which identified the mosquito *Aedes aegypti* as the single agent in the transmission of yellow fever. Further impetus was provided by the successful U.S. campaign against the disease during the construction of the Panama Canal.

The launching of systematic international sanitary information in the hemisphere was another accomplishment. The third convention called on the member countries to establish sanitary information committees under direct supervision by the PASB to collect and transmit data on public health on their territories.

In 1910, the change of the term from sanitary convention to conference marked a shift in the agenda. After that date, the gatherings were no longer concerned solely or even primarily with quarantine issues but began to consider the promotion of health as a whole, including such matters as smallpox vaccination, campaigns against malaria and tuberculosis, national health legislation, scientific study of tropical diseases, and food and water safety. For several years, however, international efforts in public health languished due to the World War I.

Consolidating Pan American Identity

The sixth sanitary conference, which was convened in 1920, elected another U.S. surgeon general, Hugh S. Cumming, as the director of the PASB. During his 27 years of service, marked by intense activity, important developments shaped its role as well as that of national sanitary authorities. The PASB's crucial role in the exchange and dissemination of information is highlighted by the publication since 1922 of the journal known today as *Pan American Journal of Public Health*, which is published in English and in Spanish.

Another milestone was the adoption in 1924 of the Pan American Sanitary Code, a legally binding international instrument. Ratified by all states in the Americas, it has provided the basis for the continuous development of the PASB as an international institution. The code specified the PASB's functions, and has remained in effect ever

since. It aims to prevent the spread of communicable diseases beyond national boundaries, promote international cooperation in health protection, standardize statistics on morbidity and mortality, facilitate exchange of health information, and streamline measures for the protection against diseases.

The PASB's first field offices were established in Guatemala and in El Paso, Texas, and extensive programs to combat infectious diseases were launched in South America under the leadership of U.S. physician Fred Soper, director of the International Health Division of the Rockefeller Foundation. They continued during World War II (1939–1945), following the 11th Pan American Sanitary Conference in 1942, which urged close collaboration between the civil and military health services.

After the UN founding conference in San Francisco in 1945, Brazil and China recommended convening a special conference that would establish an international health organization. At the conference, which met the following year, the United States advocated the principle of dual allegiance, meaning that PASB should not only promote regional health programs in conjunction with the general policies of the international body, but would also serve as its regional committee in the Western Hemisphere.

In January 1947, delegates from 21 states of the Western Hemisphere met in Caracas, Venezuela, to consider the implications. Although all of them had been among the 61 signatories of the WHO founding constitution, they were unwilling to integrate PASB into the organization if this meant absorption, much less to abandon it. They decided to consolidate its separate identity by creating its governing bodies, as they exist today, including the transformation of PASB into the secretariat of what would become PAHO (initially called PASO, for Pan American Sanitary Organization).

In 1947 the organization adopted its constitution, which with minor adaptations remains in effect. Its agreement with WHO, approved by the First World Health Assembly in 1948 and signed the year after, specified the relationship between the two organizations. The PASB started serving as the regional office of WHO while maintaining its own Pan American identity, while the Directing Council also started functioning as the regional committee of WHO, a dual arrangement which has continued until today. In 1950, an agreement was also signed with the OAS that would make PAHO a specialized autonomous agency within the Inter-American system.

Eradication and Elimination of Diseases

For a decade the organization, under the directorship of Soper, continued to focus on the eradication of diseases. It supported a highly successful campaign in Haiti against the tropical disease yaws with the use of penicillin

Pan American Health Organization (PAHO)

Vector-Borne Diseases in the PAHO Countries

	Chagas	Chikungunya	Dengue	Leishmaniasis	Lymphatic Filariasis	Malaria	Onchocerciasis	Plague	Schistosomiasis	Yellow Fever
Anguilla		X	X							
Antigua and Barbuda		X	X							
Argentina	X		X	X		X				X
Aruba		X	X							
Bahamas		X	X							
Barbados		X	X							
Belize	X	X	X			X				
Bermuda			X							
Bolivia	X		X	X		X		X		X
Bonaire		X	X							
British Virgin Islands		X	X							
Brazil	X	X	X	X	X	X	X	X	X	X
Cayman Islands		X	X							
Chile	X									
Colombia	X	X	X	X		X				X
Costa Rica	X	X	X	X		X				
Cuba			X							
Curaçao		X	X							
Dominica		X	X							
Dominican Republic		X	X	X	X	X				
Ecuador	X		X	X		X	X	X		X
El Salvador	X	X	X	X		X				
French Guiana	X	X	X	X		X				X
Grenada		X	X							
Guadeloupe		X	X							
Guatemala	X	X	X	X		X	X			
Guyana	X	X	X	X	X	X				X
Haiti		X	X		X	X				
Honduras	X	X	X	X		X				
Jamaica		X	X							
Martinique		X	X							
Mexico	X	X	X	X		X	X			
Montserrat			X							
Nicaragua	X	X	X	X		X				
Panama	X	X	X	X		X				
Paraguay	X		X	X		X				X
Peru	X		X	X		X		X		X
Puerto Rico		X	X							
Saint Barthelemy		X	X							
Saint Kitts and Nevis		X	X							
Saint Lucia		X	X						X	
Saint Martin		X	X							
Saint Vincent and the Grenadines		X	X							
Suriname	X	X	X			X			X	X
Trinidad and Tobago		X	X							X
Turks and Caico Islands		X	X							
United States of America		X	X					X		
United States Virgin Islands		X	X							
Uruguay	X									
Venezuela	X	X	X	X		X	X		X	X

SOURCE: Adapted from "Presence of vector-borne diseases ordered by frequency and prevalence," Pan American Health Organization. Data from PAHO-CHA-CD Annual country reports to PAHO. Country or Territory reporting VT in the Americas between 2000–2013, PAHO-CHA-IR Epidemic Alert and Response, and Water Borne Diseases (IR) Reports from Member States IHR NFPs, and/or through Member States websites 2000–2014.

The countries covered in the PAHO region have contended with a variety of infectious, vector-borne diseases in the years since it was founded. Though strides have been made against many such diseases with eradication campaigns over the years, many such diseases still remain endemic in the region.

that became the model for the subsequent eradication campaigns throughout Latin America, most famously against malaria. This ambitious effort, which involved the spraying of dwellings with DDT and treatment of patients with new drugs, was carried out nationally in five- to eight-year intervals. Academic centers, funded by the Rockefeller Foundation in Brazil, Mexico, and Venezuela, besides the United States, developed research and training programs to build the necessary capacity. A smallpox eradication initiative was approved in 1950, but the massive vaccination campaigns did not start until the early 1960s. The Pan American Sanitary Code helped enforcement by providing for mandatory reporting of cases and strict surveillance.

The first Latin American director of the organization, Abraham Horwitz of Chile, who was elected in 1958, not only presided over its final change of name into PAHO but also ensured continuity of the eradication programs. Most important, the eradication of malaria was moving forward on the recognition than no vertical program could work without the integration and strengthening of health services. This was the time PAHO changed directions by focusing on health services and the development of human resources.

From 1958 to 1961, with support from the W.K. Kellogg and Rockefeller Foundations, PAHO awarded 2,098 scholarships. In 1967, to increase access to scientific journals, it created the Regional Library of Medicine and Health Sciences (known by its Spanish acronym BIREME), which then developed a Pan American network of biomedical and health information based in São Paulo, Brazil, incorporating data banks from the U.S. National Library of Medicine. By early 1966, PAHO mobilized resources for building health services infrastructure and, with support from loans by the recently created Inter-American Development Bank, developed projects for environmental sanitation, hospital construction, and the improvement of schools of medicine and public health.

By the early 1970s, PAHO aimed to support the health of women of childbearing age and children—a group that made up two-thirds of the region's population. PAHO expanded immunization programs and prenatal and perinatal services. PAHO educated mothers on the benefits of breast-feeding and securing safe water. The correlation of malnutrition with child mortality and mental retardation was the foundation for the Ten-Year Health Plan to combat malnutrition in the hopes of minimizing its effects and eliminating it in its severe form. In a landmark accomplishment in 1971, the Western Hemisphere became the first region in the world to eradicate smallpox.

⊕ Impacts and Issues

PAHO adopted as a goal the slogan "Health for All" after the 1978 International Conference on Primary Health Care in Alma-Ata (now Almaty, Kazakhstan) in 1978. Cosponsored by WHO, the organization issued a declaration urging priority be given to primary health care—a call endorsed by 134 governments and 67 international organizations, as well as by the World Health Assembly in 1979. In adopting the principles of primary health care, PAHO engaged the countries of its region to discuss a strategy creating and technically supporting local health systems (SILOS in Spanish). The ensuing strategy called for decentralization of the health services and their increased coverage in underserved urban and rural areas. While primary health team workers were trained throughout the region, community participation was a key element in ensuring their local support.

During late 1970s, maternal and child health programs were becoming central in the expansion of services at the local level. Of all PAHO programs inspired by the primary health-care strategy, immunization was arguably the most successful. Despite raging civil wars in several parts of the region, by the end of the 1980 the majority of the countries had vaccinated more than 50 percent of all children. In Central America, thanks to PAHO's Health: A Bridge for Peace program, the coverage was above 70 percent despite the armed conflict.

In 1991, the last case of polio in Peru marked its eradication in the Americas, and in 1994 the disease was certified as eliminated. Again, the Western Hemisphere was the first region to make the accomplishment.

Equity in Health

In the 1980s, Latin America experienced the worst economic crisis since the Great Depression. When neoliberal economics brought about cuts in public spending, poverty and inequalities increased, casting doubt on the relevance of development to the solution of health problems and lending support to social medicine, with its emphasis on social and economic determinants. Reforms weakened regulatory powers of the governments, with severe effects on public health programs. Emblematic of the deterioration of living conditions was the return of cholera to Peru, from where it spread rapidly across the continent.

PAHO responded by sponsoring a series of studies on the relationship between health and economic growth and between inequity in health and the gap dividing the rich and the poor. PAHO generated data on inequities within countries among social, ethnic, and gender groups, which were made available on a web-based clearing house on health equity—today's Regional Observatory of Human Resources in Health. The studies led to major investment in health, sustained by a dialogue that had been established with financial institutions as the Common Agenda of the Inter-American Development Bank, the World Bank, and PAHO. During the last decade of the 20th century, PAHO also launched several programs addressing gender inequities that have since been integrated under the rubric of Gender Equality, Cultural Diversity, and Human Rights.

PAHO as a Guardian and Guarantor of International Health

PAHO can take credit for achieving many targets of the Millennium Development Goals (MDGs), eight goals set in 2000 targeted to be achieved by the UN by 2015. In a major accomplishment, the region achieved a 51 percent decrease in infant mortality, the lowest in the developing world. This was made possibly largely because of a substantial increase of access to drinking water and thanks to PAHO's leadership in the elimination of vaccine-preventable diseases, which resulted in more than 93 percent vaccination coverage for children below five years of age. The last endemic case of measles in the region was reported in 2002, and the last endemic case of rubella in 2009.

The incidence of malaria declined by 20 percent between 2000 and 2006, while mortality from the disease decreased by 70 percent. The incidence of tuberculosis has been declining steadily since the 1990s, at the rate of up to 4 percent a year. Important progress has been made in containing and reversing the human immunodeficiency virus (HIV) epidemic, indicating a substantial reduction of new cases. Several Latin American countries, particularly Argentina, Brazil, Chile, and Costa Rica, had significantly lower mortality rates after the introduction of antiretroviral therapy. Mother-to-child HIV transmission has declined rapidly thanks to the early diagnosis and treatment of pregnant women.

However, the average health conditions at regional and national levels conceal a motley assortment of gender, ethnic, and social inequities, both within and among countries. Regrettably, the region has continued to suffer from the highest degree of unjust inequalities in the world, a condition inevitably reflected in the state of health. The health sector and available services have not been sufficient to cope with their complexity. In the increasingly interconnected and globalized world, international action on health is indispensable not only to facilitate trade and development but also to ensure human and national security.

In this respect, PAHO is particularly well placed to perform effectively in its region. It is able to exercise leadership in facilitating dialogue between governments and other actors and stakeholders, both national and regional. It is poised to serve as a broker in forging partnerships linking governmental agencies, local authorities, the private sector, academia, and civil society. It can foster closer cooperation among countries with the formation of regional cooperation networks.

⊕ Future Implications

Poverty and inequity have been persistent problems in the Americas, as in several countries the gap between the rich and the poor has widened regardless of economic growth. In 2013, the poverty rate in Latin America was 28 percent. The number of poor has remained constant, but the number of people living in extreme poverty increased by 3 million during that year. The problem is rife as well in the United States, where the income gap

has been increasing, and the average rate of poverty in 2007–2009 was 13.4 percent, up from 12 percent in 2000.

While access to health care among higher income groups has been nearly universal in most countries of the region, the majority of the poor cannot get care when they need it. Evidence suggests that approximately 30 percent of the region's population cannot access health care for financial reasons, whereas 21 percent are deterred from seeking it because of geographic barriers. Moreover, health services in most countries remain highly fragmented, which translates into the lack of continuity in care that fails to fulfill the needs and expectations of the populations the services are supposed to serve.

Universal access to health care is one of the greatest challenges the region will continue to face in the years to come. PAHO's leadership is crucial in advancing this agenda by encouraging not only the enhancement of primary care services but also by formulating coherent policies to reduce poverty and inequality in health.

Into the New Century

PAHO's centenary in 2002 was an occasion for taking stock of what had been accomplished and what was to be done next. In response to the proclamation in 2000 of the UN MDGs, the organization took action by developing strategies on goals particularly related to health and by establishing a special unit to coordinate its activities with other MDG efforts in the region.

In the first decade of the 21st century, both international governmental assistance and public expenditure for health increased, creating new opportunities for forming alliances and partnerships to meet the MDG challenges. PAHO took the lead in launching with the UN, Inter-American agencies, national and local governments, nongovernmental organizations, and universities such initiatives as Safe Motherhood, Vaccination Week in the Americas, Partnership for Maternal, Newborn and Child Health, Elimination of Mother-to-Child Transmission of HIV initiative, and Pan American Alliance for Nutrition and Development.

At the same time, PAHO opened space for dialogue and collaboration with churches, civil society groups, and nongovernmental organizations. It invested in the new modes of collaboration, such as South-South Cooperation and horizontal partnerships in different fields of health. The onset of the new century gave impetus to forms of collaboration between and within nations, more adaptable to the region's new realities.

Sustaining and Advancing Past Accomplishments

It is as difficult to sustain goals, and advance beyond them when scientific and technological progress makes this possible, as it is to achieve them. Among the different goals of the regional health agenda, that of ensuring

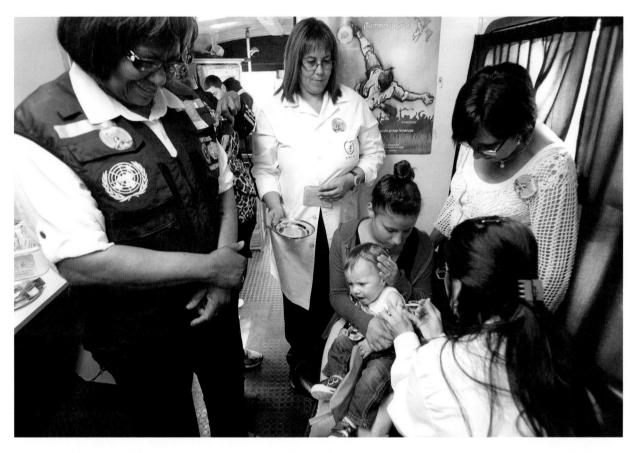

Pan American Health Organization (PAHO) Director Carissa Etienne (left) and Uruguayan Public Health Minister Susana Muñiz (right) participate in the launching of the Vaccination Week of the Americas in Montevideo, Uruguay, on April 26, 2014. Getting health plans to the entire population of Latin America and the Caribbean is the "great challenge" that faces the region, Etienne said.   © *epa european pressphoto agency b.v. / Alamy*

elimination of vaccine-preventable diseases by introducing new vaccines stands out.

Women's and maternal health will require increased efforts to reduce maternal mortality, which despite its decrease remains high in parts or all of some PAHO countries. Another necessary advance is the reduction of mother-to-child HIV transmission by at least 1 percent and the containment of the HIV/AIDS epidemic. The challenges include region-wide commitment to universal access to the diagnosis and treatment of HIV, as well programs for its prevention. Further goals include the elimination of malaria and sustained reduction of tuberculosis.

The protection of the health of students follows the WHO initiative of a health-promoting schools network and includes services for adolescents, emphasizing sexual and reproductive health as part of healthy growth. Further response by PAHO in support of community-based primary services on mental health, prevention of domestic violence, and the use of illicit drugs will be necessary.

Responding to New Challenges

The epidemic of noncommunicable diseases, such as cardiovascular and chronic respiratory diseases, cancer, and diabetes, was responsible for an estimated 5 million deaths in the Americas in 2012.

Since the policies of combating noncommunicable diseases vary in complexity, as also do the risk factors—tobacco, physical inactivity, unhealthful food consumption, and obesity, among others—they require joint action by public sectors and the private sectors linked with industry, commerce, social media. Programs promoting physical activities and the creation of secure public spaces in the cities also demand close cooperation with municipalities and local governments. Increasingly, not only national but also regional and global health security have become matters of collective responsibility.

Global Health Security Such processes of globalization as increased travel and trade, as well as climate change, have been altering the pattern and speed of the transmission of diseases prone to creating epidemics. In April 2009, the variant of influenza A (H1N1) emerged in Mexico as the century's first global pandemic. The outbreak spread worldwide, resulting in over 600,000 diagnosed cases and over 18,000 deaths. Its concentration was in the Americas where the disease was responsible for 8,500 deaths out of the approximate 190,000 cases

Global Homicide Rates per 100,000, by Country, in 2012 (Or Latest Data Available)

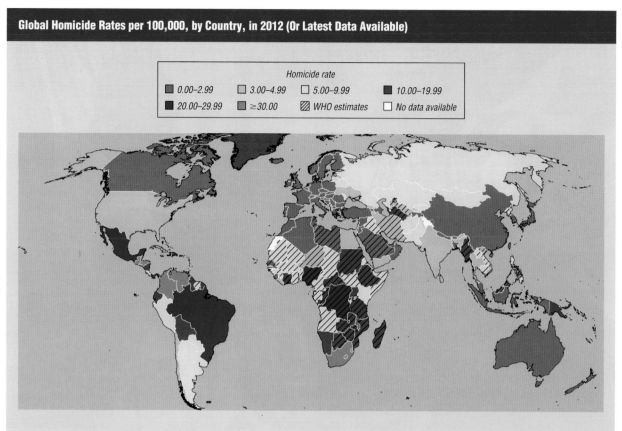

Homicide rate

■ 0.00–2.99   □ 3.00–4.99   □ 5.00–9.99   ■ 10.00–19.99
■ 20.00–29.99   ■ ≥30.00   ▨ WHO estimates   □ No data available

SOURCE: Adapted from "Map 1.1: Homicide rates, by country or territory (2012 or latest year)," in *Global Study on Homicide 2013*, United Nations Office on Drugs and Crime, 2014, p. 23, http://www.unodc.org/documents/gsh/pdfs/2014_GLOBAL_HOMICIDE_BOOK_web.pdf (accessed January 14, 2015). Data from UNODC Homicide Statistics, 2013.

diagnosed. To meet the demand in such emergencies, it is necessary to strengthen information management and improve the development of institutional capacity while using a multi-sectoral approach.

Violence and Homicides Urban violence, which affects mostly male young adults, has been the leading cause of mortality and disability in the group of 15- to 44-year-olds and a major challenge to human security in the region, which has the highest rates of homicides in the world. In the graphic, global homicide rates are shown worldwide, with PAHO countries including Chile, Colombia, El Salvador, Guatemala, Honduras, Venezuela, and Mexico, and Brazil showing rates over 20 per 100,000 citizens.

No less tragic has been the high incidence of violence against women and children, with severe consequences for their mental health and well-being. Thanks to the ubiquity of advocacy groups and substantial social pressure in the region, however, these problems are better identified there than elsewhere in the developing world, although they are still far from a solution.

Environmental Risks Extreme weather situations, such as drought, inundation from heavy rain, hurricanes, and other natural disasters attributable to climate change

have started to make a severe impact. The impact has been not only on food production but is also evident in epidemic outbreaks of diseases that used to be relatively under control in the region, such as cholera, dengue, and yellow fever. Additionally, the contamination of soil, water, and air has created more and more problems for human and health security.

Scientific and technological advances bear promise that these problems can be overcome. They include new forms of dialogue and participation, which have opened thanks to information and communication technology, facilitating transparency and accountability. Access to health information by the people is bound to benefit health throughout the hemisphere. In bringing the promise to fulfillment, PAHO will remain indispensable.

SEE ALSO *Child Health; Climate Change: Health Impacts; Conflict, Violence, and Terrorism: Health Impacts; Drug/Substance Abuse; Epidemiology: Surveillance for Emerging Infectious Diseases; Food Security and Hunger; Global Health Initiatives; Health as a Human Right and Health-Care Access; Health in the WHO Americas Region; Health-Related Education and Information Access; HIV/AIDS;*

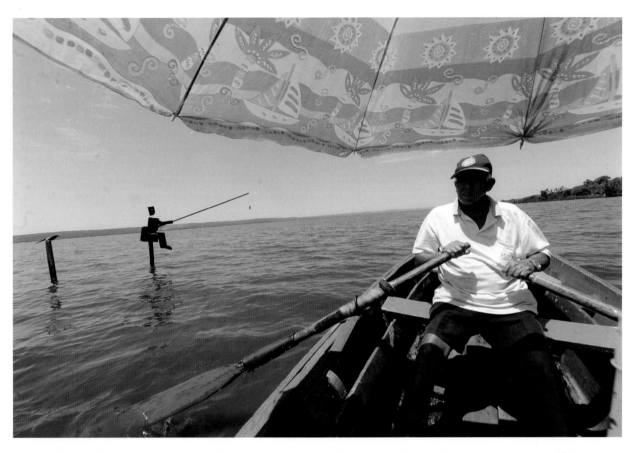

A man paddles on his boat across the Ypacaraí Lake, declared not suitable for bathing, in Ypacaraí, Paraguay. Paraguay's Health Minister Antonio Corbo said that water samples from the lake in 2012 and analyzed in São Paulo, Brazil, with the backing of the Pan American Health Organization determined that the bacteria found in the lake's waterweeds present a high level of neurologic and liver toxicity. © *Norberto Duarte/AFP/Getty Images.*

Influenza; Insect-Borne Diseases; International Health Regulations, Surveillance, and Enforcement; Malnutrition; Maternal and Infant Health; Neglected Tropical Diseases; NGOs and Health Care: Deliverance or Dependence; Noncommunicable Diseases (Lifestyle Diseases); Pandemic Preparedness; Water Supplies and Access to Clean Water; World Health Organization: Organization, Funding, and EnforcementPowers

BIBLIOGRAPHY

Books

Cueto, Marcos. *The Value of Health: A History of the Pan American Health Organization,* Scientific and Technical Publication No. 600. Washington, DC: Pan American Health Organization, 2006.

Evans, Timothy, et al., eds. *Challenging Inequities in Health: From Ethics to Action.* New York: Oxford University Press, 2001.

Howard-Jones, Norman. *The Pan American Health Organization: Origins and Evolution.* Geneva: World Health Organization, 1981.

Howard-Jones, Norman. *The Scientific Background of the International Sanitary Conferences (1851–1938).* Geneva: World Health Organization, 1975.

Oldstone, Michael B. A. *Viruses, Plagues, and History: Past, Present, and Future,* rev. ed. New York: Oxford University Press, 2010.

Pan American Health Organization. *Basic Documents of the Pan American Health Organization,* Official Document No. 341, 18th ed. Washington, DC: Pan American Health Organization, 2012.

Pan American Health Organization. *Health in the Americas,* 12th ed. Washington, DC: Pan American Health Organization, 2012.

Periodicals

Alleyne, G.A.O. "The Challenge and Prize for International Health Organizations in the Americas." *Salud Pública de México* 39, no. 5 (September–October 1997): 480–485.

Bustamante, M. "Los primeros cincuenta años de la Oficina Sanitaria Panamericana." *Boletín de la Oficina Sanitaria Panamericana* 33, no. 6 (1952). (Reprinted).

Campbell, N. R. C., D. T. Lackland, and M. L. Niebylski. "2014 Dietary Salt Fact Sheet of the World Hypertension League, International Society of Hypertension, Pan American Health Organization Technical Advisory Group on Cardiovascular Disease Prevention through Dietary Salt Reduction, the World Health Organizaton Collaborating Centre on Population Salt Reduction, and World Action on Salt and Health." *Journal of Clinical Hypertension* 17, no. 1 (2015): 7–9.

Cueto, Marcos. "International Health, the Early Cold War and Latin America." *Bulletin of Medical History* 25, no. 1 (2008): 17–41.

Cueto, Marcos. "The Origins of Primary Health Care and Selective Primary Health Care." *American Journal of Public Health* 94, no. 11 (2004): 1864–1874.

Etienne, Carissa F. "Countries Pledge Action to Reduce Child Obesity in the Americas." *The Lancet* 384 (December 6, 2014): 2021.

Jamison, Dean T., et al. "International Collective Action in Health: Objectives, Functions, and Rationale." *The Lancet* 351, no. 9101 (1998): 514–517.

Stern, Minna A. "The Public Health Service in the Panama Canal: A Forgotten Chapter of U.S. Public Health." *Public Health Reports* 120, no. 6 (2005): 675–679.

"Un siglo de la Salud Pública en las Américas." *Perspectives in Health Magazine* 7, no. 1 (2002): 11–19.

Websites

"Celebrating 110 Years of Health." *Pan American Health Organization (PAHO).* http://issuu.com/paho2012/docs/paho110_album3_screen/1?e=6477936/5775595 (accessed March 5, 2015).

"Declaration of Alma-Ata International Conference on Primary Health Care, Alma-Ata, USSR, 6–12 September 1978." *World Health Organization (WHO).* http://www.who.int/publications/almaata_declaration_en.pdf?ua=1 (accessed March 5, 2015).

"The Great Fever." *American Experience (PBS).* http://www.pbs.org/wgbh/amex/fever/index.html (accessed March 5, 2015).

"PAHO Director's Gallery 1902–2013." *Pan American Health Organization (PAHO).* http://www.paho.org/director/?page_id=166 (accessed March 5, 2015).

Rebecca De Los Rios

Pan-American Interoceanic Highway or Transoceanic Highway: Health Impacts

🌐 Introduction

The Pan-American Interoceanic Highway, or Transoceanic Highway, is a transcontinental road in South America that connects the Atlantic and Pacific Oceans. The highway cuts through desert, mountains, dense jungle, and other terrain, bisecting the countries of Peru and Brazil. The route stretches 3,358 miles (5,404 kilometers) from the Peruvian port of San Juan de Marcona on the Pacific Ocean to the Brazilian port of Santos on the Atlantic Ocean.

Completed in 2011, the international construction effort has paved the way for further economic development in South America and increased trade with countries around the world. Of particular importance, the highway opens a trade route for Brazilian exports to Asia through Peruvian ports on the Pacific. The highway is a shipping alternative to circumnavigating the continent or traveling through the Panama Canal.

The Pan-American Interoceanic Highway project is part of the larger Initiative for the Integration of Regional Infrastructure in South America (IIRSA) that hopes to thread the continent with transportation and communication infrastructure. IIRSA has planned more than 500 development projects and several transportation corridors that will bisect the continent.

An international development project of the scope of the Pan-American Interoceanic Highway is bound to bring consequences, some adverse. There exist both positive and negative health impacts of an infrastructure project on such a massive scale. Positive health impacts include penetration of health-care access into remote regions of South America. This ostensibly includes better caregiving, more medicine, and the construction of new clinics. Adverse health impacts associated with the Pan-American Interoceanic Highway include prostitution and violence, environmental degradation and pollution, drug use and trafficking, and road accidents.

🌐 Historical Background

The Incas were responsible for pioneering the first major transportation network on the South American continent. They built more than 25,000 miles (40,000 kilometers) of roads, mostly in the north–south direction. The Incan roads ran along the backbone of the Andes Mountains through what today are the countries of Ecuador, Peru, Chile, and Argentina. Traveling perpendicular to the Andes has always been a challenge. The near impenetrability of the Andes Mountain range and Amazon rain forest made intercontinental travel and trade both dangerous and slow for centuries.

The dream of a networked system for trade in South America was revived with the early European colonists. Realizing the commercial importance of a continental transportation system, European merchants and government officials set out to map the continent's geography and river systems. This led to the charting of the Amazon, Orinoco, Paraguay, and Paraná Rivers, among others. One of these European visionaries was the Prussian explorer Alexander von Humboldt (1769–1859), who explored the South American continent from 1799 to 1804. Humboldt, after whom the Humboldt Current in the Pacific Ocean is named, imagined a system of Pan American canals to facilitate trade.

In 1925, the Pan American Congress of Highways convened delegates from 19 countries in Buenos Aires, Argentina, to "survey and select possible routes for a system of paved highways in Latin America," writes Howard Erlichman in his book *Camino del Norte*. Following the summit, U.S. Secretary of State Frank Kellogg (1856–1937) outlined the reasons for opening a system of highways in South America in his report to U.S. President Calvin Coolidge (1872–1933), stating: "This undeveloped hinterland is the storehouse of incalculable resources in raw materials, the exploitation of which would bring wealth to the individuals and nations owning them, labor for the unemployed and new impetus to foreign trade."

ENVIRONMENTAL DEGRADATION AND POLLUTION

The environmental impacts of the Pan-American Interoceanic Highway are myriad: the loss of biodiversity, loss of plant and animal habitat, loss of forest cover, and disruption of riverine systems and hydrological basins, among others. Critics say the environmental impact assessments of the highway were insufficient and irresponsibly expedited. "One weak point of the construction of this highway consists of the lack of environmental studies that to date have not identified specific situations of risk to the environment that could result from the construction of the highway," says a study from Peru's National Institute of Civil Defense.

The agricultural and extractive industries already have taken advantage of the Pan-American Interoceanic Highway. The road has paved the way for the clearing of forest to plant crops such as soybean, corn, and wheat, and to raise livestock. Though tied to the economic development of the South American interior, the agricultural industry has had a profound effect on the environment surrounding the Pan-American Interoceanic Highway. Likewise, extractive industries such as gold mining and logging, much of which is illegal and unregulated, have affected the environment to a great extent. There exist public health risks associated with the informal settlements that have cropped up around these agricultural and extractive industries.

The construction of the Pan-American Interoceanic Highway has exacerbated deforestation due to extractive industry activity. The areas along the highway in the Madre de Dios region of Peru, which is rife with gold mining, experienced a deforestation rate of 4,732 acres (1,915 hectares) per year between 2006 and 2009, up from 722 acres (292 hectares) per year between 2003 and 2006. In his book *The Impact of the IIRSA Road Infrastructure Programme on Amazonia*, Pitou van Dijck writes, "The sixfold increase [in deforestation] was due to the inflow of miners that was facilitated by improved access to this remote and sparsely populated region over secondary roads radiating from the Interoceanic Corridor."

Vehicle pollution and runoff are harmful to the environment and human health. "Automobile and truck use contributes to water pollution in several ways beside runoff from roadways and parking lots," write Howard Frumkin and colleagues in the book *Urban Sprawl and Public Health*. Nitrogen and petroleum compounds from vehicles can contaminate ground water and some compounds are carcinogens. The Pan-American Interoceanic Highway is associated with vehicle pollution and runoff harmful to human health.

The extractive industries have leached substances into the environment that are harmful to human health. In addition to the formal mining industry in Peru, around 60 illegal mines operate in Madre de Dios region. One serious problem, especially with illegal small-scale mining operations, is contamination with the mercury used to extract gold. Some estimates put the amount of mercury released yearly in Peru at 33 to 44 tons (30 to 40 metric tons), according to a 2014 article in *Forbes*.

The mineral wealth of the Amazon basin has been estimated at US$3 trillion worth of gold, tin, copper, uranium, iron ore, rare earth metals, bauxite, and others. The extraction of these minerals and metals no doubt will be expedited by the construction of the Pan-American Interoceanic Highway. Though this will mean an economical boon for Amazonian countries such as Peru and Brazil, at least in the short term, scientists have not assessed adequately the environmental degradation and effect on human health due to pollution.

One major consequence of these agricultural, extractive, transportation, and informal settlement activities will be the impact on water in the Amazon. "Clean water is fundamental to the maintenance of the Amazon's unique aquatic ecosystems and to the health of its people, who rely on surface water to satisfy their household water needs and to provide fish and other aquatic plants and organisms for their nutritional needs," writes Michael McClain of Florida International University in his book *The Biogeochemistry of the Amazon Basin*.

By 1963, most of the Pan-American Interoceanic Highway, which runs 30,000 miles (48,000 kilometers) from Alaska to Tierra del Fuego, was complete save for one major interruption at the border of Panama and Colombia. As of 2013, a highway bridging the so-called Darién Gap had not been connected due to pushback from local governments and environmentalists. Today, the Pan-American Interoceanic Highway runs roughly north–south and parallel to the Rocky and Andes Mountains. This leaves vast expanses of Latin America still lacking paved access to urban hubs and trade networks.

In the 1970s, Brazilian President General Emílio Garrastazu Médici (1905–1985) promised to open up the country's interior to development. Seeing the effects of a severe drought in Brazil's remote Northeast, Médici announced the ambitious National Integration Plan (PIN). Brazil received financial help from the U.S. Agency for International Development (USAID). The Trans-Amazon Highway was cut through the hinterlands between Brazil's Atlantic coast and the Peruvian border. This 3,082-mile (4,960-kilometer) segment would later form part of the Pan-American Interoceanic Highway. By 1984, Brazil had finished paving a road connecting its capital São Paulo to the state of Rondônia on the border with Bolivia and Peru.

In 2000, 12 South American countries made it a priority to complete the Pan-American Interoceanic Highway at a cost that was estimated at US$2.6 billion. Four years later, Peruvian President Alejandro Toledo (1946–) and Brazil's President Luiz Inácio Lula da Silva (1945–) agreed to complete the remaining 711 miles (1,144 kilometers) of highway needed to connect the two countries. The Peruvian segment of the Pan-American Interoceanic Highway cost approximately US$2.8 billion to complete, according to the investigative journalism outfit Connectas. Brazil, the region's economic powerhouse, agreed to finance much of the construction

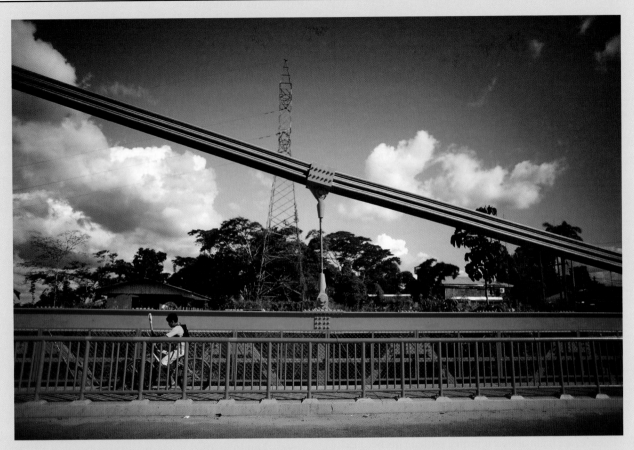

A man crosses a recently built bridge on the Pan-American Interoceanic Highway, in the capital of the Madre de Dios region, a boom-town located at the confluence of two rivers, on November 13, 2013, in Puerto Maldonado, Peru. The biologically diverse Madre de Dios (Mother of God) region has seen deforestation from gold mining in the area triple since 2008, when gold prices spiked during global economic turmoil. Small-scale miners are drawn to the area in hopes for higher pay but often face abysmal conditions. Gold is usually amalgamated with mercury during the process of informal mining in the region, which is discharged into the water supply and air, poisoning fish and sickening people in the area. Peru is the largest producer of gold in Latin America and the sixth largest in the world. Informal mining accounts for roughly 20 percent of the gold production in Peru. © *Mario Tama/Getty Images.*

on the Peruvian side. With the completion in 2011 of the Billinghurst Bridge in Peru, the Pan-American Interoceanic Highway was completed.

⊕ Impacts and Issues

The Pan-American Interoceanic Highway is hastening the development of the South American hinterland, which includes the construction of informal settlements. Informal settlements occur on the periphery of urban and semi-urban areas and along new transportation and trade routes such as highways. Informal settlements have grown along the trajectory of the Pan-American Interoceanic Highway. Previously isolated towns have seen their populations swell due to the influx of trade and people. New towns, many supporting extractive industries, have sprung up along the Pan-American Interoceanic Highway.

The Pan-American Interoceanic Highway's construction has led to the transformation of this frontier, the urban development of which is mostly informal in its planning. Due to their lack of governance and civic planning, informal settlements are associated with prostitution, violence, drug use and trafficking, limited access to health care, and poor sanitation.

The city of Puerto Maldonado in the Peruvian Amazon is a prime example of the development of the South American hinterland. With the completion of the Pan-American Interoceanic Highway came a major influx of colonists from Peru's highlands in search of jobs in logging, oil drilling, and gold mining, as well as informal economies to support these extractive industries. The result has been explosive population growth in Puerto Maldonado, from 25,000 in 1998 to more than 200,000 in 2014.

Puerto Maldonado is one of the largest cities along the Pan-American Interoceanic Highway. Yet it did not have a sewage treatment plant when the highway was finished. This poses a public health risk in addition to an environmental problem. Puerto Maldonado also had limited medical services. A report from the Peruvian National Institute of Civil Defense showed the city had 114 hospital beds for a population that exceeded 200,000. Dozens of other smaller cities along the Pan-American Interoceanic Highway similarly lack basic services such as sanitation and access to health care.

There are significant health impacts associated with the informal settlements along the Pan-American Interoceanic Highway. These health impacts are exacerbated by the informal nature of these settlements and the ineffective governance and security of these areas. Prostitution and human trafficking, particularly with children, have been a problem that coincides with economic development and expanding infrastructure. In Brazil, the 116 Highway that runs along the eastern coast from Fortaleza to São Paulo has earned itself the name "highway to hell" for the underage prostitution it has spurred. In his book *Highway to Hell: The Road Where Childhoods Are Stolen*, journalist Matt Roper writes about the "pain and turmoil for thousands of innocent young girls" on Brazilian Highway 116. The United Nations estimates the number of child prostitutes in Brazil to be in the hundreds of thousands. Studies on child prostitution on the Pan-American Interoceanic Highway are lacking.

Drug use and drug trafficking, and their associated violence, are hallmarks of informal settlements because of limited policing, border control, and governance. Drug trafficking has increased with the construction of highways connecting Brazil and Peru and neighbors such as Colombia and Bolivia. In 2013, Peru surpassed Colombia as Latin America's top coca and cocaine producer, with the capability to produce up to 340 tons of cocaine per year.

Brazil is the region's largest market for this cocaine, and lax border control has led to an uptick in drug trafficking. "I wouldn't be surprised if this road became one of main drug-trafficking routes in the next few years," said the Peruvian governor of Madre de Dios region in an interview with Dan Collyns and Tom Phillips published in 2011 in the *Guardian*, in the article "Pacific-Atlantic Route Drives Up Fears of Crime and Destruction."

Informal settlements lack many of the basic health-care services a city provides. Though the economic development of the South American hinterland has reduced child mortality rates and fertility, basic services such as sanitation, education, and access to health care are lacking in many remote regions and informal settlements around existing towns and cities. The lack of these services along the Pan-American Interoceanic Highway and its informal settlements will have a serious impact on the welfare of people living and working along the 3,357-mile (5,404-kilometer) stretch of highway. The health of

indigenous communities in the South American hinterland is also at risk from limited health-care services.

In recent years, Brazil has made a concerted effort to populate its remote cities with doctors and health-care services with varied success. Indeed, it offers universal health-care coverage that purports to cover every citizen in the vast country. One program dubbed More Doctors has recruited Cuban health professionals to work in Brazil's interior cities such as Manaus, due mostly to a lack of Brazilian doctors willing to work in these places. Health-care penetration into the Brazilian hinterland has been a challenge due to constrained resources and the distance from Brazil's coast, where most of the population lives.

In Peru, programs such as Basic Health aim to rehabilitate the health sector and provide access to the rural poor. Without increased investment in health-care services, however, access to medicine, doctors, and primary, diagnostic, and advanced care will remain limited along the Pan-American Interoceanic Highway. "Despite significant economic progress, infrastructure gaps and inequalities in education, health and access to basic amenities including water and sanitation still prevail," according to a 2013 report on Peru from the World Health Organization.

Infectious Diseases

Population growth in the hinterlands of Peru and Brazil likely will lead to more cases of tropical diseases such as dengue fever and malaria. Both mosquito-borne viral diseases—dengue and malaria—have been implicated in several hundreds of thousands of cases per year in the tropical regions of those countries. As the Pan-American Interoceanic Highway leads to the urbanization of the interior, there is greater opportunity for humans to come into contact with disease-carrying mosquitoes and other pathogens. Tuberculosis, leishmaniasis, leprosy, schistosomiasis, Chagas disease, yellow fever, and cholera also are found in the region.

Sexually transmitted diseases such as the human immunodeficiency virus (HIV) have become a concern along the Pan-American Interoceanic Highway due to the increase in prostitution, drug use, and other factors. Brazil is currently experiencing an HIV resurgence. With more than 650,000 estimated to be HIV-infected in 2012, Brazil has the highest number of adults living with HIV/AIDS in Latin America. Tuberculosis-HIV co-infections also have become a problem in Brazil. Access to medical services is essential in controlling these diseases. Providing these services along the entire stretch of the Pan-American Interoceanic Highway poses a challenge.

⊕ Future Implications

The Pan-American Interoceanic Highway is paving the way for the economic development of the South American hinterland. This infrastructure will have both positive and negative effects on the health of the people living in and moving to the communities that exist along the highway network. From a public health standpoint, the highway will bring benefits such as access to medicine and health care. Simultaneously, the highway will introduce and exacerbate adverse health effects such as prostitution and violence, environmental degradation and pollution, drug use and trafficking, and road accidents, among others.

Ensuring the delivery of health care to mitigate these adverse impacts along the Pan-American Interoceanic Highway will be of chief concern to the municipal, state, and federal governments of Peru and Brazil. The environmental impacts of the extractive industries, informal economies, and inputs of the highway facilitates will continue to be a cost to the development of the South American hinterland and the economic growth of countries such as Peru and Brazil.

Carlos Eduardo Huertas sums up the potential ramifications of the Pan-American Interoceanic Highway in the article "The Amazon Is Opening Up." He writes: "Projects of this magnitude are a good space for symbolic transformations on the continent. Not repeating the mistakes Latin America has made in the past is key to preventing inequality and deepening poverty. Doing things with the lowest possible budget means losing opportunities for real leaps in the development of the region and can render large interventions like the Interoceanic Highway a spearhead with pitiful social and environmental devastation."

SEE ALSO *Health in the WHO Americas Region; Pan American Health Organization (PAHO); Vulnerable Populations; Water Supplies and Access to Clean Water*

BIBLIOGRAPHY

Books

Erlichman, Howard J. *Camino del Norte: How a Series of Watering Holes, Fords, and Dirt Trails Evolved into Interstate 35 in Texas.* College Station: Texas A&M University Press, 2006.

Frumkin, Howard, Lawrence Frank, and Richard Jackson. *Urban Sprawl and Public Health: Designing, Planning, and Building for Healthy Communities.* Washington, DC: Island Press, 2004.

Meinig, Donald William. *The Shaping of America: A Geographical Perspective on 500 Years of History,* Vol. 2: *Continental America, 1800–1967.* New Haven, CT: Yale University Press, 1993.

McClain, Michael. "The Relevance of Biogeochemistry to Amazon Development and Conservation," in *The Biogeochemistry of the Amazon Basin.* Michael E. McClain, Reynaldo L. Victoria, and Jeffrey E. Richey, eds. New York: Oxford University Press, 2001.

Rice, Herbert Howard. *Pan American Congress of Highways, Buenos Aires, October 5–16, 1925: Report of the Delegates of the United States Designated by the President in Pursuance of a Joint Resolution of Congress Approved March 4, 1925.* Washington, DC: U.S. Government Printing Office, 1927.

Roper, Matt. *Highway to Hell: The Road Where Childhoods Are Stolen.* Oxford: Monarch Books, 2013.

Schroth, Götz, et al., eds. *Agroforestry and Biodiversity Conservation in Tropical Landscapes.* Washington, DC: Island Press, 2004.

Stoddard, Richard Henry. *The Life, Travels and Books of Alexander von Humboldt.* New York: Rudd & Carleton, 1859.

van Dijck, Pitou. *The Impact of the IIRSA Road Infrastructure Programme on Amazonia.* New York: Routledge, 2013.

Websites

Collyns, Dan, and Tom Phillips. "Pacific-Atlantic Route Drives Up Fears of Crime and Destruction" *Guardian,* July 14, 2011. http://www.theguardian.com/environment/2011/jul/14/pacific-atlantic-route-brazil-peru (accessed March 6, 2015).

"El largo recorrido de la Interoceánica suramericana." *Connectas.* http://www.connectas.org/amazonas/es/vias1.html (accessed September 28, 2014).

Huertas, Carlos Eduardo. "The Amazon Is Opening Up." *International Consortium of Investigative Journalists,* September 11, 2012. http://www.icij.org/blog/2012/09/jungle-highway (accessed May 31, 2015).

Initiative for the Integration of Regional Infrastructure in South America. http://www.iirsa.org/ (accessed September 28, 2014).

"Integrating Conservancy and Sustainable Development in Interoceanic Highway." *Inter-American Development Bank.* http://www.iadb.org/en/projects/project-description-title,1303.html?id=pe-m1056 (accessed September 28, 2014).

"La carretera Interoceánica: Un repaso de su histórica construcción." *La República,* September 12, 2012. http://www.larepublica.pe/12-09-2012/la-carretera-interoceanica-un-repaso-de-su-historica-construccion (accessed March 6, 2015).

Leahy, Joe. "Cuban Doctors Fill the Gap in Brazilian Interior." *Financial Times,* December 27, 2013. http://www.ft.com/cms/s/0/66a41bc4-6c91-11e3-ad36-00144feabdc0.html#axzz3TolXrWdA (accessed March 8, 2015).

Létourneau, Alex. "Illegal Mining Severely Impacting Peruvian Environment." *Forbes,* July 4, 2014. http://www.forbes.com/sites/kitconews/2014/07/04/illegal-mining-severely-impacting-peruvian-environment/ (accessed March 8, 2015).

Reel, Monte. "Traveling from Ocean to Ocean across South America." *New York Times*, February 19, 2014. http://www.nytimes.com/2014/02/23/magazine/south-america-road-trip.html?_r=0 (accessed March 8, 2015).

Smith, Jennie Erin. "A State of Nature: Life, Death, and Tourism in the Darién Gap." *New Yorker*, April 22, 2013. http://www.newyorker.com/magazine/2013/04/22/a-state-of-nature (accessed March 8, 2015).

"Success Factors in Women's and Children's Health: Mapping Pathways to Progress." *Parternership for Maternal, Newborn and Child Health, World Health Organisation*, November 2013. http://www.paho.org/nutricionydesarrollo/wp-content/uploads/2014/03/Success-Factors-in-Womens-and-childrens-Health.-Mapping-Pathways-to-Progress.pdf (accessed May 26, 2015).

Aleszu Bajak

Pandemic Preparedness

⊕ Introduction

Pandemic preparedness enables countries to recognize and manage a pandemic (when an infectious disease becomes prevalent over an entire region or the world) through the use of established plans, preparations, and protocols. According to the "Checklist for Influenza Pandemic Preparedness Planning," prepared by the World Health Organization (WHO) in 2005, the goals of pandemic preparedness are to "help reduce transmission of the pandemic virus strain; to decrease the number of cases, hospitalizations, and deaths; to maintain essential services; and to reduce the economic and social impact of a pandemic."

Pandemics are unpredictable but recurring events that cause severe social, economic, and political stress. To mitigate the severity of that stress, advanced planning and preparedness are crucial. In the 21st century, this concept primarily has concerned existing and potential global outbreaks of the deadly influenza A strain, such as H1N1 (swine flu) and H5N1 (avian flu). However, historically a variety of diseases have gotten out of control and led to pandemics including measles, tuberculosis, plague, smallpox, human immunodeficiency virus/acquired immune deficiency syndrome (HIV/AIDS), and cholera.

A pandemic occurs when an infectious disease, such as a new subtype of a virus, emerges for which no one has an immunity. This typically triggers multiple simultaneous epidemics around the world, with many cases and many deaths. Outbreaks of various diseases happen all the time, and they may even carry a high death toll, but what causes a disease to become a pandemic is how quickly it spreads to large groups via chains of transmission. In the case of flu, this is from person to person. With the ease of global transportation and urbanization, epidemics such as the flu virus can travel rapidly around the world.

The WHO has recommended that countries develop national preparedness plans, specifically to lay out a strategies for handling a flu pandemic. Over the years, more than 140 countries have created national plans for flu pandemics, but according to the WHO, many of these plans will work for outbreaks of other highly transmissable diseases as well. The WHO also has urged countries to adopt its suggested framework for pandemic preparedness.

Pandemic preparedness plans sometimes take years to draft and are supposed to be detailed and comprehensive. This is because the most effective plans take what the WHO calls a "multisectoral" approach, meaning the plan involves "many levels of government, and people with various specialties including policy development, legislative review and drafting, animal health, public health, patient care, laboratory diagnosis, laboratory test development, communication expertise, and disaster management," according to its 2005 "Checklist."

⊕ Historical Background

History is replete with pandemics that struck fast, hard, and without warning. This historically has left governments and communities ill prepared to handle the catastrophic effects of these pandemics. Many of the worst events killed millions, sickened and left vulnerable millions more, ravaged economies, and shook social and political structures. Some even may have altered the course of history.

One of the first reported pandemics struck the Mesopotamian city of Seleucia (in modern-day Iraq) in 165 CE and spread to Rome. At one point the scourge, which scholars believe may have been either smallpox (an acute contagious viral disease, with fever and pustules usually leaving permanent scars) or measles (an infectious viral disease causing fever and a red rash on the skin), killed an estimated 2,000 Romans per day and even claimed the lives of Roman emperor Marcus Aurelius Antoninus (121–180) and co-regent Lucius Verus (130–169).

The next deadliest pandemic struck the Byzantine Empire in 541 and was likely the first recorded case of the bubonic plague, a bacterial disease transmitted by

RESPONSE TO 2009 SWINE FLU PANDEMIC

Pandemics, particularly of influenza, are generally fast moving and can take governments, health agencies, and the public by surprise. However, in theory, a properly formulated preparedness plan can help mitigate the effects of these events.

This was evident with the H1N1, "swine flu" outbreak in 2009. This was the first pandemic under the International Health Regulations, an international legal framework passed in 2005 and enacted in 2007, that legally bound World Health Organization (WHO) member countries to uphold certain obligations to prevent and mitigate a pandemic.

The first report of swine flu came from Veracruz, Mexico, in February 2009 where the virus had been circulating for months before it was noticed. A short time later, April 15, 2009, the first U.S. case of H1N1 (swine flu) was diagnosed, setting in motion a response by the Centers for Disease Control and Prevention (CDC) to start working on a vaccine for the new virus. Just 11 days after that first report, the U.S. government declared H1N1 a public health emergency. Several U.S. states as well as the countries of Canada, Spain, the United Kingdom, New Zealand, Israel, and Germany had reported cases by the end of April.

At first, distribution of the vaccine was slow, and there was not enough of it, so the people at highest risk of complications were given priority for receiving it. By June 2009, 74 countries were affected by the pandemic. Before the pandemic was over, its reach was truly global, with all countries reporting cases.

Beyond distribution of the vaccine, the international community responded quickly with other measures. The European Union health commissioner urged people to postpone any nonessential travel to the United States and Mexico. The Public Health Agency in Canada mapped the genetic code of H1N1, the first time that had been done. The United Kingdom's national health service created a website that allowed people to self-assess symptoms and get antiviral medication in an attempt to alleviate the burden on healthcare providers.

In November 2009, cases were starting to decline, and more vaccination doses were available. Roughly 80 million people in the United States alone were vaccinated. On August 10, 2010, the WHO declared an end to the global H1N1 flu pandemic. The CDC estimates that 43 million to 89 million people had H1N1 between April 2009 and April 2010. They also estimated that there were between 8,870 and 18,300 H1N1-related deaths.

In the years since the pandemic, public health agencies and governments have worked to fix the shortcomings the event highlighted. Some of the changes include efforts at earlier detection of a potentially pandemic disease through access to online field reports, a renewed commitment from WHO member states to share vaccines, and continued work toward faster production and distribution of vaccines.

the bite of infected fleas (or, in its pneumonic from, person to person), characterized by fever, delirium, and the formation of buboes (swollen, inflamed lymph nodes in the armpit or groin). Known as the plague of Justinian, the event quickly killed roughly 25 million and sickened Emperor Justinian (483–565), although he survived. In the capital city of Constantinople, as many as 5,000 people were dying per day. The plague of Justinian lasted just one year, and by its end about 40 percent of the city's population and roughly one-fourth of the eastern Mediterranean population were dead.

Yet this was nothing compared to the bubonic plague that devastated Europe and Asia from 1339 to 1351. At the time the plague hit, the global population has been estimated to be about 450 million. By its end, about 75 million people, including half the population in Europe, had died. Scientists and scholars believe the disease, also known as the Black Death, originated in China and was carried via infected fleas on shipboard rats along the Silk Road (a network of trade routes that linked the regions of the ancient world in commerce) to Sicily where it quickly spread.

Ensuing centuries would bring more waves of disease. Smallpox from 1775 to 1782 devastated North and Central America; tuberculosis (an infectious bacterial disease characterized by the growth of nodules in the tissues, especially the lungs) ravaged Europe and North America from 1800 to 1922; and seven cholera (an infectious and often fatal bacterial disease of the small intestine) pandemics since 1817 have killed millions globally.

That said, nothing prepared the world for what would become known as the deadliest pandemic in history. In its first 25 weeks, the Spanish flu that began in 1918 killed on average 1 million people per week worldwide and about 40 million by the time it ended abruptly in 1919. The flu spread quickly, exacerbated by close living quarters among troops fighting in World War I (1914–1918).

The disease came on quickly, with people feeling perfectly fine in the morning only to die by nightfall. Those who did not die from the flu itself often succumbed to complications caused by bacteria, such as pneumonia. Furthermore, whereas most flu strains are deadly primarily for the very old and the very young, this flu killed healthy adults mostly between the ages of 20 to 50 years old.

Flu viruses are so common there is a new pandemic at least once per generation. Since the 1918 pandemic there have been three major flu pandemics including the 2009–2010 H1N1 pandemic. Also known as the "swine flu" because of the strain's resemblance to a virus that afflicts pigs, this flu was particularly virulent. Before it subsided, between 43 million and 89 million people had H1N1 between April 2009 and April 2010, according to the U.S. Centers for Disease Control and Prevention (CDC). There were an estimated 8,870 to 18,300 H1N1-related deaths, reports the CDC.

Among the recent global pandemics is HIV/AIDS. This retrovirus (a family of enveloped viruses that replicate in a host cell through the process of reverse transcription) is transmitted through bodily fluids and breaks down the body's immune system. Scientists think the virus first infected people in Africa sometime before 1937 but was not identified until the early 1980s. The disease initially spread slowly, but an epidemic among homosexual men in Western countries at the end of the 1970s eventually caught the attention of scientists and public health professionals. There is no cure for HIV/AIDS, although antiretroviral drugs seem to temper the disease, allowing those infected to live longer.

HIV/AIDS is an ongoing pandemic. The virus has infected more than 75 million people, killed more than 39 million, and remains a major global health concern. According to the WHO, there were approximately 35 million people living with HIV at the end of 2013, with 2.1 million people becoming newly infected with the virus that year. Sub-Saharan Africa accounts for almost 70 percent of the global total of new HIV infections.

⊕ Impacts and Issues

There are myriad diseases that could cause a pandemic. For example, one that scientists and public health officials are watching is the coronavirus, which causes severe acute respiratory syndrome (SARS, a severe form of pneumonia). This disease first appeared in China in 2002 and quickly caused 8,096 cases and 774 deaths. It spread to 26 countries before that wave fizzled out in 2003 because infection control procedures prevented further spread.

One of the most difficult viruses to contain is the influenza virus because of its ability to spread and mutate quickly, rendering vaccines developed to fight it ineffective. Outbreaks of flu occur annually, but occasionally a strain emerges that causes a worldwide pandemic, such as the Spanish flu of 1918. But even a typical flu year can cause seasonal outbreaks that sicken as many as 5 million and kill 500,000. Furthermore, the virus is endemic in several species, including humans, birds, and pigs.

The concern in the 21st century has been several avian influenza A viruses that have emerged, including H5N1 virus, first detected in 1997, and the H7N9 and

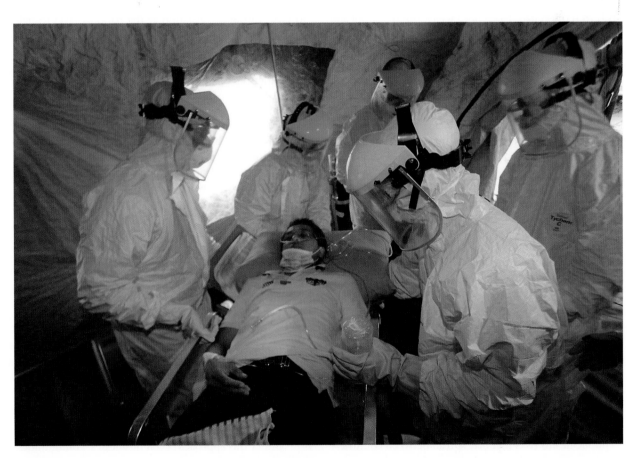

Indonesian health officials conduct simulation exercises for Ebola preparedness involving mock plane passengers during the Ministry of Health's 50th anniversary celebrations near the National Monument, Jakarta, Indonesia, on November 12, 2014. The World Health Organization on October 13, 2014, urged East Asian and Pacific countries to strengthen defenses against the Ebola outbreak. The region of 1.8 billion has been a hot spot for many emerging diseases, including severe acute respiratory syndrome (SARS) and avian influenza. © *Sagarmata/Anadolu Agency/Getty Images.*

H10N8 viruses, first reported in 2013. Any of these could hold potential for pandemic, but that is what frustrates scientists, public health officials, and the public: these diseases are unpredictable, with the only certainty being not if there will be a pandemic, but when.

This is particularly worrisome because pandemics share some common characteristics and challenges, including a rapid spread with a global reach among populations with little or no immunity to the disease. Because of this, health systems can become overwhelmed quickly. Most nations are not likely to have the staff, facilities, equipment, and hospital beds needed to cope with the sheer number of sick people coming through the doors. Putting plans in place to accommodate for such events is called surge capacity, which requires preparing to have enough staff, hospital beds, ventilators, medications, vaccines, coffins, morgue space, and so forth, in place if a pandemic occurs. For diseases where a vaccine is available and antivirals necessary, the supply is likely to be much smaller than the demand. In addition, if past pandemics are any indication, these viruses tend to spread globally in two or three waves of illness. Moreover, pandemics disrupt the economy and the regular function of society. From travel bans to event cancellations to school and business closings, pandemics can cause major financial and functional damage in a community.

Successful implementation of a comprehensive plan for addressing a pandemic can save many lives, although the unpredictability and rapid spread of pandemics will still exact a global toll. According to the WHO in its 2005 "Checklist for Influenza Pandemic Preparedness Planning," "even in one of the more conservative scenarios, it has been calculated that the world will face up to 233 million outpatient visits, 5.2 million hospital admissions, and 7.4 million deaths globally, within a very short period."

The international community had long recognized the need for coordination between countries in order to contain disease. Following cholera epidemics in Europe in the early 19th century, an 1851 conference in Paris produced the International Sanitary Regulations. These were revised and renamed the International Health Regulations (IHR) in 1969. By 1995, it had become clear that the IHR needed revision again, both to account for emerging infectious diseases and to better increase communication and coordination between countries in response to diseases. The revised version of IHR was completed in 2005 and went into force in 2007. The IHR is an international law that binds the WHO and its 194 member countries to uphold certain obligations when it comes to the prevention, control, and response to public health risks that may spread between countries. In addition to having a preparedness plan in place, member states also are obligated to notify the WHO, which the IHR establishes as the lead agency during an international public health crisis, of incidents that may affect public health. Other regulations govern international travel, including health measures for travelers and sanitary procedures at points of entry into a country.

The first test of this law came during the 2009–2010 swine flu outbreaks. While this framework created mechanisms for good communication, information sharing, and a recommended chain of command, it broke down in some key areas, according to Dr. Harvey V. Fineberg, in his 2014 review of the process for the *New England Journal of Medicine* titled "Pandemic Preparedness and Response—Lessons from the H1N1 Influenza of 2009."

Among the challenges, Fineberg found, was that different countries had plans at varying levels of completion. Some countries and even the WHO did not have the budget or resources to implement certain mandated portions of the law, and the law lacked financial penalties or punitive trade sanctions should member states violate any portion of the law. Efforts to address these shortcomings are ongoing.

Moreover, the WHO states that another problem with the law is that different countries have different legislations, policies, regulations, and requirements that support IHR implementation to varying degrees. To that end, the WHO has been working with member countries to push through legislation at the national level to help smooth this process.

When it comes to the creating the plans themselves, the countries have to at minimum establish a procedure and leadership protocol to address preparing for an emergency, surveillance, case investigation and treatment, preventing spread of the disease in the community, maintaining essential services, and researching, evaluating, and implementing testing and revision of the national plan. To implement these plans, the WHO recommends what is called a "Whole of Society" approach, which emphasizes the importance of involving everyone—not just the health sector—in helping to contain the spread of a pandemic.

For example, national governments need to lead the overall coordination for preparedness. It is the governments' responsiblity to enact or modify legislation and policies in support of pandemic preparedness while also ensuring that resources are properly allocated. Governments are also best equipped to coordinate efforts across agencies both in the public and private sector to mobilize a broad response to a pandemic should the need arise.

Meanwhile, the health sector's responsibilities include providing reliable information on the risk, severity, and progression of a pandemic; prioritizing and continuing health care during a pandemic; enacting steps to reduce the spread of the disease in the community and in health-care facilities; and protecting and supporting health-care workers during a pandemic.

Under this approach, even businesses, communities, individuals, families, and civil society organizations have roles to play in mitigating the effect of a pandemic. For example, if electrical or water services are disrupted during a pandemic, the service providers are supposed to have a contingency plan so that if nothing else, they can

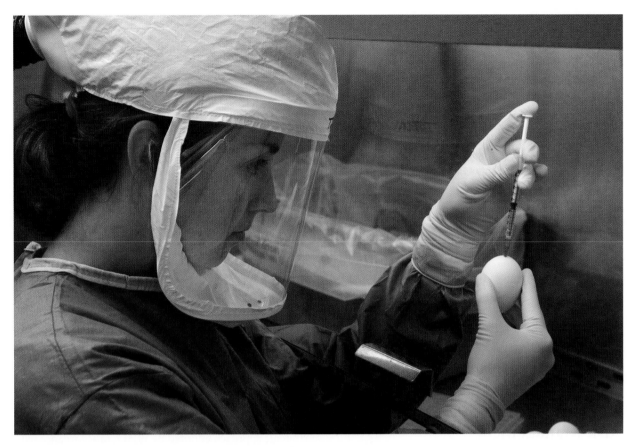

A microbiologist in the Influenza Branch at the Centers for Disease Control and Prevention conducts an experiment inside a biological safety cabinet (BSC) within the Biosafety Level 3–enhanced laboratory. The airflow within the BSC helps prevent any airborne virus from escaping the confines of the cabinet, and as part of her personal protective equipment, she wears a powered air purifying respirator. She is inoculating 10-day-old embryonated chicken eggs with a specimen containing an H5N1 avian influenza virus as part of a study to investigate the pathogenicity and transmissibility of newly emerging H5N1 viruses. Identification of genetic markers affecting the ability of H5N1 viruses to transmit efficiently helps in the early identification of emerging H5N1 viruses with pandemic potential, which is important for pandemic preparedness. © *Greg Knobloch/U.S. Centers for Disease Control and Prevention.*

get power and water to medical facilities to ensure the facilities can continue to operate and provide care.

Furthermore, civil society organizations are expected to harness their various expertise and their close and direct relationship with the public to offer support as well as raise awareness and communicate accurate information to the public. For individuals and families, their primary responsibilities include making sure that they have access to accurate information, food, water, and medicines and are self-quarantining if necessary.

⊕ Future Implications

One of the major challenges outlined by Fineberg in the 2014 article analyzing the global response to the 2009 H1N1 epidemic was the failure of many member states to fulfill the requirements for pandemic preparedness mandated by the IHR. A WHO questionnaire distributed to member states in 2011 received only a 66 percent response rate, or 128 members of a total of 194.

Of those who responded, only 58 percent had developed blueprints for achieving pandemic preparedness, and less than 10 percent reported having fully implemented the recommendations of the IHR.

Still, one of the biggest limitations in preparedness remains how little is known about pandemics. Fineberg notes that "the annals of influenza are filled with overly confident predictions based on insufficient evidence." In reality, it is impossible to know which virus will emerge as the next pandemic, and how severe it will be, but more research can help mitigate the uncertainty.

Although information and even vaccine sharing between countries is improving, the traditional methods of vaccine production, particularly when it comes to the flu, cannot respond quickly enough to an emerging pandemic. The traditional model relies on growing vaccine viruses in eggs, which requires a large amount of eggs as well as time for the viruses to grow and replicate in the eggs. In 2013 the U.S. Food and Drug Administration approved a method of vaccine production that involves a "recombinant" vaccine virus (meaning that its genetic material comes from different sources) that can replicate in insect cells. The fact that this methodology is not reliant on the egg supply or the availability of the influenza virus means that production can ramp up far more quickly.

Fineberg's analysis of the 2009 H1N1 epidemic acknowledged the challenges of readiness, including insufficient resources, the need for international coordination, and the difficulty inherent in making quick and measured decisions when a pandemic arises. Beyond better research and vaccine production, pandemic preparedness requires the full commitment to pandemic preparedness on the part of government and health agencies, including the provision of adequate funding for research and preparedness initiatives, proper staffing of public health leadership and analysis positions, and better coordination and information sharing between countries. Fineberg also offered this warning: "Whenever the next influenza pandemic arises, many more lives may be at risk. By heeding the lessons from the 2009 H1N1 pandemic, the international community will be able to cope more successfully the next time."

PRIMARY SOURCE

Pandemic Influenza Risk Management

SOURCE *"Introduction," from* Pandemic Influenza Risk Management: WHO Interim Guidance. *Geneva: World Health Organization (WHO), 2013, 3. http://www.who.int/influenza/ preparedness/pandemic/GIP_PandemicInfluenz aRiskManagementInterimGuidance_Jun2013. pdf (accessed January 25, 2015).*

INTRODUCTION *This primary source is the introduction section from a World Health Organization (WHO) document providing guidance on pandemic preparedness for global leadership. WHO states that "Advance planning and preparedness are critical to help mitigate the impact of a pandemic."*

1. INTRODUCTION

The influenza A(H1N1) 2009 pandemic was the first to occur since WHO had produced preparedness guidance. Guidance had been published in 1999, revised in 2005 and again in 2009 following advances in the development of antivirals and experiences with influenza A(H5N1) infections in poultry and humans. The emergence of the influenza A(H1N1)pdm09 virus provided further understanding of influenza pandemics and requirements for pandemic preparedness and response. The report of the Review Committee on the Functioning of the International Health Regulations (2005) in relation to Pandemic (H1N1) 2009

concluded: "The world is ill-prepared to respond to a severe influenza pandemic or to any similarly global, sustained and threatening public-health emergency."

The Review Committee recommended that WHO should revise its pandemic preparedness guidance to support further efforts at the national and subnational level. Revisions recommended included: simplification of the pandemic phases structure; emphasis on a risk-based approach to enable a more flexible response to different scenarios; reliance on multisectoral participation; utilization of lessons learnt at the country, regional and global level; and further guidance on risk assessment. The Review Committee's report reflected the broad experiences of Member States during the influenza A(H1N1) 2009 pandemic—and the key point that previous pandemic planning guidance was overly rigid. Member States had prepared for a pandemic of high severity and appeared unable to adapt their responses adequately to a more moderate event. Communications also proved to be of immense importance during the influenza A(H1N1) 2009 pandemic, within the health and non-health sectors and to the public. Provision of clear risk assessments to decision-makers placed significant strain on ministries of health, and effective communication with the public was challenging.

This 2013 guidance is based on the principles of all-hazards emergency risk management for health (ERMH), thereby aligning pandemic risk management with the strategic approach adopted by WHO, in accordance with World Health Assembly resolution 64.10. Commensurate with this approach, this guidance promotes building on existing capacities—in particular those under the International Health Regulations (2005) (IHR [2005]) core capacities, in order to manage risks from pandemic influenza. Certain aspects of implementation of ERMH for national pandemic preparedness may therefore be linked with the core capacity strengthening activities required by the IHR (2005). This guidance can therefore be used as a model to illustrate how the mechanisms required for response to and recovery from pandemic influenza can be applied, as appropriate, to the management of all relevant health emergencies.

A risk-based approach to pandemic influenza management is emphasized and Member States are encouraged to develop flexible plans, based on national risk assessments. This guidance also places pandemic planning in the whole-of-society context. This 2013 revision therefore (1) reflects the approach taken at national level where pandemic influenza planning often rests with national disaster management authorities and (2) introduces or promotes all-hazards ERMH at Ministry of Health level, including mechanisms for wider national engagement.

This guidance also summarizes the roles and responsibilities of WHO relevant to pandemic preparedness, in terms of global leadership and support to Member States.

SEE ALSO *Cholera and Dysentery; Influenza; Tuberculosis (TB); Viral Diseases; World Health Organization: Organization, Funding, and Enforcement Powers*

BIBLIOGRAPHY

Books

Knobler, Stacey L., et al., eds. *The Threat of Pandemic Influenza: Are We Ready?: Workshop Summary.* Washington, DC: National Academies Press, 2005.

Lemon, Stanley M., et al. *Ethical and Legal Considerations in Mitigating Pandemic Disease: Workshop Summary.* Washington, DC: National Academies Press, 2007.

Pandemic Influenza Preparedness and Response: A WHO Guidance Document. Geneva: World Health Organization, 2009.

Periodicals

Fineberg, Harvey V. "Pandemic Preparedness and Response—Lessons from the H1N1 Influenza of 2009." *New England Journal of Medicine* 370, no. 14 (April 3, 2014): 1335–1342.

Morens, David M., Gregory K. Folkers, and Anthony S. Fauci. "What Is a Pandemic?" *Journal of Infectious Diseases* 200, no. 7 (August 2009): 1018–1021.

Websites

"The 2009 H1N1 Pandemic: Summary Highlights, April 2009–April 2010." *U.S. Centers for Disease Control and Prevention (CDC).* http://www.cdc.gov/h1n1flu/cdcresponse.htm (accessed March 20, 2015).

"About Pandemics." *Flu.gov.* http://www.flu.gov/pandemic/about/ (accessed March 20, 2015).

Chan, Margaret. "Influenza A (H1N1): Lessons Learned and Preparedness: Keynote Speech at a High-Level Meeting." *World Health Organization (WHO),* July 2, 2009. http://www.who.int/dg/speeches/2009/influenza_h1n1_lessons_20090702/en/ (accessed March 20, 2015).

"Comparative Analysis of National Pandemic Influenza Preparedness Plans." *World Health Organization (WHO),* January 2011. http://www.who.int/influenza/resources/documents/comparative_analysis_php_2011_en.pdf (accessed March 20, 2015).

"The Five Deadliest Outbreaks and Pandemics in History." *Culture of Health.* http://www.rwjf.org/en/blogs/culture-of-health/2013/12/the_five_deadliesto.html (accessed March 20, 2015).

"H1N1 (Originally Referred to as Swine Flu)." *Flu.gov.* http://www.flu.gov/about_the_flu/h1n1/ (accessed March 20, 2015.

"Humanitarian Pandemic Preparedness Programme." *International Federation of Red Cross and Red Crescent Societies.* http://www.ifrc.org/en/what-we-do/health/diseases/pandemic-influenza/humanitarian-pandemic-preparedness-programme/ (accessed March 20, 2015).

"Informal Consultation on Influenza Pandemic Preparedness in Countries with Limited Resources." *World Health Organization (WHO).* http://www.who.int/influenza/resources/documents/CDS_CSR_GIP_2004_1.pdf (accessed March 20, 2015).

"Influenza: Public Health Preparedness." *World Health Organization (WHO).* http://www.who.int/influenza/preparedness/en/ (accessed March 20, 2015).

"International Health Regulations: Safeguarding Health in Emergencies through Legislation." *World Health Organization (WHO), Regional Office for South-East Asia (SEARO).* http://www.searo.who.int/entity/ihr/topics/IHR_legislation/en/ (accessed March 20, 2015).

"Pandemic Flu History." *Flu.gov.* http://www.flu.gov/pandemic/history/index.html (accessed March 20, 2015).

"Pandemic Influenza." *CIDRAP: Center for Infectious Disease Research and Policy.* http://www.cidrap.umn.edu/infectious-disease-topics/pandemic-influenza#overview&1-4 (accessed March 20, 2015).

"PREPARE: Pandemic Preparedness Project." *International Medical Corps.* https://internationalmedicalcorps.org/prepare#.VM2OqC6YTXS (accessed March 20, 2015).

Rowe, Janet. "Deadly Pandemics through History." *University of Toronto Magazine,* Winter 2013. http://janet297.rssing.com/browser.php?indx=15829647&item=7 (accessed March 20, 2015).

"What Is a Pandemic?" *World Health Organization (WHO),* February 24, 2010. http://www.who.int/csr/disease/swineflu/frequently_asked_questions/pandemic/en/ (accessed March 20, 2015).

"WHO Checklist for Influenza Pandemic Preparedness Planning." *World Health Organization (WHO),* 2005. http://www.who.int/csr/resources/publications/influenza/WHO_CDS_CSR_GIP_2005_4/en/ (accessed March 20, 2015).

Melanie R. Plenda

Parasitic Diseases

🌐 Introduction

The U.S. Centers for Disease Control and Prevention (CDC) define a parasite as "an organism that lives on or in a host organism, and gets its food from or at the expense of its host." Parasites can have complicated life cycles that include multiple hosts. People can get parasites from contaminated food or water, insect bites, or sexual contact. Some parasites can infect humans and cause no symptoms at all, however, a small percentage can cause mild to severe illness and even death if contracted.

There are two primary disease-causing parasites in humans: protozoa (a type of microbe) and helminths (wormlike parasites, including tapeworms and flukes). The most common parasitic diseases are transmitted via contaminated food or water, through person to person contact, or via vectors (carriers) such as sand flies or mosquitos. Among the more common food-borne and waterborne parasitic diseases are giardiasis, cryptosporidiosis, and cyclosporiasis. The most common vector-borne diseases are malaria and leishmaniasis. Helminths are typically transmitted when an infected host defecates directly on to the ground, generally in areas where there is poor sanitation; the parasite's eggs present in the feces then contaminate the soil.

Symptoms vary depending on the disease; some parasites cause no symptoms at all. Symptoms of protozoa-induced infections can include fever, flulike symptoms, nausea, vomiting, abdominal pain, rectal bleeding, bloating, weight loss, and diarrhea. Untreated helminth infections can lead to a host of problems including subcutaneous nodules, conjunctivitis, retinitis, blindness, dysentery, urticarial vasculitis, diarrhea, cough, hepatosplenomegaly, fever, and abdominal pain.

According to the CDC, diseases caused by protozoan and helminth parasites are among the leading causes of death and disease in tropical and subtropical regions of the world. Part of the reason for this is the difficulty of controlling the vectors (carriers) of disease, primarily due to pesticide resistance, concerns about the environment, and lack of adequate support to apply existing vector control methods.

There are no vaccines at this time to help prevent or control the spread of parasitic diseases, resulting in a significant reliance on treatment drugs. However, according to the CDC, most existing treatments are either not completely effective or toxic to humans.

Even safe drugs that work will not work forever, given the emergence and spread of drug-resistant types of parasites. The best example of this is the global proliferation of drug-resistant *Plasmodium falciparum*, the protozoan responsible for the most lethal form of malaria, according to the CDC. Many global health agencies, nongovernmental organizations, and charities have been calling for quick development of more and better treatment options.

🌐 Historical Background

Many of today's parasites are souvenirs from humans' hominid days, according to F. E. G. Cox in his article, "History of Human Parasitology," published in the journal *Clinical Microbiology Reviews* in October 2002. While many of the parasites that can potentially cause problems in humans are rare, a small portion cause significant disease in the world.

Worms in calcified helminth eggs have been discovered in mummies dating from 1200 BCE. Coprolites (fossilized dung) found in North America reveal hookworm ova dating to somewhere between 3500 BCE and 480 CE.

Though protozoa would not be discovered until after the microscope was invented, historic records describing what was most likely amoebic dysentery (bloody diarrhea) date back to at least 1000 BCE. Several of these epidemics are described throughout history, including reports during the Middle Ages of "bloody flux" in Europe, Asia, Persia, and Greece.

However, the first written evidence of these tiny passengers comes from Egyptian writings known as the Ebers papyrus. Named for Georg Ebers, a German Egyptologist who discovered the tome in Thebes in 1873, the document is known as the medical papyrus of herbal knowledge and dates back to 1500 BCE. In it, what are very likely intestinal parasites are described. Other civilizations seem to have been aware of them as well, as there are written records of what most likely were parasites coming from China (3000 to 300 BCE), India (2500 to 200 BCE), Rome (700 BCE to 400 CE), and the Arab Empire in the latter part of the first millennium, according to Cox.

During the Renaissance (1300–1700), Antonie van Leeuwenhoek first discovered tiny one-celled organisms he called animalcules in his homemade microscopes. This was a critical piece of the foundation needed for future discoveries in parasitology. Leeuwenhoek is known today as the first microbiologist.

By the 19th century, some very exciting discoveries were leading to major strides in parasitology, Cox writes, and two major breakthroughs made this possible. The first came when scientists finally disproved spontaneous generation, which was the idea that living organisms could be produced from nonliving matter. The second advance took place over time; it was the acceptance of germ theory, which is the idea that microscopic organisms cause infectious diseases.

These ideas surely helped Friedrich Lösch, who first discovered the amoeba *Entamoeba histolytica* in Russia in 1873 and established its relationship to disease. A few years later, Greek physician Stephanos Kartulis discovered that dysentery was likely caused by an amoeba. However, according to Cox, the definitive work on what was known about the pathology of amoebiasis at the end of the 19th century was an 1891 report from William Thomas Councilman and Henri Lafleur who were working for Johns Hopkins Hospital in Baltimore, Maryland, in the United States. Much of their work is still valid today.

Helminthology also gained validity in the 18th and 19th centuries. It was during this time that Swedish botanist, physician, and zoologist Carolus Linnaeus (1707–1778) described and named six helminth worms. By the beginning of the 20th century, 28 species had been recorded in humans. Since then, Cox estimates that the number has grown to about 300 parasitic worms and 70 species of helminths.

⊕ Impacts and Issues

Parasitic infections tend to have the most detrimental effect in developing countries, where there is generally less access to clean water or adequate sanitation. However, parasitic diseases affect people living in developed countries as well. Protozoa and helminths are the

PALEOPARASITOLOGY

For the past century—a relatively short time when it comes to science—there has been a growing interest in the field of paleoparasitology and archaeoparasitology.

Paleoparasitology is the science that uses parasitological techniques for diagnosing parasitic diseases in history. Traditionally this has referred only to study of parasites in non-human, ancient materials; archaeoparasitology is the study of parasites in humans and hominids in the past. However, many of the most recent scientific writings in this area use the term paleoparasitology to refer to the study of parasites in ancient humans, as this writing will do.

Paleoparasitology got its start in the early 1900s. In 1910, Sir Marc Armand Ruffer, an experimental pathologist and bacteriologist, first described calcified *Schistosoma hematobium* (flatworm) eggs in the kidney tissues of two Egyptian mummies. *S. hematobium* is the cause of urinary schistosomiasis. In 1944, Professor Lothar Szidat published the first record of the presence of *Ascaris lumbricoides, Trichuris trichiura*, and *Diphyllobothrium latum* eggs in the intestinal contents of 5th-century corpses found in an East Prussian bog.

These were the first seeds of what would become paleoparasitology. It would take another 40 years before researchers took an interest in seeking out eggs by examining archaeological sediment and coprolites (desiccated feces). Before this, parasitic infection in prehistoric humans was based mostly on observation of mummified remains. But once researchers began actively looking for the eggs and collecting samples, they started seeing the value to studying ancient disease.

Over the years, the study of parasites has evolved. In the beginning, work was largely dependent on whether the parasite could be seen through a microscope. More recently, molecular biology has helped advance the study of paleoparasitology. Scientists now use DNA, even hybrids of DNA and ancient DNA sequencing methods, to identify parasites and learn more about their findings.

As the field has grown, researchers have been able to answer fundamental questions at the heart of several fields. Scientists have gained insight and knowledge into health, diet, and farming of the past; they have learned about migration patterns, climate change, cultural contacts, and sanitary practices, among many other things. Scientists have also been better able to understand the origins and evolution of parasites, as well as the relocation of parasites as a result of globalization, all of which can have profound value when it comes to future study of parasites.

main causes of parasitic infections, many of which can be avoided with access to safe food and water as well as proper sanitation and hygiene.

Several of the most common protozoa-related diseases cause severe diarrhea, including amoebiasis, cryptosporidiosis, and giardiasis. About 88 percent of the 4 billion diarrhea cases reported worldwide annually are linked to unsafe water, inadequate sanitation, or insufficient hygiene. Roughly 2 million people die each year from diarrheal diseases; of those, more than 600,000 are children. The World Health Organization (WHO) estimates that 94 percent of diarrheal cases can be prevented by increasing the availability of clean water, improving sanitation, and providing instruction on proper hygiene.

Many parasitic infections fall within the category of neglected tropical diseases (NTDs), a diverse group of tropical infections that are endemic among low-income populations in developing regions of Africa, Asia, and the Americas. Parasitic NTDs include lymphatic filariasis, onchocerciasis, and guinea worm disease. These NTDs affect more than 1 billion people, or one-sixth of the world's population, according to the CDC. These diseases have a tremendous impact on the populations they affect, including disfigurement, lost ability to attend school or work, stunted growth in children, cognitive impairment in young children, and the economic burden of medical treatment and lost income for governments.

Protozoan Illnesses

Protozoa are microscopic, one-celled organisms that can be free-living or parasitic in nature. The ability of protozoa to multiply in humans contributes to their survival and allows serious infections to result from just a single organism. Protozoa can live in the intestines or the blood and tissues. Those that live in the intestines are typically transmitted to others via a fecal-oral route; for example, when a person consumes contaminated food or water, or through person-to-person contact. Protozoa that live in the blood or tissue, however, are transmitted by vector, such as through the bite of a mosquito or sand fly.

Entamoeba

Amoebiasis is caused by the parasitic protozoa *Entamoeba histolytica*. The parasites are transmitted through contaminated food or water or through person-to-person contact. Severe cases cause ulcerative colitis and amoebic dysentery, the hallmark of which is bloody diarrhea with mucous. The parasites can also leave the gut and infect the liver, which causes what is known as hepatic amoebiasis (abscess on the liver). Amoebiasis occurs worldwide, but is more common in areas or countries with poor sanitation, particularly in the tropics.

Cryptosporidium

Cryptosporidium, also known as Crypto, is the parasite that causes the diarrheal disease cryptosporidiosis. Crypto can be spread in a variety of ways but the most common is by contaminated drinking water. Cryptosporidiosis occurs worldwide, and it is one of the most frequent causes of waterborne disease among people in the United States, according to the CDC. There are an estimated 748,000 cases of cryptosporidiosis each year in the United States.

Giardia

Giardia is a microscopic parasite that causes the diarrheal illness known as giardiasis. The parasites, *Giardia intestinalis*, *Giardia lamblia*, or *Giardia duodenalis*, are found on surfaces, in soil, food, or water that has been contaminated with feces from infected humans or animals, according to the CDC. The most common transmission for *Giardia* is through ingesting contaminated water. According to the CDC, giardiasis infects nearly 2 percent of adults and 6 to 8 percent of children in developed countries worldwide. However, the CDC notes, nearly 33 percent of people in developing countries have had giardiasis at least one point in their lives.

Leishmania

Leishmania is a parasite transmitted by the bite of infected sand flies; the parasite causes the disease leishmaniasis. There are three main forms of this disease. Visceral leishmaniases, also known as kala-azar, is the most serious and is fatal if left untreated; cutaneous, the most common form, causes ulcers on exposed parts of the body, leaving lifelong scars and serious disability; and mucocutaneous, which leads to partial or total destruction of mucous membranes of the nose, mouth, and throat. An estimated 1.3 million new cases and 20,000 to 30,000 deaths occur annually.

Plasmodium

Plasmodium is the parasite that causes malaria. There are four species of parasites that cause malaria in humans including *Plasmodium falciparum*, *Plasmodium vivax*, *Plasmodium malariae* and *Plasmodium ovale*. According to the WHO, *Plasmodium falciparum* and *Plasmodium vivax* are the most common, and *Plasmodium falciparum* is the most deadly. Some human cases of malaria in recent years have also been found to be caused by *Plasmodium knowlesi*, a species that causes malaria among monkeys and occurs in certain forested areas of southeast Asia.

These parasites are transmitted to humans through the bite of infected female *Anopheles* mosquitoes. Malaria is a life-threatening disease that is both preventable and curable. About 3.2 billion people are at risk of malaria. According to the WHO, there were about 198 million cases of malaria in 2013 and an estimated 584,000 deaths. Most deaths occur among children living in Africa. However, mortality rates among children in Africa have been reduced by an estimated 58 percent since 2000.

Toxoplasma gondii

Toxoplasma gondii is the parasite that causes toxoplasmosis. It is one of the most common parasites and causes no symptoms in most people. However, this parasite is particularly dangerous to pregnant women because of transmission to the fetus and people with an immunodeficiency. More than 6 billion people have been infected with *T. gondii*.

The parasite is usually transmitted by consuming contaminated meat, particularly pork, lamb, and venison,

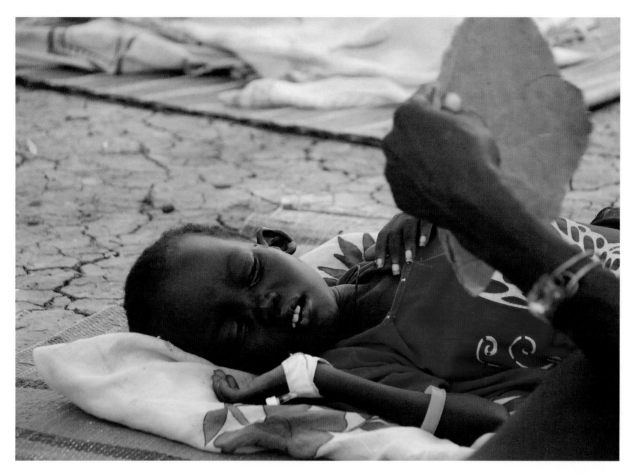

A South Sudanese child recovers from kala-azar (visceral leishmaniasis) disease at a hospital in Malakal, the capital of Upper Nile State. Kala-azar is a serious, systemic form of the parasitic disease leishmaniasis, which is transmitted by the bite of small insects called sand flies. It is usually fatal without treatment. © *Peter Martell/AFP/Getty Images.*

or by coming into contact with cat feces infected with *T. gondii*. Those who do present symptoms typically complain of flulike illness and may have swollen lymph glands or muscle aches and pains that last for a month or more. During severe infections, *Toxoplasma* can cause damage to the brain, eyes, and other organs.

Helminths

In their adult form, helminths are large, multicellular organisms. Helminths, the name for which is derived from the Greek word for "worm," can either be free-living or parasitic.

Three groups of helminths affect humans. Flatworms (platyhelminths) are one group and include the trematodes (flukes) and cestodes (tapeworms). Thorny-headed worms (acanthocephalans), which in their adult forms live in the gastrointestinal tract, are another group. Scientists think these worms are the intermediate between cestodes and nematodes (roundworms). The third group is roundworms, which also reside in the gastrointestinal tract as adults, as well as in the blood, lymphatic system, or subcutaneous tissues. The larval states of roundworms can cause disease by infecting various body tissues.

Many helminth infections are soil-transmitted and caused by a variety of different species of parasitic worms. The main species that infect humans are the roundworm *Ascaris lumbricoides*, the whipworm *Trichuris trichiura*, and the hookworms *Necator americanus* and *Ancylostoma duodenale*.

Adult worms living in the intestines can produce thousands of eggs each day, which then are transmitted out of the host's body when the host defecates. These eggs end up contaminating the soil in areas with poor sanitation, where open defecation is practiced, or where human feces are used as fertilizer. According to the WHO, once in the soil, the helminth eggs can be ingested when people eat vegetables that have not been carefully cooked, washed, or peeled (all of which would remove the eggs attached to the food) or drink from contaminated water sources. They can also be ingested by children when they play in dirt and put their hands in their mouths without washing. Other parasites, such as the hookworm, hatch in the soil and then develop into a form that can penetrate the skin. When a person walks barefoot in infested soil, he or she can become infected by a hookworm.

Estimated Deaths per 100,000 Population, by Country, from Malaria in 2013

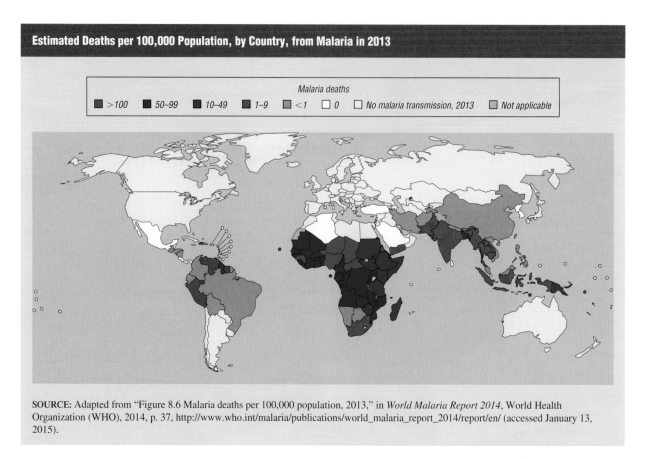

Malaria deaths

■ >100   ■ 50–99   ■ 10–49   ■ 1–9   ■ <1   □ 0   □ No malaria transmission, 2013   □ Not applicable

SOURCE: Adapted from "Figure 8.6 Malaria deaths per 100,000 population, 2013," in *World Malaria Report 2014*, World Health Organization (WHO), 2014, p. 37, http://www.who.int/malaria/publications/world_malaria_report_2014/report/en/ (accessed January 13, 2015).

The World Health Organization estimates that in 2013, there were 198 million cases of malaria worldwide resulting in more than 580,000 deaths.

The WHO estimates that over 1.5 billion people—or 24 percent of the world's population—suffered from soil-transmitted helminth infections as of 2014. The WHO identified the need to treat and educate the more than 270 million preschool-age children and more than 600 million school-age children living in parasite-prevalent areas as a high priority since the parasites' affect on the physical, nutritional, and cognitive development of children is particularly detrimental. The worms deprive the body of iron and protein as they feed on the tissues and blood. Further, the worms make it much more difficult for the host's body to absorb nutrients from the food he or she takes in. The result of this nutritional deprivation is stunted growth and physical development. More severe infections can lead to loss of appetite, diarrhea, abdominal pain, general malaise, weakness, and anemia.

⊕ Future Implications

A major public health question concerns the effect climate change will have on parasites. Many researchers predict that though some species will die out as temperatures rise and the environment changes, others will simply adapt or change environs. This could potentially cause serious infection in new populations without immunities to protect them against parasites.

One of the challenges in quantifying the effect of climate change on parasites and habits and life cycles is the lack of an effective model for studying the subject. One of those better models may be on the horizon. In 2013, Peter K. Molnár and colleagues developed a model, described in "Metabolic Approaches to Understanding Climate Change Impacts on Seasonal Host-Macroparasite Dynamics" in *Ecology Letters*, that aims to determine the range of most disease-causing parasites, even if little is known about them, into the future. The method takes the projected temperature change for an area and then calculates how it might alter the organism's metabolism and life cycle. The model determines a "fundamental thermal niche," the highest and lowest temperatures at which parasites can live, given the need for balance between body size and body temperature. The model suggests that as temperatures rise, some organisms at the top of their temperature range will die off, but others at the lower end of their range may encroach on new areas.

Great strides are also being made when it comes to one of the greatest parasitic killers: malaria. In recent years, there have been increased prevention and control measures that have led to a 47 percent reduction in malaria mortality rates globally and 54 percent in the WHO African Region since 2000. Four countries have been certified by the WHO director-general as having eliminated malaria: the United Arab Emirates (2007), Morocco (2010), Turkmenistan (2010), and Armenia (2011). The WHO plans to continue its efforts along with nongovernmental and charitable organizations.

However, health organizations recommend the continued use of insecticide-treated mosquito nets, indoor spraying with residual insecticides, and taking antimalarial medicines as prevention. The challenge for health agencies is to continue to monitor the presence of drug-resistant strains of malaria. The WHO recommends quick development of alternative insecticides for use when mosquitos become immune to those currently in use.

Soil-transmitted helminths continue to be an issue for developing countries, but efforts are underway to lower the rate of infection through the periodic drug treatment of those considered to be part of at-risk populations, including children, women of childbearing age (including pregnant women in the second and third trimesters and breast-feeding women), and adults in certain high-risk occupations, such as tea pickers or miners, living in endemic areas. The WHO recommends providing this treatment even when no symptoms of infection exist, and combining it with efforts to raise awareness of the importance of good health and hygiene, and improvements to sanitation whenever possible. The WHO estimated that diseases caused by helminths could be eliminated in children by 2020 if 75 percent of children (roughly 873 million) in affected areas could receive this treatment.

PRIMARY SOURCE

Neglected Parasitic Infections in the United States: Chagas Disease

SOURCE Neglected Parasitic Infections in the United States: Chagas Disease, *Fact Sheet. U.S. Centers for Disease Control and Prevention (CDC). http://www.cdc.gov/parasites/resources/pdf/npi_chagas.pdf (accessed January 25, 2015).*

INTRODUCTION *This primary source is a fact sheet compiled by the Division of Parasitic Diseases and Malaria at the U.S. Centers for Disease Control and Prevention (CDC). It describes Chagas disease, related public health concerns, and CDC's response to the problem.*

NEGLECTED PARASITIC INFECTIONS IN THE UNITED STATES

Chagas Disease

Chagas disease is a preventable infection caused by the parasite *Trypanosoma cruzi* and spread by infected insects called triatomine bugs. The initial infection usually does not cause severe symptoms and is often not even diagnosed. After years of chronic infection, some people develop heart diseases such as abnormal rhythms, heart failure, and an increased risk of sudden death. Chagas disease can also cause gastrointestinal problems, such as severe constipation and difficulty swallowing.

Infection is typically spread by contact with the triatomine bug, most commonly found in rural parts of Mexico, Central America, or South America. However, the disease can also be transmitted from mother to baby (congenital), through organ transplant, or through blood transfusion. Chagas disease is considered a Neglected Parasitic Infection, one of a group of diseases that results in significant illness among those who are infected and is often poorly understood by health care providers.

Who is most at risk for Chagas disease?

People in the United States are at higher risk of acquiring Chagas disease if they have emigrated from rural Mexico, Central America, or South America, have lived in a house made with mud walls and a thatched roof (where triatomine bugs hide), and have been in contact with the bug.

Chagas disease primarily affects individuals from endemic areas (Mexico, Central America, or South America) who acquired the infection before arriving in the United States. Children born to infected mothers are at risk for congenital transmission of Chagas disease.

Why be concerned about Chagas disease in the U.S.?

- An estimated 300,000 infected people are living in the United States, nearly all of whom were originally infected in endemic areas. These persons often do not know they are infected and are at risk for the severe cardiac or gastrointestinal problems from the disease. Diagnosis and treatment can reduce this risk.

- Donor screening to detect *T. cruzi* in the blood supply began in early 2007. As of June 2013, more than 1,800 confirmed positive infections among blood donors had been reported to AABB (formerly American Association of Blood Banks) by blood centers. While these efforts have likely reduced the risk of acquiring Chagas disease from blood products, the large number of positive donors identified indicates that many people with Chagas disease do not know they are infected and could benefit from diagnosis and treatment.

- Infected triatomine bugs and wild animals that harbor *T. cruzi* infection have been found in the United States for decades. There are some reports of vectorborne (spread by contact with the bug) infection originating in the United States.

CDC is currently working to address Chagas disease by:

- Partnering with state and local healthdepartments to educate and advise health professionals to help them better care for patients with Chagas disease

- Supporting physicians and patients in the United States with confirmatory diagnostic testing and release of treatment drugs available under investigational protocols

- Increasing provider awareness of Chagas disease, including publishing free, Web-based Continuing Medical Education (CME) and Continuing Nursing Education (CNE) programs

- Conducting studies that assessed Chagas disease perception, awareness, and understanding among patients and health care providers to help direct education outreach and address barriers to care for Chagas disease patients

- Developing, in collaboration with a number of other groups including academic institutions and partner organizations, improved diagnostic tests for Chagas disease and ways to determine if treatment has been successful

- Collaborating with investigators to determine the congenital risk of Chagas disease among at-risk mothers living in the United States

Additional work needed includes:

- Improve outreach to healthcare providers so they can better care for patients with Chagas disease

- Determine the risk of transmission of *T. cruzi* in the United States to help prevent new infections from bugs and from mothers with Chagas disease to their unborn babies

- Quantify the number of people with heart disease caused by Chagas disease

SEE ALSO   *Centers for Disease Control and Prevention (CDC); Food Preparation and Food Safety; Global Health Initiatives; Health-Related Education and Information Access; Insect-Borne Diseases; Malaria; Neglected Tropical Diseases; NGOs and Health Care: Deliverance or Dependence; Sanitation and Hygiene; Vulnerable Populations; Water Supplies and Access to Clean Water; Waterborne Diseases; World Health Organization: Organization, Funding, and Enforcement Powers; Zoonotic (Animal-Borne) Diseases*

BIBLIOGRAPHY

Books

Boireau, Pascal, Food and Agriculture Organization of the United Nations, World Health Organization. *Multicriteria-Based Ranking for Risk Management of Food-Borne Parasites.* Rome: Food and Agriculture Organization of the United Nations, 2014.

Caffrey, Conor R. *Parasitic Helminths: Targets, Screens, Drugs and Vaccines.* Weinheim, Germany: Wiley-Blackwell, 2012.

Hotez, Peter J. *Forgotten People, Forgotten Diseases: The Neglected Tropical Diseases and Their Impact on Global Health and Development,* 2nd ed. Washington, DC: ASM Press, 2013.

Lamb, Tracey J., ed. *Immunity to Parasitic Infections.* Chichester, UK: Wiley, 2012.

Petersen, Eskild, Lin H. Chen, and Patricia Schlagenhauf-Lawlor, eds. *A Geographic Guide to Infectious Diseases.* Chichester, UK: Wiley-Blackwell, 2011.

McGuire, Robert A., and Philip R. P. Coelho. *Parasites, Pathogens, and Progress: Diseases and Economic Development.* Cambridge, MA: MIT Press, 2011.

Periodicals

Cox, F. E. G. "History of Human Parasitology." *Clinical Microbiology Review* 15, no. 4 (October 1, 2002): 596–612. Available online at http://cmr.asm.org/content/15/4/595.full.pdf%20html (accessed January 23, 2015).

Faulkner, Charles T., and Karl Reinhard. "A Retrospective Examination of Paleoparasitology and Its Establishment." *Journal of Parasitology* 100, no. 3 (2014): 253–259.

Furtado, João M., Justine R. Smith, Rubens Belfort, Devin Gattey, and Kevin L. Winthrop. "Toxoplasmosis: A Global Threat." *Journal of Global Infectious Diseases* 3, no. 3 (July 2011): 281–284.

Hubert Jaeger, Lauren, and Alena Mayo Iñiguez. "Molecular Paleoparasitological Hybridization Approach as Effective Tool for Diagnosing Human Intestinal Parasites from Scarce Archaeological Remains." *PLOS ONE* 9, no. 8, (August 27, 2014): e105910.

Kim, Myeong-Ju, Dong Hoon Shin, Mi-Jin Song, Hye-Young Song, and Min Seo. "Paleoparasitological Surveys for Detection of Helminth Eggs in Archaeological Sites of Jeolla-do and Jeju-do." *Korean Journal of Parasitology* 51, no. 4 (2013): 489–492.

Molnár, Peter K., Susan J. Kutz, Bryanne M. Hoar, and Andrew P. Dobson. "Metabolic Approaches to Understanding Climate Change Impacts on Seasonal Host-Macroparasite Dynamics." *Ecology Letters* 16, no. 1 (January 2013): 9–21.

Patz, Jonathan A., Thaddeus K. Graczyk, Nina Geller, and Amy Y. Vittor. "Effects of Environmental Change on Emerging Parasitic Diseases." *International Journal for Parasitology* 30, nos. 12–13 (2000): 1395–1405.

Websites

"10 Facts on Malaria." *World Health Organization (WHO).* http://www.who.int/features/factfiles/malaria/en/ (accessed January 23, 2015).

"About Parasites." *U.S. Centers for Disease Control and Prevention (CDC).* http://www.cdc.gov/parasites/about.html (accessed January 23, 2015).

"Amoebiasis." *World Health Organization (WHO).* http://www.who.int/ith/diseases/amoebiasis/en/ (accessed January 23, 2015).

"Climate Change and Human Health—Risks and Responses." *World Health Organization (WHO).* http://www.who.int/globalchange/summary/en/index5.html (accessed January 25, 2015).

"Ectoparasitic Infections." *U.S. Centers for Disease Control and Prevention (CDC).* http://www.cdc.gov/std/treatment/2010/ectoparasitic.htm (accessed January 23, 2015).

"Parasitic Diseases." *U.S. National Institutes of Health (NIH).* http://www.nlm.nih.gov/medlineplus/parasiticdiseases.html (accessed January 23, 2015).

"Soil-Transmitted Helminth Infections." *World Health Organization (WHO).* http://www.who.int/mediacentre/factsheets/fs366/en/ (accessed January 23, 2015).

"Toxoplasmosis Frequently Asked Questions (FAQs)." *U.S. Centers for Disease Control and Prevention (CDC).* http://www.cdc.gov/parasites/toxoplasmosis/gen_info/faqs.html (accessed January 23, 2015).

Melanie R. Plenda

Pharmaceutical Dumping (Drug Dumping)

⊕ Introduction

Pharmaceutical dumping or drug dumping is the improper disposal of medications and medicinal products. A growing body of scientific evidence shows that environmental contamination by very small amounts of medical compounds has become ubiquitous throughout the world's waterways, although usually only in amounts that are in the parts per billion or trillion. In addition to contamination that occurs when unmetabolized drugs are flushed by consumers, pharmaceuticals also enter into the environment through dumping by pharmaceutical manufacturers or hospitals, eventually finding their way into surface, ground, and drinking water.

Pharmaceutical manufacturers, utilities, and government officials maintain that such trace levels of medical compounds are far below the threshold for having any adverse effects on human beings. However, a number of studies have been conducted that show that drug pollution has severe adverse effects on wildlife. In addition, studies indicate drug pollution may play a role in the evolution of antibiotic resistant microbes. Furthermore, not enough research has been done on adverse effects that may arise as a result of interactions between different pharmaceutical compounds in the waste environment, or on the effects of long-term and continuous exposure to the mixtures. But due to the high cost of the technology required for the removal of pharmaceutical contamination from the environment, manufacturers and regulators have for the most part chosen to await further scientific evidence before action is considered necessary.

⊕ Historical Background

The presence of pharmaceuticals in the environment was first speculated about in scientific reports in the 1960s that questioned whether many of the synthetic chemicals produced and used by humans could break down naturally and, if not, be accumulating in waste. In the 1970s, the first scientific tests to detect pharmaceuticals in water systems were conducted in the United States. These tests found molecular by-products of aspirin and cholesterol drugs in sewage at wastewater treatment plants. Since then, the body of scientific knowledge on the subject has grown significantly, with tests for detecting pharmaceuticals in surface, estuary, ocean, ground, and tap water conducted by scientists in the Brazil, Canada, Denmark, Finland, France, Germany, Japan, the Netherlands, Switzerland, South Korea, the United Kingdom, and United States.

In 1998, two European scientific reports brought significant attention to the issue of pharmaceutical waste. One was a study on the large number of male fish in water downstream from wastewater treatment plants in the United Kingdom, which stated that male fish were developing egg yolks normally found in female fish. The change is thought to have been caused by types of pharmaceutical chemical known as endocrine disruptors, also known as steroid hormones, synthetic molecules that mimic the chemicals that control growth and reproduction, among other biological processes. That same year, a report was also published that found the molecular by-products of a heart medication in the middle of the North Sea. According to the U.S. Geological Survey (USGS), "detectable concentrations of a drug in such a large body of water suggested the need for further research."

In 1999 and 2000, the USGS sampled water from 139 streams in 30 U.S. states as part of a National Stream Reconnaissance research initiative that found 80 percent of the streams studied were contaminated by on average 7 and at most 38 different types of pollutants normally found in residential, industrial, or agricultural wastewater, including human and veterinary drugs and steroid hormones. The reports claimed that contaminants were found at levels that did not exceed drinking-water guidelines or health advisories, though guidelines for some compounds were not yet established. It also warned of the potential adverse effects of the exposure to

PHARMACEUTICAL WASTE AND ANTIBIOTIC RESISTANCE

Antibiotics and other pharmaceutical waste are discharged into the environment at higher rates when manufactured in developing countries such as India where environmental regulations are not as thoroughly enforced and treatment facilities not as advanced. In the past decade, scientists have established a link between pharmaceutical dumping and the evolution of multidrug-resistant superbugs. A Swedish study published in 2009 found that an amount equivalent to 45,000 doses of the antibiotic ciprofloxacin was discharged into the Isakavagu stream around Hyderabad by pharmaceutical manufacturers every day. Ciprofloxacin was once considered an antibiotic so powerful it was used as a last resort, but its discharge into the environment has given bacteria the kind of exposure needed to mutate and gain resistance.

India is host to over 5,000 pharmaceutical manufacturers that produce close to one-third of the world's antibiotics. The antibiotics produced are low-cost, generic medications, and Indian doctors had a tendency to overprescribe them, giving opportunities for bacteria to accumulate more resistance. Due to inadequate sanitation, this liberal use of antibiotics gradually helped undermine the drugs' effectiveness, as waterborne antibiotics mixed with bacteria in sewage and entered into drinking water, helping the evolution of superbugs as the antibiotics traveled in India's waterways. Animals and people drinking the contaminated water are at risk of becoming colonized by the drug-resistant bacteria.

As a result of the unregulated consumption and disposal of antibiotics in India, a mutation called NDM-1 occurred that allowed antibiotic resistance to be spread easily among different types of bacteria. NDM-1, or New Delhi metallo-beta-lactamase-1, was named after the Indian capital, where a Swedish man in 2007 first got an infection resistant to all standard antibiotics. Bacteria with the NDM-1 gene were found in 51 of 171 open drains and 2 of 50 samples of public tap water in samples taken in 2010 from sites in New Delhi.

In response to the international uproar over the possible global health implications of the NDM-1 mutation, the Indian government began the difficult task of regulating antibiotic use and disposal of a population of 1.2 billion. Most of the time, antibiotics can be obtained in India without a prescription, so India began requiring pharmacists to keep records for up to two years for audits and inspection. In 2010, a pipeline to a modern sewage treatment plant was built to divert further contamination of the waters surrounding Hyderabad. And in 2011, the use of antibiotics began to be tracked in India's over 100,000 hospitals.

With its densely populated cities, over consumption of antibiotics, and lack of adequate sanitation and environmental regulation, scientists are concerned India's rivers and streams have become a fertile breeding ground for antibiotic resistance. India only treats 30 percent of the 10.1 billion gallons of sewage it generates every day. Without modern underground drainage systems, open drains overflow during the rainy season. An estimated 100 million Indian people carry germs with the NDM-1 gene, as of 2012.

the complex mixtures that form from the interaction of different pollutants. Between 2002 to 2008, the USGS conducted over 160 more studies assessing water quality in U.S. streams, wells, sediment, and soil.

In March 2008, the issue of pharmaceuticals in the environment received a large dose of media attention when the Associated Press (AP) published a three-part investigative report on pharmaceuticals in the drinking water of 41 million Americans, reprinted as front-page news in publications worldwide. The first part summarized a survey of the water providers for the 50 largest U.S. cities as well as small communities from all 50 states.

Through interviews with over 230 officials, academics, and scientists, as well as reviews of scientific articles and analysis of federal drinking water databases, the report presented a comprehensive profile of the extent of drug pollution in U.S. water that included 24 major metropolitan areas and contamination of 36 of 62 watersheds of major U.S. water providers. In the second part, the report presented the sides of the debate over the potential long-term effects of small amounts of pharmaceuticals, with an overview of studies on their effects on aquatic organisms and also the secrecy in which studies on water quality must be conducted under, out of fears by U.S. officials that disclosure could cause an unwarranted public panic or even be a national security threat. The third part identified both consumers and manufacturers as sources of the contamination, and explains how pharmaceuticals that reach wastewater require an expensive, technologically advanced treatment process called reverse osmosis in order to be removed, or in some cases cannot be removed at all.

The report also explained how the chlorine typically used to treat wastewater may actually chemically transform the compounds into something that may potentially be more toxic, and that while the effects of individual compounds are known, the interactions in the cocktail of medical compounds found in wastewater have not sufficiently been studied.

In April 2008, a month after the publication of the AP report on pharmaceuticals in U.S. water, a congressional hearing was held in which U.S. senators questioned the U.S. Environmental Protection Agency (EPA) about why water providers were not required to test for pharmaceuticals, and, if federal scientists have known about the contamination, why they insisted on shrouding the issue in secrecy while still maintaining that the water is safe to drink. The EPA's answer was that, due to the lack of conclusive evidence of the contamination having any adverse effects on humans, it would be unreasonable and expensive to require testing by utilities, and that they should only test for pharmaceuticals if they are financially and technically capable. Some experts' testimonies disagreed with the EPA's method of "wait and see," and senators strongly urged them to do more. However, the EPA still does not require water providers to test for pharmaceuticals and the U.S. Food and Drug Administration (FDA) has never rejected a new drug application based on environmental impact, as of early 2015.

⊕ Impacts and Issues

Pharmaceutical compounds also enter into the environment through a variety of methods, including dumping by pharmaceutical manufacturers. In a 2004–2009 study of 26 wastewater treatment plants by the USGS, the muscle relaxant metaxalone, the pain reliever oxycodone, the opioid methadone, the sedative butalbital, and other pharmaceuticals were found in wastewater at two treatment plants downstream of pharmaceutical manufacturers. In 2009, the AP also reported that at least 271 million pounds (122.9 million kilograms) of pharmaceuticals were legally released by U.S. manufacturers and drugmakers into waterways that provide drinking water. Approximately 249 million pounds (112.9 million

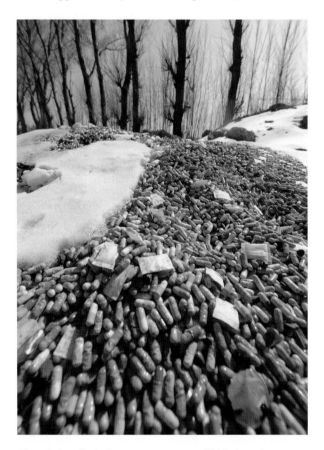

Discarded medical pills are strewn over a rubbish dump in a suburb of Beijing, China. © Gou Yige/AFP/Getty Images.

kilograms) were the antiseptics phenol and hydrogen peroxide; 8 million pounds (3.6 million kilograms) were a skin bleaching cream; 3 million pounds (1.4 million kilograms) were nicotine from patches; and the rest were an assortment of 18 other compounds identified as both industrial chemicals and active pharmaceutical ingredients including treatments for head lice, worms, and the antibiotic tetracycline hydrochloride.

Agribusiness and veterinary practices are some of the largest consumers of pharmaceuticals such as antibiotics and steroid hormones, which are used to keep animals healthy and promote growth. Approximately 70 percent of all antibiotics used globally are given to livestock, and usually only 10 percent of the antibiotic can be absorbed into their bodies. The rest is excreted as manure that, if used as a fertilizer, may pass traces of pharmaceuticals to crops, as in a 2005 study that showed a fractional but significant amount of antibiotics absorbed by corn, lettuce, and potatoes. The pharmaceuticals can also seep through the soil into aquifers that provide drinking water or contaminate surface water through runoff. Some of it may also spread through the environment when livestock are eaten by predators, as was the case of the collapse of vulture populations in Pakistan due to residue of diclofenac, a common anti-inflammatory medication, in cattle carcasses in early in the first decade of the 21st century.

Another way pharmaceutical compounds reach public waterways and drinking supplies is through use by consumers. When drugs are used, what is not absorbed by the body is excreted in urine and flushed. Some drugs are absorbed better than others: the common pain reliever acetaminophen is absorbed up to 80 percent, while only half of the antibiotic ciprofloxacin can be absorbed, and only 20 percent of the medication metformin for diabetes is absorbed. Although some medical compounds do break down in the treatment process, few water treatment facilities have the advanced and expensive technology required to completely remove pharmaceutical contaminants, so trace levels of pharmaceutical compounds eventually make their way into drinking water and waterways. Because the use or improper disposal of illicit drugs is also more common in urban areas, trace levels of illicit substances make their way into the drinking water of cities, though some are also found in rural areas. In all cases, pharmaceutical mixture compositions found in drinking water are linked to usage patterns of a particular area.

Expired drugs also make their way into the environment through improper disposal in toilets or sinks. Flushing of expired drugs down the toilet is common, in households as well as hospitals and nursing homes. The AP also estimated that 250 million pounds (113.4 million kilograms) of pharmaceuticals and contaminated packaging are disposed of improperly into garbage bins, sinks, and toilets at hospital and nursing homes. The EPA, which does not regulate the disposal of hazardous

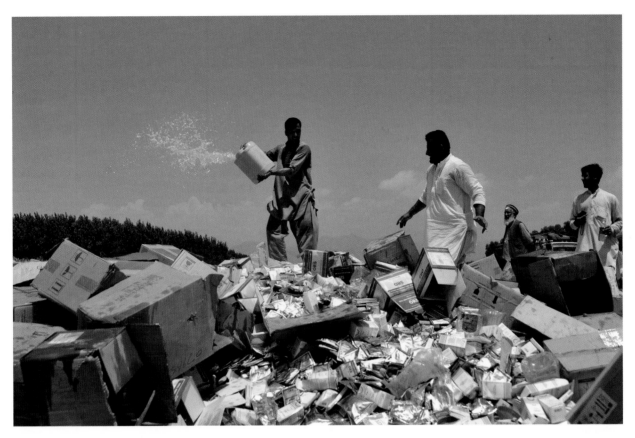

Health workers from the Afghanistan Health Ministry pour fuel over expired medicines collected from various hospitals and pharmacies before setting them alight on the outskirts of Jalalabad in Nangarhar Province. © *Noorullah Shirzada/AFP/Getty Images.*

waste from hospitals, advises that unwanted medications be put into garbage bins rather than toilets or sinks, so they might be contained in landfills and possibly incinerated rather than being discharged into the sewage system where removal is more difficult. However, even if contained in landfills, pharmaceuticals may still reach waterways through runoff.

Expired drugs are also being dumped in massive quantities into nations appealing for humanitarian assistance under the guise of charitable donations. Many countries that accept charitable donations of pharmaceuticals lack the infrastructure to hold or disseminate them.

An audit conducted by the World Health Organization (WHO) of charitable donations to Albania in May 1999 revealed that 50 percent of the drugs donated by nonmedical organizations were either inadequately labeled, improperly packaged, irrelevant to the crisis, or expired, ultimately ending up as waste. In another study of drugs donated during the crisis in Bosnia and Herzegovina between 1992 and 1996, the authors estimate that more that more than 50 percent of the 55 million to 68 million pounds (25 million to 30.8 million kilograms) of medical supplies donated during the crisis were also inappropriate. By shifting the burden of disposal of pharmaceutical waste onto countries that lack modern facilities,

the negative effects on the environment can be amplified, prompting the WHO to publish "Guidelines for Safe Disposal of Unwanted Pharmaceuticals in and after Emergencies" in 1999.

Endocrine Disrupting Compounds

Environmental contamination by endocrine disrupting compounds (EDCs) have always been of particular concern due to the powerful effect they have on the hormone systems, and thus many aspects of an organism's biology, reproduction in particular. In addition to plastic and pesticides, pharmaceutical waste is another large source of EDCs, as the active ingredients in birth control, hormone therapies, and skin creams. Nonmedical exposure to EDCs has been shown to cause reproductive abnormalities, cancer, and birth defects. In some well-documented cases, even medical exposure can have unintended effects. For example, the use of diethylstilboestrol (DES) for breast cancer treatment and to prevent miscarriage in pregnant women throughout the mid-20th century was widespread until children exposed to DES in the womb developed reproductive abnormalities upon puberty, and the drug was quietly phased out.

Because of the possible human health implications, the effects of EDCs on wildlife have been the subject of intense research. Contamination of the environment by EDCs was long suspected but first detected in the water of U.S. rivers in 1984. Following the discovery of feminized male fish that produced egg yolks normally found in females downstream from wastewater treatment plants in the United Kingdom in the late 1990s, studies on EDCs and other pharmaceuticals' effect on aquatic organisms increased exponentially.

Some of the most cited research on the topic was done by the USGS in collaboration with the U.S. Fish and Wildlife Service on aquatic life in Lake Mead, the largest reservoir in the United States and main source of drinking water for Las Vegas and Southern California. The fish studied live in an environment contaminated by the 180 million gallons (681.4 million liters) of wastewater discharged into it every day, and fish populations have lower amounts of sex hormones, smaller reproductive parts, and decreased sperm count. In comparison of water before and after it mixes with wastewater, the contaminated water was found to have 646 more times the amount of EDCs.

In similar studies, EDCs' effect on wildlife has also been documented in waterways throughout North America and the world. In a seven-year Canadian study, the active ingredient of birth control pills was dripped at levels found in contaminated aquatic habitats into a pristine lake in Ontario. After seven weeks, male fathead minnows began to be feminized, and eventually stopped reproducing altogether, leading to a near extinction of the species, leading scientists to believe that similar die-offs occur in the wild. Severely impaired reproductive function has also been found in Japanese zebrafish and Atlantic salmon in the North Sea off the coast of Norway, as well as shortened life spans of fish and prawns living in Chinese wastewater and stunted oysters in waters off the coast of Singapore. In a study conducted in the United Kingdom in 2004, 86 percent of male fish sampled in 51 sites were found to be feminized. All 160 wastewater treatment plants tested in another 2012 study done in the United Kingdom had more EE2, the active hormonal ingredient in birth control, than the current recommended European Union (EU) guidelines, with over 80 treatment plants with 13 times the maximum amount.

Regulation

Without conclusive scientific evidence that trace levels of EDCs or other pharmaceuticals have any harmful effects on human health, their disposal has gone largely unregulated until the early 2010s. Rather than the costly removal of all pharmaceutical pollutants, the current strategy to mitigate potential harmful effects is the prioritization of medical compounds with largest potential risk to human health. For example, in 2013, the EU added pharmaceuticals for the first time to its "pollutant watch list" of the Water Framework Directive, by adding EE2 and E2, the

two active EDCs in birth control, as well as diclofenac, a pain medication. However, the legislation only requires member states to monitor levels of pollutants without any obligations for their phaseout or removal except to keep levels below maximums by enforcement date. Enforcement, which was set for 2015, may not occur until 2018. In addition, due to a compromise with the pharmaceutical industry, the deadlines for complying to the standards were extended from 2021 to 2027.

As outlined by the WHO in their information sheet on "Pharmaceuticals in Drinking Water," the logic for the lack of urgency for regulation of pharmaceutical waste is due to the extremely low amounts in which pharmaceuticals occur in the environment, often less than one part per billion. Because these trace levels of individual medical compounds are 10 to 1,000 times lower than the standard minimum dosage for any clinical effects to be observed, the WHO and other regulatory organizations maintain that the compounds pose no threat to human health. However, the document does acknowledge the gaps in knowledge concerning the issue, such as whether the complex mixtures of trace amounts of pharmaceuticals might be producing more subtle, synergistic effects.

⊕ Future Implications

As the consumption of pharmaceuticals is likely to continue increasing due to aging populations and developing markets, the issue of how to dispose of pharmaceutical waste is likely to grow in both relevance and severity. The value of the global pharmaceutical market is projected to reach $1.1 trillion to $1.2 trillion by 2017. Over one-third of this market is controlled by the 10 largest drug companies, 6 based in the United States and 4 in Europe. In 2017, over 50 percent of all pharmaceuticals will be in emerging markets, primarily in Brazil, Russia, India, and China.

As of early 2015, the lack of conclusive evidence on the adverse health risks that pharmaceutical waste poses to humans is used as justification for manufacturers and regulators to avoid the high cost of removing the pollutants. In a comparison done by the AP in 2008, the only treatment process shown to remove all pharmaceutical contaminants, reverse osmosis, can cost as much as 15 times more per month for the average U.S. family than the next best treatment, granular activated carbon filtering, while another treatment, ozonation, is cheaper though even less effective. In 2012, during the debate about whether to regulate levels of the birth control hormone EE2 found in the water in the EU, the cost for building a treatment plant for a UK town with a population of 250,000 was estimated at US$10.3 million and approximately US$1.3 million a year to operate, with a total cost of US$51.5 million for the treatment of water in Wales alone.

Because of these high costs, most water treatment facilities still use the standard procedure of filtration and disinfection with chlorine, even though studies show this may actually transform some pharmaceutical compounds, like the common pain reliever acetaminophen, into a more toxic substance.

SEE ALSO *Antibiotic/Antimicrobial Resistance; Drug/ Substance Abuse; Life Expectancy and Aging Populations; Methicillin-Resistant* Staphylococcus aureus *(MRSA); NGOs and Health Care: Deliverance or Dependence; Pharmaceutical Research, Testing, and Access; Sanitation and Hygiene; Waterborne Diseases; Water Supplies and Access to Clean Water; World Health Organization: Organization, Funding, and Enforcement Powers*

BIBLIOGRAPHY

Books

American Chemical Society, and Rolf U. Halden, ed. *Contaminants of Emerging Concern in the Environment: Ecological and Human Health Considerations.* Washington, DC: American Chemical Society, 2010.

Brooks, Bryan W., and Duane B. Huggett, eds. *Human Pharmaceuticals in the Environment Current and Future Perspectives.* New York: Springer, 2012.

Donohoe, Martin, ed. *Public Health and Social Justice.* San Francisco, CA: Jossey-Bass, 2013.

Eldridge, J. Charles., and James T. Stevens, eds. *Endocrine Toxicology*, 3rd ed. New York: Informa Healthcare, 2010.

Larsen, Laura, ed. *Environmental Health Sourcebook: Basic Consumer Health Information about the Environment and Its Effects on Human Health*, 3rd ed. Detroit, MI: Omnigraphics, 2010.

Roig, Benoit, ed. *Pharmaceuticals in the Environment: Current Knowledge and Need Assessment to Reduce Presence and Impact.* London: IWA, 2010.

Shadlen, Kenneth C. *Intellectual Property, Pharmaceuticals and Public Health: Access to Drugs in Developing Countries.* Cheltenham, UK: Edward Elgar, 2011.

Pharmaceuticals in the Nation's Drinking Water: Assessing Potential Risks and Actions to Address the Issue. Washington, DC: Government Printing Office, 2014.

Periodicals

Arnold, Kathryn, et al. "Assessing Risks and Impacts of Pharmaceuticals in the Environment on Wildlife and Ecosystems." *Biology Letters* 9, no. 4 (August 23, 2013). Available online at http://rsbl.royalsocietypublishing.org/content/9/4/20130492.full (accessed March 27, 2015).

Owen, Richard, and Susan Jobling. "Environmental Science: The Hidden Costs of Flexible Fertility." *Nature* 485, no. 7399 (2012): 441.

Websites

Donn, Jeff. "Tons of Released Drugs Taint U.S. Water." *U.S. News & World Report*, April 19, 2009. http://www.usnews.com/science/articles/2009/04/19/tons-of-released-drugs-taint-us-water?PageNr=1 (accessed April 9, 2015).

Donn, Jeff, Martha Mendoza, and Justin Pritchard. "Health Care Industry Sends Tons of Drugs into Nation's Wastewater System." *Associated Press*, March 9, 2008. http://hosted.ap.org/specials/interactives/pharmawater_site/sept14a.html (accessed March 27, 2015).

"Emerging Contaminants in the Environment" *U.S. Geological Survey (USGS).* http://toxics.usgs.gov/regional/emc/ (accessed March 16, 2015)

Gale, Jason, and Adi Narayan. "Drug-Defying Germs from India Speed Post-antibiotic Era." *Bloomberg Business*, May 7, 2012. http://www.bloomberg.com/news/articles/2012-05-07/drug-defying-germs-from-india-speed-post-antibiotic-era (accessed March 27, 2015).

"Guidelines for Safe Disposal of Unwanted Pharmaceuticals in and after Emergencies." *World Health Organization (WHO).* http://www.who.int/water_sanitation_health/medicalwaste/unwantpharm.pdf (accessed March 17, 2015).

"Information Sheet: Pharmaceuticals in Drinking-water." *World Health Organization (WHO)*, 1999. http://www.who.int/water_sanitation_health/medicalwaste/unwantpharm.pdf (accessed March 17, 2015).

"National Stream Reconnaisance." *U.S. Geological Survey (USGS).* http://toxics.usgs.gov/regional/emc/streams.html(accessed March 16, 2015)

"Pharmaceuticals and Personal Care Products (PPCP)." *U.S. Environmental Protection Agency (EPA).* http://www.epa.gov/ppcp/ (accessed March 16, 2015).

Josh Phillip Cabrido

Pharmaceutical Research, Testing, and Access

⊕ Introduction

The research and testing of safe and effective pharmaceutical therapies is important, so it is critical that tests of drugs yield reliable evidence on the effectiveness, safe dosage, and possible harms. Medical interventions also are a finite resource, making the time spent identifying the proper drugs and doses an equally important commodity.

The development, manufacturing, and distribution of medications is a costly endeavor for pharmaceutical companies due to the many steps involved in ensuring safety. In 2013, Pharmafile, a UK-based news service for the pharmaceutical industry, estimated that the pharmaceutical industry invested approximately US$1.3 billion to bring a new drug to market, and a significant portion of research funding is spent on basic "bench sciences" to identify target sites and the synthesis of new compounds. Research spending also includes testing different combinations of medications together, adjusting their chemistry to make them adaptable to a variety of climate conditions or environments, improving their delivery methods, and reverse-engineering existing drugs that have come off patent. In addition, pharmaceutical companies must adhere to strict ethical guidelines when completing their research. All of these factors go into how much pharmaceutical companies decide to charge for the pharmaceuticals they produce.

⊕ Historical Background

The discovery of natural compounds and synthetic pharmaceutical drugs has played a critical role in improving overall health and life expectancy throughout human history. Around 3000 BCE, the Chinese Yan Emperor found that the herb *ma huang* could be used to treat coughing spells. In approximately 300 BCE, the Greeks documented a process for extracting morphine from damaged poppy seeds in the form of opium.

Centuries later, thousands of 17th-century British Royal Navy sailors were afflicted with scurvy, a disease causing bleeding gums, jaundice, and ultimately death if left untreated. Scurvy results from a diet lacking in vitamin C, an essential nutrient typically found in vegetables and citrus fruits. The human body requires vitamin C to make connective tissue; without it, weak connective tissues can result in hemorrhages and capillary bleeding. In 1747, Scottish naval physician James Lind (1716–1794) performed one of the first controlled trials to test several of the commonly used scurvy treatment methods. Lind's experiment involved assigning 12 afflicted soldiers to one of six possible treatments: apple cider; oranges and lemons; vinegar; diluted oil of vitriol; seawater; or a mixture containing garlic, mustard seed, and other ingredients. Lind then observed the soldiers receiving oranges and lemons (both high in vitamin C) were the first to recover from the disease, followed by the soldiers receiving apple cider. Captain James Cook (1728–1779) implemented these findings in his three-year voyage around the world, during which not a single sailor died from scurvy. Unfortunately, the Royal Navy did not require all British ships to have an adequate provision of lemon juice until nearly 1800.

It is not uncommon to observe delays between research, testing, and access to pharmaceutical breakthroughs. Discoveries are not necessarily followed by their widespread adoption and as a result, those most in need of new drugs and treatments are not always the first to receive them. And although pharmaceutical interventions exist for an ever-increasing number of conditions, there is still a demand for many basic, lifesaving, medicines in developing countries. The World Health Organization (WHO) refers to the drugs and medications that satisfy the priority health-care needs of a population as essential medicines, whereas drugs that are used to address non-life-threatening conditions generally are termed lifestyle medicines. The WHO recommends that all essential medicines "are available at all times in adequate amounts, be affordable, and have a proven efficacy, quality and safety." Lifestyle medicines are costly and generally available only to the more-affluent echelons within a given society.

The experiment on Royal Navy soldiers carried out by Lind had many of the elements of the modern clinical trial, but it lacked sufficient numbers of participants (and statistical power) to be applicable to the general population. The first clinical trial in modern times to use the experimental techniques; randomization, double-blinding, and placebo control occurred in 1943, when researchers identified streptomycin as a novel antibiotic treatment for life-threatening infections. The medication was moderately effective when it was used on U.S. Army soldiers near the end of World War II (1939–1945). Merck & Co. manufactured a limited supply of streptomycin and exported it to the United Kingdom in 1946. The Medical Research Council (MRC) decided to test the effectiveness of streptomycin in the treatment of pulmonary tuberculosis.

Randomization was a statistical concept introduced by mathematician R. A. Fisher (1890–1962) in 1926. The vital element of randomized medical experiments is the unpredictability of the next assignment. The physician's interpretation of treatment effects are not enough to provide reliable evidence. Randomization can remove the subjective biases that might be introduced into the experiment by the investigators. Randomly assigning study subjects to treatment conditions also increases the chances that each group will be relatively balanced with respect to unmeasured characteristics. Following an ideal randomization procedure yields treatment groups that are comparable in terms of age, sex, race, socioeconomic status, and other factors. A randomized clinical trial often is a study comparing the effects of a particular intervention against an alternative treatment, control, or placebo.

A placebo is an inactive substance with no therapeutic effect that the study subject believes is a medical treatment. Pharmaceutical placebos usually are pills or injections that have the identical appearance to the substance being investigated but lack the active ingredient. The intention of including placebos in medical research is to separate the specific treatment effects from the clinical setting effect. Context, healing expectations, and the treatment environment can influence study subjects considerably, especially when an outcome is difficult to quantify, such as changes in pain or mood. Use of a placebo successfully conceals the treatment to which the subject has been randomly assigned.

This combination of random assignment, balanced groups, and use of placebos are important for obtaining reliable information on drugs and medicines. For example, Thomas Karlowski conducted a clinical trial in 1975 to test the effects of vitamin C on the common cold. The investigators were pressed to begin the trial in order to capitalize on the regional "cold season," and as a result were unable to obtain an adequate placebo for comparison. Vitamin C (also known as ascorbic acid)

has a distinct bitter taste, whereas the placebo pill the investigators used was made of lactose (the sugar found in milk). The study subjects reportedly "tasted the contents of their capsules and professed to know whether they were taking the ascorbic acid or the placebo," and a significant proportion of the subjects correctly identified which treatment they had received. As for the efficacy of vitamin C against the common cold? The data suggested that vitamin C reduced the duration of cold symptoms, provided the subjects thought they had taken vitamin C. Conversely, there was a higher rate of colds among subjects who thought they were receiving the placebo but actually were receiving the vitamin C.

The vitamin C experiment is an example of the placebo effect—the improvement or worsening of symptoms after taking an inactive drug or treatment. For example, in a study on chronic low back pain, half of the patients in the experiment were told the activity they would be performing (simple leg-flexion) might cause them to experience an increase in back pain. The other half of the participants were told the same activity would have no overall effect on back pain. The group receiving the negative information about the leg-flexion task were more afraid to perform the activity and also reported experiencing more pain than the other treatment group.

Because of the placebo effect, many studies are conducted "blinded." Blinded study subjects are unaware of the treatment group to which they have been assigned. Investigators or researchers also may be blinded. Blinding the investigators attempts to remove biases that might occur during the analysis and interpretation of the study results. When both subjects and investigators are blinded the study is referred to as "double blinded."

In the streptomycin trial, the results of the treatment groups (presented via x-ray "films") were assessed by an independent panel of experts who did not know which condition the patient had been assigned. The passage from the original paper outlining this method reads: "The films have been viewed by two radiologists and a clinician, each reading the films independently and not knowing if the films were of C (control) or S (streptomycin) cases."

The Development of the Pharmaceutical Industry

Early pharmaceuticals were derived primarily from plant sources. Given the relatively unrefined methods typically used to procure these substances, their purity and effectiveness tended to be inconsistent and unreliable. These unpredictable variations in potency made individual dosages almost impossible to determine. Drug quality could be either too concentrated and hazardous or too dilute to induce any treatment effects. Swiss-German physician and scientist Philippus Theophastrus Bombast von Hohenheim (1493–1541) often is referred to as the founder of toxicology for establishing the adage "the dose makes the poison." During this period, medical and therapeutic substances were prepared by apothecaries, a role now reserved for pharmacists or chemists.

As the science of chemistry gained interest and investors, apothecary companies began to mass-produce drugs such as morphine, quinine, and strychnine. In 1826, French pharmacists Pierre-Joseph Pelletier (1788–1842) and Joseph-Bienaimé Caventou (1795–1877) isolated quinine, a substance used in the treatment of malaria. Native to Peru, quinine originally was derived from cinchona tree bark and used to treat shivering in cold climates. In their laboratory in Paris, Pelletier and Caventou processed 150 tons of imported cinchona bark into pure quinine in what could be described as the first large-scale pharmaceutical manufacturing endeavor. Within a few years, Emanuel Merck (1794–1855) established the E. Merck chemical factory and began producing pills, syrups, and powders for commercial and wholesale purchases. Merck (now known as Merck, Sharp & Dohme) remains one of the largest pharmaceutical companies in the world.

Pharmaceutical companies continued to discover new forms of treatment throughout the 19th century. Rudolf Buchheim (1820–1879) and Oswald Schmiedeberg (1838–1921) introduced the scientific method and experimentation to the pharmacy discipline. Buchheim published the seminal textbook of pharmacology in 1856. Schmiedeberg became his successor and in 1872 created the first Institute of Pharmacology in eastern France. This period witnessed German physician Robert Koch (1843–1910) formulating his famous "four postulates" on the establishment of steps for determining the cause of a particular infectious disease. Renowned physician Paul Ehrlich (1854–1915) later asserted that disease-causing organisms could be targeted selectively with specific medicines. Major developments in the pharmaceutical sciences in the 19th century include the developments of tablets, gelatin capsules, and the hypodermic syringe.

The number of new pharmaceutical companies and drugs grew steadily in the beginning of the 20th century. Hormones (estrogen, testosterone, and progesterone) were discovered in the 1920s and 1930s, along with vaccines and vitamins. The antibiotic revolution in medicine initially began with the release of Prontosil from Bayer laboratories. Prontosil was a sulfa drug used to treat a wide range of bacterial conditions, including streptococcus. Unfortunately, there were not sufficient regulatory mechanisms in place to oversee the development and safety of new medications in the United States. As a result, 105 deaths occurred in 1937 when the S.E. Massengill Company manufactured and distributed "Elixir Sulfanilamide" throughout the southern United States. The elixir was made using the poisonous solvent diethylene glycol, and the company had not conducted any tests for toxicity or safety. Not long after, Alexander Fleming (1881–1955) stumbled onto penicillin, and the antibiotic was mass produced by Charles Pfizer & Co. during World War II.

After the war, the pharmaceutical industry had the ability to mass-produce and distribute newly developed substances. This era saw progressions in the use of diuretics (drugs that promote urination) and antihypertensives (drugs that lower blood pressure) for cardiovascular disease. Researchers also identified Paclitaxel, one of the first cancer medicines. Paclitaxel was extracted from the bark of the Pacific yew tree after scientists discovered it possessed antitumor effects. During this period drugs that acted on the central nervous system were introduced, and psychopharmacology (the study of the effect of drugs on the mind and behavior) flourished.

Ethical Guidelines

The atrocities committed during World War II under the guise of Nazi science resulted in the construction of the Nuremberg Code. Originally drafted by Dr. Leo Alexander (1905–1985) in 1947 as a set of standards for conducting legitimate research, these ethical principles consist of 10 points addressing the use of human subjects in medical experimentation. Included among them are the requirements for informed consent, proper experimental design that provides useful information for the good of society, and the judicious reduction of unnecessary risks. In 1948, the World Medical Association drafted the Geneva Declaration, expanding ethical guidance and providing a collection of moral precepts for health-care providers, commonly referred to as the "Physician's Oath." These articles later would be codified in the Declaration of Helsinki, the document generally viewed as the centerpiece for research ethics.

Despite explicitly addressing what was considered appropriate ethical behavior for clinicians and scientists, these edicts were not law, so violations had no legal repercussions. This lack of regulatory framework was exposed when the German pharmaceutical company Chemie Grünenthal marketed and sold the substance thalidomide. Beginning in 1957, thalidomide was advertised as a treatment for morning sickness during pregnancy. This so-called wonder drug was prescribed and sold in almost 50 different countries around the world. In 1961, Australian obstetrician William McBride (1927–) suspected thalidomide of causing birth defects. These findings later were confirmed by German pediatrician Widukind Lenz (1919–1995). Thalidomide caused thousands of deformities and deaths of children across Europe, Asia, and Australia. Chemie Grünenthal stopped manufacturing and distributing the drug as a result of the overwhelming evidence provided by McBride and Lenz. Thanks to the diligent work of Dr. Frances Oldham Kelsey (1914–), the U.S. Food and Drug Administration (FDA) halted the distribution of thalidomide due to a lack of scientific evidence regarding its safety and efficacy.

The FDA had been created at the dawn of the 20th century with the intention of regulating foods. However, prompted by the Elixir Sulfanilamide catastrophe in 1937, the U.S. Congress passed the Food, Drug, and Cosmetic Act a year later. Congress approved an amendment to the Food, Drug, and Cosmetic Act in 1962 that included the provision that drugs must not only be safe but also effective. The amendment also stipulated the pharmaceutical companies must conduct testing on new drugs and substances by qualified personnel, and that subjects must provide informed consent before participating in any drug studies. The agency continues to adapt its regulatory ability in the constantly shifting landscape of pharmaceutical sciences.

The international medical and scientific community was shocked by the thalidomide calamity in the 1960s. At the 16th World Health Assembly in 1963, the WHO called for "ways and means of ensuring that drugs exported to a producing country comply with the drug control requirements which apply in that country for domestic use." In 1968, the WHO also launched a Pilot Research Project for International Drug Monitoring. This project sought to develop an international system to maintain records on adverse side effects and drug reactions. Eventually it would become the WHO's Programme for International Drug Monitoring.

⊕ Impacts and Issues

The standards for ethical clinical research continued to evolve as the pharmaceutical market expanded across the globe. In response, the European Medicines Agency (EMA) was established in 1995 to supervise and evaluate human and veterinary medicines. This agency is a decentralized network of approximately 4,500 experts located throughout the European Union. Pharmaceutical companies must apply for marketing authorization to advertise medicines in the European Economic Area. Upon obtaining access, drugs and medications are monitored continuously.

By 1996, the International Conference on Harmonisation of Technical Requirements for Registration of Pharmaceuticals for Human Use (ICH) convened to establish an international set of clinical research guidelines. The goal of this organization was to synthesize the collection of ethical standards established in Europe, Japan, and the United States. The standards developed by the ICH, referred to as Good Clinical Practices (GCPs), have been criticized for failing to address many of the ethical concerns addressed by the Helsinki Declaration and failing to respond to input from many national medical organizations.

The 1997 U.S. Food and Drug Administration Modernization Act (FDAMA) established the first clinical trial registry with the intention of increasing transparency and public knowledge about clinical trials involving human subjects (ClinicalTrials.gov). A report published by the U.S. Institute of Medicine in 2007 raised concerns about the agency's ability to regulate the pharmaceutical industry. Although the FDAMA stipulated that registration was a requirement for clinical research, most trial investigators initially failed to comply with this proviso. In 2004, the pharmaceutical giant GlaxoSmithKline was sued for failing to report the adverse effects of Paxil, a popular antidepressant drug. Within months, the International Committee of Medical Journal Editors declared they would no longer publish the results of unregistered trials. This prompted the WHO to establish the International Clinical Trials Registry Platform in 2006. Although participation in the international registry is voluntary, the U.S. Congress passed the FDA Amendments Act in 2007, unequivocally requiring compliance and penalizing insubordinate trial investigators. Trial registries also were launched in Europe and Canada.

As the science of pharmaceutical research and clinical trials evolves, medical professionals continue to monitor the ethical and societal ramifications. In 2008, the FDA discontinued the use of the Helsinki Declaration and adopted the set of Good Clinical Practices (GCP) issued by the ICH. Health-care providers have expressed concern about this change in policy. As Jonathan Kimmelman, Charles Weijer, and Eric Meslin wrote in "Helsinki Discords: FDA, Ethics, and International Drug Trials" in *The Lancet* 2009, "the Declaration of Helsinki has a breadth and depth that GCP lacks. For sure, GCP covers similar topics to the [Helsinki] Declaration, but the focus of GCP is regulatory harmonisation, not the articulation of ethical commitments."

Costs of New Drugs

As pharmaceutical companies continue to research innovative drugs and therapies, questions remain about the cost effectiveness of novel medicines. Increases in global health-care costs have been driven partially by pharmaceutical drug spending. New medications typically are more expensive and therefore account for a significant portion of the rising costs for essential medicines. Cost-effectiveness comparisons generally are required for existing versus new drugs in countries providing universal health care, such as the United Kingdom. Pharmaceutical companies also face additional challenges, such as the relative decrease in the number of genuinely innovative drug patents since 2005. Drug patents exist to prevent competing companies or manufacturers from producing a generic competitor to a particular chemical formula. A typical drug patent lasts for 20 years following the date of the original application. When patents expire, pharmaceutical companies usually need to discover new means of securing revenue.

Developing nations face additional challenges in providing basic, lifesaving medicines to their citizens.

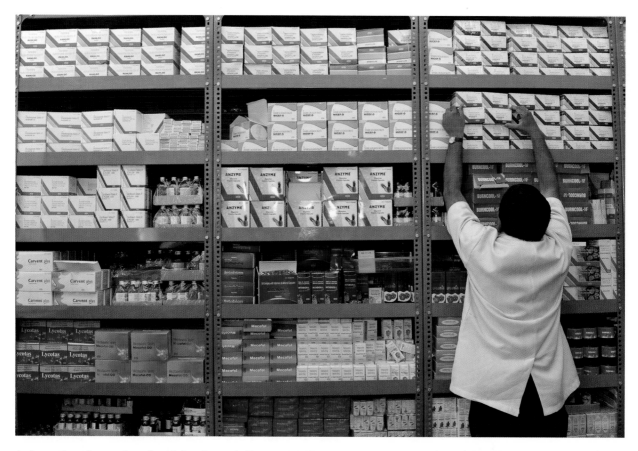

A pharmacist pulls out a box of medicines from a shelf at a generic-drug store at the Victoria Hospital in Bangalore, India. The generic-drug store, which was opened in Bangalore in 2012 by the medical education department in association with the Karnataka State Cooperative Consumer Federation, sells generic drugs that are priced less than 50 percent of the maximum retail price so that they are more affordable.   © *Manjunath Kiran/AFP/Getty Images.*

The barriers to access to essential medicines for low- and middle-income countries (LMICs) include cost, poor quality, and knowledge of their appropriate use. In the inaugural *Medicine in Health Systems* WHO 2014 report, the authors outline many of the struggles and successes involved in ensuring that LMIC populations receive essential medicines. The "health system" approach assumes there will be both foreseeable and unanticipated consequences for delivering essential pharmaceutical interventions to LMIC populations. The goal of this report was to address the equitable access to all essential medicines, ensuring that essential medicines are affordable, and ensuring that essential medicines are used appropriately.

The WHO updates the list of essential medicines every two years, adding those interventions that demonstrate "due regard to public health relevance, evidence on efficacy and safety, and comparative cost-effectiveness." The affordability of medicine is a difficult concept to determine, but the minimum criteria generally include reasonable out-of-pocket expenses that do not require individuals to incur financial hardships such as borrowing money or selling assets to pay for essential medicines

and treatments. The appropriate use of essential medicines considers overuse, underuse, and misuse such as the use of antibiotic treatment for viral infections. Barriers to access may include limited or nonexistent health-care human resources and infrastructure and the level of training health-care workers have received as well as political instability and corruption.

Pharmaceutical companies are encouraged to invest in research and development of new medicines used to treat conditions such as human immunodeficiency virus/acquired immune deficiency syndrome (HIV/AIDS), tuberculosis, malaria, and other neglected diseases that affect LMICs disproportionately. The lack of research on innovative pharmaceutical treatments has been a continued area of concern for the WHO. During 2000–2011, less than 5 percent of the 850 new therapies registered were used for treating neglected diseases. Pharmaceutical companies have proposed a variety of initiatives that could be used to help bridge the gap between essential medicines and LMICs. For example, tiered-pricing or reduced payment options might improve access for some populations. Pharmaceutical companies also have offered to conduct pro bono (work performed for the public

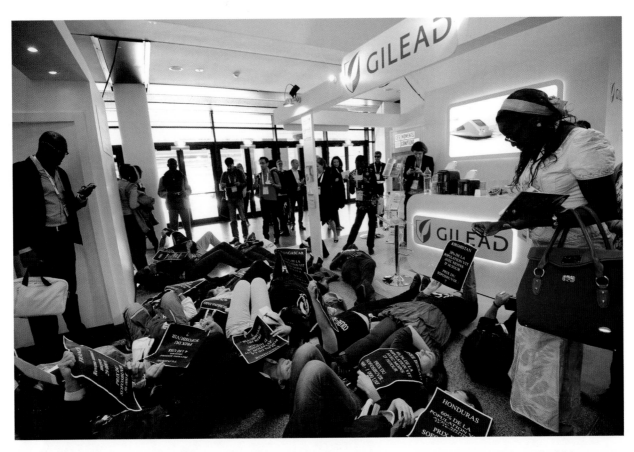

Members of the association Act Up hold signs as they lie on the floor in front of a stand of U.S. pharmaceutical giant Gilead Sciences to denounce the high price of a new drug, Sofosbuvir, to treat hepatitis C, on April 29, 2014 in Montpellier, southern France. The World Health Organization estimates there are 184 million people infected with hepatitis C worldwide through sources such as transfusions, with the disease causing half a million deaths annually. © *Sylvain Thomas/AFP/Getty Images.*

good without charge) trials and public/private partnerships for investing in research and development.

Case study comparisons of four countries and their health-care financing schemes provides a wealth of relevant information. For example, the New Cooperative Medical Scheme (NCMS) in rural China covers socioeconomically disadvantaged citizens with primarily private donor providers. The NCMS pays 100 percent of the costs of covered essential medicines after patients pay a deductible (a specified amount of money that must be paid before coverage begins), whereas the National Health Insurance Scheme in Ghana, the Jamkesmas in Indonesia, and the Seguro Popular in Mexico do not require patients to pay a deductible. The NCMS also is the only program that discontinues coverage after a maximum amount has been reached. All four schemes generally limit coverage to essential medicines prescribed by accredited health-care providers.

The WHO advocates implementing pharmaceutical policies that satisfy the four decision-making conditions in the "accountability for reasonableness" framework. The four conditions are:

1. Publicity: Policies regarding both direct and indirect limits on the provision and reimbursement of medicines and their rationales should be publicly accessible.

2. Relevance: The rationale for decisions should provide a reasonable explanation of how the varied health needs of a defined population are met under reasonable resource constraints. An explanation is "reasonable" if it is grounded in principles and evidence that are accepted as relevant by fair-minded people who are disposed to finding mutually justifiable terms of cooperation.

3. Revision and appeals: All decisions and policies must be subject to mechanisms for challenge and dispute resolution, and more broadly, provide opportunities for revision and improvement in light of new evidence and arguments.

4. Regulation or enforcement: There must be voluntary or public regulation to ensure that the conditions set out above are met.

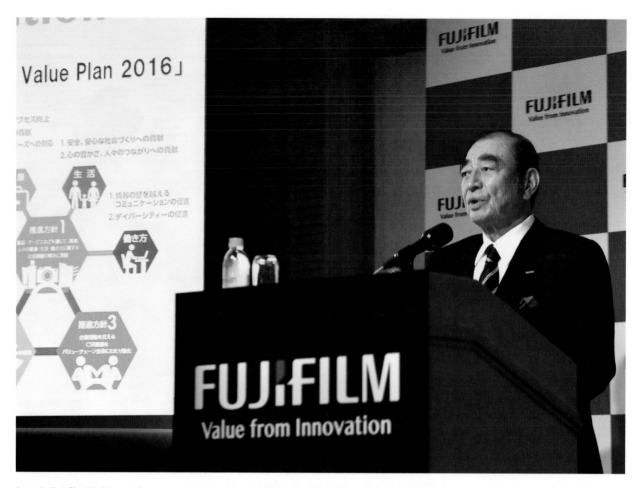

Japan's Fujifilm Holdings Chairman and CEO Shigetaka Komori announces the company's three-year business strategy in Tokyo on November 11, 2014, as the imaging company expands its health-care business sector. Fujifilm said the company's Avigan anti-influenza drug would be formally approved by World Health Organization in early 2015 for treating patients infected with the Ebola virus, though it was still in the preliminary stages of testing.   © *Yoshikazu Tsuno/AFP/Getty Images.*

🌐 Future Implications

In 2014, the WHO published a report intended to enhance the capacity of national pharmaceutical monitoring centers to identify, analyze, and, it was hoped, reduce medication errors. This approach, referred to as "pharmacovigilance," is defined as "the science and activities relating to the detection, assessment, understanding and prevention of adverse effects or any other drug-related problem." The WHO Programme for International Drug Monitoring maintains a database with individual case safety reports from member states in the Swedish Uppsala Monitoring System. The database (Vigimed) is a web-based information exchange system built for communication between health organizations, nongovernmental organizations, and regulatory agencies around the world.

Additional international organizations that assist in monitoring pharmaceutical use include The World Alliance for Patient Safety and the International Medication Safety Network. Founded in 2004 by the WHO, the World Alliance for Patient Safety addresses such challenges as medication safety such as correctly prescribing and dispensing pharmaceuticals as well as preventing fraudulent drugs from entering the market. The International Medication Safety Network was created in 2006 to prevent medication errors, develop a common international terminology, and share information related to reducing medical errors between countries and regulatory authorities.

SEE ALSO *Antibiotic/Antimicrobial Resistance; Global Health Initiatives; Health as a Human Right and Health-Care Access; Pharmaceutical Dumping (Drug Dumping); Vaccines*

BIBLIOGRAPHY

Books

Baciu, Alina, Kathleen P. Stratton, and Sheila Burke, eds. *The Future of Drug Safety: Promoting and Protecting the Health of the Public.* Washington, DC: National Academies Press, 2007.

Evans, Imogen, Hazel Thornton, Iain Chalmers, and Paul Glasziou. *Testing Treatments: Better Research for Better Healthcare*, 2nd ed. London: Pinter & Martin, 2011.

Kestenbaum, Bryan. *Epidemiology and Biostatistics: An Introduction to Clinical Research*. New York: Springer, 2009.

Raviña, Enrique. *The Evolution of Drug Discovery: From Traditional Medicines to Modern Drugs*. Weinheim, Germany: Wiley-VCH, 2011.

Sneader, Walter. *Drug Discovery: A History*. Hoboken, NJ: Wiley, 2005.

Periodicals

Dickersin, Kay, and Rennie Drummond. "The Evolution of Trial Registries and Their Use to Assess the Clinical Trial Enterprise." *JAMA* 307, no. 17 (May 2, 2012): 1861–1864.

Gøtzsche, Peter, and Anders Jørgensen. "Opening Up Data at the European Medicines Agency." *British Medical Journal* no. 342 (May 10, 2011): d2686.

Herder, Matthew. "Unlocking Health Canada's Cache of Trade Secrets: Mandatory Disclosure of Clinical Trial Results." *Canadian Medical Association Journal* 184, no. 2 (February 2012): 194–199.

Kimmelman, Jonathan, Charles Weijer, and Eric M. Meslin. "Helsinki Discords: FDA, Ethics, and International Drug Trials." *The Lancet* 373, no. 9657 (January 3, 2009): 13–14.

Kinch, Michael S., Austin Haynesworth, Sarah L. Kinch, and Denton Hoyer. "An Overview of FDA-Approved New Molecular Entities: 1827–2013." *Drug Discovery Today* 19, no. 8 (August 2014): 1033–1039.

Wadman, Meredith. "US Lawsuit Extends Thalidomide's Reach: Drug Blamed for a Broader Range of Harmful Effects." *Nature News*, November 9, 2011.

Zumla, Alimuddin, Payam Nahid, and Stewart Cole. "Advances in the Development of New Tuberculosis Drugs and Treatment Regimens." *Nature Reviews Drug Discovery* 12, no. 5 (May 2013): 388–404.

Websites

"2013 Cost to Bring Drug to Market: $1.3 Billion." *Healthcare Economist*. http://healthcare-economist.com/2013/12/09/2013-cost-to-bring-drug-to-market-1-3-billion/ (accessed March 8, 2015).

"Development of Country Profiles and Monitoring of the Pharmaceutical Situation in Countries." *World Health Organization*. http://www.who.int/medicines/areas/coordination/coordination_assessment/en/ (accessed January 20, 2015).

"Guidance for Industry E6 Good Clinical Practice: Consolidated Guidance." *U.S. Food and Drug Administration*. http://www.fda.gov/downloads/Guidances/ucm073122.pdf (accessed January 20, 2015).

"Medicines in Health Systems: Advancing Access, Affordability and Appropriate Use." *World Health Organization*. http://www.who.int/alliance-hpsr/resources/flagshipreports/en/index1.html (accessed January 20, 2015).

"Pharmaceutical Access in Least Developed Countries: On-the-Ground Barriers and Industry Successes." *Essential Medicines and Health Products Information Portal: A World Health Organization resource*. http://apps.who.int/medicinedocs/documents/s17815en/s17815en.pdf (accessed January 20, 2015).

"Proceedings of the Eighth International Conference of Drug Regulatory Authorities (ICDRA)." *World Health Organization (WHO)*. http://apps.who.int/medicinedocs/en/d/Js4924e/4.html (accessed January 20, 2015).

"Sixteenth World Health Assembly." *World Health Organization*. http://apps.who.int/iris/bitstream/10665/136208/1/WHA16_PB-22_eng.pdf?ua=1 (accessed January 20, 2015).

"Trials of War Criminals before the Nuremberg Military Tribunals under Control Council Law No. 1." *United States Library of Congress*. http://http://www.loc.gov/rr/frd/Military_Law/pdf/NT_war-criminals_Vol-II.pdf (accessed January 20, 2015).

Martin James Frigaard

Pneumonia and Pneumococcal Diseases

🌐 Introduction

Pneumonia is an inflammatory response in the lungs to an infection or a foreign material in the airways.

Many different pathogens (microorganisms that cause disease) can cause pneumonia. Its origin may be bacterial, fungal, or viral, though noninfective irritants also can cause pneumonia. According to the American Lung Association, the noninfective irritants that may cause pneumonia include inhaled food, liquid, gases, or dust. Pneumonia often follows on the heels of influenza (flu) or even a common cold, but it also can arise independently.

Of the infectious causes of pneumonia, among the most important are viruses such as influenza, adenovirus, and respiratory syncytial virus, and bacteria such as *Streptococcus pneumoniae*, *Chlamydia pneumoniae*, *Haemophilus influenzae* type b (Hib), *Klebsiella pneumoniae*, and *Pseudomonas aeruginosa*. Historically, however, bacteria have caused the most deadly types of pneumonia. Many of the bacteria that cause pneumonia naturally occur in the throat and nasal passages, especially in children. When they are inhaled into the lungs, they can cause pneumonia.

The most common type of viral pneumonia, sometimes referred to as walking pneumonia, is respiratory syncytial virus (RSV). According to the American Lung Association, viruses cause about half of pneumonia cases. These illnesses tend to be slightly less severe than bacterial pneumonias. Young children seem to be the most susceptible to viral pneumonia; RSV is one of the most common childhood pneumonias.

There are more than 90 kinds of known pneumococcal bacteria in existence. Worldwide, the most common type of bacterial pneumonia in children is caused by *Streptococcus pneumonia*, followed closely by Hib. The myriad illnesses caused by *S. pneumoniae* are known together as pneumococcal disease and (aside from pneumonia) can cause bacteremia (blood infections), meningitis, sinus infections, and middle ear infections, among many others. Bacteremia and meningitis are considered invasive forms of the disease, because the infection starts when the bacteria enter areas of the body (the blood, or in the case of meningitis, the fluids and tissues surrounding the brain and spinal cord) that are typically sterile.

Each of the bacteria that can cause pneumonia tends to occur in a specific setting or in a certain type of patient. For example, *Pseudomonas* generally infects patients in hospitals or nursing homes, while in community settings, people are more likely to contract *Streptococcus*.

Fungal pneumonias are most often caused by *Pneumocystis jirovecii*. This fungus is common and typically not harmful, but for those with compromised immune systems, such as people—particularly infants—with human immunodeficiency virus (HIV), the fungus causes pneumonia. About one-quarter of deaths in HIV-infected infants can be attributed to this form of pneumonia. Another fungal pneumonia is caused by *Pneumocystis carinii*, an opportunistic fungi that mostly affects people with acquired immune deficiency syndrome (AIDS). The debut of *Pneumocystis carinii* alerted researchers in the early 1980s to a new disease.

Viral, bacterial, and fungal pneumonia may be contracted from droplets spread through the air when an infected person sneezes or coughs. Pneumonia can also be spread through the blood, particularly during and after childbirth. The World Health Organization (WHO) observes that in order to develop effective prevention and treatment programs, more research is needed to determine the various pathogens that cause pneumonia and how they are transmitted.

When a person has pneumonia, the alveoli (small sacs in the lungs) react to invading infectious organisms or foreign particles with an inflammatory response that results in excess fluid secretions. Breathing becomes difficult, limiting the amount of oxygen a person is able to intake, and the infected person will often cough to try to discharge the fluid from the lungs. Symptoms of viral and bacterial pneumonia are very similar, although viral pneumonia tends not to be as severe at first. A fever as high as 105 degrees Fahrenheit (40.6 degrees Celsius) is not uncommon with bacterial pneumonia, accompanied by excessive sweating and rapid breathing and pulse. Cases of pneumonia range from mild to life-threatening.

Other symptoms of many pneumonias include a productive cough that brings up greenish or yellow mucus or possibly bloody mucus; shaking chills; shortness of breath, especially when climbing stairs; sharp or stabbing chest pain that worsens with deep breathing or coughing; headache; excessive sweating; clammy skin; low appetite; low energy; and fatigue. Along with a fever and dry cough, people with viral pneumonia also suffer from muscle pain and weakness. Over the course of 12 to 36 hours, breathlessness increases and the cough worsens.

Older adults with pneumonia may also experience confusion. Infants who become severely ill may become too weak to eat or drink and could also experience unconsciousness, hypothermia (dangerously low body temperature), and convulsions (seizures).

Anyone can contract pneumonia, but those at greatest risk for severe bouts or complications arising from the disease are the very old, the very young, and persons with other underlying health conditions. Because their immune systems are not as strong, viral pneumonia is more common in young children and older adults than it is in young and middle-aged adults. Others with compromised immune systems, such as babies born prematurely, children with heart and lung disorders, persons with HIV, patients undergoing cancer chemotherapy, and people who have had organ transplants are also at increased risk of developing viral pneumonia.

Pneumonia is also often a complication of other diseases such as flu and measles. Complications of pneumonia can include pericarditis, which is an inflammation of the sac around the heart, as well as abscesses and lesions in the lungs.

A medical examination to diagnose pneumonia involves listening to the lungs using a stethoscope to detect rapid breathing and bubbling, crackling, or rumbling chest sounds called rhonchi, which indicate the presence of fluid in the alveoli. A chest x-ray or computed

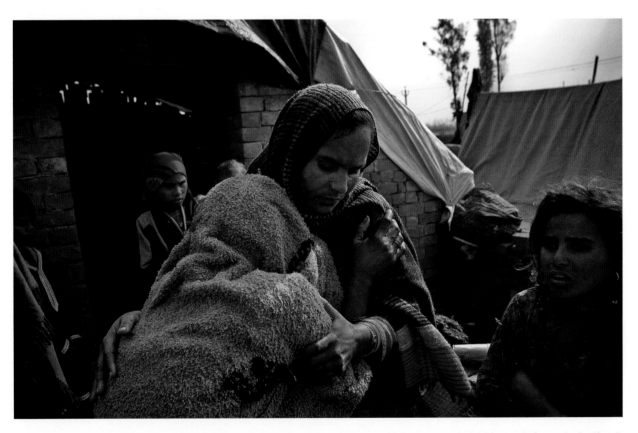

A woman is held by a relative while she cries during the funeral of her seven-month-old daughter, in the Malakpur relief camp in the Shamli District of Uttar Pradesh, India. Her daughter was on medicine for a week for pneumonia but died despite the treatment. The cold winter led to the death of over 34 children in the relief camps between September 2013 and January 2014. Pneumonia is the biggest killer of children in India, killing almost 400,000 children under age five in India every year, according to the Indian Academy of Pediatrics in 2014. © Getty Images.

tomography (CT) scan reveal the shadows or opacities on the affected lung(s) that characterize pneumonia.

Though the development of effective antibiotic treatment for bacterial pneumonia has dramatically reduced the death rate from this disease, according to the WHO, pneumonia was the single-largest infectious cause of death in children worldwide as of 2015. In 2013, the disease killed roughly 935,000 children younger than five years old and accounted for 15 percent of all childhood deaths of children younger than five years. While pneumonia is common all over world, it is most prevalent in South Asia and sub-Saharan Africa. The map shows the higher rates of pneumonia in children under age 5 in South Asia and sub-Saharan Africa compared with North America, Europe, and Australia.

Some types of pneumonia can be prevented. Vaccines are available to prevent infection with several strains of viruses and bacteria that cause pneumonia, including Hib, influenza, pertussis (whooping cough), measles, varicella (chicken pox), and pneumococcal bacteria. The U.S. Centers for Disease Control and Prevention (CDC) recommends that all children younger than 5 years old, all adults 65 years or older, and people age 6 and older with certain risk factors, such as compromised immune systems, receive a pneumococcal vaccination. Once acquired, pneumonia is treated with medication and supportive care to relieve symptoms and promote recovery.

⊕ Historical Background

Pneumonia has long afflicted humankind. It is described in writings of the Greek physician Hippocrates (c. 460 BCE– c. 377 BCE) that are more than 2,400 years old, with reference to even earlier occurrences. However, it was not until 1881 that the bacteria causing the most common pneumococcal disease, *Streptococcus pneumonia*, was first isolated. French chemist Louis Pasteur (1822–1895) isolated the bacteria using the saliva of a rabies patient. However, it would be another three years before the German pathologist and microbiologist Carl Friedlander (1847–1887) and French physician Charles Talamon (1850–1929) were able to describe the connection between the bacteria and lobar pneumonia (the form of the disease that affects one or more lobes of the lungs). Despite this discovery, however, there was still some confusion when it came to distinguishing the various types of pneumonia.

However, in 1884, Hans Christian Gram (1853–1938), a Danish bacteriologist, developed Gram's stain, a test that uses red and purple dyes to determine the presence of bacteria. The years between 1915 and 1945 were active ones for discovery. Scientists were able to determine the chemical structure of the pneumococcal capsular polysaccharide (when the bacteria encapsulates itself in a chain of sugars), its virulence, and the role bacterial polysaccharides play in human disease. By 1940,

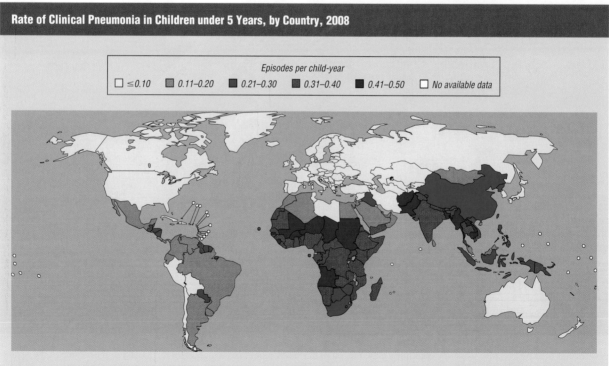

Rate of Clinical Pneumonia in Children under 5 Years, by Country, 2008

Episodes per child-year

☐ ≤0.10   ▨ 0.11–0.20   ▨ 0.21–0.30   ▨ 0.31–0.40   ■ 0.41–0.50   ☐ No available data

SOURCE: Adapted from "Fig. 1. Incidence of childhood clinical pneumonia at the country level," in Ruden, Igor, et al., "Epidemiology and Etiology of Childhood Pneumonia," *in Bulletin of the World Health Organization* 86, no. 5, May 2008, World Health Organization (WHO), http://www.who.int/bulletin/volumes/86/5/07-048769/en/ (January 13, 2015).

the CDC says, more than 80 strains of pneumococci had been described.

Vaccine research began in earnest around 1911. In 1929, Scottish biologist Alexander Fleming (1881–1955) discovered the medicinal benefits of "mold juice" from the *Pencicillium* fungi, which was effective against certain bacteria, but he was never able to create a successful purified version of the mold to use against bacteria. In 1939, scientists at the Sir William Dunn School of Pathology at Oxford University, led by Australian pharmacologist and pathologist Howard Florey (1898–1968) and British biochemist Ernst Chain (1906–1979), were able to successfully purify the antibiotic penicillin from the mold.

The first patient was treated with penicillin in 1942. By 1944, clinical trials among military and civilian populations were showing that the drug was effective against streptococcal, staphylococcal, and gonococcal diseases. The U.S. pharmaceutical company Pfizer began to produce penicillin on a larger scale when it opened its first commercial plant for production in 1944. Between 1943 and 1944, production of penicillin grew from 21 billion units to 1,663 billion units and was up to more than 6.8 trillion units in 1945, according to the American Chemical Society.

Once penicillin was in widespread use, interest in a vaccine waned, but there were still many deaths attributable to pneumonia. In the late 1960s, vaccine research ramped up and eventually bore fruit. The first pneumococcal vaccine for adults was licensed in the United States in 1977 and protected against 14 different strains of pneumonia. That number expanded to 23 strains in 1983. The first pneumococcal vaccine for use on children was licensed in 2000 and protected against seven strains; it was expanded in 2010 to address 13 strains.

One of the most common types of viral pneumonia, RSV, was first isolated after it was discovered in a colony of chimpanzees. Though there is no specific treatment for this particular form of pneumonia, some drug treatment may help very young children. A vaccine has not yet been developed to prevent RSV.

⊕ Impacts and Issues

Most healthy people can effectively combat pneumonia with their immune system defenses. However, those living in developing countries, children in particular, are often vulnerable. Children are at higher risk of developing the disease because they often already have compromised immune systems due to malnutrition, recurring disease, or chronic diseases like HIV infection. Further, children living in crowded homes, homes with cigarette smokers, or in conditions where the air is polluted as a result of cooking with wood or dung, are at an even higher risk.

Though there are drugs and vaccines that can treat and prevent some forms of pneumonia, globally

EVOLUTION OF A DRUG-RESISTANT SUPERBUG

Researchers are developing new classes of antibiotics to combat multidrug-resistant (MDR) bacteria, however, both existing and new drugs must be used sparingly because too much use promotes the development of new MDR strains. This happens because as antibiotics kill off susceptible strains, they allow MDR strains to displace the other susceptible strains, and in the process the antibiotics lose their effectiveness. Along with new drug development, researchers are learning more about how bacteria become drug resistant.

In 2011, an international team of scientists was able to decipher the genetic code of 240 samples of *Streptococcus pneumoniae*, a strain of bacteria that frequently causes pneumonia and death, particularly among children. In doing this, they were able to see just how the bacteria were able to change over time, which provided insight into how bacteria become drug resistant.

The researchers reported the study results in an article, "Rapid Pneumococcal Evolution in Response to Clinical Interventions," published in the journal *Science* in 2011. They concluded that both vaccinations and overuse of antibiotics contributed to the evolution of these bacteria.

To conduct the study, the researchers collected *Streptococcus pneumoniae*, known as the pneumococcal molecular epidemiology network clone 1 (PMEN1) from infected patients in 22 countries. It is believed this particular strain first showed up in 1970, after penicillin was already in widespread use, and its resistance to many antibiotics gave it a competitive advantage over those bacteria easily killed by antibiotics.

The team of researchers isolated samples of this strain from 1984 to 2008. One of the things they noticed is that this particular strain of pneumonia changes one letter of its DNA sequence every 15 weeks. Furthermore, the strain recombines its DNA with other bacteria (which in turn brings about an average of 72 individual letter changes) and can occasionally introduce new genes or gene variations. In short, it is constantly rearranging its DNA.

The bacteria is also able to trick the immune system by encasing itself in a polysaccharide capsule, which is an outer covering made of sugar, in this case referred to as 23F. This capsule was one of the targets of the 2000 vaccine known as PCV7. Then the bacteria changed again, this time wrapping themselves in a different sugar, 19A.

So while the vaccine was addressing 23F, the new variation not only developed but also had no competition anymore from 23F, thanks to the vaccine. Although understanding the reconfigurations of the strain does not necessarily reveal future variations, researchers have learned more about how bacteria acquire drug resistance and the ability to evade vaccines.

it remains the leading infectious cause of death among children younger than five years of age. The majority of these deaths are in low- and middle-income countries, with more than half occurring in South Asia and sub-Saharan Africa.

There are about 3,000 cases of pneumococcal meningitis in the United States each year, and of those from 10 to 30 percent of infected patients die. Symptoms include a stiff neck, light sensitivity, fever, and disorientation.

Pneumococcal bacteremia occurs in about 25 percent of all pneumococcal infections and affects more than 50,000 people in the United States each year. Both of these invasive diseases can be fatal. About 20 percent of patients with pneumococcal bacteremia die. The death rate is much higher in the older adults, at about 60 percent. The disease causes chills and fever, and can complicate infections. Those who survive may sustain permanent injury such as hearing loss, seizures, or brain damage.

About 175,000 people are hospitalized each year in the United States alone as a result of pneumococcal pneumonia. Further, the CDC estimates that pneumococci are responsible for as much as 36 percent of adult community-acquired pneumonia (an acute respiratory illness contracted through social interaction outside a hospital setting) and 50 percent of hospital-acquired pneumonia (an acute respiratory illness contracted in a hospital setting or as a result of a hospital stay).

Pneumococcal diseases caused by bacteria are treated with antibiotics, usually amoxicillin. However, there are some strains of bacteria that have developed drug resistance. Drug resistant pneumonias usually require longer hospital stays and are associated with more severe complications.

While antibiotics are readily available in developed countries, this is not always the case in the developing world. According to the WHO, only about one-third of children who need antibiotics in the developing world have access to them. The cost of diagnostics and antibiotic treatment for these children is an estimated US$109 million per year.

Antibiotics do not cure viral pneumonia. However, according to the U.S. National Institutes of Health, the flu vaccine can prevent pneumonia caused by the flu virus and the drug palivizumab can be given to children younger than two years of age in order to prevent pneumonia caused by respiratory syncytial virus.

There is a pneumococcal vaccine that protects against 23 strains of pneumonia, but it is generally most effective in adults. There is a vaccine for children known as PCV13, which protects against 13 strains of the most severe pneumococcal infections. According to the CDC, since this vaccine was added to the recommended childhood vaccination schedule in the United States in 2000, when it only protected against seven strains, invasive pneumococcal disease in children has dropped by nearly 80 percent.

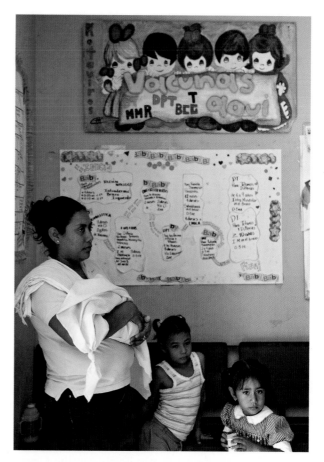

A woman waits to have her daughters vaccinated against pneumococcus-caused pneumonia at a health-care center in Managua, Nicaragua. In 2011, Nicaragua, Honduras, and Guyana received an important provision of pneumococcal vaccines from the Global Alliance for Vaccines and Immunization (Gavi), an organization backed by the World Bank, World Health Organization, and UNICEF, among other donors.
© *Elmer Martinez/AFP/Getty Images.*

🌐 Future Implications

Because many factors contribute to contracting pneumonia, no single prevention, treatment, or control method alone is effective. There are, however, ways to mitigate the severity of these diseases and reduce the number of cases. In an ideal scenario, vaccinations used in combination with basic prevention methods such as consistent hand washing and using tissues to capture coughs and sneezes, along with early diagnosis and treatment, can help to reduce the occurrence of these infectious diseases. However, in developing countries where basic nutrition and hygiene may be severely lacking and indoor air pollution is widespread, preventing, treating, and controlling the spread of pneumonia is especially challenging.

The WHO has several recommendations aimed at reducing infectious diseases in general and pneumonia specifically. Among these is increasing the number of new mothers who exclusively breast-feed their children. Research demonstrates that exclusive breast-feeding in the first six months of a child's life not only provides the child with needed nutrition but also assists to prevent pneumonia and reduce the duration of the illness in affected infants.

The WHO also estimates that deaths caused by pneumonia could decrease as much as 30 percent in a short time across the 75 countries with the greatest number of deaths if the pneumonia interventions in these countries were raised to the level of the richest 20 percent of households in each country. To that end, the WHO and the United Nations Children's Fund (UNICEF) created the Integrated Global Action Plan for the Prevention and Control of Pneumonia and Diarrhoea to promote interventions that protect, prevent, and treat pneumonia in children. These interventions include promoting breast-feeding and complementary nutrition; increasing access to qualified health-care workers, facilities, medicine, and oxygen; vaccinations; providing education about the importance regular hand washing with soap; reducing indoor air pollution; HIV prevention; and drug treatments for HIV-infected and exposed children. By 2015, many countries, including Bangladesh, India, Uganda, and Zambia, had implemented plans to increase to reduce the occurrence of pneumonia.

Another alarming trend is the rise of multidrug-resistant bacteria as a primary cause of hospital-acquired pneumonia. This suggests that many of the most commonly used antibiotics will become ineffective to treating infections. Antibiotic resistance is also a concern in community-acquired pneumonia, which is increasingly penicillin-resistant.

PRIMARY SOURCE

Ending Preventable Child Deaths from Pneumonia and Diarrhoea by 2025

SOURCE *"Executive Summary," from* Ending Preventable Child Deaths from Pneumonia and Diarrhoea by 2025: The Integrated Global Action Plan for Pneumonia and Diarrhoea (GAPPD). *Geneva: World Health Organization (WHO)/United Nations Children's Fund (UNICEF), 2013, 5–6. http://apps.who.int/iris/bitstream/10665/79200/1/9789241505239_eng.pdf (accessed January 25, 2015).*

INTRODUCTION *This primary source is taken from a publication detailing the United Nations Children's Fund (UNICEF) and World Health*

Organization's full action plan on eliminating child deaths from two major illnesses, pneumonia and diarrhea.

EXECUTIVE SUMMARY

Ending two major preventable causes of child death

Stopping the loss of millions of young lives from pneumonia and diarrhoea is a goal within our grasp. The *integrated Global Action Plan for the Prevention and Control of Pneumonia and Diarrhoea (GAPPD)* proposes a cohesive approach to ending preventable pneumonia and diarrhoea deaths. It brings together critical services and interventions to create healthy environments, promotes practices known to protect children from disease and ensures that every child has access to proven and appropriate preventive and treatment measures.

The goal is ambitious but achievable: to end preventable childhood deaths due to pneumonia and diarrhoea by 2025.

…

Closing the gap: reaching all children with existing interventions

Pneumonia and diarrhoea remain major killers of young children. Together, these diseases account for 29% of all deaths of children less than 5 years of age and result in the loss of 2 million young lives each year.

The solutions to tackling pneumonia and diarrhoea do not require major advances in technology. Proven interventions exist. Children are dying because services are provided piece-meal and those most at risk are not being reached. Use of effective interventions remains too low; for instance, only 39% of infants less than 6 months are exclusively breastfed while only 60% of children with suspected pneumonia access appropriate care. Moreover, children are not receiving life-saving treatment; only 31% of children with suspected pneumonia receive antibiotics and only 35% of children with diarrhoea receive oral rehydration therapy.

Using interventions that work

Research shows that these interventions and activities work:

- Exclusive breastfeeding for six months and continued breastfeeding with appropriate complementary feeding reduces the onset and severity of diarrhoea and pneumonia.

- Use of vaccines against *Streptococcus pneumonia* and *Haemophilus influenzae* type b, the two most common bacterial causes of childhood pneumonia, and against rotavirus, the most common cause of childhood diarrhoea deaths, substantially reduces the disease burden and deaths caused by these infectious agents. In response, an increasing number of countries are introducing these vaccines.

- Use of vaccines against measles and pertussis substantially reduces pneumonia illness and death in children.

- Use of simple, standardized guidelines for the identification and treatment of pneumonia and diarrhoea in the community, at first-level health facilities and at referral hospitals, such as those for integrated management of childhood illness (IMCI), substantially reduces child deaths.

- Oral rehydration salts (ORS), and particularly the low-osmolarity formula, are a proven life-saving commodity for the treatment of children with diarrhoea. Use of zinc supplements with ORS to treat children with diarrhoea reduces deaths in children less than five years of age.

- Innovative demand creation activities are important for achieving behaviour change and sustaining long-term preventive practices.

- Water, sanitation and hygiene interventions, including access to and use of safe drinking-water and sanitation, as well as promotion of key hygiene practices provide health, economic and social benefits.

- Reduction of household air pollution with improved stoves has been shown to reduce severe pneumonia. Safer and more efficient energy in the home prevents burns, saves time and fuel costs, and contributes to better development opportunities.

SEE ALSO *Antibiotic/Antimicrobial Resistance; Bacterial Diseases; Methicillin-Resistant* Staphylococcus aureus *(MRSA)*

BIBLIOGRAPHY

Books

Fein, Alan, et al. *Diagnosis and Management of Pneumonia and Other Respiratory Infections.* Caddo, OK: Professional Communications, 2012.

Marrie, Thomas J., ed. *Community-Acquired Pneumonia.* New York: Kluwer Academic, 2001.

U.S. Centers for Disease Control and Prevention. *Manual for the Surveillance of Vaccine-Preventable Diseases.* Atlanta: U.S. Centers for Disease Control and Prevention, 2012.

World Health Organization. *Essential Drugs and Medicines Policy, Priority Medicines for Europe and the World: A Public Health Approach to Innovation.* Geneva: World Health Organization, 2012.

Periodicals

Croucher, N. J., et al. "Rapid Pneumococcal Evolution in Response to Clinical Interventions." *Science* 93, no. 884 (2011): 430–434.

Musher, Daniel M., and Anna R. Thorner. "Community-Acquired Pneumonia." *New England Journal of Medicine* 371, no. 17 (October 23, 2014): 1619–1628.

Wyrwich, Kathleen W., Holly Yu, Reiko Sato, David Strutton, and John H. Powers. "Community-Acquired Pneumonia: Symptoms and Burden of Illness at Diagnosis among US Adults Aged 50 Years and Older." *Patient* 6, no. 2 (June 2013): 125–134.

Websites

"Active Bacterial Core Surveillance (ABCs)." *U.S. Centers for Disease Control and Prevention (CDC).* http://www.cdc.gov/abcs/index.html (accessed March 30, 2015).

"Discovery and Development of Penicillin." *American Chemical Society.* http://www.acs.org/content/acs/en/education/whatischemistry/landmarks/flemingpenicillin.html (accessed March 30, 2015).

"Pneumococcal Disease." *National Foundation for Infectious Disease.* http://www.nfid.org/idinfo/pneumococcal (accessed March 15, 2015).

"Pneumococcal Disease." *National Institutes of Health.* http://www.niaid.nih.gov/topics/pneumococal/pages/pneumococcaldisease.aspx (accessed March 30, 2015).

"Pneumococcal Disease." *World Health Organization (WHO).* http://www.who.int/immunization/topics/pneumococcal_disease/en/ (accessed March 15, 2015).

"Pneumococcal Disease and the Vaccine (Shot) to Prevent It." *U.S. Centers for Disease Control and Prevention (CDC).* http://www.cdc.gov/vaccines/vpd-vac/pneumo/fs-parents.html (accessed March 15, 2015).

"Pneumococcal Disease Epidemiology and Prevention of Vaccine-Preventable Diseases." *U.S. Centers for Disease Control and Prevention (CDC).* http://www.cdc.gov/vaccines/pubs/pinkbook/pneumo.html (accessed March 20, 2015).

"Pneumonia." *Mayo Clinic.* http://www.mayoclinic.org/diseases-conditions/pneumonia/basics/definition/con-20020032 (accessed February 9, 2015).

"Pneumonia." Fact Sheet No. 331. *World Health Organization (WHO),* Updated November 2014. http://

www.who.int/mediacentre/factsheets/fs331/en/ (accessed February 9, 2015).

"Pneumonia—Adults (Community Acquired)." *National Institutes of Health.* http://www.nlm.nih.gov/medlineplus/ency/article/000145.htm (accessed February 9, 2015).

"Pneumonia Can Be Prevented—Vaccines Can Help." *U.S. Centers for Disease Control and Prevention (CDC).* http://www.cdc.gov/features/pneumonia/ (accessed February 9, 2015).

"Pneumonia Fact Sheet." *American Lung Association.* http://www.lung.org/lung-disease/influenza/in-depth-resources/pneumonia-fact-sheet.html (accessed November 22, 2014).

Melanie R. Plenda

Poliomyelitis (Polio)

⊕ Introduction

Poliomyelitis, or polio, is a highly contagious viral infection that can lead to paralysis, breathing problems, and death. Once known as infantile paralysis, polio was a feared disease and a pervasive killer prior to the turn of the 21st century, particularly of children. In the 2010s it has been eradicated from most of the planet due to widespread vaccination. Polio is endemic only in Afghanistan, Nigeria, and Pakistan, although outbreaks do occur elsewhere, particularly in war zones when vaccination campaigns are disrupted. Polio was endemic in more than 125 countries in 1988. Eradication is close, but, as noted by the World Health Organization (WHO), as long as one child remains infected, children everywhere are at risk. According to the WHO, failure to eradicate the disease completely could result in as many as 200,000 new cases every year around the world.

The vast majority of cases of polio cause no symptoms. In the 5 percent or so of cases where symptoms are present, there are two kinds of polio: non-paralytic polio is a mild disease, whereas paralytic polio can be severe and even fatal. There are three kinds of paralytic polio. In spinal polio, the poliovirus attacks motor neurons in the spinal cord, causing paralysis in the arms and legs and breathing difficulties. In bulbar polio, the neurons responsible for sight, vision, taste, swallowing, and breathing are affected. Finally, bulbospinal polio is a combination of both the spinal and bulbar forms of the disease. Many people with non-paralytic polio go on to make a full recovery, but those with the paralytic form of the disease generally become permanently paralyzed.

The causative agent of polio, the poliovirus, is an enterovirus of the *Picornaviridae* family. Poliovirus is highly contagious and is spread by fecal-oral contact. It may enter the water supply via the feces of an infected person. Where sanitation is poor, the virus then spreads rapidly through contaminated food and water.

The disease mainly affects children under the age of five. However, pregnant women, those with impaired immunity, and those who have not been vaccinated are also at risk of contracting polio.

Polio has an incubation period of 7 to 10 days, after which time around a quarter of those infected will experience flulike symptoms and possibly arm and leg stiffness and back and leg pain. The paralytic form of the disease, which affects less than 1 percent of those infected, starts with similar symptoms and then progresses to loss of muscle reflexes, muscle pain and spasms, and loose or floppy limbs. Around 5 to 10 percent of those with paralytic polio will die from immobilization of the breathing muscles. Diagnosis of polio is by detection of poliovirus in throat secretions, stool samples, or cerebrospinal fluid.

There is no actual cure for polio, so treatment focuses upon managing the symptoms, which includes bed rest, painkillers, and physiotherapy. The iron lung was a device that aided breathing by pulling and pushing on the chest muscles in those whose respiratory function was affected. This has been superseded by portable ventilators.

In countries where polio has been eradicated, doctors may have little or no experience of the disease. Even where the disease can still occur, it may not be recognized or seen as a priority because symptoms may be mild and mortality relatively rare. Meanwhile, many of those who have recovered from polio may go on to develop a condition known as post-polio syndrome, characterized by fatigue, muscle and joint pain, respiratory problems, and other symptoms. Post-polio syndrome occurs an average of 35 years after the initial polio infection and is poorly understood, although it is known not to be a resurgence of the original infection. Patients with post-polio syndrome may be dismissed or misunderstood by their doctors, given the lack of understanding around polio and the long time lag between the original infection and the new symptoms.

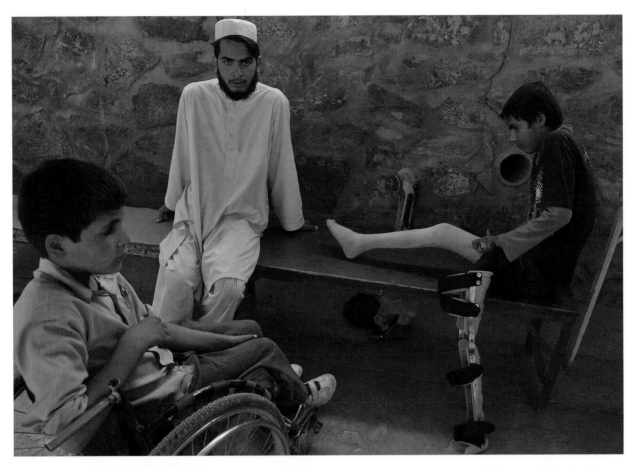

Fifteen-year-old Mustafa (right), from Logar Province, tries to adjust his artificial leg as other patients look on in one of the International Committee of the Red Cross hospitals for war victims and the disabled in Kabul, Afghanistan. Mustafa lost his left leg due to polio when he was younger. © *Massoud Hossaini/AFP/Getty Images.*

⊕ Historical Background

Polio is an ancient viral disease that actually was represented in Egyptian art around 3,000 years ago. It first was described in literature at the end of the 18th century, and one famous victim was the Scottish writer Sir Walter Scott (1771–1832). Toward the end of the 19th century, polio reached epidemic proportions, raising particular concerns when what had been seen as primarily a children's disease began to affect adults.

Later, scientists realized that it was actually improvements in sanitation that were causing an upsurge in polio. Children had been naturally immunized by exposure to the disease itself, until improvements in hygiene made transmission of polio by the fecal-oral route less likely. Up to 50,000 people per year in the late 19th and early 20th centuries were affected by polio in the United States, including President Franklin D. Roosevelt (1882–1945), who was paralyzed by polio in 1921.

Scientific Understanding of Polio

Early in the 20th century, American pathologist Simon Flexner (1863–1946) carried out experiments in which monkeys who had been injected with nasal secretions of polio patients developed the disease. In 1935, the charity the March of Dimes began raising money to research the disease. By 1949, scientists had grown the poliovirus in the lab. The life-threatening paralysis of the respiratory muscles led to the invention of the iron lung by American physiologist Cecil Kent Drinker (1887–1956). This also paved the way toward the development of critical care medicine, in which support of respiration is often necessary.

These scientific developments led to the introduction of vaccines against polio starting in 1955. By 1994, intensive vaccination campaigns led to the eradication of polio from the Western Hemisphere. This success, and that of the global eradication of smallpox, led the WHO to propose the elimination of polio from the planet also.

⊕ Impacts and Issues

There are three strains of the poliovirus, none of which can survive for long outside the human body. The virus dies out unless it infects an unvaccinated person. Furthermore, oral polio vaccine is cheap and can be delivered by

POLIO VACCINES

Having poliovirus infection and recovering from it does provide lifelong immunity against the disease. However, this is limited to the type of poliovirus involved. Being infected with poliovirus 1 will not protect against poliovirus 2 or poliovirus 3. Therefore, the development of effective vaccines against paralytic polio was a major scientific breakthrough. There are two different vaccines in use as of 2015. One is an inactivated (killed) polio vaccine and the other is a live, attenuated oral polio vaccine. Immunization against all three strains of polio remains necessary, even in countries where the disease has been eradicated. Most people will have been immunized as children but if they have missed out, for whatever reason, they can still receive the vaccine. Those who are considering travel to an area where polio remains endemic will need to take advice on protection with a booster dose of vaccine.

Inactivated Polio Vaccine

American virologist Jonas Salk (1914–1995) developed the first polio vaccine in 1955. This was produced from live poliovirus from all three strains. During manufacture, the virus is killed with formalin, a chemical disinfectant, so it carries no risk of infecting those being immunized. The inactivated vaccine is injectable, and it can be administered either on its own or in combination with other vaccines against other diseases, such as diphtheria, tetanus, hepatitis B, and *Haemophilus influenzae* disease (including Hib).

Experience with the Salk vaccine over many years has shown that it can stop transmission of the poliovirus. It has been used to eradicate polio in many countries. Side effects associated with its administration are mild and transient. Polio-free countries generally use inactivated vaccine to maintain their eradication status. However, an obvious drawback is that because the Salk vaccine is injectable, it requires either a health-care professional or trained volunteer to administer it. Where mass vaccination was required

and the health-care infrastructure was weak or nonexistent, this was not a practical proposition as part of the eradication campaign.

Oral Polio Vaccine

Albert Sabin (1906–1993), a Russian American pediatrician and microbiologist, developed a live attenuated polio vaccine for oral use in the mid-1950s. However, early experience with this vaccine was problematic because, being live, it could produce paralytic polio in healthy volunteers. Later trials, following further development of the vaccine, were more successful, and the oral vaccine came into use in the 1961, superseding the use of the Salk vaccine. It was easier to organize a mass vaccination campaign based upon an oral vaccine because it could be administered by people with no special training.

As researchers began to learn more about the poliovirus, they were able to develop strains for use in the vaccine that were less likely to attack the nervous system and less likely to be transmitted. The original oral polio vaccine was a trivalent vaccine against the three strains. However, monovalent vaccines, which act against only type 1 or type 3 poliovirus have been licensed for use in various countries since 2005. There is also a monovalent vaccine against type 2 poliovirus.

The oral polio vaccine produces a local immune response in the lining of the intestines. This is the site where the poliovirus reproduces after infection. Because this response decreases the shedding of the virus, it provides a barrier to its transmission to others. This ability, together with its ease of administration and low cost, has made the oral polio vaccine the first choice for global eradication of the disease. As the disease is reduced within a population, however, oral vaccine use is generally decreased in favor of the inactivated (injectable) vaccine.

anyone because no injection is needed. Therefore, the global eradication of polio by mass vaccination is a reasonable objective.

However, when someone is immunized with the oral polio vaccine, it replicates in the intestine and also is excreted. Where sanitation is poor, the vaccine-derived virus can spread. As it circulates in the environment, it may acquire genetic mutations that make it infectious. This form of virus is called circulating vaccine-derived poliovirus (cVDPV). If vaccination coverage in the area is poor, the population will be susceptible to infection with cVDPV.

The WHO and its partners already had demonstrated that another disease, smallpox, could be eradicated through a mass vaccination campaign taking place over a number of years. Eradicating an infectious disease requires meeting a number of challenges. An effective vaccine must be available on a large scale, and it must be affordable. There must also be an infrastructure of transport, and people to deliver the immunization shots. Conflict

zones and remote areas can make it difficult to access those who need the vaccine. Finally, the whole operation must be financed. Nevertheless, lessons were learned from the smallpox eradication campaign, so the scene was set for a similar initiative to eradicate polio from the world.

The Global Polio Eradication Initiative

Set up in 1988, the Global Polio Eradication Initiative (GPEI) is the largest ever public-private partnership for global health. It brings together national governments, the WHO, Rotary International, the U.S. Centers for Disease Control and Prevention (CDC), the United Nations Children's Fund (UNICEF), and charitable foundations such as the Bill & Melinda Gates Foundation. Its stated goal is a polio-free world.

The success of the initiative can be measured by the fact that polio cases are down by 99 percent since it was set up. From 350,000 children paralyzed by polio in 125 countries in GPEI's first year, the number of cases had declined to 416 in 2013, of which 160 were in the

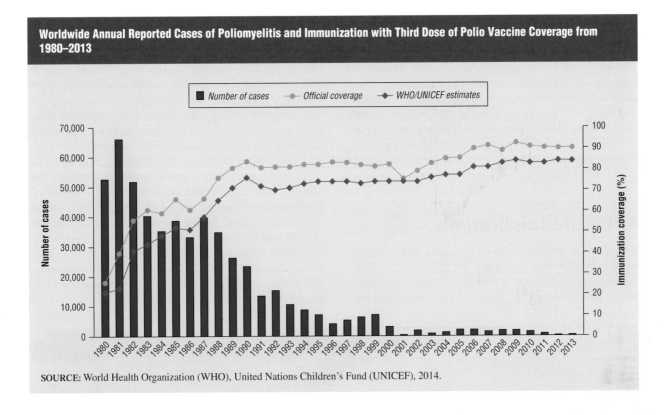

Worldwide Annual Reported Cases of Poliomyelitis and Immunization with Third Dose of Polio Vaccine Coverage from 1980–2013

SOURCE: World Health Organization (WHO), United Nations Children's Fund (UNICEF), 2014.

three remaining endemic countries. The initiative has involved 200 countries and 20 million volunteers, who have immunized around 2.5 billion children over the lifetime of the campaign. The work has required funding of US$10 billion.

Polio was eradicated in the United States in 1979 and from the WHO Region of the Americas in 1994. Other countries soon followed, and by 2002, polio was endemic only in India, Nigeria, Pakistan, Somalia, Egypt, Afghanistan, and Niger. By 2008, Nigeria was the only African country still affected by polio. In 2011, India reported the eradication of polio. In the mid-2010s, polio is endemic only in Nigeria, Afghanistan, and Pakistan. Eighty percent of the world's population live in certified polio-free regions and more than 10 million cases of polio, some of which would have been paralytic polio, have been avoided.

The GPEI has a four-point strategy. First, there is routine immunization that aims to deliver three doses of oral polio vaccine to 80 percent of children in a country during the first year of life. Second, National Immunization Day campaigns, also known as Supplementary Immunization, are intended to catch children not routinely immunized or who have been only partly immunized. The campaigns also boost immunity against polio among those who have been immunized. Third, a thorough surveillance program is needed to identify new cases of polio and test the water for the presence of poliovirus. Finally, targeted mop-up campaigns involve door-to-door immunization in places where polio is known or suspected to

be present. Such campaigns helped finally eliminate the disease from Peru, Colombia, and Cambodia.

Polio and Politics

Getting the polio vaccine to children in war-torn areas has always been one of the biggest challenges faced by the GPEI. But left without immunization, pockets of polio can grow and spread, threatening the whole campaign. This is why in May 2014 the WHO declared polio to be a public health emergency of international concern. There has been a significant increase in the number of cases, particularly in the Middle East and Central Asia, which are affected by conflict.

Of particular concern is how polio is being seen again in areas where it was previously considered to be eradicated. For instance, Syria had been free of polio for 14 years, and then an outbreak occurred there in 2013.

Once polio reappears, it can spread to other countries. At the end of 2013, 60 percent of polio cases were from the international spread of poliovirus. Nine states were affected: Afghanistan, Cameroon, Equatorial Guinea, Ethiopia, Israel, Nigeria, Pakistan, Somalia, and Syria. The main priority is for these countries to interrupt the spread of wild polio within their borders. In particular, those who are intending to travel must be immunized. As of May 2014, the WHO states that Pakistan, Cameroon, and Syria pose the greatest threat of export of wild polio.

Polio immunization can be used both as a tool for peace and a weapon of war. The tradition of National

Immunization Days, where millions of children can be immunized in a one-day campaign, often repeated after a short time, has become well-established. These campaigns sometimes are accompanied by a cease-fire, known as a campaigns of Tranquility, in war zones. The campaigns have occurred in many countries, including Angola, El Salvador, and Peru, and more recently, in Pakistan and Afghanistan. However, the Taliban banned polio immunization in parts of Pakistan in 2012, believing the vaccine to be part of a Western plot. Some polio workers have been attacked, and even killed, while trying to deliver the vaccine.

⊕ Future Implications

The status of eradication as of late 2012 was that there were only 223 wild poliovirus (WPV) cases in 2012. According to GPEI it was the "fewest polio cases in the fewest countries ever." However, the disease surged back to 416 cases in 2013, mainly due to an increase in cases in Pakistan and cases from Pakistan exported to Syria. That news was countered in 2014 with the encouraging news that India, long regarded as the most difficult place to end polio, had not recorded a single case for more than three years, and polio was no longer considered endemic in the country. Outbreaks in countries where there had been reinfection had nearly all been stopped. In particular, there was only one case of WPV in Syria in 2014.

The Polio Eradication and Endgame Strategic Plan 2013–2018 is a comprehensive, long-term strategy that aims to deliver the global eradication of the disease. It has been developed by the GPEI with "national health authorities, global health initiatives, scientific experts, donors and other stakeholders," under the direction of the World Health Assembly. As well as eliminating both wild and vaccine-derived polio, the plan aims to continue the work of the GPEI to deliver other health services to children around the world. The eradication effort has

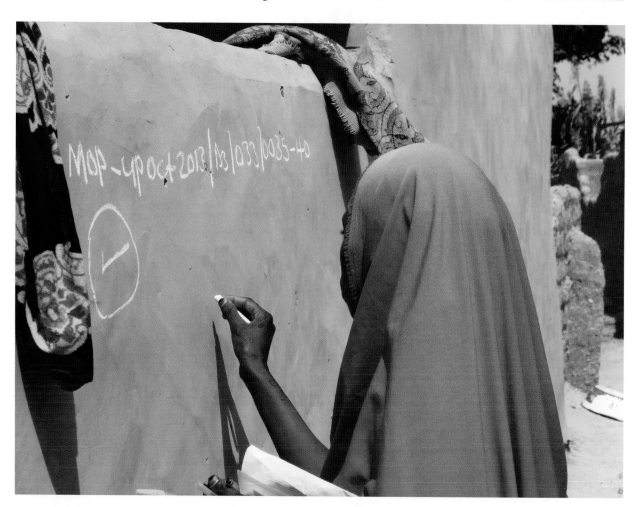

A polio vaccinator marks a house indicating the under-five children have been given oral polio drops in the Dawanau district of Kano, northern Nigeria, during a polio immunization campaign in six local government areas found to harbor poliovirus. The Bill & Melinda Gates Foundation is funding a high-tech electronic tracking of vaccination in eight high-risk states in the region as part of global effort to eradicate polio. The Gates have vowed to help end the scourge of polio in Nigeria, Africa's most populous nation, still blighted by the debilitating disease. © *Aminu Abubakar/AFP/Getty Images.*

expanded capacity to deal with other infectious diseases, through the development of surveillance and immunization systems.

The plan has a four-point strategy. First, there is to be detection and interruption of all poliovirus transmission. To this end, lessons will be taken from the campaign in India and in the three countries where it remained endemic in 2014 (Afghanistan, Pakistan, and Nigeria) and where innovation and emergency plans have been employed. Second, immunization will be improved by phasing out the oral vaccine and replacing it with inactivated polio vaccine. There will also be the introduction of new polio vaccines.

Third, the plan will contain poliovirus and certify the interruption of transmission. This means that all regions must go for three years without a case of polio before they can be certified polio-free. This is important because there may be gaps in surveillance and polio cases occurring. This means the infection could be transmitted to anyone who has not been immunized. Finally, there is a legacy plan that will transfer the polio program's experience to other areas of health care. All four strands of the plan will be pursued in parallel until 2018. The cost of the plan, which will be covered by existing and new donors, will be US$5.5 billion. It will be a worthwhile investment, however, because infectious-disease experts have estimated that eradication of polio will save the world $40 billion to $50 billion.

The Legacy Plan

Since 1988, the GPEI has trained and mobilized millions of volunteers and health-care workers. They have reached households and locations not previously involved in health initiatives in many parts of the world. The GPEI also put in place a real-time globalized surveillance and response capacity. All of these resources could be put to work in the service of other health initiatives in the future. This is why a legacy plan has been put in place by the Polio Eradication and Endgame Strategic Plan 2013–2018. A global framework, which is to be considered by the World Health Assembly in 2015, is to be set up to deliver the legacy plan. Other diseases that are in the process of being eradicated include dracunculiasis (guinea worm disease), lymphatic filariasis (also known as elephantiasis), measles, mumps, rubella, and pork tapeworm. The approach is similar to that being used for polio, involving surveillance, immunization, and case finding.

Phase out of the Oral Vaccine

According to the WHO, since 2000, more than 10 billion doses of oral polio vaccine had been administered to 3 billion children as of 2014. During this time, there have been 20 outbreaks of cVDPV in 20 countries, and 758 cases of associated polio. Generally such outbreaks have been stopped by giving two to three rounds of immunization, as for the transmission of WPV. Although the risk of cVDPV is very small compared with the benefit of preventing millions of cases of wild polio with the vaccine, it is unacceptable within the context of a global eradication target, especially after the incidence of polio is greatly reduced in a population. That is why the oral vaccine is set to be phased out by 2019.

PRIMARY SOURCE

Global Health: Polio

SOURCE *"Updates on CDC's Polio Eradication Efforts—CDC Continues to Support the Global Polio Eradication Effort." Centers for Disease Control and Prevention (CDC), January 23, 2015. http://www.cdc.gov/polio/updates/index .htm (accessed January 25, 2015).*

INTRODUCTION *This primary source is a January 23, 2015, update on the global efforts of the U.S. Centers for Disease Control and Prevention (CDC) to eradicate polio, in conjunction with partner organizations. The website is updated periodically. With the goal of eradicating polio finally in sight, the CDC stresses the need for successful completion.*

UPDATES ON CDC'S POLIO ERADICATION EFFORTS

January 23, 2015

CDC Continues to Support the Global Polio Eradication Effort

The eradication of polio is an important priority for the Centers for Disease Control and Prevention (CDC). We are closer than we have ever been to eradicating polio and it is critical that we take advantage of this opportunity.

On December 2, 2011, CDC Director Thomas R. Frieden, MD, MPH, activated CDC's Emergency Operations Center (EOC) to strengthen the agency's partnership engagement through the Global Polio Eradication Initiative (GPEI) External Web Site Icon, which is committed to completing the eradication of polio. On December 14, 2011, Dr. Frieden enlisted the support of the entire CDC community to become active participants in an intensified effort to eradicate polio worldwide.

CDC's Involvement

In the final push toward global polio eradication, CDC continues its close collaboration with partners, including the World Health Organization (WHO), the United Nations Children's Fund (UNICEF), Rotary International, and the Bill and Melinda Gates Foundation to ensure a coordinated global and country-level response.

CDC polio eradication activities and staff have moved into the EOC operational structure to ensure maximum use of CDC resources to support polio eradication, and to scale up timely technical expertise and support for polio-infected countries (Afghanistan, Cameroon, Equatorial Guinea, Ethiopia, Iraq, Nigeria, Pakistan, and Syrian Arab Republic) and for countries at risk of polio outbreaks, in coordination with GPEI partners.

Since December 2, 2011, approximately 545 workers have supported CDC's polio eradication efforts in the EOC and in the field. Of these, 170 workers have completed 823 field deployments to Angola, Chad, Côte d'Ivoire, and other areas. Each day an average of 40 people are working on polio eradication in CDC's EOC.

Activation of the EOC has provided enhanced capacity for CDC's STOP Transmission of Polio (STOP) program, which trains public health volunteers in the United States and globally to improve polio surveillance and help plan, implement, and evaluate vaccination campaigns. Since December 2, 2011, 537 individuals have been deployed on more than 1140 assignments to work with the STOP program in dozens of countries, including Chad, Haiti, and Kenya.

In addition, the EOC has provided enhanced capacity to scale up in-country technical expertise and support for—polio surveillance, planning, implementation, and monitoring of polio vaccination campaigns—strengthening routine immunization, strengthening management and accountability.

A few additional examples of CDC polio eradication activities include:

- An in-depth review of priority countries' polio eradication plans to assess program gaps and training needs, and elaboration of plans for CDC's engagement in those countries.

- Publication of several joint World Health Organization Weekly Epidemiologic Record/CDC Morbidity and Mortality Weekly Reports (MMWR) highlighting polio eradication progress related to Nigeria, Afghanistan, Pakistan, risk assessment for polio outbreaks, possible eradication of wild poliovirus type 3, polio-free certification in SEARO, and progress towards worldwide eradication.

- Collaboration with GPEI partners on detailed country-plans for expanded technical and management support, including assistance with outbreak responses, surveillance reviews, vaccination campaign planning and monitoring, and data management.

- The development of indicators for monitoring polio vaccination campaign performance in the areas of planning, implementation, and evaluation.

Review of WHO proposed outbreak response protocols for all polio-affected and at risk countries.

The Global Push toward the Finish Line

Polio incidence has dropped more than 99 percent since the launch of global polio eradication efforts in 1988. According to global polio surveillance data from January 21, 2015, 356 polio cases have been reported to date in 2014 from Afghanistan, Cameroon, Equatorial Guinea, Ethiopia, Iraq, Nigeria, Pakistan, and Syria. So far in 2015, 1 case has been reported from Pakistan.

On March 27, 2014, Dr. Frieden and senior CDC immunization staff were present when India, along with the other 10 countries of the South East Asia Region, was certified polio-free. The country was once considered the most complex challenge to achieving global polio eradication. Four of the six regions of the World Health Organization have been certified polio-free: the Americas (1994), Western Pacific (2000), Europe (2002) and South East Asia (2014). 80% of the world's people now live in polio-free areas.

While no polio cases have been detected in India for more than three years, poliovirus transmission is ongoing in the three endemic countries—Afghanistan, Nigeria, and Pakistan. GPEI's Independent Monitoring Board considers Nigeria and Pakistan to be the greatest challenges for eradicating polio. On May 5, 2014, after receiving advice from an Emergency Committee of independent experts and in order to protect progress toward eradication, WHO Director-General Margaret Chan declared the recent international spread of wild poliovirus a "public health emergency of international concern," and issued Temporary Recommendations under the International Health Regulations (2005) to prevent further spread of the disease.

It is therefore imperative that we make this final push toward eradication one of our highest priorities. As Dr. Frieden has stated, "If we fail to get over the finish line, we will need to continue expensive control measures for the indefinite future…, More importantly, without eradication, a resurgence of polio could paralyze more than 200,000 children worldwide every year within a decade." Now is the time, we must not fail.

SEE ALSO   *Child Health; Global Health Initiatives; Sanitation and Hygiene; Vaccine-Preventable Diseases; Vaccines; Viral Diseases*

BIBLIOGRAPHY

Books

Kluger, Jeffrey. *Splendid Solution: Jonas Salk and the Conquest of Polio.* New York: G.P. Putnam's Sons, 2004.

Oshinsky, David. *Polio: An American Story.* New York: Oxford University Press, 2005.

Williams, Gareth. *Paralysed with Fear: The Story of Polio.* Basingstoke, UK: Palgrave Macmillan, 2013.

Wilson, Daniel. *Polio.* Santa Barbara, CA: Greenwood Press, 2009.

Periodicals

World Health Organization. "Polio Vaccines: WHO Position Paper January 2014, Recommendations." *Vaccines* 32, no. 33 (July 2014): 4117–4118.

Websites

Chan, Margaret. "WHO Director General Reports to Panel on Polio Situation." *World Health Organization,* September 22, 2014. http://www.who.int/dg/speeches/2014/unga-polio/en/ (accessed January 16, 2015).

"Poliomyelitis," Fact Sheet No. 114. *World Health Organization (WHO),* Updated October 2014. http://www.who.int/mediacentre/factsheets/fs114/en/ (accessed April 14, 2015).

"Poliomyelitis (Polio)." *World Health Organization (WHO).*http://www.who.int/topics/poliomyelitis/en/ (accessed January 16, 2015).

Rothberg, Daniel. "Southeast Asia Is Polio-Free, World Health Organization Rules." *Los Angeles Times,* March 27, 2014. http://articles.latimes.com/2014/mar/27/world/la-fg-wn-southeast-asia-india-polio-free-world-health-organization-20140327 (accessed January 16, 2015).

"What Is Vaccine-Derived Polio?" Online Q & A. *World Health Organization (WHO),* Updated October 2014. http://www.who.int/features/qa/64/en/ (accessed April 14, 2015).

World Health Organization (WHO). "Polio Eradication and Endgame Strategic Plan 2013–2018." *Global Polio Eradication Initiative (GPEI),* 2013. http://www.polioeradication.org/Resourcelibrary/Strategyandwork.aspx (accessed January 16, 2015).

Susan Aldridge

Population Issues

⊕ Introduction

As of July 2014, the United Nations (UN) stated that the world population was 7.244 billion, and it was predicted to reach 7.325 billion by July 2015. The U.S. Census Bureau estimates that there is one birth every eight seconds and one death every 12 seconds, which means that there is a net gain in the world population of one person every 14 seconds.

Global population is increasing at about 1.14 percent a year. In the 1960s, this rate reached a peak of over 2 percent and has been in decline ever since. This growth in the world's population has both positive and negative implications. The presence of more people, especially the young, can contribute to economic development and higher living standards for all. At the same time, each human on the planet creates a demand on resources of food, water, and energy and also creates waste. Moreover, demand for natural resources, and particularly for fossil fuels, is creating climate change and other environmental problems.

The largest countries in the world in terms of population are China and India. These are the only countries with over 1 billion people each. The population of the United States is nearly 319 million, as of 2014. According to the World Population Review, over half of the world's current population lives in 10 countries. These are: China, India, the United States, Indonesia, Brazil, Pakistan, Nigeria, Bangladesh, Russia, and Japan. India is set to surpass China as the world's country with the largest population by around 2030. More than 100 million people live in the world's largest cities, most of which are in Asia, and the largest of which is Shanghai, China. A total of just under 300,000 people live in the world's smallest countries, by population, of which the smallest is Vatican City, home to just 500 residents.

As well as absolute numbers, the structure, or demographics, of the world's population is important. Of note, there has been a shift in the age profile of the population. Reduced child mortality, coupled with high fertility, has led to an increase in the number of young people, particularly in Africa. In developed countries, there has also been an increase in the number of older people, thanks to high standards of living, which promote higher life expectancy. This trend is also being seen in some emerging economies like Vietnam and Bangladesh. Moreover, the world's population is increasingly concentrated in cities. These demographic shifts offer both opportunities and challenges.

It should be borne in mind that these population figures are estimates, rather than exact numbers. When the last milestone was passed and world population exceeded 7 billion, on October 31, 2011, according to the UN, it is not known who the seven billionth person actually was or where he or she was born. There is not even agreement on when the milestone actually happened, with the U.S. Census Bureau and the World Bank believing that the date when the human population reached 7 billion was in March or April 2012. Data on population comes from estimates prepared by most national governments, which may be based upon censuses taken at periodic intervals and also on mortality and fertility data. The UN also collects population data, which is published each year. When looking at how the world population will change in the future, researchers make projections based upon various kinds of analyses.

⊕ Historical Background

Estimates of the growth of world population over time begin with the start of the agricultural era, around 10,000 years ago. At this time, world population was about 5 million people. Over the next 8,000 years, it grew to 200 million at the most conservative estimate, and to 600 million according to the most generous estimate. The growth rate during this period was likely less than 0.05 percent per year. It took until around 1800 for the human population to reach 1 billion.

The Industrial Revolution was a great landmark in human population history. The global population experienced a sharp increase during this period, doubling by around 1930, to reach 2 billion. It then took only another 30 years to reach 3 billion, in 1959. Thereafter, time to reach the next billion got ever shorter, with 4 billion reached in 1974, 5 billion in 1987, and 6 billion in 1999. This means that during the 20th century, world population grew from 1.65 billion to 6 billion. Looking back over the entire course of human history, from the emergence of modern man around 50,000 years ago, at a rough estimate, around 106 billion people have been born.

Overpopulation Fears

In 1798, Thomas Malthus (1766–1834) made a famous prediction that the population would grow more rapidly than its ability to feed itself. Eventually, food would run out and people would starve. He believed that the global population would grow geometrically following the mathematical series: 1, 2, 4, 8, 16, 32, and so on, while food production could only grow arithmetically, following the series: 1, 2, 3, 4, 5. Food supply would not be able to keep up with the expanding population's needs, according to this theory. Although it is true that more than 800 million people in the world do not have enough to eat, the predicted mass starvation has not yet occurred. This is mainly because the food supply has been able to grow faster than Malthus ever envisaged, thanks to the use of fertilizers and modern plant-breeding techniques.

However, more recent thinkers have also proposed that the rapid expansion of the human population could lead to disastrous results. One is the Stanford University population biologist Paul R. Ehrlich (1932–). Like Malthus, he warned of mass starvation in his 1968 book *The Population Bomb*. Later, he pointed to other problems associated with increased population. These stem from the threefold increase in human activity since the end of World War II (1939–1945) and include expansion of agriculture, deforestation, damming of rivers, and the vast increase in the use of motor vehicles. Added to these is the increase of methane and carbon dioxide levels in the atmosphere that has come from the escalating use of fossil fuels to support the demands of the human population. All these issues came to the forefront in the 1970s, with the growth of the Green politics movement in Europe.

⊕ Impacts and Issues

The size of the human population, the numbers of children people have, and how and where people live all have an impact on important aspects of the planet, from air and water quality to wildlife habitats, weather, and climate. In the early 1970s, Ehrlich, together with John Holdren (1944–), later President Barack Obama's (1961–) science adviser, and Barry Commoner (1917–2012), a founding member of the modern environmental movement, put forward a formula to measure the impact of a growing human population on Earth.

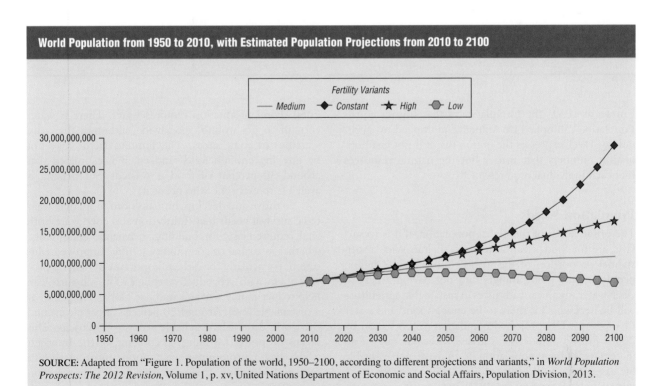

World Population from 1950 to 2010, with Estimated Population Projections from 2010 to 2100

SOURCE: Adapted from "Figure 1. Population of the world, 1950–2100, according to different projections and variants," in *World Population Prospects: The 2012 Revision*, Volume 1, p. xv, United Nations Department of Economic and Social Affairs, Population Division, 2013.

URBANIZATION

A marked demographic trend in recent years has been the shift of people from rural to urban locations. In 1950, more than two-thirds of the world's population lived in rural settings, according to the United Nations Population Division. Today, just over half the world's population lives in cities. By 2050, it is estimated that the 1950 situation will be reversed, with two-thirds of the world's population living in cities.

In 1950, the global urban population was 0.7 billion; in 2014, this had risen to 3.9 billion. In 2050, it is projected to rise again to 6.3 billion. In contrast, the rural population is predicted to remain about the same. In 2020, it is likely to peak at just under 3.4 billion and to decline to 3.2 billion by 2050. At a national level, this means that many countries now have the majority of their population resident in cities rather than in the countryside. The number of predominantly rural countries is decreasing.

The most urbanized regions of the world are North America, Latin America, and the Caribbean. Here, 80 percent or more of the population lives in cities. In Europe, 73 percent of the population are city dwellers, and this is likely to reach more than 80 percent by 2050. Africa and Asia remain predominantly rural, with 40 percent and 43 percent of their populations, respectively, living in urban areas in 2014. Both regions are projected to urbanize rapidly, respectively reaching 56 percent and 64 percent urban by 2050. However, they will still be the two least urbanized regions of the world, according to the United Nations Population Division.

In Africa, there will be variation in level of urbanization. Nearly half of African countries are likely to be at least 60 percent urban by 2050. However, nine countries will remain less than 40 percent urban; this includes countries that have some of the highest overall populations, such as Uganda and Ethiopia. In Asia, one-quarter of countries are already at least 80 percent urban. The urbanization trend will continue in Asia, and by 2050, only Cambodia, Nepal, and Sri Lanka will be less than 40 percent urban. By 2050, half of countries in Europe, and the whole of North America will be at least 80 percent urbanized. In Latin America and the Caribbean, nearly half of countries will be 80 percent urbanized.

Thus, there will be 2.5 billion new city dwellers by 2050. Most of these will be living in Africa and Asia. It is these urban areas that are going to absorb most of the projected growth in the world's population. This growth will be particularly marked in India, China, and Nigeria, which will account for more than one-third of global urban population growth. Another 20 percent of this growth will occur in the Democratic Republic of the Congo, Ethiopia, Tanzania, Bangladesh, Indonesia, Pakistan, and the United States.

As far as the rural population is concerned, 36 percent of countries saw a decline in recent years, while 61 percent saw an increase. Around two-thirds of countries will see a decrease in their rural populations between 2014 and 2050, according to UN estimates. The biggest rural loss will occur in Japan, where there will be a 71 percent reduction. However, many countries in sub-Saharan Africa will see an increase in their rural populations, particularly in Chad, Malawi, Zambia, Burundi, Niger, and Uganda. This is because of an overall population increase in these countries.

Urbanization offers both opportunities and challenges. Cities drive forward development, both economic and social. They are a focus for government, business, transportation, education, and communication. However, unplanned and rapid urban growth leads to slum conditions, poverty, unemployment, and crime. Thus, policy makers should plan the growth of cities in a sustainable way. This means building the infrastructure for water, sanitation, transport, energy, and communications. There should be ample opportunity for employment and access to services. Only in this way can living standards of both urban and rural dwellers be improved.

Known as IPAT, the formula states that Impact equals Population multiplied by Affluence multiplied by Technology. IPAT expresses the notion that it is not just population numbers that matter but the natural resources that each individual requires.

Population Needs

The prime needs of the global population, if it is to survive, are for food, clean water, and shelter. With a substantial proportion of the world's more than 7 billion people already going hungry and not having access to clean water, significant advances in sustainable agriculture will be necessary for there to be enough food and water to support a UN projected population of 9.6 billion by 2050. Equally important is access to health care, if an increasing human population is to have a reasonable life expectancy and quality of life. Demand for food will increase by 50 percent by 2030 and by 70 percent by 2050. Food production requires water. There is water enough to go around, worldwide, although there are scarcities in some areas. The limiting factor may not be growing enough food—indeed, it is estimated that around 30 percent of food is wasted—but making it available to everyone who needs it.

To thrive and develop, humans need more than their basic survival needs met. Education and energy are both vital requirements for building a dynamic community, whether in a rural or community setting. Improved education, particularly for girls, is important in helping provide them with reproductive choice. This, in turn, can help reduce family size and stabilize global population at a sustainable level. Around 20 percent of people around the world do not have reliable access to electricity. This means no power for lighting, cooking, or the Internet, which has a profound impact upon nutrition, health care, and education. It also severely limits transportation possibilities.

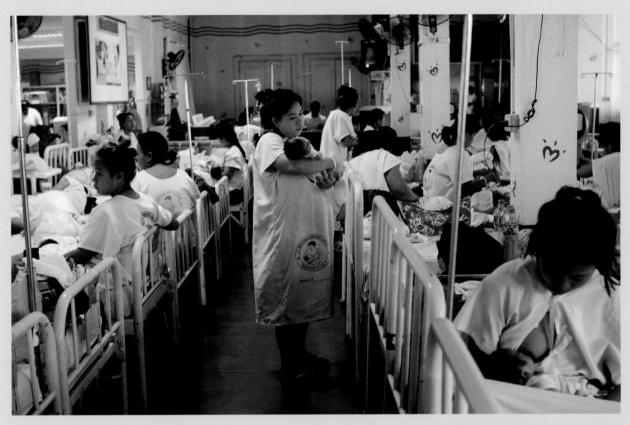

Indigent mothers tend to new born infants at a government-run hospital ward on August 11, 2014, in Manila, Philippines. The Philippines has one of the fastest-growing populations in Southeast Asia with around 100 million people. At least 12 million people live in the capital city of Manila alone, making it one of the most densely populated and largest cities in the world. Lack of space and economic opportunities has pushed around 4 million people to live informally along waterways, bridges, and even cemeteries, further straining the already weak infrastructure and limited resources of the city. *© Dondi Tawatao/Getty Images.*

Impact on the Environment

Unfortunately, the demands of an increasing human population are having a deleterious effect upon the environment. This, in turn, can make it harder to meet the demands of this population. For instance, human activity related to a growing population and its needs has resulted in the emission of greenhouse gases into the atmosphere. The resulting climate change has lowered crop yields and caused extreme weather events, such as flooding, which destroy homes and cost lives.

Demand for energy for transportation and electricity has not only increased the use of fossil fuels, driving climate change, but has also had a negative impact upon air quality. Growth in traffic has led to emissions of nitrogen oxides, particulate matter, and ozone into the air, which has been linked to increased heart and lung disease, and premature mortality. In China, for instance, cities regularly exceed the safe particulate matter levels set by the World Health Organization, owing to the traffic increase

that has accompanied the country's economic development. This is putting the health of China's urban population at risk.

As the global population grows, so does the amount of solid waste it produces, particularly in cities. The amount of solid waste produced by the human population has increased 10-fold since the beginning of the 20th century. An analysis by Canadian scientists, published in the journal *Nature*, estimates that 6.61 tons (6 billion metric tons) of solid waste will be produced by 2025. Landfill sites in emerging cities like Seoul, Shanghai, Mexico City, and Rio de Janeiro are fast filling up. Their presence can cause an environmental threat as leakage may contaminate water and land. Burning waste in incinerators can release pollutants to the air. Worst of all, in some places such as India, waste is merely dumped waste on vast, unmanaged open mountains, attracting local residents who scavenge and put their health at risk. It is likely that solid waste production will begin to slow

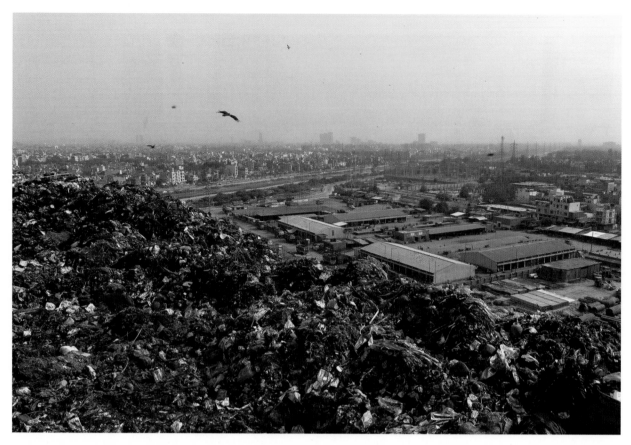

Birds fly over the garbage at the Ghazipur landfill site overlooking housing east of New Delhi, India. The population of New Delhi, which is predicted to reach close to 21 million by 2015, generates 8,000 tons of garbage per day. The trash is not separated between organic and inorganic materials—everything from leftover food to batteries and beverage cans goes into Indian bins—causing massive pollution and raising toxic emissions. With 1.26 billion people, India was the world's second-most-populous nation after China (1.37 billion) in 2014, but was expected to surpass China by 2025. © *Chandan Khanna/AFP/Getty Images.*

down as living standards rise and people become more aware of waste reduction and recycling efforts. But waste production is likely to remain an environmental problem well into the next century.

Global Population Structure

The three dimensions of population structure used by demographers to analyze the impact of populations are fertility, mortality, and migration. Information on these dimensions generates patterns and trends that policy makers can use to formulate sustainable plans for human development in the future. Fertility is the number of children a woman bears during her lifetime. Mortality is how long an individual lives, while migration looks at the movements of people across the globe, both within and between countries.

The current global fertility rate is 2.5 children per woman, with marked variation between countries. The replacement level, beyond which a population will shrink, is currently 2.1 children per woman. There has been a global decline in fertility from around five children per woman to 2.5, which can be attributed to increased

female education and better access to family planning. Fertility continues to be high in sub-Saharan Africa, at an average of 4.6 children per woman. According to the World Bank, fertility rates are highest in Niger, Mali, and Somalia, at 7.6, 6.9, and 6.7 children per woman respectively. Several other African nations have fertility rates in excess of 6 children per woman. In many countries, however, fertility has decreased, sometimes below replacement level, as is so in the United States. In Brazil, average family size has decreased from 6.3 children to 1.9 children per woman over just two generations.

Falling child mortality, coupled with continuing high fertility, has meant that there is a high population of young people in Africa. However, this growth has not been matched by a corresponding increase in education and employment. These are investments that need to be made if the potential of these young people is to be harnessed for development and improved standards of living. Nongovernmental organizations like Young People We Care are setting up projects to equip young people in Africa with useful skills. More should also be done to ensure that policy makers connect with young people.

Developed countries and so-called advanced developing countries have a different demographic issue in their shift toward an increasingly aging population. The number of people aged over 60 is rising dramatically, with a corresponding increase in the incidence of noncommunicable diseases, such as cancer, diabetes, and dementia. This means that the cost to health and social care budgets will soar, unless more is done to ensure that a long life is also a healthy one. For instance, more monitoring of blood pressure could make a huge contribution, as undiagnosed hypertension is responsible for more preventable deaths and disability through heart disease, kidney disease, and stroke than any other risk factor.

People have always migrated in search of a better life. Migration can benefit the recipient country by adding to the numbers of people with skills who can enhance economic productivity. However, it may also create social tensions if native residents feel that immigrants are depriving them of employment opportunities or failing to integrate into the nation's culture and values. The export of those with vital skills, such as health-care workers and researchers, may also have a detrimental effect upon the emigrants' country of origin.

According to a 2013 report from the Pew Research Center, the number of international migrants rose from 154 million in 1990 to 232 million in 2013. Because of global population growth, the overall proportion of migrants has remained constant at 3 percent of the population. The most notable trend is an increase of migration from middle-income countries, like India and China, to high-income regions, such as Europe and North America. In 1990, 57 percent of migrants went to high-income countries; by 2013, this had increased to 69 percent. Meanwhile, 48 percent of international migrants originated in middle-income countries in 1990; by 2013, this had increased to 58 percent. The United States remains the country of choice for international migrants, with one migrant in five living there. European countries are also attractive destinations for migration.

Focus on Family Planning

Providing global access to sexual and reproductive health as well as contraception is key to ensuring that population growth is stable and sustainable. A report from the Copenhagen Consensus, a group of economists specializing in development, suggests that each dollar spent on providing universal sexual and reproductive health by 2030 and making modern contraception available to all women by 2040 gives a return of $120. Fewer children born to a woman means reduced infant and maternal mortality. Overall, a lower population means less pressure on resources locally, nationally, and internationally, and more opportunities for education and economic productivity.

Successful family planning technology, allowing women to limit the size of their families or space out their children more, already exists. The issue now is to make it available to women who want to benefit from it.

This means overcoming prejudice and taboo that exists still in some regions and also improving health-care infrastructures to ensure fulfillment of contraceptive needs.

Old Age: The New Normal

The most recent figures from the UN, presenting world mortality data for 2005–2010, show that half of all deaths now occur in the over-65 age group. In the period 1950–1955, 22 percent of deaths occurred in old age. This increase in the percentage of old-age deaths applies to both developed and less-developed countries. Overall, the increase in the percentage of deaths in old age is due to reduction in child mortality, which refers to deaths between birth and four years of age. The percentage of mid-age deaths, occurring between the ages of 5 and 64, has remained relatively stable since the mid-1960s.

Within this broad statistic, there are some important variations. In less-developed regions, overall, the main reason for the shift to an older-age demographic is because of a decline in childhood mortality. However, in the least-developed countries within this region, there has been an important influence of an increase in mid-age deaths, owing to high prevalence of human immuno-deficiency virus/acquired immune deficiency syndrome (HIV/AIDS). In 1950–1955, the percentage of mid-age deaths in these countries was 34 percent; in 2005–2010 it had risen to 40 percent. In more developed countries, the percentage of mid-age deaths declined from 34 percent in 1950–1955 to 25 percent in 2005–2010. The main cause of this decrease is a reduction of deaths from noncommunicable disease, such as heart disease, which can be attributed to improvements in health care. In 2005–2010, the countries with the highest percentage of old-age deaths were Italy (86 percent), Sweden (86 percent), and Greece (85 percent). The three nations with the lowest percentage of old-age deaths were the Democratic Republic of the Congo (13 percent), Chad (12 percent), and Angola (11 percent).

⊕ Future Implications

Experts disagree on both the maximum future size of the total human population and when this maximum figure will be reached. A 2013 study from the UN and University of Washington researchers suggests that population growth will not level off without a rapid decrease in birthrates among women in sub-Saharan Africa. World population could reach between 9.6 billion and 12.3 billion by 2100. The study used government data and expert forecasts for mortality rates, fertility rates, and international migration. Previously, however, population experts had said that world population would peak at 9 billion in 2045 and then start to level off. This estimate is based on the assumption that as living standards rise around the world, average family size would start to decrease and people will live longer. Therefore, growth would slow and eventually stop.

According to the 2013 study, it is likely that the population of Africa will be between 3.5 billion and 5.1 billion people at the end of the 21st century. The population of Asia, at 4.4 billion in 2014, would likely peak at 5 billion around the middle of the 21st century, and then start to decline. The populations of North America, Europe, Latin America, and the Caribbean were likely to remain at below 1 billion each.

PRIMARY SOURCE

World Population Prospects: The 2012 Revision

SOURCE *United Nations Department of Economic and Social Affairs Population Division (2013). "Executive Summary," from* World Population Prospects: The 2012 Revision, Highlights and Advance Tables. *Working Paper No. ESA/P/ WP.228, xv–xvi. http://esa.un.org/unpd/ wpp/Documentation/pdf/WPP2012_HIGH- LIGHTS.pdf (accessed January 25, 2015).*

INTRODUCTION *This primary source summarizes global population estimates and projections. It is an excerpt from a report prepared in 2012 by the Population Division of the Department of Economic and Social Affairs of the United Nations Secretariat.*

EXECUTIVE SUMMARY

The *2012 Revision* is the twenty-third round of official United Nations population estimates and projections, prepared by the Population Division of the Department of Economic and Social Affairs of the United Nations Secretariat. The *2012 Revision* builds on the previous revision by incorporating the results of the 2010 round of national population censuses as well as findings from recent specialized demographic surveys that have been carried out around the world. These sources provide both demographic and other information to assess the progress made in achieving the internationally agreed development goals, including the Millennium Development Goals (MDGs). The comprehensive review of past worldwide demographic trends and future prospects presented in the *2012 Revision* provides the population basis for the assessment of those goals.

According to the *2012 Revision* of the official United Nations population estimates and projections, the world population of 7.2 billion in mid–2013 is projected to increase by almost one billion people within the next twelve years, reaching 8.1 billion in 2025, and to further increase to 9.6 billion in 2050 and 10.9 billion by 2100.

These results are based on the medium-variant projection, which assumes a decline of fertility for countries where large families are still prevalent as well as a slight increase of fertility in several countries with fewer than two children per woman on average.

Small differences in the trajectory of fertility during the next decades will have major consequences for population size, structure, and distribution in the long run. The "high-variant" projection, for example, which assumes an extra half of a child per woman (on average) compared to the medium variant, implies a world population of 10.9 billion in 2050 and 16.6 billion in 2100. The "low-variant" projection, where women have half a child less, on average, than under the medium variant, would produce a population of 8.3 billion in 2050. Thus, a constant difference of only half a child above or below the medium variant would result in a global population in 2050 of around 1.3 billion more or less compared to the medium variant of 9.6 billion.

Compared with the results from the previous revision, the projected global population total in this revision is higher, particularly after 2075, for several reasons. First, fertility levels have been adjusted upward in a number of countries on the basis of recently available information. In the new revision, the estimated total fertility rate (TFR) for 2005–2010 has increased in several countries, including by more than 5 per cent in 15 high-fertility countries from sub-Saharan Africa. In some cases, the actual level of fertility appears to have risen in recent years; in other cases, the previous estimate was too low. The cumulative effects of these higher estimates of current fertility levels will play out over several decades and are responsible for significant upward adjustments in the projected population size of certain countries between the two revisions. Second, slight modifications in the projected fertility trajectories of some very populous countries have yielded important differences in long-run forecasts. Third, future levels of life expectancy at birth are slightly higher in several countries within this latest projection; longer survival, like higher fertility, generates larger populations. Lastly, a small portion of the difference between revisions is attributable to changes in the projection methodology used for this revision.

Almost all of the additional 3.7 billion people from now to 2100 will enlarge the population of developing countries, which is projected to rise from 5.9 billion in 2013 to 8.2 billion in 2050 and to 9.6 billion in 2100, and will mainly be distributed among the population aged 15–59 (1.6 billion) and 60 or over (1.99 billion), as the number of children under age 15 in developing countries will hardly increase. Growth is expected to be particularly dramatic in the least developed countries of the world, which are projected to double in size from 898 million inhabitants in 2013 to 1.8 billion in 2050 and to 2.9 billion in 2100.

In contrast, the population of the more developed regions is expected to change minimally, passing from

1.25 billion in 2013 to 1.28 billion in 2100, and would decline were it not for the net increase due to migration from developing to developed countries, which is projected to average about 2.4 million persons annually from 2013 to 2050 and 1 million from 2050 to 2100.

At the country level, much of the overall increase between 2013 and 2050 is projected to take place in high-fertility countries, mainly in Africa, as well as countries with large populations such as India, Indonesia, Pakistan, the Philippines and the United States of America.

The results of the *2012 Revision* incorporate the findings of the most recent national population censuses, including from the 2010 round of censuses, and of numerous specialized population surveys carried out around the world. *The 2012 Revision* provides the demographic data and indicators to assess trends at the global, regional and national levels and to calculate many other key indicators commonly used by the United Nations system.

SEE ALSO *Family Planning; Life Expectancy and Aging Populations; Vulnerable Populations; World Health Organization: Organization, Funding, and Enforcement Powers*

BIBLIOGRAPHY

Books

Relethford, John H. *Human Population Genetics*. Hoboken, NJ: Wiley-Blackwell, 2012.

Swanson, David A., and Jeff Tayman. *Subnational Population Estimates*. Dordrecht, Netherlands: Springer, 2010.

United Nations Population Fund. *Population Situation Analysis: A Conceptual and Methodological Guide*. New York: United Nations Population Fund, 2010.

Periodicals

Cumberland, Sarah, and Adrienne Germain. "From Population Control to Human Rights." *Bulletin of the World Health Organization* 90, no. 2 (February 2011): 77–156.

Gerland, Patrick, et al. "World Population Decline Unlikely This Century." *Science* 346, no. 6206 (October 10, 2014): 234–237.

Myrskylä, Mikko, et al. "Advances in Development Reverse Fertility Declines." *Nature* 460 (August 6, 2009): 741–743.

Reijnders, Lucas, and Sam Soret. "Quantification of the Environmental Impact of Different Dietary Protein Choices." *American Journal of Clinical Nutrition* 78, no. 3 (September 2003): 668S–668S.

Websites

Behrman, Kohler. "Post-2015 Consensus: Population and Demography Assessment." *Copenhagen Consensus.* http://www.copenhagenconsensus.com/publication/post-2015-consensus-population-and-demography-assessment-kohler-behrman (accessed March 31, 2015).

Connor, Phillip, D'Vera Cohn, and Ana Gonzalez-Barrera. "Changing Patterns of Global Migration and Remittances." *Pew Research Center*, December 17, 2013. http://www.pewsocialtrends.org/2013/12/17/changing-patterns-of-global-migration-and-remittances/ (accessed March 31, 2015).

Hoornweg, Daniel, Perinaz Bhada-Tata, and Chris Kennedy. "Environment: Waste Production Must Peak This Century." *Nature*, October 30, 2013. http://www.nature.com/news/environment-waste-production-must-peak-this-century-1.14032#/ref-link-2 (accessed March 31, 2015).

McElroy, Molly. "UW Research: World Population Could Be Nearly 11 Billion by 2100." *UW Today*, June 13, 2013. http://www.washington.edu/news/2013/06/13/uw-research-world-population-could-be-nearly-11-billion-by-2100/ (accessed March 31, 2015).

"Population Facts." *United Nations, Department of Economic and Social Affairs, Population Division*, August 2014. http://www.un.org/en/development/desa/population/publications/pdf/popfacts/PopFacts_2014-3.pdf (accessed March 31, 2015).

"State of World Population." *United Nations Population Fund (UNFPA)*, 2014. http://www.unfpa.org/swop (accessed March 31, 2015).

"Title X Family Planning" *U.S. Department of Health and Human Services, Office of Population Affairs.* http://www.hhs.gov/opa/title-x-family-planning/index.html (accessed March 31, 2015).

"Urban Population Growth." *World Health Organization (WHO)*. http://www.who.int/gho/urban_health/situation_trends/urban_population_growth_text/en/ (accessed March 31, 2015).

"USAID's Family Planning Guiding Principles and U.S. Legislative and Policy Requirements" *USAID*. http://www.usaid.gov/what-we-do/global-health/family-planning/usaids-family-planning-guiding-principles-and-us-0 (accessed March 31, 2015).

"World Population Prospects—The 2012 Revision." *United Nations Department of Economic and Social Affairs Population Division*, 2012. http://esa.un.org/wpp/ (accessed March 31, 2015).

Susan Aldridge

Post-Traumatic Stress Syndrome

⊕ Introduction

Post-traumatic stress syndrome, more frequently called post-traumatic stress disorder (PTSD), is the product of a person experiencing a traumatic event that is beyond the range of the normal human experience. In a normal reaction to danger, the body prepares a fight or flight response that recedes after the danger has passed. In extreme cases this acute natural reaction can cause the sufferer to feel stressed, frightened, anxious, and irritable long after the danger has passed. This condition is considered PTSD.

There is no way of telling whether, once subjected to a traumatic event, a person will develop post-trauma stress symptoms, but there are risk factors that psychologists have identified. If a person has experienced childhood abuse or neglect in advance of another traumatic event, has other mental health problems, or lacks a stable support network of family and friends, that person could be at risk. If a person has a job that increases the risk of repetitive exposure to trauma, such as first responders or police officers, that person's risk of developing the disorder can be compounded. PTSD is associated most closely with the war veterans but can result from any range of traumatic events such as accidents, physical or sexual assault, or natural disasters.

Not all people who are subjected to traumatic events end up with the disorder, even when similar risk factors are present. Brain anatomy, a person's history with trauma, culture, and individual personality characteristics are all currently being studied so that one day there will be a better understanding of how trauma affects the brain and how stress disorders can be prevented.

⊕ Historical Background

PTSD has not always been known by that name, but symptoms of the kind that exist today have been known and described in literature throughout history. *Gilgamesh*, the first known piece of human literature; *The Iliad* by Homer; and the Bible all contain descriptions of the psychological casualties that occurred in countless past wars. In conflicts prior to the Vietnam War (1954–1975), the manifestations of similar symptoms were termed soldier's heart, shell shock, and war neurosis.

The first known medical descriptions of *névrose de guerre* (war neurosis), as it was called in France until the 20th century, was in a classical French treatise on illnesses, *Nosographie Philosophique* (1798), by Philippe Pinel. PTSD was named cardiorespiratory neurosis because of rapid heart rate and hyperventilation of the sufferers.

It was not until after the Industrial Revolution, when mechanical accidents such as train crashes produced similar symptoms in survivors, that physicians began to see a link between the two groups. The hypothesis that people were suffering from a disorder, and not just a hysteria or insanity, was met with considerable criticism, especially in Western countries. It was a Russian psychiatrist at the start of the 20th century who first started providing psychiatric treatment to soldiers after the Russo-Japanese War (1904–1905). He emphasized the similarities between the psychological states of the returning veterans with the diagnoses descriptions of train crash survivors.

Shell Shock

The Industrial Revolution mechanized transportation and industry, but also mechanized war. World War I (1914–1918) was the first to be waged with planes, bombs, and chemical warfare. The industrial nature and brutality of the war, which could never have been anticipated by its participants, is considered contributory to the extraordinarily high percentage of psychiatric patients the war produced. Hospitals were overwhelmed by soldiers without physical wounds but experiencing psychological trauma. Robert Gaupp (1870–1953), a German psychologist, reported that "the main causes are the fright and anxiety brought about by the explosion of enemy shells and mines."

The resulting reactions—deafness, muteness, inability to stand or walk, and tremors with no physical basis—were termed shellshock. Doctors found that treating the soldiers immediately, near the front lines, and among their comrades had the effect of preventing the symptoms from becoming chronic. By the end of World War I, a universal therapy doctrine had been established. But by the start of World War II (1939–1945), the principles that had been applied in the previous conflict had been forgotten and had to be discovered anew. Shell shock became the term that remained in the American and European lexicon until the United States entered the Vietnam War.

The Seed of Stigma

Despite the reactions of soldiers, and victims, it was not completely accepted that the symptoms people described were real. Many people accused soldiers of faking the symptoms as a way to be removed from the front lines of battle or taking advantage of the possibility they might be discharged with a lifetime pension. Even now, medals for being wounded in combat, such as the Purple Heart in the United States, are awarded only to those who sustain physical injury; there is no corresponding award for sustaining psychological damage during combat. In one less than compassionate episode, in 1917, UK officials executed 306 British soldiers by firing squad when they were accused of cowardice and desertion because of the trauma symptoms they had experienced. In 2006, the British government issued posthumous pardons to the soldiers' families. The idea that the soldiers suffering from psychological injury during war were somehow weaker or more cowardly than their counterparts is a pervasive reason why, even today, there is strong resistance to seeking treatment.

Community as Prevention

The resistance to seeking treatment increased after the Vietnam War. American veterans came home to a country protesting the war, and a community unsupportive of veterans' involvement. In World Wars I and II, the onset of symptoms was immediate and benefited from quick intervention at the front lines. Whereas some front line interventions were used to help veterans in Vietnam, the treatment did nothing to prevent a delayed onset of PTSD. Most researchers blame the hostile environment to which the veterans returned and the lack of support structures at home for the late onset of symptoms. For American soldiers, the delayed PTSD was considered new, but late onset of symptoms had been seen before: a small subset of soldiers drafted unwillingly in World War I into the German Army from the Alsatian region of France also experienced abnormally high rates of PTSD with a delayed onset. The Alsatian region lies across the border of both France and Germany and possesses a unique cultural identity

with elements of both countries. Because the soldiers were from across the French border, they were considered untrustworthy by the Germans during the conflict. They were treated as traitors once they returned to France. In both these instances, the soldiers returned from horrifying experiences to a hostile atmosphere, where they lacked emotional support from society. In both cases the trauma did not cause chronic damage until after they returned home.

PTSD in Civilian Life

However, it is important to realize that PTSD is not just a soldier's syndrome. For example, in 1994, Rwanda suffered a genocide, during which officials estimated that more than a million people died in less than four months. Women were subjected to brutal sexual assaults; friends became each other's executioners, and the country's structure crumbled. As a result of the genocide, no working psychiatric hospital existed, and most of the staff had been killed. It was reported that even a decade later only a single psychiatrist resided in all of Rwanda. Rates of PTSD in Rwanda have not been studied exhaustively, but among the few studies that do exist, results seem to be similar to other studies cross-culturally indicating a mixture of factors contributing to the occurrence of PTSD symptoms.

⊕ Impacts and Issues

Veterans and civilians experiencing the U.S. wars in Iraq (2003–2011) and Afghanistan (2001–) are among the most recent populations to develop PTSD en masse, with experts estimating that the disorder occurs in almost 20 percent of the returning U.S. veteran population. Men are more likely to experience a major trauma (about 60 percent) than women (50 percent), but women are more likely to develop the disorder. About 5.2 million people in United States suffer from PTSD.

As noted however, trauma is not limited to soldiers and can occur in many settings. Countries across the globe have refugees, victims of genocide, sexual assault, and countless other individuals experiencing events that can cause trauma. Many times these events destroy the infrastructure and medical facilities necessary to provide adequate care. Relief efforts have concentrated heavily on physical injury rather than psychological health. However, in 2013, the World Health Organization (WHO) released guidelines for primary care health-care workers dealing with trauma-related mental disorders following traumatic events such as conflicts and natural disasters.

Symptoms

Studies show that brain function can be changed by severe or repetitive trauma. Severe or repetitive trauma can trick the mind into believing that the experience is

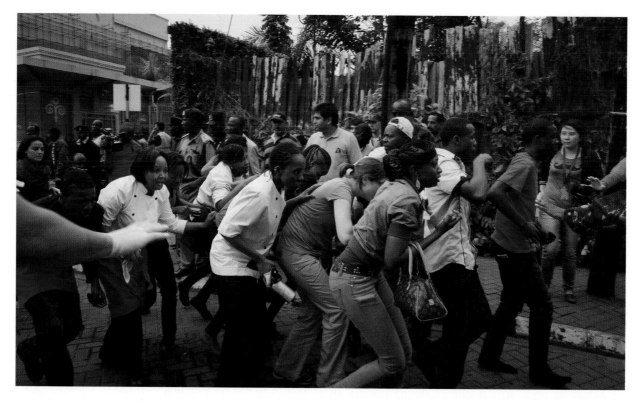

Civilians flee after hiding during a gun battle in the Westgate Mall in Nairobi, Kenya. Gunmen threw grenades and opened fire at the upscale mall. Some people who were caught up in the Westgate Mall terrorist attack are showing signs of post-traumatic stress disorder according to psychologist Katie McLaughlin of the University of Washington in Seattle, and children caught up in the attack seem to be especially vulnerable. © *Jonathan Kalan/AP Images.*

happening over and over again. Those repetitive intrusive memories are one of the three categories in which psychiatrists group PTSD symptoms. The other two categories are dissociative symptoms and hyperarousal.

The category of intrusive memories can cover a wide range of experiences including flashbacks in which the sufferer relives the experience in vivid detail. Dreams that can mimic or remind that dreamer of the event are common. Although less common, unrelated but similar physical experiences can remind the person of the trauma. For example, if the individual was running at the time of the initial trauma, running could reproduce the same emotional and psychological state even though there is no impending danger in the current situation.

Dissociative symptoms can be less obvious to the outside world but no less detrimental to the psychological state of the traumatized person. Many PTSD sufferers avoid thinking about the event and avoid the places, people, or activities that could in some way be related to the trauma. Patients report not being comfortable with downtime and unable to relax. For example, a person could choose to work long hours as a way to avoid thinking about the event. A feeling of numbness and lack of connection to the world around them, sometimes described as "watching life from the outside" is called

dissociation and is common among those who have survived trauma. Dissociation can make a person incapable of connecting with other individuals and contribute to mental health issues such as depression.

Hyperarousal symptoms include jumpiness, irritability, and a sense of always being on guard. Outbursts of uncontrollable emotion are common. Any of these symptoms can make it difficult for sufferers to maintain close relationships or to experience positive emotions.

Treatment

Treating PTSD can be dependent highly on the individual, and the circumstances surrounding the trauma. As with the front line treatment on the battlefield, treatment needs to be maintained by a positive environment and supportive relationships. People living with PTSD often see a primary physician first. Talking to a patient about whether PTSD could be a possible cause is important. Traditional psychotherapy can be most helpful when the therapy sessions are goal oriented and structured, rather than just supportive.

Evidence-based practices of therapies that have been statistically proven to be effective are tailored to the individual. Cognitive behavior therapy (CBT) is an evidence-based practice utilized to treat a variety of mental health issues. CBT slowly increases exposure to the traumatic event so that, in time, the anxiety and symptoms eventually can be reduced. With technological advances CBT is beginning to employ computer simulations to increase exposure to the trauma while providing a safe place for patients to confront their fears.

The brain must relearn how to process information during therapy for PTSD. There have been successful efforts at a stimulating the brain while using an exposure treatment such as CBT. This is called eye movement desensitization reprocess (EMDR). Results of several research studies reveal that a combination of trauma-based CBT and EMDR is very effective as first-line, nonmedication therapy for PTSD. Further study is needed to determine if the alternating movements of the eyes are related to the success of the treatment, or if the exposure treatment alone would have the same effects.

Other alternative methods of treatment, including the employment of service dogs or other animals, regular yoga practice, or meditation can supplement traditional therapies and are becoming increasingly popular. Service dogs are a 24-hour-per-day therapy that can teach the person to rely on a dog's instincts as a break from the constant vigilance that accompanies PTSD. The use of these supplementing therapies such as service dogs usually are studied in relation to veterans, but there is reason to believe that persons suffering from nonwar-related trauma would benefit from alternative methods of therapy as well.

Finally, there are a variety of medications that treat the symptoms of PTSD. It is important to understand that these medications also need to be tailored to the individual. Selective serotonin reuptake inhibitors are used most commonly as antidepressants to help to reduce symptoms. Mood stabilizers often are utilized to treat individuals with dissociative symptoms. For individuals with frequent sleep disturbances, the restoration of a normal sleep pattern can be vital to recovery. Sleep medications can be prescribed or bought over the counter at a physician's suggestion to assist in a full night's sleep. What is not suggested is self-medicating with alcohol or illegal substances. Although they may numb anxiety briefly, prolonged use can exacerbate symptoms and increase the intensity of depression. See the sidebar for more information on self-medication, drug abuse, and suicide prevention.

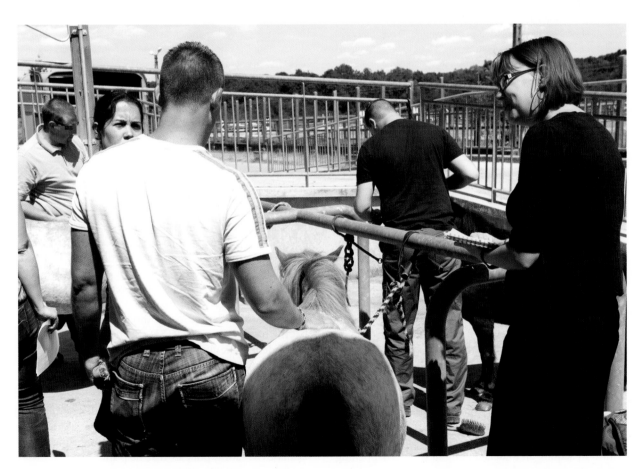

An officer suffering from post-traumatic stress disorder stands next to a pony during a session of horse therapy at the military horse riding school of Moulins-les-Metz, eastern France. The horse therapy sessions are organized and supervised by the Hospital Instruction Armies of Metz. © *Jean-Christophe Verhaegen/AFP/Getty Images.*

ALCOHOLISM, DRUG USE, AND SUICIDE

Post-traumatic stress disorder (PTSD) often is found to be a factor in illegal drug use, and alcoholism is a common avoidance mechanism and an effort to self-medicate. Self-medication occurs when an individual takes illicit drugs or alcohol in order to cope with painful emotions. Dissociative symptoms, the feeling of being outside one's body, also contribute to drug use and danger-seeking habits such as irresponsible driving that can cause the dissociative symptoms to abate temporarily.

The medicinal properties of alcohol and illegal substances are only temporary and actually can make it harder to cope with the stress and anxieties that are exacerbated by PTSD. Because sufferers sometimes have difficulty sleeping, some use alcohol as a sleep aid. Sufferers fail to realize that alcohol fundamentally changes the nature and quality of their sleep, making it less restful. They medicate the less restful sleep with more alcohol, and the cycle continues.

Up to 75 percent of the survivors of abuse or violent trauma report drinking heavily and regularly, but even this number could be low. The stigma of mental illness and substance abuse makes people less likely to report their drinking and drug habits honestly. Unfortunately, 34 percent of all men and 27 percent of all women with PTSD also will suffer from drug addiction. An estimated 28 percent of women and 52 percent of men with PTSD eventually will be classified as alcoholics. It should be noted that these percentages do not differentiate between substance use disorders that were already present before a traumatic event and those that developed after the trauma occurred. Both situations likely are present in these percentages. Some researchers suspect that the genetic factors associated with a higher likelihood of substance use disorders also could be related to a genetic predisposition for stress disorders.

Individuals who suffer from both substance use disorders and PTSD should seek treatment for the substance use first. This helps determine which symptoms are related to the substance use and which are exclusive to the post-traumatic stress. Abstaining from drugs or alcohol once addiction is present is difficult and can produce significant withdrawal symptoms such as shaking, nausea, hallucinations, and seizures. The depressant quality of alcohol coupled with the overwhelming symptoms of PTSD creates an increased risk for suicide.

Suicide is the greatest risk posed for a person with PTSD. It is a perilous problem for veterans returning from war. Suicidal thoughts can start with what is called survivor's guilt. Having witnessed the deaths of friends and colleagues, the person who is already struggling with the anxiety and depression of PTSD can start to believe that suicide is inevitable. The returning veteran may even believe that suicide is deserved because he or she survived when others did not. Suicide ideation becomes dangerous at this point. As a result of veteran's military training and combat experience, the fear that accompanies the idea of pain or death which prevents others from contemplating suicide is less prominent in veterans.

The U.S. Army suicide rate increased from 12.4 to 18.1 per 100,000 between 2003 and 2008 during the wars in Iraq and Afghanistan. The rate increased 30 percent between 2008 and 2014. That is approximately one suicide by a veteran in the United States every 65 minutes. The phenomenon is not isolated to the United States: in Great Britain, more Falklands War veterans died by taking their own lives by 2002 than actually died in the 1982 conflict. Suicide prevention is critical in helping people suffering from PTSD and substance use disorders.

With more study, physicians hope to be able to prevent PTSD from occurring and create personalized treatment if prevention fails. One of the first steps toward personalizing treatment is discovering the parts of the brain that trauma affects. In one study, participants were given a PET scan (high-resolution positron-emission tomography), which shows the brain as it is working. After patients ingested a tracer that acts as a highlighter for specific stress chemicals, researchers were able to see which parts of the brain were highlighted in persons suffering from the dissociative symptoms of PTSD. The researchers learned that under chronically stressful conditions, the targeted chemicals stop working properly. This study helped to point researchers toward more personalized treatment for persons with different varieties of symptoms. Because a significant and growing portion of the population is becoming afflicted with PTSD, it is critical to acquire an understanding of what is happening within the brain, and how this change in brain chemistry contributes to the way people with PTSD interact in society.

🌐 Future Implications

It is clear that trauma can change a person's biology, chemistry, and personality. Trauma can cause long-term damage by increasing the risk for substance use disorders, violence, and suicide. It has become known that people have exhibited symptoms of PTSD throughout recorded history, and current knowledge is the basis for a unique opportunity to help those suffering in the modern world. Assuming that the baseline cause of PTSD (the trauma itself) cannot be avoided in the future, the goal must be to establish a cohesive way to treat people who develop chronic trauma disorders as well as inhibit the condition's delayed onset.

Addressing the stigma that is attached to mental health issues and substance use disorders is the first step toward helping patients come forward and request help. Governments play pivotal roles in breaking down stigma by creating policies that help those persons who are seeking mental health treatment of all kinds. The sort of front line treatment established in World War I should be extended to current and future conflicts, but veterans should also be able to a return to a supportive environment so that a delayed onset of PTSD can be prevented.

Until recently in the United States, health insurance providers were not required to provide the same benefits for mental health treatments as they did for physical ailments. Equal treatment in health care is called parity. In 2008 the Mental Health Parity and Addiction Equity Act, later amended as a part of the 2010 Patient Protection and Affordable Care Act, required that financial requirements (such as co-pays and deductibles) achieve parity with the benefits afforded for physical ailments. In addition, treatment limitations (such as visit limits) applicable to mental health or substance use disorder benefits could be no more restrictive than the limitations applied to substantially all medical/surgical benefits. The implementation of this law is still underway. It is hoped that it will provide those in need of mental health care financial relief and equal treatment when looking for care. In countries experiencing or rebuilding from large-scale trauma, equal attention needs to be paid to relief effort in treatment and recovery from both mental and physical trauma. Finally, technological advances should be utilized in therapy as well. Pilot programs have been developed to harness the power of therapy over the Internet for people to learn about PTSD, track their symptoms, and practice coping skills.

SEE ALSO *Conflict, Violence, and Terrorism: Health Impacts; Mental Health Treatment Access*

BIBLIOGRAPHY

Books

American Psychiatric Association DSM-5 Task Force. *Diagnostic and Statistical Manual of Mental Disorders*, 5th ed. Washington, DC: American Psychiatric Association, 2013.

Foa, Edna B., et al., eds. *Effective Treatments for PTSD: Practice and Guidelines from the International Society for Traumatic Stress*, 2nd ed. New York: Guilford Press, 2009.

Krippner, Stanley, Daniel B. Pitchford, and Jeannine Davies. *Post-Traumatic Stress Disorder*. Santa Barbara, CA: Greenwood Press, 2012.

Periodicals

Crocq, Marc-Antoine. "From Shell Shock and War Neurosis to Posttraumatic Stress Disorder: A History of Psychotraumatology." *Dialogues in Clinical Neuroscience* 2, no. 1 (March 2000): 47–55.

Da Costa, Jacob Mendez. "On Irritable Heart: A Clinical Study of a Form of Functional Cardiac Disorder and Its Consequences." *American Journal of the Medical Sciences* 121, no. 1 (January 1871): 2–52.

Khadra, C., et al. "Symptoms of Post Traumatic Stress Disorder among Battered Women in Lebanon: An Exploratory Study." *Journal of Interpersonal Violence* 30, no. 2 (January 2015): 295–313.

Nijdam, M. J., B. P. Gersons, J. B. Reitsma, A. de Jongh, and M. Olff. "Brief Eclectic Psychotherapy v. Eye Movement Desensitization and Reprocessing Therapy for Post-Traumatic Stress Disorder: Randomised Controlled Trial." *British Journal of Psychiatry* 200, no. 3 (March 2012): 224–231.

Pham, Phuong N., Timothy Longman, and Harvey M. Weinstein. "Trauma and PTSD Symptoms in Rwanda: Implications for Attitudes toward Justice and Reconciliation." *JAMA* 292, no. 5 (August 2004): 602–612.

Websites

"Posttraumatic Stress Disorder." *National Alliance on Mental Illness (U.S.).* http://www.nami.org/Template.cfm?Section=posttraumatic_stress_disorder (accessed March 5, 2015).

"Post-Traumatic Stress Disorder (PTSD)." *U.S. National Institute of Mental Health (NIMH).* http://www.nimh.nih.gov/health/topics/post-traumatic-stress-disorder-ptsd/index.shtml (accessed March 5, 2015).

"PTSD: National Center for PTSD." *U.S. Department of Veterans Affairs.* http:// www.ptsd.va.gov (accessed March 5, 2015).

Margaret Loraine Scott

Pregnancy Termination

🌐 Introduction

Termination of pregnancy, also commonly known as abortion, is the interruption of a pregnancy, with loss of the fetus, before it has gone to term and generally before the fetus is able to survive on its own outside the mother's body. An abortion may be induced, by a medical process, or it may happen spontaneously. Often, induced abortion is known simply as abortion or a termination, while a spontaneous abortion may be termed a miscarriage. Worldwide, the World Health Organization (WHO) estimates around 20 percent of pregnancies end in termination.

Termination of pregnancy is done for many reasons. A single woman who becomes pregnant may fear social stigma in less liberal countries, or a married woman may feel she already has enough children and cannot afford or cope with another one. Prenatal testing can reveal both the sex of an embryo and whether it carries a genetic disorder. Sex selection abortion is quite common in some countries where the birth of a male child is highly favored, so a female fetus may be discarded. Some genetic disorders, such as thalassaemia and hemophilia, can be detected at a very early stage and affected embryos aborted rather than be born with the condition. All of the above relate to unwanted pregnancy, but a wanted pregnancy may also end spontaneously. This happens for a variety of reasons, relating either to a woman's health or to some abnormality in the fetus.

Induced abortion can be carried out by a number of methods. The important issue is whether it is done safely, with no adverse effects on a woman's health and fertility. The WHO defines safe abortion as a procedure that is carried out by trained health-care professionals, with the appropriate equipment and techniques under hygienic conditions. Unsafe abortion is a procedure where any of the above conditions is lacking. It is essential that the abortion includes provision for follow-up care and treatment of any complications such as sepsis or hemorrhage. In the context of unsafe abortion, these complications lead to a mortality rate for women that is 100 times greater than for safe abortion. Thus, unsafe abortion has a major impact on women's health worldwide.

Often, the need for abortion arises from a failure of contraception. In some places, including Japan and Eastern Europe, abortion is even used as a form of contraception. However, even safe abortion procedures are potentially more risky to a woman's health than a reliable form of contraception. Therefore, family planning advice and access to contraception should be part of post abortion care to avoid the need for future abortion procedures.

🌐 Historical Background

Termination of pregnancy has a very long history and is referred to in early Greek and Roman medical texts. It is believed that the first recorded abortion occurred in ancient Egypt, around 1550 BCE. Various methods were used to achieve an abortion. Many herbs have abortifacient properties, including silphium, a now extinct member of the fennel family, and common rue. More dangerous was the use of sharp instruments inserted into the womb.

Abortion was not generally disapproved of in ancient times. The Greek philosopher Aristotle (384–322 BCE) believed that the fetus did not develop a soul until 40 days, if male, or until 90 days, if female. Thus, early abortion did not kill an actual person, he said. The Greek physician Hippocrates (c. 460– c. 377 BCE) wrote about abortion, believing it to be a safe and acceptable medical practice, although his recommendation of jumping up and down to achieve a termination was unlikely to be effective. However, Hippocrates was aware of the potential dangers of abortion for the woman, for he forbade the use of vaginal pessaries, believing these could cause injury.

Abortion Law

Termination of pregnancy has always been an issue influenced by social, cultural, and religious beliefs. This means that abortion has, at certain times, been made illegal in many countries. Until the 19th century, in many cultures it was believed that the life of the fetus began only when the mother could feel the baby move in her womb. After 1875, scientists began to describe the process of conception (fertilization; the fusion of male and female nuclei combining both the genes and genetic traits of the mother and father). Some people then began to use the act of conception as a marker for the start of "life," allowing them to further argue that if life began at conception, in some cases abortion might be considered murder. One philosophical counter to this argument was that spontaneous abortion is a natural phenomenon that occurs in a small but consistently significant percentage of pregnancies (with the woman often not knowing she was pregnant). In response some people began to establish later horizons for the start of life (e.g., implantation, organogenesis, or a heartbeat).

The American Medical Association began to campaign against abortion, and by 1900 the practice was banned in every state in the United States. Similarly, the British government banned abortion in 1861. Nevertheless, the practice continued, with advertisements in the press promising to treat what were euphemistically called female irregularities or obstructions. Some abortionists were jailed under the new law but women who had abortions were rarely prosecuted. However, abortionists were neither licensed nor necessarily medically qualified at this time, so many women were harmed or even lost their lives after a termination.

Attitudes toward termination of pregnancy began to change in the 20th century, partly because of the growing recognition of women's rights and also with the advent of safer methods of abortion, such as vacuum aspiration. In the United States, the landmark case *Roe v. Wade* in the Supreme Court made abortion legal in 1973. In the United Kingdom, the Abortion Act 1967 was passed, allowing termination where continuing the pregnancy posed a risk to the mother's mental

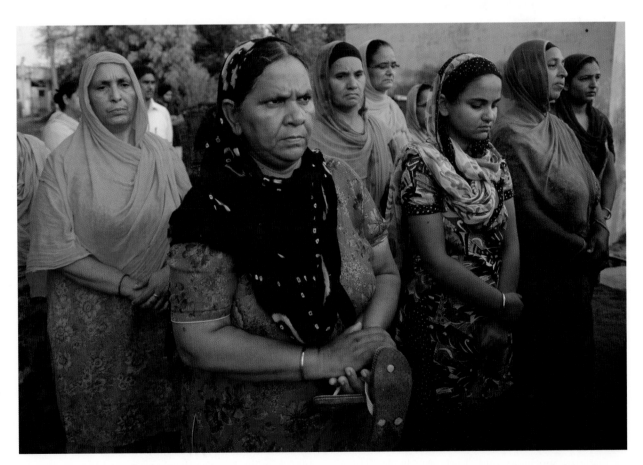

Members of the Upkar Co-ordination Society, a local Indian nongovernmental organization that works with the district administration to stop abortions on gender grounds, holds a march to raise awareness in Nawanshahr. In 2004, Nawanshahr, in the northern state of Punjab, was notorious for its abysmal sex ratio, recording just 795 female births for every 1,000 male births annually. The years from 2004 to 2011, however, witnessed a radical turnaround, with Nawanshahr recording 949 female births for every 1,000 male births in 2011, just shy of the naturally occurring rate of 952:1,000. © *Narinder Nanu/AFP/Getty Images.*

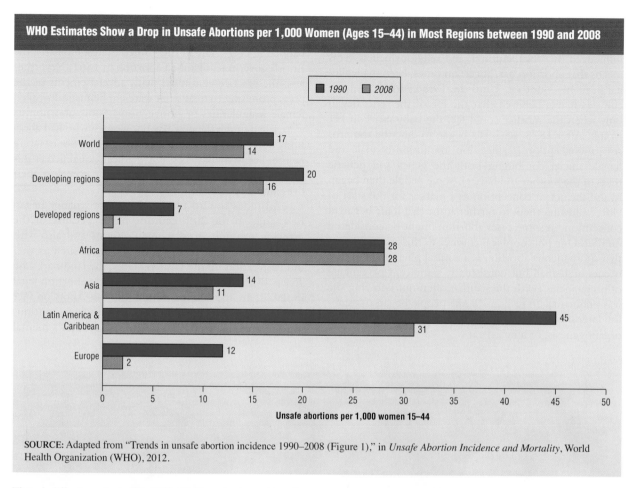

WHO Estimates Show a Drop in Unsafe Abortions per 1,000 Women (Ages 15–44) in Most Regions between 1990 and 2008

Legend: ■ 1990   ■ 2008

Region	1990	2008
World	17	14
Developing regions	20	16
Developed regions	7	1
Africa	28	28
Asia	14	11
Latin America & Caribbean	45	31
Europe	12	2

Unsafe abortions per 1,000 women 15–44

SOURCE: Adapted from "Trends in unsafe abortion incidence 1990–2008 (Figure 1)," in *Unsafe Abortion Incidence and Mortality*, World Health Organization (WHO), 2012.

Though difficult to obtain, World Health Organization estimated statistics on the number of unsafe abortions performed per 1,000 women illustrate that globally there has been a slight decrease in the number of unsafe abortions from 1990 to 2008. However, the number remains unchanged in Africa.

or physical health (except in Northern Ireland). This effectively allowed women who had approval from two doctors to have legal abortions until the fetus was 24 weeks of age.

Elsewhere, abortion law varies widely. For instance, China made abortion illegal during the 1950s, but relaxed the law by the 1980s. In India abortion was banned until 1971. However, concern over the number of women dying as a result of illegal abortions led to the legalization of termination of pregnancy.

⊕ Impacts and Issues

A safe abortion carries a very low mortality rate. Unsafe abortion, on the other hand, contributes significantly to maternal morbidity and death worldwide. Therefore, monitoring abortion rates globally is a crucial step toward achieving the United Nations Millennium Development Goal (MDG) 5, whose goal is to improve maternal health. The target of MDG 5 is to reduce

maternal mortality by 75 percent by 2015, based upon 1990 figures.

It can be more difficult to acquire abortion data compared with other health data because figures are not collected where abortion is banned or stigmatized. Nevertheless, public health researchers have collected data on abortion from a variety of sources around the world for 1995, 2003, and 2008, detailed in an article by Gilda Sedgh and colleagues in *The Lancet* in 2012. Their study shows that there were 43.8 million abortions carried out in 2008, compared with 41.6 million in 2003 and 45.6 million in 1995. In 1995, 78 percent of all abortions took place in the developing world, and this increased to 86 percent in 2008. Since 2003, the number of abortions in the developed world fell by 0.6 million, but the number of abortions increased by 2.8 million in the developing world, according to a 2012 publication by the World Health Organization and the Guttmacher Institute.

The absolute numbers of terminations are affected by population growth, so the real trends may be more easily detected by looking at abortion rates per 1,000 women of childbearing age. In 2008, this rate was 28 per 1,000, almost unchanged from 29 per 1,000 in 2003, and down from the rate of 35 per 1,000 reported in 1995. There are variations in the abortion rate between countries. The lowest is in Western Europe, at 12 per 1,000 and the highest in Eastern Europe, at 43 per 1,000. In Africa, the rate in southern Africa is 15 per 1,000, which rises to 38 per 1,000 in eastern Africa. In Asia, rates varied from 26 in south-central and western Asia to 36 in south-eastern Asia.

Research shows that 49 percent of abortions done in 2008 were unsafe. This is an increase from 44 percent in 1995. In Africa, nearly all abortions carried out were unsafe. In Asia, the proportion of unsafe abortions varies widely from negligible in eastern Asia to 65 percent in south-central Asia. In Europe, the proportion of safe abortions is 91 percent, with unsafe abortions being found mainly in Eastern Europe.

Abortion Law and Unsafe Abortions

Eighty-four countries have abortion laws that can be considered liberal and where women can thus obtain a safe abortion. However, this does not lead to more abortions occurring where the law is liberal and fewer where it is restricted. In general, the reverse is true, with the abortion rate being lower where the process is permitted and higher where it is not. This is likely because where the law is liberal, access to contraceptives is also easier, so there is less need for abortion. Where women have abortions outside the law, these abortions are likely to be unsafe ones.

Sometimes unsafe abortions occur even when the law is liberal. In India, for instance, many abortions still take place outside the health service, even though abortion has been legalized. Some of these are said to be safe, some unsafe. In Cambodia, abortion is available on demand during the first three months of pregnancy, yet half of all abortions take place in the woman's home and must be deemed to be unsafe. In Africa, the abortion law is liberal in South Africa and Zambia and legal, if more restrictive, in seven other African countries. However, the laws are not widely implemented, so most abortions are still unsafe. Clearly, any benefit to women's health by liberalizing abortion law can only be realized if there is also the health-care infrastructure necessary to deliver safe abortion.

In the developing countries where abortion law is liberal, there are fewer adverse health consequences from unsafe abortion. This has been shown to be the case in South Africa and Nepal, following liberalization of abortion law. In Ethiopia, there was a relaxing of the law in 2005 and, while it is too soon to assess countrywide impact on maternal health, one study in a large hospital has shown a decrease in the ratio of abortion complications to live births between 2003 and 2007.

Pregnancy Termination and Maternal Health

Unsafe abortion carries many risks to a woman's health. Lack of education, fear, or shame may lead a woman to attempt the abortion herself by drinking bleach or inserting sticks into the vagina in the belief that this will expel the fetus. The dangers are compounded when this is attempted later in pregnancy. If she goes to an unlicensed practitioner, there is no guarantee of hygiene or safety. Common complications of unsafe abortion include major hemorrhage and life-threatening infection. Long-term consequences include chronic inflammation of the reproductive tract, anemia, weakness, and infertility.

There are around 20 million unsafe abortions every year, most of them occurring in poorer countries and the highest number in Africa. In the United States, legalized (safe) abortion is associated with 0.6 deaths per 100,000 procedures. In contrast, unsafe abortion has a far higher mortality rate of 220 per 100,000 procedures. The number of deaths arising from these procedures is estimated at between 47,000 and 70,000, while between 5 million and 8 million will need hospital treatment afterward. This post abortion care may not be sought by the woman soon enough where abortion is illegal or stigmatized. Furthermore, the medical facilities needed may not even be available. Therefore, 3 million do not get the attention they need, according to the WHO.

The costs associated with treating the consequences of unsafe abortion are considerable, where the facilities are available. One study from 2008, cited by the WHO, puts the cost in developing countries at a minimum of US$341 million per annum. Countries that have the least access to family planning services and therefore higher demand for abortion also tend to be less likely to offer safe abortions and therefore bear the highest health-care costs for the consequences of unsafe abortion.

The WHO states that unsafe abortion accounts for 13 percent of all pregnancy-related deaths worldwide. A 2010 report on the MDGs from the United Nations suggests that the gap between developed and developing countries is greatest with respect to maternal health. A major contributor to this gap must be the marked difference in unsafe abortion rates between developed and developing countries. Thus, death from unsafe abortion is an important and largely avoidable cause of maternal mortality.

⊕ Future Implications

The MDG milestone of 2015 has now been reached, and it has been clear for some time that progress on MDG 5 has fallen a long way short in comparison with the other MDGs. This is likely because, although there have been some notable achievements, women still suffer

METHODS OF PREGNANCY TERMINATION

There are several effective ways of terminating a pregnancy. These are classified as either medical or surgical. The method of choice generally depends upon how far advanced the pregnancy is. In early pregnancy medical methods, involving drugs, will be favored. Later on, a surgical termination, perhaps in combination with drugs, will generally be used.

While all the abortion methods described here are safe, complications may still arise. That is why post abortion care is an essential part of the procedure. If the woman bleeds heavily, or develops an infection, medical advice should be available at short notice. Even if there are no complications, the clinic will need to check that the termination is complete. Similarly, pre-abortion counseling is also important to make sure the procedure complies with legal requirements and to provide an opportunity for the woman to discuss her options.

Medical Abortion

Medical abortion is sometimes known as nonsurgical abortion and involves the use of drugs given either orally or into the vagina. These medications are hormone like compounds that can interrupt the establishment of a pregnancy. Although these "abortion pills" can be self-administered, and the woman can have the termination in the comfort of her own home, they should still be issued under medical supervision, as they are powerful drugs.

Mifepristone and misoprostol, also known as RU486, are two pills taken in combination for termination of a pregnancy up to 12 weeks. If the pregnancy is very early, then one dose of mifepristone, taken in the clinic, followed by a single dose of misoprostol taken at home up to 24 to 72 hours later, may be sufficient to achieve termination. If the pregnancy is more advanced, then the regime may be more complicated and require more medical supervision.

Mifepristone blocks the hormone progesterone, which is needed to maintain the pregnancy. This action causes the uterine lining to be shed. The second medication, misoprostol, causes the uterus to contract. The pregnancy will then usually be expelled from the woman's body within six to eight hours. Bleeding from the vagina can be heavy and, rarely, a blood transfusion may be needed. Therefore, medical abortion should always take place within easy reach of emergency medical facilities.

Surgical Abortion

There are two methods of surgical termination of pregnancy. Vacuum aspiration involves applying gentle suction to the vagina to remove the pregnancy. This takes between five and ten minutes. In early pregnancy, up to 12 weeks, the aspiration procedure is generally done under a local anesthetic. Later terminations, however, are more likely to be carried out using a general anesthetic. Generally, an aspiration abortion requires just one clinic visit and the woman can go home on the same day.

Later abortions, between 15 and 24 weeks, are performed using a procedure called dilation and evacuation. It is always carried out with general anesthetic. The doctor inserts a narrow pair of forceps through the cervix and then removes the pregnancy from the womb using gentle suction. With earlier pregnancies, the woman can go home the same day. With a later pregnancy, complications are more likely, and the woman may have to stay under medical supervision overnight or return for a further visit to check that the procedure is complete.

from discrimination in many parts of the world. There is still much to be done in the areas of women's education and equality, where lack of progress has impacted on still unacceptably high level of maternal mortality, including that from unsafe abortion.

Abortion itself remains controversial in many countries. Nevertheless, women will always seek termination. They may not have access to effective contraception or they may not be able to successfully negotiate use of contraception with their partner. Moreover, any contraceptive method may fail, even if used correctly. If safe legal abortion is not available, then a woman will likely seek an abortion outside the law, which, by definition, is likely to be unsafe and puts her health at risk.

The problem of unsafe abortion will be compounded, unless services are dramatically expanded, by the fact that there will be an increase of 5 percent in the number of women of reproductive age to 1.63 billion by 2020. Most of the increase will occur in sub-Saharan Africa. The charity Marie Stopes International (MSI) has produced estimates of the number of unsafe abortions that will occur in 2020 in different countries, based upon current trends. These range from 7,300 in Papua New Guinea to 4.36 million in India.

Reducing Unsafe Abortions

To achieve the vision that no woman should die from unsafe abortion requires a comprehensive plan. The most important component of this plan is to make sure women have access to the full range of family planning, wherever they live and at an affordable cost. Where abortion is legal, services for safe abortion should be freely available and women should be made aware of their rights. Where the law is more restrictive, at least access to safe post-abortion services to deal with complications should be made available.

These services need to be developed in a broader context that enables women to make free choices about their sexual and reproductive health. This means tackling discrimination, stigma, violence against women, and

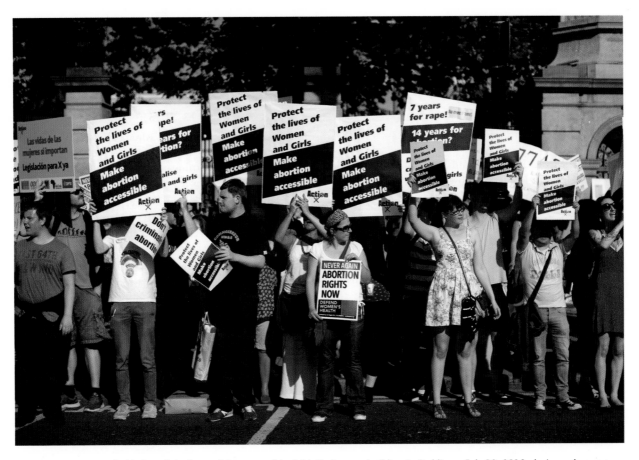

Pro-choice supporters hold placards in front of the gates of the Irish Parliament building in Dublin on July 10, 2013, during a demonstration ahead of a vote to introduce legalized abortion in limited cases where the mother's life is at risk. The bill follows a 2010 European Court of Human Rights ruling that found Ireland failed to implement properly the constitutional right to abortion where a woman's life is at risk. © *Peter Muhly/AFP/Getty Images.*

early marriage. Such changes require wider social and political change than improving the health system infrastructure in order to provide contraception and abortion.

For many women in developing countries, long-acting and permanent methods of contraception may be the preferred choice. Access to these methods has already been expanded by MSI and its partners. If, by 2020, unmet need for contraception was to be met, then 81,000 lives could be saved, according to the charity.

Even if contraceptive need was fully met, however, there will still be a need for safe abortion services, including post abortion care, around the world. Again, MSI estimates that if there was full access to safe abortion, where legal, and full access to post abortion care where needed, then another 31,000 women's lives could be saved. Thus, if a comprehensive range of contraception and abortion services was offered, this would save a total of 112,000 women's lives in 2020.

Expansion of these services should focus on those places where the problem of unsafe abortion is the most acute. The countries with the largest burden of unsafe abortions are India and Nigeria. Meanwhile, women face

the highest risks from unsafe abortion in Sierra Leone and South Sudan. A major barrier to developing abortion services has been the lack of health-care workers to deliver them. Overcoming this means training non-physician health-care professionals in termination procedures and postabortion care. A 2013 report from the WHO states that the world needs 7 million more health workers, concentrated in Africa and Asia, where unsafe abortion mortality is high. Such initiatives are already underway in Nepal, India, Pakistan, Nigeria, and Bangladesh.

SEE ALSO *Family Planning; Gender and Health; Maternal and Infant Health; Population Issues*

BIBLIOGRAPHY

Books

Kaczor, Christopher. *The Ethics of Abortion: Women's Rights, Human Life, and the Question of Justice*, 2nd ed. New York: Routledge, 2014.

Berlatsky, Noah, ed. *Abortion.* Detroit: Greenhaven Press, 2011.

World Health Organization. *Unsafe Abortion: Global and Regional Estimates of the Incidence of Unsafe Abortion and Associated Mortality in 2008*, 6th ed. Geneva: World Health Organization, 2011.

Periodicals

Kapp, Nathalie, et al. "A Review of Evidence for Safe Abortion." *Contraception* 88, no. 3 (September 2013): 350–363.

Moore, A. M., R. Kibombo, and D. Cats-Baril. "Ugandan Opinion-Leaders' Knowledge and Perceptions of Unsafe Abortion." *Health Policy & Planning* 29, no. 7 (October 2014): 893–901.

Sedgh, Gilda, et al. "Induced Abortion: Incidence and Trends Worldwide from 1995 to 2008." *The Lancet* 379 (February 18, 2012): 625–632.

Storeng, K., and F. Ouattara. "The Politics of Unsafe Abortion in Burkina Faso: The Interface of Local Norms and Global Health Practice." *Global Public Health* 9, no. 8 (September 2014): 946–959.

Websites

Guttmacher Institute and World Health Organization. "Facts on Induced Abortion Worldwide." *World Health Organization (WHO)*, January 2012. http://www.who.int/reproductivehealth/publications/unsafe_abortion/induced_abortion_2012.pdf (accessed March 13, 2015).

Mayo Clinic Staff. "Morning After Pill: Why It's Done." *Mayo Clinic.* http://www.mayoclinic.org/tests-procedures/morning-after-pill/basics/definition/prc-20012891 (accessed May 31, 2015).

"Preventing Unsafe Abortion," Fact Sheet No. 388. *World Health Organization (WHO)*, March 2014. http://www.who.int/reproductivehealth/publications/unsafe_abortion/es/ (accessed March 13, 2015).

"Safe Abortion and Post-abortion Care." *Marie Stopes International.* http://mariestopes.org/what-we-do/safe-abortion-and-post-abortion-care (accessed March 5, 2015).

Susan Aldridge

Prion Diseases

⊕ Introduction

Prion diseases, also known as transmissible spongiform encephalopathies (TSEs), are a family of rare, progressive, and fatal conditions that impair the central nervous system in both animals and humans. These diseases, as the name suggests, are caused by prions. Short for proteinaceous infectious particle, this pathogen is a unique type of infectious agent composed only of protein.

Prion diseases have long incubation periods and are characterized by the small round or oval holes the disease creates in the dense network of neurons and glia in the central nervous system. This damage causes symptoms that vary depending on the prion strain, but that generally include behavior changes, communication problems, memory and cognitive deficits, trouble swallowing, visual impairment, seizures, immobility, and eventually death. After onset, prion diseases are usually rapidly progressive and always fatal, according to the U.S. Centers for Disease Control and Prevention (CDC).

Exactly how a prion functions in the body has long been debated by scientists. However, it is generally accepted that the pathogenic prions are able to induce abnormal folding of specific normal cellular proteins called prion proteins, which are found throughout the body, but are most abundant in the brain, according to the CDC.

Human prion diseases include Creutzfeldt-Jakob disease (CJD), variant Creutzfeldt-Jakob disease, (vCJD), Gerstmann-Sträussler-Scheinker syndrome, fatal familial insomnia, and kuru. Animal prion diseases include bovine spongiform encephalopathy (BSE); chronic wasting disease, scrapie, transmissible mink encephalopathy, feline spongiform encephalopathy, and ungulate spongiform encephalopathy.

One of the most recognizable of the TSEs is vCJD due to its association with BSE, commonly known as mad cow disease. While the cause of transmission is still debated, this fatal human neurodegenerative condition has been strongly linked to the consumption of bovine meat contaminated with BSE, a degenerative, neurological cattle disease.

Between 1996 and 2014, there were 220 confirmed victims of vCJD. The majority of the reports came from the United Kingdom, but others were reported in Canada, France, Ireland, Italy, Japan, the Netherlands, Portugal, Saudi Arabia, Spain, Taiwan, and the United States. The number of cases of vCJD in the United Kingdom peaked in 2000 with 28 deaths but has since declined since measures to control the spread of the disease were implemented, according to the World Health Organization (WHO). That said, given the long incubation of this disease, that number could rise as a result of people who unknowingly consumed tainted meat decades ago.

⊕ Historical Background

Prion diseases have been making their way through animal populations for centuries. But it was scrapie, a neurodegenerative disease found in sheep, that was first recorded in 1732 in flocks of Spanish merino sheep in England. The name scrapie is Scottish and refers to the way sheep would scrape their fleece against hard objects to relieve the severe itching caused by the disease. In addition to the skin irritation, the disease caused weight loss, unsteady gait, tremors, and ultimately the death of the sheep.

For decades, the disease ravaged sheep populations across trade lines. British sheep farmers eventually petitioned Parliament to stop the movement of sheep across borders because importation had introduced scrapie to so many of the sheep flocks in the United Kingdom and elsewhere. The economic impact on the British wool industry was hard hitting and long lasting; the British government included funds for scrapie research in its first grant to the Royal Veterinary College in London in 1910. By the 1940s and 1950s, many countries banned imports of British sheep until they were proved scrapie-free.

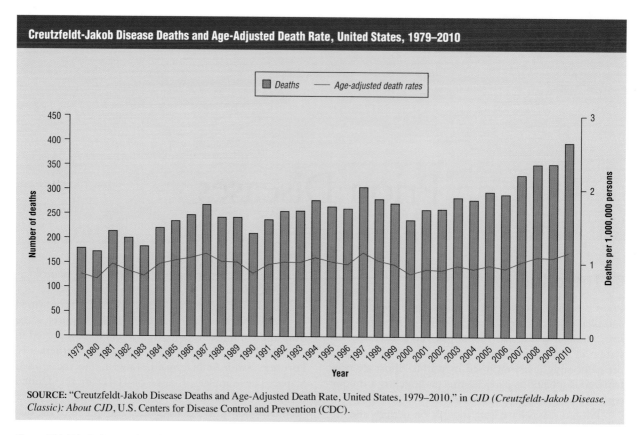

Creutzfeldt-Jakob Disease Deaths and Age-Adjusted Death Rate, United States, 1979–2010

SOURCE: "Creutzfeldt-Jakob Disease Deaths and Age-Adjusted Death Rate, United States, 1979–2010," in *CJD (Creutzfeldt-Jakob Disease, Classic): About CJD*, U.S. Centers for Disease Control and Prevention (CDC).

Creutzfeldt-Jakob disease, though rare, still kills hundreds of Americans every year and thousands worldwide.

Human TSEs did not start to catch the attention of scientists until the early 1920s, when the first case of CJD was reported. German neuropathologist Walther Spielmeyer first introduced the term Creutzfeldt-Jakob disease in 1922 to describe a strange neurological condition that caused loss of control of body movements, progressive jerking of the muscles, and dementia. The disease name was a nod to earlier case reports written independently by German neuropathologist Hans G. Creutzfeldt in 1920 and German neurologist Alfons Jakob in 1921. At first, this name was used to describe a variety of conditions that today likely would not fit the criteria for CJD.

In 1957, pediatrician and virologist D. Carleton Gajdusek stumbled onto another TSE, hidden in the highlands of New Guinea. There he found a strange encephalitis-like disease making its way through the isolated Fore tribe. The disease caused emotional instability (marked by fits of hysterical laughter), tremors, involuntary movements, intermittent rigidity, and death.

The disease, called kuru (the Fore word for "shiver"), is a degenerative TSE caused by a prion found in humans. It is commonly held that the Fore became infected with the disease through cannibalism. For years, the Fore practiced a religious ritual of eating the brains of dead loved ones, but with an incubation period of as long as 50 years, kuru was slow to develop in the tribe. Eventually the connection between the disease and cannibalism was made, causing the New Guinea government to urge the Fore to stop the practice. Once they did, the disease virtually disappeared.

The discovery of kuru eventually led to significant strides in the study of TSEs. Within a decade, scientists went on to learn that not only could TSEs be inherited and spontaneous, but that they could also be transmitted horizontally between species.

In February 1985, a cow in Great Britain that had been suffering head tremors, weight loss, and lack of coordination died. It was reported at that time as a new spongiform encephalopathy in cattle. Two years later, government officials were told about the disease, by then named BSE.

In 1988, the British government started putting several policies in place that it hoped would stem the spread of BSE. This included slaughtering animals showing signs of BSE and eventually the slaughter of all infected herds. Other measures included banning the export of British cattle older than 30 months, as well as a ban on the use of high-risk parts of the cow for human consumption (including the brain, spinal cord, and spleen).

It was also around this time that Dr. Stanley Prusiner, a U.S. biologist and neurologist, named the protein that causes TSEs prion, and hypothesized that prions are infectious self-replicating proteins. This was a revolutionary idea, considering the common belief that a cell needs genetic matter to replicate, which prions lack.

ECONOMIC IMPACTS OF BSE

Bovine spongiform encephalopathy (BSE) is a neurodegenerative prion disease that affects cattle (and is also called mad cow disease). So when an outbreak of mad cow disease occurs, it has a significant impact on the beef industry not only in the affected country but, due to the growing global economy, around the world.

In 1995, prior to the outbreak of mad cow disease, the United Kingdom was exporting 169.7 million pounds (77,000 metric tons) of beef and veal around the world. By 2000, it was closer to 4.4 million pounds (2,000 metric tons), according to a report written by Cory Pickelsimer and Thomas Wahl for the Washington State University International Marketing Program in Agricultural Commodities and Trade (IMPACT) Center information series.

This was the case throughout Europe. Between 1995 and 2000, France saw exports of beef and veal plummet from 339.5 million pounds (154,000 metric tons) to roughly 123.2 million pounds (55,000 metric tons), according to Pickelsimer and Wahl.

Consumer demand also plummeted all across Europe. The same was happening in Germany, which went from 467.4 million pounds (212,000 metric tons) in 1998 to 286.6 million pounds (130,000) in 2000. In fact, the European Union as a whole saw a drop in exports in that same five-year period, from 2.1 billion pounds (934,000 metric tons) to 286.6 million pounds (130,000 metric tons). Further, consumption of beef dropped dramatically across Europe; in places such as France and Germany, by as much as 50 percent.

But it was not just the exports that left the industry struggling. The disease decimated herds. By early in the first decade of the 21st century, more than 170,000 infected cattle had been found in the United Kingdom, but 4.4 million cattle had been slaughtered as a precaution. It is estimated that the cumulative budgetary cost of BSE for the UK government in just the first few years of the crisis was roughly £3.5 billion (US$5.28 billion).

Meanwhile, by 1992, Britain reached the peak of its BSE cases with more than 100,000 confirmed. Though the numbers for BSE started to decline at that point, the reports of CJD started to come in. Between 1993 and 1995, CJD was diagnosed in four farmers in Britain known to have BSE in their herds. On May 21, 1995, the first known victim of vCJD, died, followed by three more victims that same year. By 2005, 150 people died in the United Kingdom from the disease. Since 1996, there have been 220 confirmed victims of vCJD worldwide, with the majority in England (177) and France (27). In 2014, the United States reported its fourth case after a Texas man fell ill and died. Tests determined he had vCJD and likely contracted it on one of his many trips to Great Britain and the Middle East.

Many countries now have surveillance mechanisms in place, and BSE is a reportable disease to entities like the WHO. Furthermore, since 1989 the World Organisation for Animal Health has kept running lists of incidents of BSE in participating countries around the world and issues risk ratings for each.

⊕ Impacts and Issues

Prions have long stymied scientists and continue to cause controversy. However, ongoing research is bringing researchers ever closer to fully understanding these proteins.

Some basics are not in dispute. Prions occur in two forms: PrP^C, which is the normally functioning protein, and PrP^{Sc}, which is the infectious protein. Both PrP^C and PrP^{Sc} are made up of amino acids (the building blocks

that make up proteins) but they differ from each other in shape; PrP^{Sc} is folded.

Normal, healthy cells produce PrP^C. These proteins are found throughout the body, but the majority are in the brain. Though scientists are not entirely sure what the function of PrP^C is, they speculate that PrP^C is involved in communication between neurons, cell death, and controlling sleep patterns.

What remains controversial is that scientists are not universally convinced that PrP^{Sc} can replicate on its own. Other infectious agents contain genetic material (DNA and RNA), and this is how they are able to replicate. But PrP^{Sc} has no genetic material and still appears to replicate. Another issue debated by scientists is that some spongiform diseases have distinct strains that differ in their incubation period, symptoms, and effects on different brain regions. Some argue that these differences occur because of mutations in nucleic acid, and so critics believe prions must have genetic material.

The prevailing hypothesis on the infection process was asserted by Prusiner and is known as the protein-only hypothesis. Prusiner said prions are able to reproduce because when the PrP^{Sc} comes into contact with PrP^C, PrP^{Sc} overcomes the PrP^C and converts it to a PrP^{Sc}. As more PrP^{Sc} comes into contact with other normal PrP^C proteins, the process repeats, resulting in multiple copies of PrP^{Sc}.

Over time, the prion molecules stack up and stick together, forming long chains called amyloid fibers, which are toxic and kill cells. Then the star-shaped glial cells of the central nervous system, called astrocytes, digest the dead neurons. This process leaves holes (spongiform) and amyloid fibers where neurons used to be.

Recent decades have produced new research that further supports the protein-only hypothesis, at least in part. In 2004, researchers were able to create synthetic prions that behaved in the same way as PrP^{Sc} behaves naturally: they self-replicated, were infectious, and came in distinct strains, according to an article titled "Prion Hypothesis: The End of the Controversy?" written by Claudio Soto and published in the journal *Trends in Biochemical Sciences* in 2011. The only question remains, Soto writes, is "whether another molecule besides the misfolded prion protein might be an essential element of the infectious agent. Future research promises to reveal many more intriguing features about the rogue prions."

Creutzfeldt-Jakob Disease and Variant Creutzfeldt-Jakob Disease

Creutzfeldt-Jakob disease (also known as classic CJD) is the most common of the known human TSEs. The form that accounts for about 85 percent of total CJD cases is sporadic CJD, occurring at a rate of about one per 1 million people. Another form, familial CJD, is associated with a gene mutation and accounts for 5 to 15 percent of CJD cases. The least common form is iatrogenic CJD, which occurs due to accidental transmission via contaminated surgical equipment, corneal or meningeal (membranes that envelop the central nervous system) transplants, or the administration of human-derived pituitary growth hormones. This method of contracting the disease accounts for less than 5 percent of CJD cases, according to the WHO.

Variant CJD has several differences from classic CJD. First, it affects younger patients. Whereas the median age of death with CJD is 68, it is 28 with vCJD. It also has a longer duration of illness at 14 months as opposed to 4.5 months. The first reported case of vCJD occurred in 1994. Most of the cases of vCJD that followed occurred among people who lived in the United Kingdom. Furthermore, many of the cases diagnosed in other countries occurred in people who were likely exposed to BSE while living in the United Kingdom, according to the WHO.

Symptoms of the illness change over its duration. Early on, patients most commonly experience a range of psychiatric symptoms, including depression, apathy, or anxiety. As the disease progresses, evidence of its effect on the brain manifest through unsteadiness, difficulty walking, and involuntary movements. These worsen over time until patients are completely immobile and mute at the time of death.

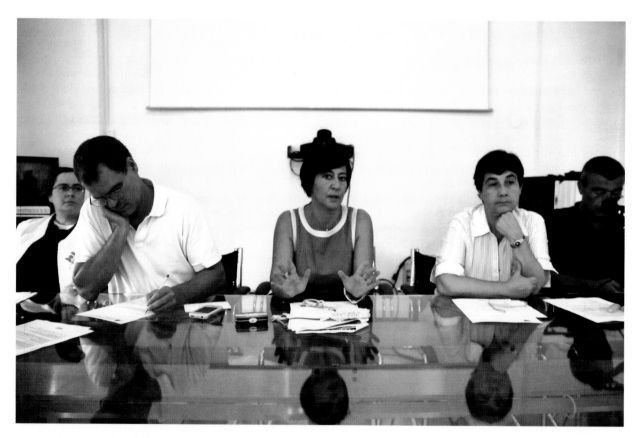

Left to right, Costanza Galli, Luca Bianciardi, Monica Calamai, Rosa La Mantia, and Marco Battaglini speak with the Italian media during a press conference in the Hospice of Palliative Care of the Hospital of Livorno on July 22, 2010, in Livorno, Italy. A 42-year old woman contracted variant Creutzfeldt-Jakob syndrome, or mad cow disease, the second human case recorded in Italy, the first being in 2002. The disease is a progressive neurological disease for which there is no treatment or cure. The patient died in 2011. © *Laura Lezza/Getty Images.*

Because the prion hypothesis is still debated by some, the exact cause of vCJD is also still in question. However, evidence strongly suggests that vCJD is linked with exposure to BSE prions found in cattle and is transmitted by eating beef.

Other TSEs

Fatal familial insomnia (FFI) is a very rare disease and is caused by an inherited mutation of the PrP gene. The disease usually strikes people between the ages of 36 and 61. The disease causes progressively worse insomnia and hallucinations, leading to delirium and dementia. In the final stages of the disease, the person is typically unresponsive and mute. The life expectancy of a person experiencing symptoms is about 18 months. There is no cure for FFI, which was first identified in 1986. As of 2013, more than 40 families are known to be affected by FFI.

Another form of TSE that is passed through families is the equally rare Gerstmann-Sträussler-Scheinker disease. Found in only a few families globally, this neurodegenerative brain disorder results from a mutant prion gene. Symptoms typically manifest sometime in adulthood and include clumsiness, unsteadiness, and difficulty walking in the early stages. The lack of muscle coordination worsens as the disease progresses, with some patients experiencing slurred speech, involuntary eye movements, rigid muscle tone, and blindness or deafness. There is no cure for the disease. Progression is slow and can last anywhere from 2 to 10 years before death.

⊕ Future Implications

Currently, the greatest threat from prions lies with vCJD and its connection to BSE. Since 1988, many countries with a history of indigenous cases of confirmed BSE, including the United Kingdom, have put public health control measures in place. These include surveillance, culling sick animals, and banning specified risk materials.

Among the strongest control measures is a UK program that excludes all animals over 30 months of age from the human food and animal feed supplies. Further, in June 2000, the European Union's BSE control measures also required the ban of mechanically recovered meat from the vertebral column of cattle, sheep, and goats for human food.

The WHO recommendations echo steps taken by the United Kingdom and other countries across the globe, but added the recommendation that pharmaceutical companies avoid use of bovine materials and those from other animal species in which TSEs naturally occur. When that is not possible, the WHO recommends that those materials be sourced from countries with a surveillance system for BSE in place reporting zero cases of BSE.

Given the incubation period of prion diseases, scientific developments in this arena are often slow. However, scientists continue to publish new findings on prions. These include the following discoveries: the infectious

prion may have a switch that makes it toxic to cells and recombinant human prion protein inhibits the propagation of infectious prions.

PRIMARY SOURCE

The Nobel Prize in Physiology or Medicine, 1997: Stanley B. Prusiner

SOURCE Pettersson, Professor Ralf F. "The Nobel Prize in Physiology or Medicine, 1997: Stanley B. Prusiner." *Nobel Prizes*, December 10, 1997. Copyright © 1998 Nobel Media AB. http://www.nobelprize.org/nobel_prizes/medicine/laureates/1997/presentation-speech.html (accessed January 25, 2015).

INTRODUCTION *This primary source is the presentation speech given by Professor Ralf F. Pettersson, announcing the award of the 1997 Nobel Prize in Physiology or Medicine to Stanley Prusiner for the discovery of prions.*

AWARD CEREMONY SPEECH

Presentation Speech by Professor Ralf F. Pettersson of the Nobel Committee at The Karolinska Institute, December 10, 1997.

Translation of the Swedish text.

Your Majesties, Your Royal Highnesses, Ladies and Gentlemen,

This year's Nobel Prize in Physiology or Medicine has been awarded to Stanley B. Prusiner for his discovery of prions - a new biological principle of infection. What is a prion? It is a small infectious protein capable of causing fatal dementia-like diseases in man and animals. It has been known for approximately a century that infectious diseases can be caused by bacteria, viruses, fungi and parasites. All these infectious agents possess a genome, the hereditary material that provides the basis for their replication. The ability to replicate is essential for the manifestation of the diseases they cause. The most remarkable feature of prions is that they are able to replicate themselves without possessing a genome; prions lack hereditary material. Until prions were discovered, duplication without a genome was considered impossible. This discovery was unexpected and provoked controversy.

Although the existence of prions was not known until the work of Stanley Prusiner, many prion diseases have been previously documented. On Iceland, scrapie, a disease affecting sheep was first described in the 18th century. In the 1920s, the neurologists Hans Creutzfeldt and Alfons Jakob discovered a similar disease in man. During the 1950s and 60s Carleton Gajdusek studied kuru, a disease that was spread through cannibalistic rituals practised by the Fore people in New Guinea. Presently attention is focused on mad cow disease, which has affected approximately 170,000 cows in Britain. These diseases exhibit common pathologies. They are inevitably fatal due to the destruction of the brains of infected individuals. The incubation times may last for several years, during which the affected regions of the brain become gradually spongy in appearance. Gajdusek discovered that kuru and Creutzfeldt-Jakob disease could be transmitted to monkeys demonstrating that these diseases are contagious. In 1976, when Gajdusek received his Nobel Prize, the nature of the infectious agent was completely unknown. At this time, these diseases were assumed to be caused by a new unidentified virus, termed a slow or unconventional virus. During the 1970s, no significant advances regarding the nature of the agent were made, that is, not until Stanley Prusiner took on the problem.

Prusiner set out to purify the infectious agent, and after 10 years of hard work he obtained a pure preparation. To his great surprise, he found that the agent consisted only of a protein, which he named prion, a term derived from proteinaceous infections particle. Strangely enough, he found that the protein was present in equal amounts in the brains of both diseased and healthy individuals. This discovery was confusing and it was generally concluded that Prusiner must have arrived at the wrong conclusion. How could a protein cause disease if it was present both in diseased and healthy brains? The answer to this question came when Prusiner showed that the prion protein from diseased brains had a completely different three-dimensional conformation. This led Prusiner to propose a hypothesis for how a normal protein could become a disease-causing agent by changing its conformation. The process he proposed may be compared to the transformation of Dr Jekyll to Mr Hyde - the same entity, but in two manifestations, a kind innocuous one, and a vicious lethal one. But how can a protein replicate without a genome? Stanley Prusiner suggested that the harmful prion protein could replicate by forcing the normal protein to adopt the shape of the harmful protein in a chain reaction-like process. In other words, when a harmful protein encounters a normal protein, the normal protein is converted into the harmful form. A remarkable feature of prion diseases is that they can arise in three different ways. They can occur spontaneously, or be triggered by infection, or occur as a consequence of hereditary predisposition.

The hypothesis that prions are able to replicate without a genome and to cause disease violated all conventional conceptions and during the 1980s was severely criticised. For more than 10 years, Stanley Prusiner fought an uneven battle against overwhelming opposition. Research during the 1990s has, however, rendered strong support for the correctness of Prusiner's prion hypothesis. The mystery behind scrapie, kuru, and mad cow disease has finally been unravelled. Additionally, the discovery of prions has opened up new avenues to better understand the pathogenesis of other more common dementias, such as Alzheimer's disease.

Stanley Prusiner,

Your discovery of the prions has established a novel principle of infection and opened up a new and exciting area in medical research. On behalf of the Nobel Assembly at the Karolinska Institute I wish to convey to you my warmest congratulations and I now ask you to step forward to receive your Nobel Prize from the hands of His Majesty the King.

SEE ALSO *Epidemiology: Surveillance for Emerging Infectious Diseases; Food Preparation and Food Safety; International Health Regulation, Surveillance, and Enforcement; Zoonotic (Animal-Borne) Diseases*

BIBLIOGRAPHY

Books

Ingram, Jay. *Fatal Flaws: How a Misfolded Protein Baffled Scientists and Changed the Way We Look at the Brain.* New Haven, CT: Yale University Press, 2013.

Max, D. T. *The Family That Couldn't Sleep: Unravelling a Venetian Medical Mystery.* London: Portobello, 2008.

Power, Christopher, and Richard T. Johnson, eds. *Emerging Neurological Infections.* Hoboken, NJ: Taylor and Francis, 2013.

Prusiner, Stanley B. *Madness and Memory: The Discovery of Prions—a New Biological Principle of Disease.* New Haven, CT: Yale University Press, 2014.

Tatzelt, Jörg, ed. *Prion Proteins.* Berlin: Springer, 2013.

Zou, Wen-Quan, and Pierluigi Gambetti, eds. *Physiology and Pathophysiology.* New York: Springer, 2013.

Periodicals

Soto, Claudio. "Prion Hypothesis: The End of the Controversy?" *Trends in Biochemical Sciences* 36, no. 3 (2011): 151–158.

Websites

"About Prion Diseases." *U.S. Centers for Disease Control and Prevention (CDC).* http://www.cdc.gov/ncidod/dvrd/prions/ (accessed February 10, 2015).

National Prion Disease Pathology Surveillance Center (U.S.). http://www.cjdsurveillance.com (accessed February 10, 2015).

"Prion Disease." *University College London.* http://www.prion.ucl.ac.uk/clinic-services/information/prion-disease/ (accessed February 10, 2015).

"Prion Diseases." *Johns Hopkins Medicine.* http://www.hopkinsmedicine.org/healthlibrary/conditions/nervous_system_disorders/prion_diseases_134,56/ (accessed February 10, 2015).

Melanie R. Plenda

Radiation Exposure

⊕ Introduction

Radiation exposure occurs any time electromagnetic rays or fast-moving particles interact with living tissue. Ionizing radiation is particularly damaging to tissue; examples include x rays, gamma radiation, and fast-moving subatomic particles such as neutrons. Biological damage caused by exposure to ionizing radiation ranges from mild tissue burns to cancer, genetic damage, and ultimately, death.

While radiation in the form of heat, visible light, and even ultraviolet (UV) light is essential to life, the word radiation is often used to refer only to those emissions that can damage or kill living things. Such harm is specifically attributed to radioactive particles as well as the electromagnetic rays with frequencies higher than visible light (UV, x rays, gamma rays). Harmful electromagnetic radiation is also known as ionizing radiation because it strips atoms of one or more of their electrons, leaving highly reactive ions called free radicals, which can damage tissue or genetic material.

There are, however, potential benefits of controlled exposures to certain kinds of radiation, which can be used for the detection, diagnosis, and treatment of certain diseases.

⊕ Historical Background

Radiation is defined as the emission of energy from an atom in the form of a wave or particle. Such energy is emitted when an atomic nucleus undergoes decay, which is associated with the radioactivity of certain naturally occurring and human-made isotopes. The radiation emitted through the radioactive decay of certain atomic nuclei consists of electromagnetic waves, or subatomic particles, or both. Electromagnetic radiation includes radio waves, infrared waves (or heat), visible light, UV radiation, x rays, and gamma rays. Radioactivity usually takes the form of a subatomic particle such as an alpha particle or beta particle, though atomic decay can also release electromagnetic gamma rays.

Measuring Exposure to Radiation

The first commonly used unit for measuring the biological effects of x-ray exposure was the roentgen. It was named after the German physicist Wilhelm Röntgen (1845–1923), who discovered x rays in 1895. A roentgen is the amount of radiation that produces a set number of charged ions in a certain amount of air under standard conditions. This unit is not, however, particularly useful for describing the potential effects of radiation on human or animal tissues. The rad unit is slightly better in this regard. It is a measure of the radiation dose absorbed by one gram of something. A rad is equal to a defined amount of energy (100 ergs) absorbed per gram.

The problem with rads as a unit of measurement for human radiation exposure is that a dose of one rad of radiation from plutonium produces a different effect on living tissue than one rad of a less harmful type of radiation. Consequently, scientists introduced the rem, which stands for "roentgen equivalent man." A rem is the dose of any radiation that produces the same biological effect, or dose equivalent, in humans as one rad of x rays.

Scientists continue to use these units, which were introduced in the 20th century, even as newer units are commonly used in some applications. The roentgen will still be the unit used to measure exposure to ionizing radiation, but the rad is being replaced with the "gray" as a measure of absorbed dose. One gray equals 100 rads. The sievert is replacing the rem as a measure of dose equivalent. One sievert equals 100 rems.

Sources of Radiation

Exposure to ionizing radiation can be divided into two categories: natural and anthropogenic (i.e., associated with human activity). Background radiation is mostly due to solar radiation in the form of cosmic rays, and also radioactivity from rocks. Exposure to background radiation is continuous, although its intensity varies. The sun is also the main source of UV radiation. Each person in the United States receives an average radiation dose per year of about one millisievert (one-thousandth sievert; this is the same as 0.1 rem). About one-half of this exposure is due to radon, a natural radioactive gas (a breakdown product of uranium) released from rocks.

Radon Environmental studies show that radon accounts for most of the radiation dose Americans receive. Released by the decay of uranium in the earth, radon can infiltrate a house through pores in block walls, cracks in basement walls or floors, or around pipes. The Environmental Protection Agency (EPA) reported estimates (in 2010) that roughly 1 in every 15 homes in the United States has elevated levels of radon. The EPA calls radon "the largest environmental radiation health problem affecting Americans." Inhaled radon may contribute to as many as 21,000 lung cancer deaths each year in the United States. The EPA now recommends that homeowners test their houses for radon gas and install a specialized ventilation system if excessive levels of gas are detected.

Anthropogenic Radiation The actual and potential sources of anthropogenic radiation include: x rays and other types of radiation used in medicine, radioactive waste generated by nuclear power stations and scientific research centers, and radioactive fallout from nuclear weapons testing. Fallout is radioactive contamination of air, water, and land following the explosion of nuclear weapons or accidents at nuclear power stations.

Radioactive waste materials are the most common source for unintentional and detrimental radiation exposure. Radioactive waste materials are produced as by-products of research, nuclear power generation, and nuclear weapons manufacture. Radioactive waste is classified by the U.S. government into five groups: high-level, transuranic (chemical elements heavier than uranium), spent fuel, uranium mill tailings, and low-level radioactive waste.

Disposal methods for radioactive wastes have varied. Since at least the 1940s, low-level wastes have been flushed down drains, dumped into the ocean, and tossed into landfills. Uranium mill tailings have been mounded into small hills at sites throughout the western United States. Over 80 percent of the total volume of radioactive waste generated in the United States is considered low-level waste. There is now a shift away from the most common disposal method of shallow land burial. Because of public demand for disposal methods that provide the greatest safety and security, disposal methods now include aboveground and belowground vaults and earth-mounded concrete bunkers.

The volatility of radioactive waste makes the cleanup of radioactive sites particularly problematic. One of the most challenging cleanup projects is the Hanford site in southeastern Washington. The site produced plutonium for more than 40 years and became the country's largest repository of nuclear waste before being shut down in the late 1980s. Decades of cleanup work requiring thousands of workers followed and was still ongoing well into the 21st century. Problem sites are a common peril of nations with nuclear power infrastructure.

Around the world, laboratories, hospitals, and nuclear power plants that produce low-level radioactive by-products are often also de facto disposal sites.

Technological improvements are resulting in much smaller exposures to radiation during medical diagnostic procedures. Efforts are also being made to reduce and better focus the radiation exposures used for therapeutic purposes (for example, to treat some kinds of cancers). Sophisticated developments, such as the three-dimensional x-ray images produced by computerized axial tomography scanners, allow health-care workers to obtain more information with less exposure to radiation.

Electromagnetic radiation from television sets and microwave ovens also has been lowered to insignificant levels in recent years, thanks to improved designs.

Radiation Injuries

The effects of radiation depend upon the type of radiation absorbed, the amount or dose received, and the part of the body irradiated. While alpha and beta particles due to radioactivity have only limited power to penetrate the body, gamma rays and x rays are far more potent. The damage potential of a radiation dose is expressed in rems, a quantity equal to the actual dose in rads (units per kilogram) multiplied by a quality factor, called *Q*, representing the potency of the radiation in living tissue.

In addition to burns to integumentary (skin) and organ systems, certain types of radiation exposure may cause mutations (DNA damage and genetic

Health Effects Caused by Radiation Exposure

Exposure (rem)	Health Effect	Time to Onset (without treatment)
5–10	Changes in blood chemistry	
50	Nausea	Hours
55	Fatigue	
70	Vomiting	
75	Hair loss	2–3 weeks
90	Diarrhea	
100	Hemorrhage	
400	Possible death	Within 2 months
1,000	Destruction of intestinal lining internal bleeding and death	1–2 weeks
2,000	Damage to central nervous system loss of consciousness;	Minutes
	and death	Hours to days

SOURCE: "Is any amount of radiation safe?" in *Radiation Protection: Understanding Radiation: Health Effects*, U.S. Environmental Protection Agency (EPA).

alterations) or accelerate the types of mutations that occur spontaneously at a very low rate. Ionizing radiation was the first mutagen that efficiently and reproducibly induced mutations in a multicellular organism. Direct damage to the cell nucleus is believed to be responsible for both mutations and other radiation mediated genotoxic effects like chromosomal aberrations and lethality. Free radicals generated by irradiation of the cytoplasm are also believed to induce gene mutations even in the nonirradiated nucleus.

There are many kinds of radiations that can increase mutations. Radiation is often classified as ionizing or nonionizing depending on whether ions are emitted in the penetrated tissues or not. X rays, gamma rays (γ), beta particle radiation (β), and alpha particle (α) radiation (also known as alpha rays) are ionizing forms of radiation.

On the other hand, UV radiation, such as that experienced by exposure to sunlight, is non-ionizing. Biologically, the differences between types of radiation effects fundamentally involve the way energy is distributed in irradiated cell populations and tissues.

Different types of radiation have different energies, and so have different effects. With alpha radiation, ionizations produce an intense but more superficial and localized deposition of energy. The energy of x rays and gamma radiation traverses deeper into tissues. This penetration leads to a more even distribution of energy as opposed to the more concentrated or localized alpha rays.

Over a lifetime, a person typically receives 7–14 rems from natural sources. Exposure to 5–75 rems causes few observable symptoms. Exposure to 75–200 rems leads to vomiting, fatigue, and loss of appetite. Exposure to 300 rems or more leads to severe changes in blood cells accompanied by hemorrhage. Such a dosage delivered to the whole body is lethal 50 percent of the time. An exposure of more than 600 rems causes loss of hair, loss of the body's ability to fight infection, and results in death. A dose of 10,000 rem will kill quickly through damage to the central nervous system.

Radiation Sickness

The symptoms that follow exposure to a harmful dose of radiation are often termed radiation sickness or radiation burn. Bone marrow and lymphoid tissue cells, testes and ovaries, and embryonic tissue are most sensitive to radiation exposure. Since the lymphatic tissue manufactures white blood cells (WBCs), radiation sickness is almost always accompanied by a reduction in WBC production within 72 hours, and recovery from a radiation dose is first indicated by an increase in WBC production.

⊕ Impacts and Issues

Significant exposure to ionizing radiation increases the risk of cancer, birth defects, and genetic damage, as well as accelerating the aging process, and causing other

HIROSHIMA AND NAGASAKI

Since their invention during World War II (1939–1945), nuclear weapons have been used only twice for non-test purposes. The United States used nuclear weapons against the Japanese cities of Hiroshima and Nagasaki near the end of the war. Although U.S. officials at the time asserted that the use of nuclear weapons shortened the war and ultimately saved lives and substantial economic cost for both sides, the decision to use the atomic bomb has long been intensely and emotionally debated. Most of the Japanese casualties were civilians.

The nuclear explosions at Hiroshima and Nagasaki demonstrated the immense power of the nuclear bomb. The effects of the explosion were immediately devastating in terms of size and scope of destruction. The radiation that was released by the explosions, however, also caused the deaths of many people weeks, months, and decades after the blasts.

Radiation released in a nuclear explosion consists of particles that have a high energy. When these particles encounter biological material, in particular deoxyribonucleic acid (DNA), they can break the DNA strands. The breakage can be so severe that a cell's repair machinery cannot compensate. Because DNA is the blueprint for the structure and all the activities that occur in cells, the radiation-induced damage to DNA is lethal to the affected cells.

Radiation exposure that does not kill cells outright can cause sub-lethal damage that alters the sequence of information contained in the DNA. As a result, when the DNA is used to make proteins, proteins that are altered from the intended forms will be made. These represent mutations.

health problems including impaired immunity. Among the chronic diseases suffered by those exposed to excessive radiation are cancer, stroke, diabetes, hypertension, cardiovascular disease, and renal disease.

Some 82 percent of the average American's radiation exposure comes from natural sources. These sources include radon gas emissions from underground, cosmic rays from space, naturally occurring radioactive elements within the human body, and radioactive particles emitted from soil and rocks. Human-made radiation, the other 18 percent, comes primarily from medical x rays and nuclear medicine but is also emitted from some consumer products (such as smoke detectors and blue topaz jewelry), or originates in the production and testing of nuclear weapons and the manufacture of nuclear fuels.

Though artificial sources of radiation contribute only a small fraction to overall radiation exposure, they remain a strong concern for two reasons. First, they are preventable or avoidable, unlike cosmic radiation, for example. Second, while the average individual may not receive a significant dose of radiation from artificial sources, geographic and occupational factors may mean dramatically higher doses of radiation for large numbers of people.

For instance, many Americans have been exposed to radiation from nearly 600 nuclear tests conducted at the Nevada test site. From the early 1950s to the early 1960s, atmospheric blasts caused a lingering increase in radiation-related sickness downwind of the site and increased the overall dose of radiation received by Americans by as much as 7 percent. Once the tests were moved underground, that figure fell to less than 1 percent.

The two most serious nuclear power accidents in history each potentially exposed hundreds of thousands of people to unacceptably high levels of radiation.

Chernobyl

In April 1986, the Chernobyl Nuclear Power Plant near Pripyat, Soviet Union (present-day Ukraine), suffered a catastrophic accident. During a planned reactor shutdown and cooling experiment, one of the facility's nuclear reactors exploded, spewing radioactive material into the air. Thirty-one people died in the explosion, and another 25 died from acute radiation sickness in attempts to contain the fire. Over 350,000 people were evacuated from an 18-mile (30-kilometer) exclusion zone around Chernobyl.

The catastrophic accident at a nuclear reactor at Chernobyl spewed radioactive contaminants into the atmosphere, affecting much of Europe. After this disaster, networks of monitors were erected in many countries to detect future radiation leaks and warn threatened populations. The largest monitoring system is in Germany, which has installed several thousand radiation sensors. These systems are able to detect radiation leaks coming from domestic or foreign sources shortly after nuclear accidents occur, allowing residents to seek shelter if necessary.

Fukushima

In northern Japan, a powerful March 2011 earthquake and resulting tsunami damaged reactor cooling systems at the Fukushima Daiichi nuclear power plant, resulting in full meltdowns in three of its six reactors. An 8-inch (20-centimeter) crack in a containment pit under one reactor also resulted in radioactive water leaking into the sea. Officials evacuated more than 70,000 people from an area within 12 miles (20 kilometers) of the facility, and advised people living within an additional 6.2-mile (10-kilometers) radius to remain indoors. Teams of workers rotated in shifts to manage the emergency, and at least 17 workers were exposed to radiation above limits considered safe. Although the reactors eventually will

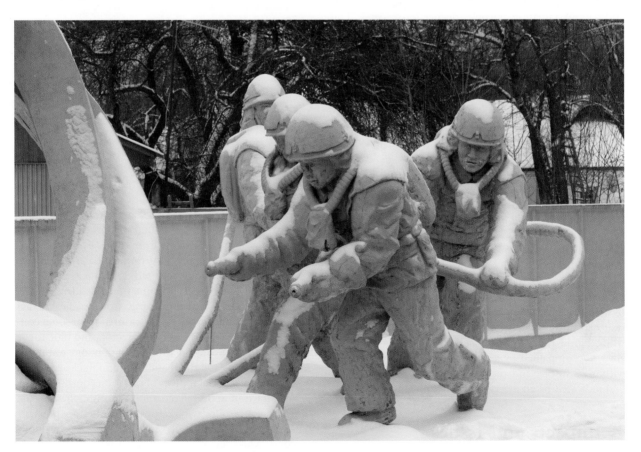

A memorial to the "liquidators" of Chernobyl, Ukraine, the firefighters and other workers who rushed to the site of the Chernobyl nuclear reactor number four explosion. Not realizing the extent of the radiation, many of those who were a part of the immediate response team did not have protective gear and died of acute radiation sickness later. © posztos/Shutterstock.com.

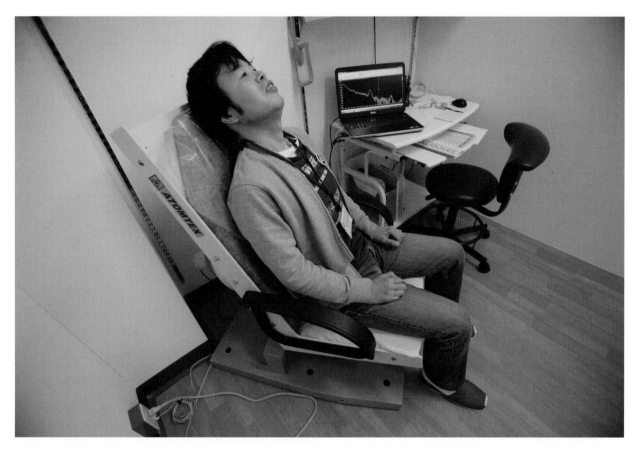

In this Saturday, February 25, 2012, photo, Hiromi Abe sits on a whole body counter to have his radiation level measured at Citizens' Radioactivity Measurement Station in Fukushima, Japan. Experts say the risks are relatively low, and people can take steps to protect themselves, such as watching what they eat and taking breaks by periodically living outside Fukushima. But risks are much higher for children, and no one can say for sure what level of exposure is safe. What is clear is Fukushima will serve as a test case that the world is watching for long-term exposure to low-dose radiation.   *© Itsuo Inouye/AP Images.*

be sealed in concrete, decontamination of the surrounding environment is expected to take decades.

In June 2011, engineers with Japan's Nuclear Emergency Response Headquarters and International Atomic Energy Agency (IAEA) officials concluded that three of the reactors at the Fukushima Daiichi nuclear power plant suffered full meltdowns following damage to cooling systems caused by the massive March 11, 2011, earthquake and tsunami. Nuclear rods in Fukushima Daiichi reactors 1, 2, and 3 reached temperatures sufficient to melt the casings, and the molten remains of the rods pooled at the bottom of the respective reactor pressure vessels.

The Chernobyl and Fukushima incidents are the only nuclear accidents to register at Level 7, signifying a major accident, on the International Nuclear Event Scale.

⊕ Future Implications

Although progress is slow, and the situation is often chaotic in the United States, the state of radioactive waste management in much of the rest of the world is even less advanced. The situation is particularly acute in Eastern Europe and the former Soviet Union, since these countries have generated huge quantities of radioactive waste. In many cases the information-gathering necessary to plan cleanup efforts has only recently begun, and much of the actual cleanup remains.

Most nations that do not already possess nuclear weapons have signed a pact to not develop them, and nations that already have them have agreed not to test them above ground (which leads to particularly intense emissions of radioactivity into the atmosphere).

Security experts continue to anticipate the use of radiation exposure as an act of terrorism (e.g., the use of "dirty bombs"—conventional explosives that release a payload of radioactive material). In 2002, an American citizen was arrested for his alleged involvement with al Qaeda to detonate a dirty bomb inside the United States. The spray of radiation in a mid-level dirty bomb could produce a relatively low level of radiation over a fairly localized area. In a densely populated city, thousands of people could be exposed to harmful levels of radiation from an explosion from a dirty bomb.

Steps are also being taken in many countries to prevent exposure resulting from anthropogenic sources of radiation in the environment.

SEE ALSO *Conflict, Violence, and Terrorism: Health Impacts; Workplace Health and Safety*

BIBLIOGRAPHY

Books

Aichinger, Horst, et al. *Radiation Exposure and Image Quality in X-Ray Diagnostic Radiology: Physical Principles and Clinical Applications*, 2nd ed. Berlin: Springer, 2012.

Balenovic, Damijan, and Emilije Stimac, eds. *Radiation Exposure: Sources, Impacts, and Reduction Strategies* Hauppage, NY: Nova Science, 2012.

Biddle, Wayne. *A Field Guide to Radiation*. New York: Penguin Books, 2012.

Clement, C. H., M. Sasaki, and International Commission on Radiological Protection. *Assessment of Radiation Exposure of Astronauts in Space*. Exeter, UK: Polestar Wheatons Ltd., 2013.

Gale, Robert Peter, and Eric Lax. *Radiation: What It Is, What You Need to Know*. New York: Knopf, 2013.

Grupen, Claus. *Introduction to Radiation Protection: Practical Knowledge for Handling Radioactive Sources*. Berlin: Springer, 2010.

Knoll, Glenn F. *Radiation Detection and Measurement*, 4th ed. Hoboken, NJ: Wiley, 2010.

Mattsson, Sören, and Christoph Hoeschen, eds. *Radiation Protection in Nuclear Medicine*. Berlin: Springer, 2013.

Mishra, K. P., ed. *Biological Responses, Monitoring and Protection from Radiation Exposure*. Hauppauge, NY: Nova Science, 2015.

NATO Advanced Training Course on Rapid Diagnosis in Population at Emergency and Risk, Antonina Cebulska-Wasilewska, Andreyan N. Osipov, and Firouz Darroudi. *Rapid Diagnosis in Populations at Risk from Radiation and Chemicals*. Edited by Antonina Cebulska-Wasilewska, Andreyan N. Osipov, and Firouz Darroudi. Amsterdam: IOS Press, 2010.

Parnell, Nicole E., ed. *Radiation Exposure in Medicine and the Environment: Risks and Protective Strategies*. New York: Nova Science, 2012.

Prince, Robert. *Radiation Protection at Light Water Reactors*. Berlin: Springer, 2012.

United Nations. *Sources, Effects and Risks of Ionizing Radiation: Levels and Effects of Radiation Exposure Due to the Nuclear Accident after the 2011 Great East-Japan Earthquake*. New York: United Nations Publications, 2014.

Periodicals

Dancause, Kelsey Needham, et al. "Chronic Radiation Exposure in the Rivne-Polissia Region of Ukraine: Implications for Birth Defects." *American Journal of Human Biology* 22, no. 5 (2012): 667–674.

Gu, G., and S. He. "Radiation Exposure." *Spine* 39, no. 19 (2014): 1628.

Mott, R. "Radiation Exposure." *Earth* 57, no. 5 (2012): 1.

Naoi, Yutaka, et al. "Internal Radiation Exposure of Ground Self-Defense Force Members Involved in the Management of the Fukushima Nuclear Power Plant Disaster." *American Journal of Disaster Medicine* 8, no. 2 (2013): 1.

Shuryak, I., R. K. Sachs, and D. J. Brenner. "Cancer Risks after Radiation Exposure in Middle Age." *Journal of the National Cancer Institute* 102, no. 21 (2010): 1628–36.

Wu, Dawei. "Radiation Exposure following Fukushima Incident." *The Lancet Oncology* 13, no. 10 (2012): e413.

Websites

"Radiation and Your Health." *U.S. Centers for Disease Control and Prevention (CDC)*. http://www.cdc.gov/nceh/radiation/default.htm (accessed March 1, 2015).

"Radiation Emergencies." *U.S. Centers for Disease Control and Prevention (CDC)*. http://emergency.cdc.gov/radiation/ (accessed March 1, 2015).

"Radiation Protection." *U.S. Environmental Protection Agency (EPA)*. http://www.epa.gov/radiation/index.html (accessed March 1, 2015).

"Radiation Sickness." *Mayo Clinic*. http://www.mayoclinic.com/health/radiation-sickness/DS00432 (accessed March 1, 2015).

K. Lee Lerner

Sanitation and Hygiene

⊕ Introduction

Sanitation is the safe disposal of waste, which can include everything from biological waste such as blood, urine, and feces to industrial and agricultural wastes. Hygiene refers to the conditions and practices that help to maintain health and prevent the spread of diseases.

Both sanitation and hygiene are vital to the health, survival, and development of a community. Most developed countries use a variety of engineering methods to prevent human contact with waste. These methods include sewerage (drainage by sewers), wastewater treatment, storm water drainage, as well as solid and excreta (urine and feces) waste management. Even simple solutions such as dry toilets (a toilet that uses aerobic bacteria to break down human waste using little or no water), pit latrines, and septic tanks can keep humans sufficiently separated from their waste. A third line of defense is basic personal hygiene practices that include hand washing with soap and bathing in uncontaminated waters.

In places where sanitation and hygiene are lacking, people are at risk for water, sanitation, and hygiene (often referred to by the acronym WASH) related diseases. These diseases can include waterborne and foodborne illnesses. For example, the 2010–2011 outbreak of cholera (a waterborne disease caused by ingesting the bacteria *Vibrio cholerae*) in Haiti sickened 500,000 people and killed 7,000, according to the U.S. Centers for Disease Control and Prevention (CDC).

Establishing and maintaining proper sanitation and hygiene practices is a challenge for some countries and communities around the globe. An estimated 2.5 billion people lack basic sanitation. That means about 38 percent of the world's population do not have access to safe disposal of human waste or the ability to maintain hygienic conditions through services such as garbage collection, industrial/hazardous waste management, and wastewater treatment and disposal, according to the CDC. Further, hundreds of millions lack soap and clean water necessary for basic hand washing, a practice that prevents the spread of diarrheal and respiratory illness. The United Nations Children's Fund (UNICEF) estimates that hand washing with soap could cut diarrheal disease by one-third.

⊕ Historical Background

Throughout human history, civilizations have attempted to bring in water and take out waste. Ruins dating back to the Neolithic and Bronze Ages indicate that people living in Egypt, Mesopotamia, and Pakistan, among other places, had some form of sanitation. In Pakistan, early systems included drainage channels and ducts. Greeks, Romans, and Mayans all discovered the benefits of indoor plumbing early in their histories. Ancient Romans, for example, built elaborate aqueduct systems that could pipe water into homes, public baths, and fountains. They also maintained massive sewers into which human waste was deposited.

When it came to human waste, early civilizations that did not practice open defecation used chamber pots; pail closets (a room where a person defecated into a bucket that was removed at regular intervals); pit toilets (a hole in the ground used for defecation); and cesspits for human waste collection.

By the early 1800s, the western world was becoming more industrialized. This meant people flocking to cities for work, which caused substandard living conditions and overcrowding. Sanitation for most people consisted of using communal facilities built over a cesspool where the waste was collected.

But the mid-19th century saw sanitation and hygiene become major public health and policy issues in Europe and the United States as a result of urbanization, immigration, industrialization, and cholera epidemics. It was an outbreak of cholera in London that led British physician John Snow to prove that the disease was caused and spread by bacteria in water contaminated with feces. His discoveries were the beginning of "germ theory," which held that disease was caused by microorganisms,

Percentage of World Population with Access to an Improved Sanitation Facility, by Country, 2012

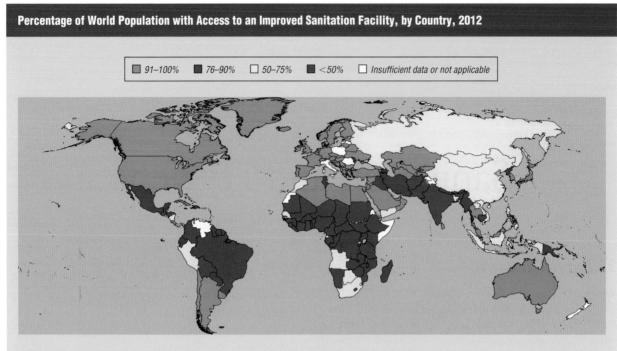

■ 91–100%   ■ 76–90%   □ 50–75%   ■ <50%   □ Insufficient data or not applicable

SOURCE: Adapted from "Fig. 9. Proportion of the population using improved sanitation in 2012," *Progress on Sanitation and Drinking-water – 2014 Update*, World Health Organization (WHO) and United Nations Children's Fund (UNICEF), 2014, p. 17, http://apps.who.int/iris/bitstream/10665/112727/1/9789241507240_eng.pdf (accessed January 13, 2015).

as opposed to miasmas (bad smells or air emanating from decaying organic matter), a popular theory at the time.

The end of the 19th century brought a new wave of sanitation systems, including the popularization and prevalence of the flush toilet. Most major urban areas had sewer systems, and indoor plumbing became more common.

In present day, most developed nations have policies and practices in place establishing proper sanitation. Globally, however, there is a dearth of sanitation in developing countries, a condition that governments, nongovernmental organizations, and charities have been working to improve.

In 2000, following the Millennium Summit of the United Nations (UN), eight international development goals (known as the Millennium Development Goals or MDGs) were set. They included the goal of halving the number of people without proper sanitation by 2015. In July 2010, the UN General Assembly explicitly recognized the human right of access to clean drinking water and sanitation. The UN further called on states and international organizations to increase financing and infrastructure help provide safe, clean, accessible, and affordable drinking water and sanitation for all.

⊕ Impacts and Issues

In developed countries, primarily in urban areas, wastewater is collected in sewers. From there, it flows to a wastewater treatment plant where it is filtered and sanitized before being discharged into a large body of water such as a lake, river, or ocean. Another method for collecting and treating waste, particularly in rural and suburban areas, is called on-site or decentralized treatment. This is a system where wastewater is collected into a receptacle, such as a septic tank; water and solids are separated before water seeps into a septic field.

It is commonly accepted that hand washing and bathing with soap and clean water lowers the risk of contracting and spreading diseases ranging from the common cold to cholera. In 2012, Americans spent more than US$3.1 billion on soap alone. In developed parts of the world, there are myriad ways to keep clean, including antibacterial cleansers, wipes, sprays, and gels.

However, in the developing world, access to proper sanitation and hygiene has proven challenging. In 2012, the World Health Organization (WHO) estimated there were "46 countries where less than half the population has access to an improved sanitation facility." The WHO estimated that globally there were 2.5 billion people living without improved sanitation (defined as hygienically separating human urine and feces from human contact). Among the world's regions, southern Asia and sub-Saharan Africa continue to have the lowest levels of coverage. In Latin America and the Caribbean, seven countries have coverage of over 90 percent including Ecuador, Honduras, and Paraguay; the lowest levels of coverage were found in Haiti and Bolivia.

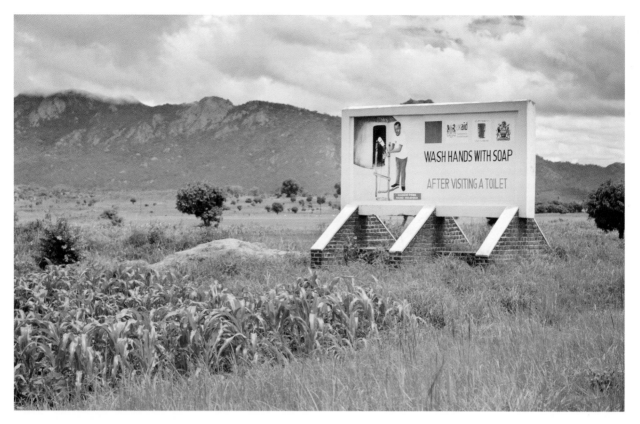

A billboard advises good hygiene practices after visiting a toilet in Dedza, Malawi.   © *Brendan Howard/Shutterstock.com.*

In 2012, more than 1 billion people worldwide still practiced open defecation, which leads to contaminated water sources and the spread of disease. Though this number has fallen 21 percent during the period in which it was monitored (1990–2012), 1 billion people have no sanitation facilities and continue to use gutters, bushes, and open water bodies for defecation. Though the majority of those practicing open defecation live in rural areas, a growing number are poorer people in urban areas. It is most prevalent in southern Asia, but also occurs in northern Africa, sub-Saharan Africa, Latin America, and the Caribbean.

According to the 2014 report "Progress on Drinking Water and Sanitation," a joint endeavor by WHO and UNICEF, "Open defecation perpetuates the vicious cycle of disease and poverty and is an affront to personal dignity." The report goes on to say that the countries with the most open defecation have the highest numbers of deaths of children younger than five, as well as high levels of undernutrition, high levels of poverty, and large disparities between the rich and poor. The practice also tends to affect girls and women the most, according to the report, since lack of safe private toilets, in close proximity to the home, leaves women and girls vulnerable to violence and can be an impediment to girls' education.

Though reliable data are scarce on this issue, best estimates indicate that as much as 90 percent of wastewater

in developing countries is discharged untreated—directly into rivers, lakes, or the ocean, according to the WHO/UNICEF 2014 Progress Report. This practice tends to place an inequitable burden on the poor because sewage removed from households of the wealthy tends to be discharged untreated or partially treated into storm drains, waterways, or landfills, polluting the residential areas inhabited by the poor.

Lack of sanitation creates just the right conditions for disease. Not only are people bathing and drinking in contaminated water, but local hospitals and schools are also failing to provide adequate sanitation and hygiene. This has meant a persistence of neglected tropical diseases (a diverse group of diseases caused by protozoa, bacteria, viruses, or parasitic worms called helminths), as well as waterborne diseases and others.

The WHO estimates that neglected tropical diseases (NTDs) affect 1.4 billion people. Symptoms of NTDs vary significantly from disease to disease; however, immediate symptoms include fever, aches, rash, sores, or swelling of the lymph nodes or at the site of infection. There are more than 300 types of NTDs. Of the 17 NTDs endemic in 149 countries, the seven most prevalent are lymphatic filariasis (a parasitic disease caused by microscopic, threadlike worms); onchocerciasis (a tropical skin disease caused by a parasitic filarial worm, transmitted by the bite of blackflies); trachoma (a contagious bacterial

MICROCREDITS AND WASH

The concept of microfinancing is not new. However, it has only been relatively recently that this model has expanded to provide small, low-cost loans to individuals and small businesses looking to bring sustainable water and sanitation systems into households and communities.

Microfinancing is the extension of small loans to borrowers who may not have collateral, credit history, or reliable employment to qualify for traditional loans from lending institutions. It is commonly accepted that the modern concept of microcredit originated in Bangladesh, India, in 1983 with the Grameen Bank. Since then, larger lending institutions as well as dedicated microfinancing institutions worldwide have been issuing these sorts of loans. Historically, these loans have been used to help impoverished people, usually women and generally in rural or developing countries, start businesses.

In recent years, the notion of using microcredits as a way of helping the poor get access to potable water and proper sanitation has been gaining some traction. Funding—particularly commercial credit—for water and sanitation projects has typically gone to the public sector. However, low tariffs and cost recovery limit credit to public utilities. This creates a situation where there is greater need than there is financing to address the lack of water and sanitation in these rural and developing communities. Further, these loans have tended to benefit communities that already had some sort of existing water and sanitation systems. This meant that the poorest and most in need were not getting access to water and sanitation.

However, with the backing of philanthropic organizations and microfinance lending institutions, there are three ways that microcredits are being used to improve the water, sanitation, and hygiene (WASH) sector. These include microcredits given at the household level that provide water connections, indoor plumbing, or on-site sanitation; credits for small business to invest in water supply; and for upgrading services in more urban areas and improving shared facilities in low income areas. While the latter has not been used widely, the other two methods have been fairly popular and relatively successful.

Statistically, the vast majority of these loans are repaid. According to water.org, a nonprofit associated with the Bill & Melinda Gates Foundation, 99 percent of the microcredit loans, dubbed WaterCredit, had been paid back between 2003 and 2014. Part of the reason for this is that households that relied on buying water, usually at a greatly inflated rate, are now paying much less with a household connection. Furthermore, members of these households are able to be more productive, both because they are not getting sick from waterborne and sanitation related diseases and because they do not have to walk for hours a day to access water.

While microcredits for water and sanitation have been helpful, there has been some criticism. Microcredits and microfinancing in general are often touted as ways to get people out of poverty and to empower women. However, critics say that these programs have fallen short of these goals and often leave the poor worse off because they have taken on a debt they cannot repay. Research into this area is ongoing.

infection of the eye); schistosomiasis (a chronic disease caused by infestation with blood flukes); and three soil-transmitted helminthic infections: hookworm, ascariasis, and trichuriasis. For people with recurring bouts of NTDs or those who do not receive proper treatment, these diseases can lead to chronic illness, disability, and in some cases death.

Waterborne illnesses also run rampant in areas lacking proper sanitation. The most common include campylobacter, cholera, *Escherichia coli* infection, giardiasis, hepatitis A, rotavirus, shigellosis, and typhoid fever. Symptoms of these diseases vary, but diarrhea and vomiting are the most commonly reported and often do the most damage. Left untreated or not treated quickly, many of these diseases lead to severe dehydration and death.

About 88 percent of the 4 billion diarrhea cases reported worldwide are linked to unsafe water, inadequate sanitation, or insufficient hygiene. Roughly 2 million people die each year from diarrheal diseases; of these, more than 600,000 are children. The WHO estimates that 94 percent of diarrheal cases are preventable through modifications to the environment, including interventions that increase the availability of clean water, improved sanitation, and hygiene.

Both NTDs and waterborne diseases are particularly common and virulent in poor, rural, and peri-urban (the communities in between rural and urban) areas. These also tend to be areas where underlying health problems such as malnutrition and human immunodeficiency virus/acquired immune deficiency syndrome (HIV/AIDS) make contracting one of these diseases worse.

Lack of sanitation and hygiene practices coupled with a lack of potable (safe to drink) water affects not only the health of a community but its educational and economic opportunities. Scientists and researchers assert that if people who currently lack access to potable water, improved sanitation, and proper tools for hygiene were equipped with these things, it would have a substantial impact on eradicating poverty and hunger, reducing child mortality, improving maternal health, combating infectious diseases, and ensuring environmental sustainability.

Researchers project that there would be "an overall estimated gain of 1.5 percent of global GDP [gross domestic product] and a USD$4.3 return for every dollar invested in water and sanitation services due to reduced health-care costs for individuals and society; greater productivity and involvement in the workplace through better access to facilities; … and opportunity for growth of new industries,"

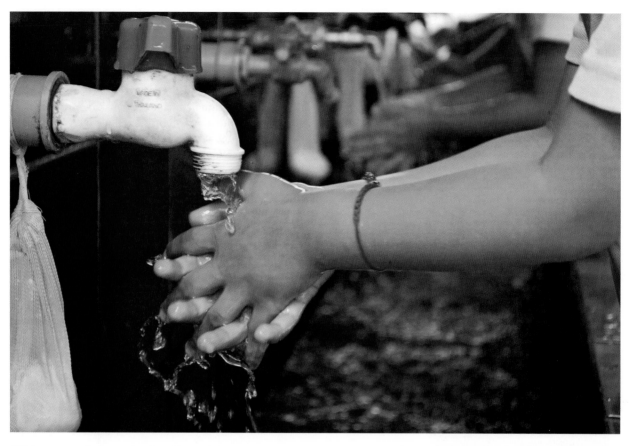

Children are taught proper hand washing techniques at school.   © *Thanamat Somwan/Shutterstock.com.*

according to the *UN-Water Global Analysis and Assessment of Sanitation and Drinking-Water (GLAAS) 2014 Report.* History bears this out. For example, the impact of clean water technologies on public health in the United States is estimated to have had a rate of return of 23 to 1 for investments in water filtration and chlorination during the first half of the 20th century, according to the U.S. National Bureau of Economic Research.

There are many impediments to providing WASH resources for people. The majority of countries where water, sanitation, and hygiene are an issue have policies in place for regulation, but not all countries fully implement, fund, or review them, according to *GLAAS 2014.* Further more, many of these nations are short on human and financial resources as well as skilled and willing graduates able to work in rural areas of these affected countries.

Monitoring is also a challenge. Many countries have policies regarding the monitoring of progress, but following through is difficult for a variety of reasons, including lack of willingness on the part of survey subjects to give information for fear of stigma and survey groups living in hard-to-reach or dangerous areas.

One of the biggest challenges is financing. International aid has increased over the past several decades; on the national level, however, funding is lacking. Furthermore, according to the *GLAAS 2014* report, the money

that is being spent on sanitation is concentrated in urban areas despite the fact that the rural population is most in need of improved sanitation. The report found that spending for rural sanitation constitutes less than 10 percent of total WASH financing.

There is political support for universal access to sanitation but fewer than one-third of the countries reviewed in the *GLAAS 2014* report have national WASH plans that are being fully implemented, funded, and regularly reviewed, including those in institutional settings such as schools and hospitals. According to the report, these are critical spaces when it comes to WASH: "Water and sanitation services in schools can ensure that children, especially girls, stay in school and learn lifelong hygiene habits. In health clinics, WASH services ensure the privacy and safety of patients, particularly expectant mothers during delivery, and are essential to prevent and respond to disease outbreaks."

⊕ Future Implications

Providing potable water and proper sanitation and hygiene has the potential to prevent at least 9.1 percent of the global disease burden and 6.3 percent of all deaths, according to the WHO. Improved sanitation reduces diarrhea morbidity by 37.5 percent and washing hands at critical times can reduce the number of diarrhea cases by as much as 35 percent, according to the UN Millennium Project. Improvement of drinking-water quality would lead to a 45 percent reduction of diarrhea episodes.

Improving sanitation would also have environmental benefits. The most obvious of these is reduction in pollution of water sources and land, which would benefit inland and coastal fisheries and land values. Systems allowing for nutrient reuse could turn fecal sludge into fertilizer or biogas generation. Improved sanitation could open up opportunities to expand tourism, offering a cleaner environment and lower health risks.

Though most countries are not yet able to reap these benefits, there has been progress. In 2012, 89 percent of the global population used an improved source of drinking water, and 64 percent used an improved sanitation facility, according to the WHO/UNICEF 2014 Progress Report. The MDG drinking water target has been met by 116 countries, and 77 have met the MDG sanitation target. Overall, open defecation decreased from 24

percent to 14 percent from 1990 to 2012. However, as of late 2014, it appeared that not all of the 116 countries participating in the goals challenge were going to reach the MDG goal of reducing the percentage of the population without improved sanitation to 25 percent by 2015.

Several countries reported that efforts are underway to reduce sanitation inequalities by making services more affordable to the poor. Methods include increasing block tariffs, reducing connection fees, supplying vouchers, offering free water tanks and water allocations, and making microfinance loans available.

According to UNICEF, eliminating open defecation is critical to accelerating progress toward halving the number of people living without improved sanitation. In May 2014, UN Deputy Secretary General Jan Eliasson launched a public campaign to end the practice and improve access to toilets and latrines. The ongoing awareness campaign focuses on breaking the taboo of talking publicly about open defecation and the diseases that occur, particularly among children, as a result. Furthermore, since 2001, November 19 has been recognized

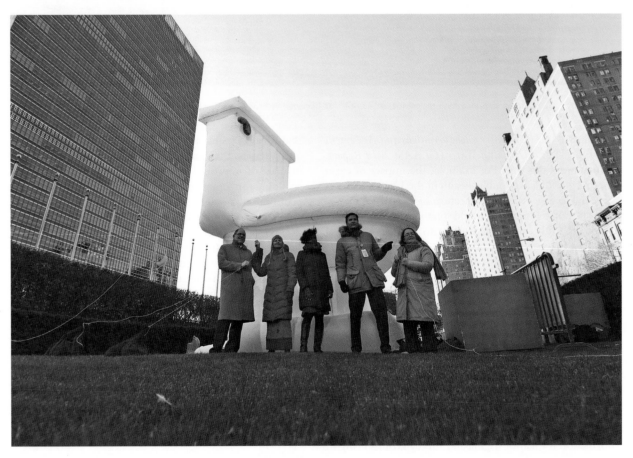

United Nations (UN) staff install a 15-door-high inflatable toilet to mark the World Toilet Day in front of the UN headquarters in New York on November 19, 2014. The UN called for an end to defecation in the open, with fears growing that it has helped spread the deadly Ebola virus ravaging West Africa. The UN estimates that 2.5 billion people do not have access to an improved sanitation facility, including toilets or latrines, with detrimental consequences on human health, dignity and security, the environment, and social and economic development. *© Jewel Samad/AFP/Getty Images.*

as World Toilet Day, an international day of action meant to draw attention to the global sanitation challenge.

The UN also established the Thematic Priority Area on Water Supply and Basic Sanitation in support of the goal to provide universal access to safe water and sanitation. The group's mission is "to foster collaboration between UN agencies, provide value added services to the UN and its member states, support initiatives that facilitate achievement of the relevant development goals, raise awareness and support UN global advocacy on water supply and basic sanitation, and coordinate with non-UN water initiatives related to water supply and basic sanitation," as posted on the UN-Water website.

The UN and WHO are working on a series of sanitation goals with the hope of reaching the targets by 2030. These goals include eliminating open defecation; achieving universal access to basic drinking water, sanitation and hygiene for households, schools, and health-care facilities; halving the proportion of the population without access at home to safely managed drinking water and sanitation services; and progressively eliminating inequalities in access. To accomplish this will take a collective effort on the part of national governments, local communities, and international agencies alike.

It will also mean securing, absorbing, and targeting international and national financing; renewing focus on health facilities; strengthening action when it comes to hygiene promotion; supporting the operation and maintenance of existing infrastructure and services; and expanding efforts in neglected rural areas.

PRIMARY SOURCE

Rural Hygiene

SOURCE *Nightingale, Florence.* Rural Hygiene. *London: Spottiswoode & Co., 1894, 7–13. Available online at http://pds.lib.harvard.edu/pds/view/7405264?n=13&printThumbnails=no (accessed January 25, 2015).*

INTRODUCTION *This primary source is taken from the writings of Florence Nightingale (1820–1910). Known for her role as a nurse during the Crimean War (1853–1856), she also contributed to the field of public health. In this excerpt from her publication* Rural Hygiene, *Nightingale describes domestic sanitary practices in rural 19th-century England. Similar conditions are still found in parts of the world today.*

2. PRESENT STATE OF RURAL HYGIENE

We will now deal with the

2. PRESENT STATE OF RURAL HYGIENE, which is indeed a pitiful and disgusting story, dreadful to tell.

For the sake of giving actual facts,—it is no use lecturing upon drainage, water-supply, wells, pig-sties, storage of excrement, storage of refuse, &c., &c., *in general*; they are dreadfully concrete,—I take leave to give the facts of one rural district, consisting of villages and one small market town, as described by a Local Government Board official this year; and I will ask the ladies here present whether they could not match these facts in every county in the kingdom. Perhaps, too, the lady lecturers on Rural Hygiene will favour us with some of their experiences.

A large number of the poor-cottages have been recently condemned as "unfit for human habitation," but though "unfit" many are still "inhabited," from lack of other accommodation.

Provision for conveying away surface and slop water is conspicuous either by its absence or defect. The slop-water stagnates and sinks into the soil all round the dwellings, aided by the droppings from the thatch. [It has been known that the bedroom slops are sometimes emptied out of window.] There *are* inside sinks, but the waste-pipe is often either untrapped or not disconnected.

It is a Government Official who says all this.

Water-supply almost entirely from shallow wells, often uncovered, mostly in the cottage garden, not far from a pervious privy pit, a pig-sty, or a huge collection of house refuse, polluted by the foulness soaking into it. The liquid manure from the pig-sty trickles through the ground into the well. Often after heavy rain the cottagers complain that their well-water becomes thick.

The water in many shallow wells has been analysed. And some have been closed; others *cleaned out*. But when no particular impurity is detected, no care has been taken to stop the too threatening pollution, or to prohibit the supply. In one village which *had* a pump, it was so far from one end that a pond in an adjoining field was used for their supply.

It may be said that, up to the present time, *practically* nothing has been done by the Sanitary Authorities to effect the removal of house refuse, &c.

In these days of investigation and statistics, where results are described with microscopic exactness and tabulated with mathematical accuracy, we seem to think figures will do instead of facts, and calculation instead of action. We remember the policeman who watched his burglar enter the house, and waited to make quite sure whether he was going to commit robbery with violence or without, before interfering with his operations. So as we read such an account as this we seem to be watching, not robbery, but murder going on, and to be waiting for the rates of mortality to go up before we interfere; we wait to see how many of the children playing round the houses shall be stricken down. We wait to see whether the filth will really trickle into the well, and whether the foul water really will poison the family, and how many will die of it. And then, when enough have died, we think it time to spend some money and some trouble to stop the murders going further, and we enter the results of our "masterly inactivity" neatly in tables; but we do not analyse and tabulate the saddened lives of those who remain, and the desolate homes in our "*sanitary*" "districts."

Storage of Excrement in These Villages.—This comes next. And it is so disgustingly inefficient that I write it on a separate sheet, to be omitted if desired. But we must remember that if we cannot bear with it, the national health has to bear with it, and especially the children's health. And I add, as a fact in another Rural District to the one quoted above, that, in rainy weather, the little children may play in the privy or in the so called "barn" or small outhouse, where may be several privies, several pigs, and untold heaps of filth. And as the little faces are very near the ground, children's diarrhœa and diseases have been traced to this miasma.

Cesspit Privies.—The *cess-pits are excavations* in the ground; often left unlined. Sometimes the privy is a wooden sentry-box, placed so that the fœcal matter falls directly into a ditch. Cess-pits often very imperfectly or not at all covered. Some privies with a cubic capacity of 18 or 20 feet are emptied from once to thrice yearly. But we are often told that all the contents "ran away," and that therefore emptying was not required!

These privies are often close to the well—one within a yard of the cottagers' pump.

Earth closets are the exception, cess-pit privies the rule. [In another place 109 cess-pit privies were counted to 120 cottages. And, as might be expected, there was hardly a pure well in the place.]

In one, a market town, there *are* water-closets, so called from being without water.

Storage of Refuse and Ashes.—Ashpits are conspicuous by their absence. Huge heaps of accumulated refuse are found piled up near the house, sometimes under the windows, or near the well, into which these refuse heaps soak. Where there *are* ashpits, they are piled up and overflowing. Privy contents are often mixed up with the refuse or buried in a hole in the refuse-heap.

As to the *final disposal*, in most cases the cottagers have allotments, but differing in distance from but a few yards to as much as two miles from their homes. Their privy contents and ash refuse are therefore valuable as manure, and they would "strongly resent" any appropriation of it by the Sanitary Authority.

And we might take this into account by passing a bye-law to the effect that house refuse must be removed at least once a quarter, and that if the occupier neglected to do this, the Sanitary Authority would do it, *and would appropriate it*. This amount of pressure is thoroughly legitimate to protect the lives of the children.

Health Missioners might teach the value of co-operation in sanitary matters. For instance, suppose the hire of a sewage-cart is l*s*. the first day, and six-pence every other

day. If six houses, adjacent to each other, subscribed for the use of the sewage-cart, they would each get it far cheaper than by single orders.

The usual practice is to wait until there is a sufficient accumulation to make worth while the hiring of a cart. The ashes, and often the privy contents too, are then taken away to the allotments. A statement that removal takes place as much as two or three times a year is often too obviously untrue.

But, as a rule, the occupiers have sufficient garden space, *i.e.* curtilage, for the proper utilisation of their privy contents. [I would urge the reading of Dr. Poore's "Rural Hygiene" on this particular point.]

Often the garden is large enough for the utilisation of ashes and house refuse too. But occupiers almost always take both privy and ashpit contents to their allotments. Thus hoarding-up of refuse matters occurs. In some cases the cost of hiring horse and cart—the amount depending on the distance of the allotment from the dwelling—is so serious a consideration that if bye-laws compelled the occupiers to remove their refuse to their allotments, say every month, either the value of the manure would be nothing, or the scavenging must be done at the expense of the Sanitary Authority. From the public health point of view, the Sanitary Authority should of course do the scavenging in all the villages.

The health Economy of the Community demands the most profitable use of manure for the land. Now the most profitable use is that which permits of least waste, and if we could only regard economy in this matter in its true and broad sense, we should acknowledge that the Community is advantaged by the frequent removal of sewage refuse from the houses, where it is dangerous, to the land, where it is an essential. And if the Community is advantaged, the Community should pay for that advantage. The gain is a double one—safety in the matter of health—increase in the matter of food, besides the untold gain, moral as well as material, which results from the successful cultivation of land.

There are some villages without any gardens—barely room for a privy and ashpit. But even in these cases the occupiers generally have allotments.

Plenty of bye-laws may be imposed, but bye-laws are not in themselves active agents. And in many, perhaps in most, cases they are impossible of execution, and remain a dead letter.

Now let us come to

3. WHAT THE WOMEN HAVE TO DO WITH IT—*i.e.*, how much the cottage mothers, if instructed by instructed women, can remedy or prevent these and other frightful evils.

And first

(1) OUR HOMES—The Cottage Homes of England being, after all, the most important of the homes of any class, should be pure in every sense. Boys and girls must

grow up healthy, with clean minds, and clean bodies, and clean skins. And the first teachings and impressions they have at home must all be pure, and gentle, and firm.

It is *home* that teaches the child after all, more than any other schooling. A child learns before it is three whether it shall obey its mother or not. And before it is seven its character is a good way to being formed.

When a child has lost its health, how often the mother says: "O, if I had only known, but there was no one to tell me!"

God did not intend all mothers to be accompanied by doctors, but He meant all children to be cared for by mothers.

(*a*) *Back Yard and Garden.*—Where and how are slops emptied? The following are some of the essential requisites: slops to be poured slowly down a drain, not hastily thrown down to make a pool round the drain; gratings of drain to be kept clean and passage free; soil round the house kept pure, that pure air may come in at the window; bedroom slops not to be thrown out of window; no puddles to be allowed to stand round walls; privy contents to be got into the soil as soon as possible—most valuable for your *garden*; cesspools not to be allowed to filter into your shallow wells; pump water wells must be taken care of, they are upright drains, so soil round them should be pure. Bad smells are danger-signals. *Pig-sties*—Moss litter to absorb liquid manure, cheap and profitable; danger from pools of liquid manure making the whole soil foul.

SEE ALSO *Bacterial Diseases; Global Health Initiatives; Health as a Human Right and Health-Care Access; International Health Regulation, Surveillance, and Enforcement; NGOs and Health Care: Deliverance or Dependence; Vulnerable Populations; Water Supplies and Access to Clean Water; Waterborne Diseases*

BIBLIOGRAPHY

Books

Ayisi, Ruth Ansah. *The Water, Sanitation and Hygiene Promotion (WASH) Programme, Malawi*. Lilongwe, Malawi: UNICEF Unite for Children, 2010.

African Conference on Sanitation and Hygiene. *Meeting Report, AMCOW: Sanitation and Hygiene Task Force*. Kigali, Rwanda: Third Africa Conference on Sanitation and Hygiene, 2011.

Bradley, Mark, ed., with Kenneth R. Stow. *Rome, Pollution, and Propriety: Dirt, Disease, and Hygiene in the Eternal City from Antiquity to Modernity*. Cambridge, UK: Cambridge University Press, 2012.

Calow, Roger, Eva Ludi, and Josephine Tucker, eds. *Achieving Water Security: Lessons from Research in Water Supply, Sanitation and Hygiene in Ethiopia*. Rugby, UK: Practical Action, 2013.

Thematic Working Group on Water, Hygiene and Sanitation. *Sanitation and Hygiene in East Asia*. Manila: World Health Organization, Regional Office for the Western Pacific, 2010.

UN-Water Global Analysis and Assessment of Sanitation and Drinking-Water (GLAAS) 2014 Report: Investing in Water and Sanitation: Increasing Access, Reducing Inequalities. Geneva: World Health Organization, 2014.

Periodicals

Hoang, Van Minh, and Hung Nguyen-Viet. "Economic Aspects of Sanitation in Developing Countries." *Environmental Health Insights* 5 (2011): 63–70.

Nicole, Wendee. "The WASH Approach." *Environmental Health Perspectives* 123, no. 1 (January 2015): A6–A14.

Song, Liang, et al. "Surveillance Systems for Neglected Tropical Diseases: Global Lessons from China's Evolving Schistosomiasis Reporting Systems, 1949–2014." *Emerging Themes in Epidemiology* 11, no. 1 (2014): 2–28.

Websites

"Global Water, Sanitation, & Hygiene (WASH)." *U.S. Centers for Disease Control and Prevention (CDC)*. http://www.cdc.gov/healthywater/global/sanitation/ (accessed March 5, 2015).

"Investing in Water and Sanitation: Increasing Access, Reducing Inequalities." *World Health Organization (WHO)*. http://www.who.int/water_sanitation_health/publications/glaas_report_2014/en/ (accessed March 5, 2015).

"Progress on Drinking Water and Sanitation, 2014 Update." *World Health Organization (WHO)/United Nations Children's Fund*. http://www.who.int/water_sanitation_health/publications/2014/jmp-report/en/ (accessed March 5, 2015).

"Thematic Priority Area: Water Supply and Basic Sanitation." *UN-Water: The United Nations Inter-Agency Mechanism on All Freshwater Related Issues, Including Sanitation*. http://www.unwater.org/activities/thematic-priority-areas/water-supply-and-basic-sanitation/en/ (accessed March 5, 2015).

"Water, Sanitation and Hygiene." *United Nations Children's Fund (UNICEF)*. http://www.unicef.org/wash/ (accessed March 5, 2015).

"Water, Sanitation, and Hygiene (WASH)." *UNHCR*. http://www.unhcr.org/pages/49c3646cef.html (accessed March 5, 2015).

"Water Sanitation Health." *World Health Organization (WHO)*. http://www.who.int/water_sanitation_health/hygiene/sanitpromotionguide/en/ (accessed March 5, 2015).

Melanie R. Plenda

SARS, MERS, and the Emergence of Coronaviruses

⊕ Introduction

A coronavirus is a common virus that typically causes mild or moderate upper-respiratory tract illnesses. The coronavirus is so named because of the crownlike spikes on its surface ("corona" being Latin for "crown"). There are specific coronaviruses that infect people and others that infect animals, but it is rare that a particular coronavirus will infect both animals and people. In the 21st century, two coronaviruses emerged that could infect both animals and people, causing the lethal and highly transmissable diseases known as severe acute respiratory syndrome (SARS) and Middle East respiratory syndrome (MERS). Both the SARS coronavirus (SARS-CoV) and the Middle East respiratory syndrome coronavirus (MERS-CoV) also have close genetic and physiological relationships with known coronaviruses afflicting bats.

⊕ Historical Background

The first known case of SARS was traced to a November 2002 case in Guangdong Province, China. By mid-February 2003, Chinese health officials tracked more than 300 cases, including five deaths in Guangdong Province, from what was at the time described as an acute respiratory syndrome.

The SARS Outbreak

In February 2003, Liu Jianlun, a 64-year-old Chinese physician from Zhongshan hospital (later determined to have been a "super-spreader," a person capable of infecting unusually high numbers of contacts) traveled to Hong Kong to attend a family wedding despite the fact that he had a fever. Epidemiologists subsequently determined that Liu passed on the SARS virus to other guests at the Metropole Hotel, where he stayed in Hong Kong. These people included American businessman Johnny Chen, three women from Singapore, two Canadians, and a Hong Kong resident. Liu's travel to Hong Kong and the subsequent travel of those he infected allowed SARS to spread from China to the infected travelers' destinations.

Chen, the American businessman, grew ill in Hanoi, Vietnam, and was admitted to a local hospital. Chen infected 20 health-care workers at the hospital, including the Italian epidemiologist Carlo Urbani (1956–2003), who worked at the Hanoi World Health Organization (WHO) office. Urbani provided medical care for Chen and first formally recognized and reported SARS as a unique disease on February 28, 2003. By early March, 22 hospital workers in Hanoi were ill with SARS.

Urbani's report did not draw much attention among epidemiologists until it was coupled with news reports in mid-March that Hong Kong health officials had also discovered an outbreak of an acute respiratory syndrome among health-care workers. Unsuspecting hospital workers admitted the Hong Kong man infected by Liu to a general ward at the Prince of Wales Hospital there under the assumption that he had a typical severe pneumonia, a fairly routine admission. The first notice that clinicians were dealing with an usual illness came from the observation that hospital staff, along with those subsequently determined to have been in close proximity to the infected persons, began to show signs of illness. Eventually, 138 people, including 34 nurses, 20 doctors, 16 medical students, and 15 other health-care workers, contracted SARS-related pneumonia.

Hong Kong authorities then decided that those suffering the flulike symptoms would be given the option of self-isolation, with family members allowed to remain confined at home or in special camps. Compliance checks were conducted by police.

One of the Canadians infected in Hong Kong, Sui-Chu Kwan, returned to Toronto, Ontario, and died in a Toronto hospital in March 2003. As in Hong Kong, because there were no initial alerts from China about the SARS outbreak, Canadian officials did not suspect that Kwan had been infected with a highly contagious virus until Kwan's son and five health-care workers showed

ISOLATION AND QUARANTINE

Before the advent of vaccines and effective diagnostic tools, isolation and quarantine were the principal tools to control the spread of infectious disease. The term quarantine derives from the Italian *quarantine* and *quaranta giorni* and dates to the plague in Europe. As a precautionary measure, the government of Venice restricted entry into the port city and mandated that ships coming from areas of plague—or otherwise suspected of carrying plague—had to wait 40 days before being allowed to discharge their cargos.

The legal basis of quarantine in the United States was established in 1878 with the passage of federal quarantine legislation in response to continued outbreaks of yellow fever, typhus, and cholera.

The public discussion of SARS-related quarantine in the United States and Europe renewed tensions between the needs for public health precautions that safeguard society at large and the liberties of the individual. During the later years of the 19th century and throughout the 20th century, the law bent toward protecting the greater needs of protecting society. The fact that the establishment of quarantine was sometimes used to contain and discourage immigration often made the use of quarantine a political, as well as medical, issue. In other cases, such as with tuberculosis (TB), quarantine proved effective, and courts wielded wide authority to isolate, hospitalize, and force patients to take medications.

Isolation and quarantine remain potent tools in the modern public health arsenal. Both procedures seek to control exposure to infected individuals or materials. Those with confirmed illnesses are kept in isolation to prevent them from infecting others. Those who are not yet ill but may become so because they had contact with an infected person or infected items may be quarantined until it is determined that they are not infected.

Isolation and quarantine both act to restrict movement and to slow or stop the spread of disease within a community. Depending on the illness, patients placed in isolation may be cared for in hospitals, specialized health-care facilities, or in less severe cases, at home. Isolation is a standard procedure for TB patients. In most cases, isolation is voluntary; however, isolation can be compelled by federal, state, and some local laws.

State governments within the United States have a general authority to set and enforce quarantine conditions. At the federal level, the U.S. Centers for Disease Control and Prevention's (CDC) Division of Global Migration and Quarantine is empowered to detain, examine, or conditionally release (release with restrictions on movement or with a required treatment protocol) individuals suspected of carrying a communicable disease.

The CDC in Atlanta recommended SARS patients be voluntarily isolated but did not recommend enforced isolation or quarantine, in 2003. Regardless, CDC and other public health officials, including the surgeon general, sought and secured increased powers to deal with SARS. On April 4, 2003, U.S. President George W. Bush (1946–) signed Presidential Executive Order 13295, which added SARS to a list of quarantinable communicable diseases. The order provided health officials with the broader powers to seek the "apprehension, detention, or conditional release of individuals to prevent the introduction, transmission, or spread of suspected communicable diseases."

Other diseases on the U.S. communicable disease list, specified pursuant to section 361(b) of the Public Health Service Act, include "Cholera; Diphtheria; infectious Tuberculosis; Plague; Smallpox; Yellow Fever; and Viral Hemorrhagic Fevers (Lassa, Marburg, Ebola, Crimean-Congo, South American, Hanta, and others yet to be isolated or named)."

similar symptoms. By mid-April, Canada reported at least 130 SARS cases and 15 fatalities.

Increasingly faced with reports that provided evidence of global dissemination, on March 15, 2003, the WHO took the unusual step of issuing a travel warning that described SARS as a worldwide health threat. WHO officials announced that SARS cases and potential cases had been tracked from China to Singapore, Thailand, Vietnam, Indonesia, the Philippines, and Canada. Although the exact cause of the illness had not, at that time, been determined, WHO officials' issuance of the precautionary warning to travelers bound for Southeast Asia about the potential SARS risk got the word out to public health officials about the possible dangers of the new disease.

Within days of the first WHO warning, SARS cases were reported in the United Kingdom, Spain, Slovenia, Germany, and the United States.

WHO officials were initially encouraged that isolation procedures and alerts were working to stem the spread of SARS, as some countries reporting small numbers of cases experienced no further dissemination to hospital staff or others in contact with SARS victims. However, in some countries, including Canada, where SARS cases occurred before WHO alerts, SARS continued to spread beyond the bounds of isolated patients. WHO officials responded by recommending increased screening and quarantine measures that included mandatory screening of persons returning from visits to the most severely affected areas in China, Southeast Asia, and Hong Kong.

Late in March 2003, Urbani, the scientist who initially reported SARS, died of complications related to the disease. In early April 2003, the WHO took the controversial additional step of recommending against nonessential travel to Hong Kong and Guangdong Province of China. The recommendation, sought by infectious disease specialists, was not controversial within the medical community but caused immediate concern regarding the potentially widespread economic impacts.

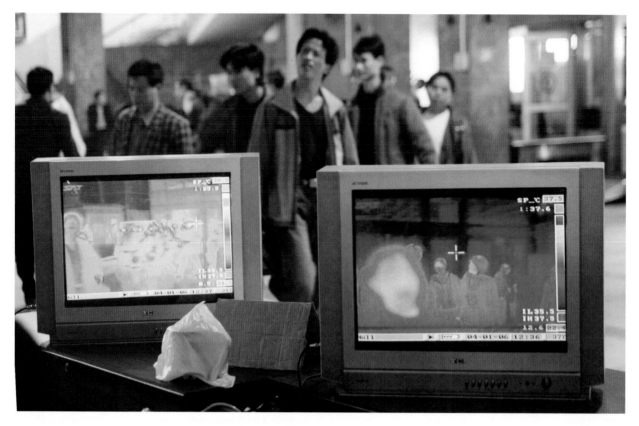

Following a confirmed SARS case in Guangzhou, China, thermal scanners check body temperatures in a Guangzhou railway station to protect travelers against SARS on January 6, 2004. © *Peter Parks/AFP/Getty Images.*

In China, fear of a widespread outbreak ultimately spurred an intensive effort in Beijing to isolate SARS victims and halt the spread of the disease. By the end of April 2003, schools in Beijing were closed, along with many public buildings and areas.

Mounting reports of SARS showed a rapid global dissemination of the virus. By April 9, 2003, the first confirmed reports of SARS cases in Africa reached WHO headquarters, and eight days later a confirmed case was discovered in India. Within months, the crisis had subsided almost as quickly as it arose. By the end of the outbreak in July 2003, 8,098 people worldwide had contracted SARS, and 774 died from complications of the disease.

Scientists scrambled to isolate, identify, and sequence the pathogen responsible for SARS. Modes of transmission characteristic of viral transmission allowed scientists to place early attention on a group of viruses termed coronaviruses—some of which are associated with the common cold. There was a global two-pronged attack on the SARS pathogen, with some efforts directed toward a positive identification and isolation of the virus, and other efforts directed toward discovering the genetic molecular structure and sequence of genes contained in the virus. The development of a genomic map of the precise nucleotide sequence of the virus would be key

in any subsequent development of a definitive diagnostic test, the identification of effective antiviral agents, and perhaps a vaccine. The development of a reliable and definitive diagnostic test was considered of paramount importance in keeping SARS from becoming a global pandemic. A definitive diagnostic test would not only allow physicians earlier treatment options, but would also allow the earlier identification and isolation of potential carriers of the virus.

The SARS virus is usually transmitted by aerosolized droplets of virus-infected material. SARS has an incubation period range of 2 to 10 days, with an average incubation of about 4 days. Much of the incubation period allows the virus to be both transported and spread by a carrier with no symptoms. The initial symptoms are nonspecific and common to the flu. After the initial period, persons with SARS typically spike a fever of at least 100.4 degrees Fahrenheit (38 degrees Celsius) as they develop a cough, shortness of breath, and difficulty breathing. SARS often fulminates (reaches its maximum progression) in a severe pneumonia that can cause respiratory failure and death in about 10 percent of its victims.

No definitive therapy has been demonstrated to have clinical effectiveness against the virus that causes SARS. Antibiotics, antiviral medications, corticosteroids, and supportive therapies such as fluids and ventilation are the mainstays of treatment for SARS. Antibiotics, because they target bacterial infections, are ineffective in treating SARS. As of mid-2015, no antiviral agents have been developed to successfully treat patients infected with the virus. In previous epidemics, patients were treated with high doses of glucocorticoids and the antiviral agent, ribavirin. However, these treatment modalities were not beneficial and were linked to immediate and late side effects.

MERS-CoV and MERS Syndrome

In September 2012, health officials in London identified the novel coronavirus (NCoV) MERS in a patient transferred from Qatar. The newly identified virus had killed one person in Saudi Arabia. MERS was first reported September 24, 2012, on ProMed Mail by an Egyptian virologist, Dr. Ali Mohamed Zaki, working in Jeddah, Saudi Arabia. Symptoms of MERS include fever, cough, and shortness of breath, often progressing to acute respiratory distress and kidney failure. Most cases require hospitalization for serious illness, but up to 20 percent of people with MERS-CoV present with milder symptoms, and some cases have also been identified in people without symptoms.

MERS is a severe respiratory illness caused by the novel coronavirus MERS-CoV. MERS-CoV is likely zoonotic in origin, meaning it originally occurred in animals.

Scientists suspect that bats are a reservoir for MERS, and as dromedary camels in Oman, Egypt, and Saudi Arabia show infection with a similar virus, they likely serve as an intermediate host and are considered the primary source of MERS zoonotic infection in humans. MERS-CoV has been called a SARS-like virus.

Reports of confirmed cases of MERS-CoV slowed during the summer of 2014. According to the WHO, by February 2015, there had been a total of over 1,000 laboratory-confirmed cases of MERS-CoV including 376 deaths. With over 50 new infections in the first three weeks of February 2015 alone, the WHO called for an increased international response to the MERS-CoV outbreak.

Uncertainty in Reporting Emerging Diseases

In early 2004, Chinese authorities reported another outbreak of SARS affecting 17 people, this time originating from six laboratory workers who were exposed to the virus. In late 2004, four more unlinked, community-acquired cases of SARS were found in Guangdong Province. Although the source of this outbreak was unconfirmed, it is suspected to have originated in wild animals, most likely those found in food markets.

Reports of cases of SARS that were suppressed by the Chinese government surfaced again in early

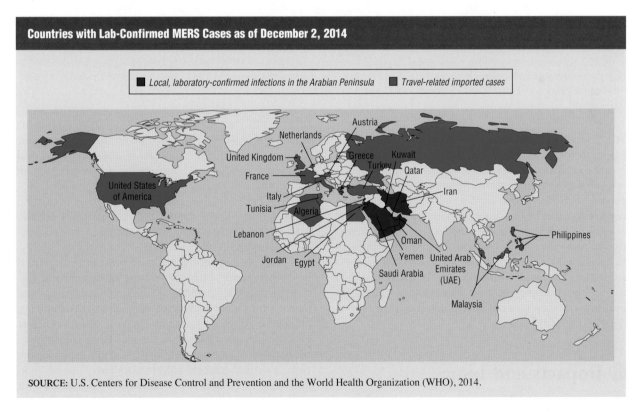

Countries with Lab-Confirmed MERS Cases as of December 2, 2014

■ *Local, laboratory-confirmed infections in the Arabian Peninsula*   ■ *Travel-related imported cases*

SOURCE: U.S. Centers for Disease Control and Prevention and the World Health Organization (WHO), 2014.

In 2012, a highly contagious human coronavirus now known as Middle East respiratory syndrome coronavirus (MERS-CoV) was identified in the Middle East. As of late 2014, cases indicate how highly transmissible the virus is and how secondary cases have shown up in health-care workers with no known travel to the Middle East.

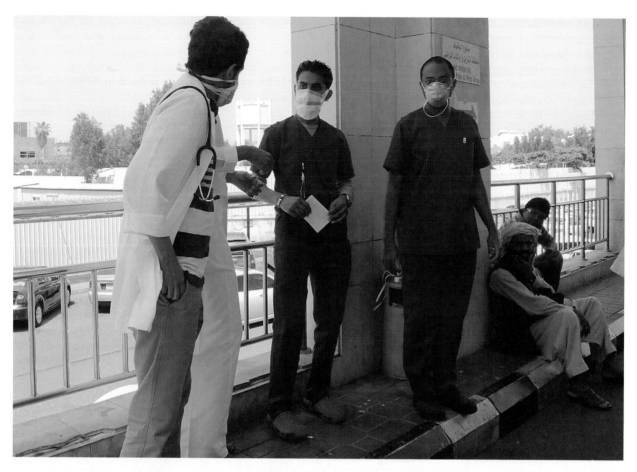

Saudi hospital employees wear mouth and nose masks as they stand outside a local hospital's emergency department, on April 22, 2014, in the Red Sea coastal city of Jeddah, Saudi Arabia. The health ministry reported more MERS cases in Jeddah, prompting authorities to close the emergency department at the city's King Fahd Hospital. The ministry said it registered 261 cases of infection across the kingdom between the discovery of the MERS in September 2012 and April 2014. © *AFP/Getty Images.*

2012. One man was subsequently arrested for spreading false information via the Internet, stating that a hospital in Baoding, Hebei Province, had confirmed a case of SARS. Concurrently, however, more than 300 people with an undisclosed respiratory illness were reportedly isolated at a military hospital in Hebei, and rumors of SARS continued to spread via the Internet. By February 24, 2012, Chinese public health authorities reported that the outbreak was caused by a severe adenovirus 55, along with cases of influenza that surged in the region during this time frame. China shared this information with international public health monitoring systems worldwide.

⊕ Impacts and Issues

The emergence of SARS demonstrated that like influenza viruses, coronaviruses can spread quickly through vulnerable human populations. Because bat populations host coronaviruses, bats became a more prominent natural animal reservoir of viruses capable of causing potentially deadly and widespread outbreaks of disease. A good deal of research funding and interest turned to the study of bat populations and their interactions with humans.

The outbreak also spurred identification of existing coronaviruses. For example, the coronaviruses HCoV-HKU1 and HCoV-NL63 were identified as causes of human respiratory tract infections.

Many flu-causing viruses have previously originated from Guangdong Province because of cultural and cuisine practices that bring animals, animal parts, and humans into close proximity. In such an environment, pathogens (disease-causing organisms) can more easily genetically mutate and make the leap from animal hosts to humans. Scientists have identified the masked palm civet, a catlike creature sold in southern Chinese food markets for its meat, as the probable incidental host for exposing the SARS virus to humans. The original hosts were probably bats that, in turn, infected the civets. The first cases of SARS showed increased prevalence among Guangdong food handlers and chefs.

Chinese health officials initially remained silent about the SARS outbreak, and no special precautions were taken to limit travel or prevent the spread of the disease. The world health community, therefore, had no chance to institute early testing, isolation, and quarantine measures that might have prevented the subsequent global spread of the disease. Eventually, under a new generation of political leadership, Chinese officials subsequently apologized for a slow and inefficient response to the SARS outbreak. Allegations that officials covered up the extent of the spread of the disease caused the dismissal of several local administrators, including China's public health minister and the mayor of Beijing.

The experience with SARS has dramatically increased pandemic readiness in many countries. For example, after a health emergency due to pandemic influenza was declared in May 2009, Lam Ping-yan, director of health for the Hong Kong Special Administrative Region of China, assured residents that the region was prepared for the next viral outbreak. Although each new virus can present resistance to specific drugs, Hong Kong has stockpiled the antiviral medicine Tamiflu for every citizen and has more than 1,000 hospital beds held in reserve in special isolation wards to combat respiratory illness.

⊕ Future Implications

Health authorities assert that the emergent virus responsible for SARS will remain endemic, or part of the natural array of viruses, in many regions of China.

SARS cases spurred reforms in the International Health Regulations (IHRs) that are designed to increase both surveillance and reporting of infectious diseases and to enhance cooperation in preventing the international spread of disease. In many regards, the SARS outbreak revealed what was effective in terms of public health responses, readiness, and resources.

SARS cases provided a test of reforms in IHRs designed to increase surveillance and reporting of infectious diseases—and to enhance cooperation in preventing the international spread of disease. Although not an act of bioterrorism, because the very same epidemiologic principles and isolation protocols might be used to both initially determine and respond to an act of bioterrorism, intelligence and public health officials closely monitored the political, scientific, and medical responses to the SARS outbreak. In many regards, the SARS outbreak provided a real and deadly test of public health responses, readiness, and resources.

Common to both responses to the SARS outbreak and a potential deliberate biological attack using pathogens such as smallpox or anthrax is the need to rapidly develop accurate diagnostic tests, treatment protocols, and medically sound control measures.

Along with the U.S. Centers for Disease Control and Prevention and other government agencies around the world, the WHO maintains constant surveillance to detect the reemergence of the virus that causes SARS. Viruses (including the SARS virus) have previously escaped high-security laboratories—often on the clothes of lab workers—and critics argue that risk analysis requirements for Bio Security Level 3 or Bio Security Level 4 labs (the most secure labs) are insufficient to ensure public safety.

PRIMARY SOURCE

Pneumonia—China (Guangdong): RFI

SOURCE *"PNEUMONIA—CHINA (GUANGDONG): RFI." ProMED-mail, February 10, 2003. Archive number 20030210.0357. Retrieved from http://www.promedmail.org (accessed February 9, 2015).*

INTRODUCTION *This primary source is a post from Program for Monitoring Emerging Diseases, or ProMED-mail, an Internet reporting system for emerging public health threats. ProMED-mail is maintained by the International Society for Infectious Diseases and the Harvard School of Public Health. The post from Stephen Cunnion was the first warning of the outbreak of SARS in China.*

PNEUMONIA—CHINA (GUANGDONG): RFI

A ProMED-mail post
<http://www.promedmail.org>
ProMED-mail is a program of the
International Society for Infectious Diseases
<http://www.isid.org>

Date: 10 Feb 2003
From: Stephen O. Cunnion, MD, PhD, MPH <cunnion@erols.com>

This morning I received this e-mail and then searched your archives and found nothing that pertained to it. Does anyone know anything about this problem?
"Have you heard of an epidemic in Guangzhou? An acquaintance of mine from a teacher's chat room lives there and reports that the hospitals there have been closed and people are dying."

Stephen O. Cunnion, MD, PhD, MPH
International Consultants in Health, Inc
Member ASTM&H, ISTM
<cunnion@erols.com>

PRIMARY SOURCE

SARS and Carlo Urbani

SOURCE *Reilley, Brigg, Michel Van Herp, Dan Sermand, and Nicoletta Dentico. "SARS and Carlo Urbani."* New England Journal of Medicine *348 (May 15, 2003): 1951–1952. Copyright © 2003 Massachusetts Medical Society. http://www.nejm.org/doi/full/10.1056/NEJMp030080 (accessed January 25, 2015).*

INTRODUCTION *This primary source, published in the* New England Journal of Medicine, *is a tribute to a heroic physician who died after contracting a deadly emergent virus. Dr. Carlo Urbani was a president of Médecins Sans Frontières (Doctors Without Borders) and, along with many public health colleagues, worked selflessly to fight pandemics and save lives.*

SARS and Carlo Urbani

On February 28, the Vietnam French Hospital of Hanoi, a private hospital of about 60 beds, contacted the Hanoi office of the World Health Organization (WHO). A patient had presented with an unusual influenza-like virus. Hospital officials suspected an avian influenza virus and asked whether someone from the WHO could take a look. Dr. Carlo Urbani, a specialist in infectious diseases, answered that call. In a matter of weeks, he and five other health care professionals would be dead from a previously unknown pathogen.

We now know that Hanoi was experiencing an outbreak of severe acute respiratory syndrome (SARS). Dr. Urbani swiftly determined that the small private hospital was facing something unusual. For the next several days, he chose to work at the hospital, documenting findings, arranging for samples to be sent for testing, and reinforcing infection control. The hospital established an isolation ward that was kept under guard. Dr. Urbani worked directly with the medical staff of the hospital to strengthen morale and to keep fear in check as SARS revealed itself to be highly contagious and virulent. Of the first 60 patients with SARS, more than half were health care workers. At a certain moment, many of the staff members made the difficult decision to quarantine themselves. To protect their families and community, some health care workers put themselves at great personal risk, deciding to sleep in the hospital and effectively sealing themselves off from the outside world.

In some ways, the SARS outbreak in Hanoi is a story of what can go right, of public health's coming before politics. First-line health care providers quickly alerted the WHO of an atypical pneumonia. Dr. Urbani recognized the severity of the public health threat. Immediately, the WHO requested an emergency meeting on Sunday, March 9, with the Vice Minister of Health of Vietnam. Dr. Urbani's temperament and intuition and the strong trust he had built with Vietnamese authorities were critical at this juncture. The four-hour discussion led the government to take the extraordinary steps of quarantining the Vietnam French Hospital, introducing new infection-control procedures in other hospitals, and issuing an international appeal for expert assistance. Additional specialists from the WHO and the Centers for Disease Control and Prevention (CDC) arrived on the scene, and Médecins sans Frontières (MSF, or Doctors without Borders) responded with staff members as well as infection-control suits and kits that were previously stocked for outbreaks of Ebola virus. The Vietnam French Hospital has been closed temporarily, and patients with SARS are cared for in two wards of the public Bach Mai Hospital, with the assistance of a team from MSF. No new cases in health care workers have been reported, and the outbreak in Vietnam appears to be contained. By dealing with the outbreak openly and decisively, Vietnam risked damage to its image and economy. If it had decided to take refuge in secrecy, however, the results might have been catastrophic.

Dr. Urbani would not survive to see the successes resulting from his early detection of SARS. On March 11, he began to have symptoms during a flight to Bangkok. On his arrival, he told a colleague from the CDC who greeted him at the airport not to approach him. They sat down at a distance from each other, in silence, waiting for an ambulance to assemble protective gear. He fought SARS for the next 18 days in a makeshift isolation room in a Bangkok hospital. Dr. Carlo Urbani died on March 29, 2003.

SARS is a pandemic of our global age. In just a few weeks, SARS had spread through air travel to at least three continents. Conversely, in the same amount of time, researchers working in no fewer than 10 countries have collaborated to identify the virus, sequence its genome, and take steps toward rapid diagnosis. It is now hoped that the large strides taken in basic research will quickly lead to therapeutic advances or a vaccine.

Health care workers continue to be on the front line. Apart from the index patient, all the patients in the Vietnamese outbreak who died were doctors and nurses. In Hong Kong, approximately 25 percent of patients with SARS have been health care professionals, including the chief executive of the hospital authority. The intensive care wards are full—a situation that is exacerbated by the staffing difficulties presented by the hundreds of SARS cases affecting medical personnel. It is becoming difficult to import additional infection-control equipment, since countries where the suits are manufactured are holding onto their stocks as they brace themselves for outbreaks of SARS within their own borders. Once effective drug therapy has been found, similar problems may arise with availability and distribution, especially if the effective treatment turns out to involve a relatively rare and expensive drug, such as ribavirin.

It remains to be seen whether the number of new SARS outbreaks will ebb or whether what we have seen to date is indeed the leading edge of a much larger pandemic. Currently, the attack rate in Hong Kong is approximately 2 cases per 10,000 population over the course of two months. This rate compares favorably with the seasonal attack rates of influenza-like illness, which reached 50 cases per 10,000 population in one week this winter in Europe.

In 1999, Dr. Urbani was president of MSF-Italy and a member of the delegation in Oslo, Norway, that accepted the Nobel Peace Prize. Although he would be gratified that so much has been accomplished with respect to SARS in such a short time, he would certainly point out that the other diseases he worked with—such as the human immunodeficiency virus and AIDS, tuberculosis, and malaria, which kill millions of people each year—deserve to be treated with similar urgency. Whatever the future direction of SARS, it is clear that Dr. Urbani's decisive and determined intervention has bought precious time and saved lives. We remember Dr. Urbani with a mixture of pride in his selfless devotion to medicine and unspeakable grief about the void his departure has left in the hearts of his colleagues around the world.

SEE ALSO *Epidemiology: Surveillance for Emerging Infectious Diseases; International Health Regulations, Surveillance, and Enforcement; Isolation and Quarantine; Viral Diseases; Zoonotic (Animal-Borne) Diseases*

BIBLIOGRAPHY

Books

Barrett, Ron, and George J. Armelagos. *An Unnatural History of Emerging Infections.* Oxford: Oxford University Press, 2013.

Calisher, Charles H. *Lifting the Impenetrable Veil: From Yellow Fever to Ebola Hemorrhagic Fever and SARS.* Red Feather Lakes, CO: Rockpile Press, 2013.

Chen, Sue, Nicole R. Wyre, and Agnes E. Rupley, eds. *New and Emerging Diseases.* Philadelphia: Elsevier, 2013.

Davis, Deborah, and Helen F. Siu, eds. *SARS: Reception and Interpretation in Three Chinese Cities.* London: Routledge, 2014.

Ding, Huiling. *Rhetoric of a Global Epidemic: Transcultural Communication about SARS.* Carbondale: Southern Illinois University Press, 2014.

Hui, David S. C., Wing-Wai Yew, and Alimuddin Zumla. *Emerging Respiratory Infections in the 21st Century.* Philadelphia: Saunders, 2010.

Lal, Sunil K., ed. *Molecular Biology of the SARS-Coronavirus.* Heidelberg, Germany: Springer 2010.

Mackenzie, John S., Martyn Jeggo, Peter Daszak, and J. A. Richt, eds. *One Health: The Human-Animal-Environment Interfaces in Emerging Infectious Diseases.* New York: Springer, 2013.

Olsson, Eva-Karin, and Lan Xue, eds. *SARS from East to West.* Lanham, MD: Lexington Books, 2011.

Serradell, Joaquima, with Hilary Babcock, consulting ed. *SARS*, 2nd ed. New York: Chelsea House, 2010.

Snodgrass, Mary Ellen. *World Epidemics: A Cultural Chronology of Disease from Prehistory to the Era of SARS.* Jefferson, NC: McFarland, 2011.

Periodicals

Chan, Engle Angela, et al. "An Evaluation of Nursing Practice Models in the Context of the Severe Acute Respiratory Syndrome Epidemic in Hong Kong: A Preliminary Study." *Journal of Clinical Nursing* 15, no. 6 (2011): 661–670.

Chan, Lucy Chen, and Jin Xu. "China's Engagement with Global Health Diplomacy: Was SARS a Watershed?" *Negotiating and Navigating Global Health: Case Studies in Global Health Diplomacy* (2011): 203–219.

Gomersall C. D., and G. M. Joynt. "Middle East Respiratory Syndrome: New Disease, Old Lessons." *The Lancet* 381, no. 9885 (2013): 2229–2230.

Hafner, S. "SARS Attacks!" *Microbes and Infection* 15, no. 2 (2013): 85–87.

Leung, C. H., and C. D. Gomersall. "Middle East Respiratory Syndrome." *Intensive Care Medicine* 40, no. 7 (2014): 1015–1017.

Websites

"Key Facts—MERS-CoV." *Public Health England.* http://www.hpa.org.uk/Topics/InfectiousDiseases/InfectionsAZ/MERSCoV/GeneralInformation/respqandanovelcoronavirus2013/ (accessed March 1, 2015).

"Middle East Respiratory Syndrome (MERS-CoV)." *U.S. Centers for Disease Control and Prevention (CDC).* http://www.cdc.gov/coronavirus/mers/index.html (accessed March 1, 2015).

"Severe Acute Respiratory Syndrome (SARS)." *U.S. Centers for Disease Control and Prevention (CDC).* http://www.cdc.gov/sars/index.html (accessed March 1, 2015).

"WHO Statement on the Third Meeting of the IHR Emergency Committee concerning MERS-CoV." *World Health Organization (WHO).* http://www.who.int/ihr/procedures/statement_20130925/en/index.html September 25, 2013. (accessed March 1, 2015).

K. Lee Lerner

Smallpox Eradication and Storage of Infectious Agents

⊕ Introduction

Smallpox, or variola major, is a highly contagious disease that is caused by the variola virus. The name smallpox comes from the Latin word for "spotted." A visual hallmark of smallpox is the raised bumps that appear on the victim's face and body. The virus spreads from contact with victims, as well as from contaminated air droplets and even from objects used by other smallpox victims (books, blankets, etc.). Smallpox is fatal in approximately 25 percent of cases.

After acquisition of the virus, there is a 12- to 14-day incubation period, during which the virus multiplies, but no symptoms appear. The onset of symptoms occurs suddenly and includes fever and chills; muscle aches; and a flat, reddish-purple rash on the chest, abdomen, and back. These symptoms last about three days, after which the rash fades and the fever drops. A day or two later, the fever returns, along with a bumpy rash starting on the feet, hands, and face. This rash progresses from the feet along the legs, from the hands along the arms, and from the face down the neck, ultimately reaching and including the chest, abdomen, and back. The individual bumps, or papules, fill with clear fluid, and, over the course of 10 to 12 days, become pus-filled. The pox eventually scab over, and when the scab falls off, left behind is a pock or pit, which remains as a permanent scar.

Death from smallpox usually follows complications such as bacterial infection of the open skin lesions, pneumonia, or bone infections. A very severe and quickly fatal form of smallpox called sledgehammer smallpox results in hemorrhage from the skin lesions, as well as from the mouth, nose, and other areas of the body.

There is no cure for smallpox, and treatment consists of making the patient feel as comfortable as possible and lessening the symptoms. Prevention of the disease by the administration of smallpox vaccine is the most effective strategy to eliminate the spread of smallpox. The vaccine for the disease is one of the most effective vaccines ever created, and the World Health Organization (WHO) declared smallpox eradicated in 1980. The last confirmed naturally occurring smallpox case was in 1977. Ali Maow Maalin, a hospital employee in Merca, Somalia, acquired the disease, but survived his bout with smallpox.

The eradication of smallpox is considered one of the greatest public health achievements of the 20th century. Following eradication, the WHO requested that all laboratories in the world either destroy their smallpox virus stocks or transfer them to one of two reference laboratories, the Institute of Viral Preparations in Moscow or the U.S. Centers for Disease Control and Prevention (CDC) in Atlanta, Georgia. The stocks of the Institute of Viral Preparations were transferred in 1994 to the State Research Center of Virology and Biotechnology of the Russian Federation in Siberia, now the WHO Collaborating Centre for Orthopoxvirus Diagnostics. Specimens of smallpox virus were still officially held in the United States and Russia as of early 2015.

Samples of variola DNA may also be recoverable from old medical samples, such as the century-old smallpox scabs discovered in an envelope tucked in a 19th-century medical textbook in a New Mexico library in 2004. In 2014, a U.S. official found more smallpox samples in a storage room on the National Institutes of Health campus in Bethesda, Maryland.

⊕ Historical Background

In China, India, and the Americas, from about the 10th century, it was noted that individuals who had had even a mild case of smallpox could not be infected again. Material from people ill with smallpox (fluid or pus from the papules, the scabs) was scratched into the skin of people who had never had the illness in an attempt to produce a mild reaction and its accompanying protective effect. These efforts often resulted in full-fledged smallpox, and probably served only to help effectively spread the infection throughout the community.

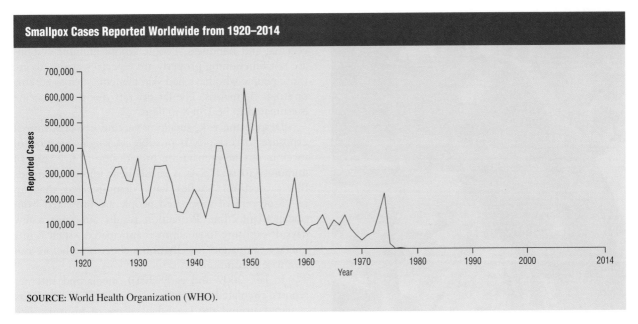

Smallpox Cases Reported Worldwide from 1920–2014

SOURCE: World Health Organization (WHO).

As the World Health Organization graph illustrates, smallpox was successfully eradicated by 1980.

In 1798, English physician Edward Jenner (1749–1823) published a paper in which he discussed his important observation that milkmaids who contracted a mild infection of the hands (called cowpox, and caused by a relative of variola) appeared to be immune to smallpox. He created an immunization against smallpox that used the infected material found in the lesions of cowpox infection. Jenner's paper led to much work in the area of vaccinations and ultimately resulted in the creation of an effective smallpox vaccine, which utilizes the vaccinia virus—another close relative of variola.

Global Eradication of Smallpox Virus

Smallpox is dangerous only to human beings. Animals and insects can neither be infected by smallpox, nor carry the virus in any form. Humans cannot carry the virus, unless they are symptomatic. These important facts entered into the 1967 decision by the WHO to attempt worldwide eradication of the smallpox virus. From 1967 to 1980, the WHO oversaw a global campaign, the WHO Intensified Smallpox Eradication Program, to eliminate smallpox entirely.

The eradication strategy had two basic features. First came mass vaccination campaigns in each target country, coordinated with that country's government. The goal was to vaccinate at least 80 percent of the population of each target country. Smallpox vaccination is a simple procedure involving multiple skin punctures in the side of the arm with a two-pronged metal tool resembling a lobster fork. The tool, termed a bifurcated needle, is dipped once into a vial containing liquid smallpox vaccine and then repeatedly stuck into the skin over a small area. The injection typically becomes sore, blisters, and

forms a scab. When the scab falls off, a distinctive scar is left. Earlier, less-convenient methods were displaced by the bifurcated-needle procedure during the global eradication campaign.

The smallpox vaccine does not contain smallpox virus but live vaccinia virus. Vaccinia virus almost never causes fatal disease; the reported death rate from smallpox vaccination is approximately a death per a million vaccinations. An immune system that has learned to recognize and attack the vaccinia virus will also recognize and attack the variola virus at its first appearance. Smallpox virus may enter the body of an immunized person but is destroyed by the immune system before it can gain a foothold.

The second aspect of the eradication strategy was termed "surveillance and containment." Since some percentage of the population in most countries remained unvaccinated even at the height of the eradication campaign, smallpox still occurred. Surveillance and containment involved keeping a lookout for outbreaks of smallpox and then selectively, intensively vaccinating people in the vicinity of the outbreak.

This two-part strategy was successful. In the United States, for example, the last case was reported in Texas in 1949. Smallpox was eliminated in Brazil in 1971 and in Indonesia in 1972. A few outbreaks in Europe were caused by travelers but were rapidly contained. The last case of the more severe form of smallpox, variola major, occurred in Bangladesh in 1975, just a few years before the last case of natural smallpox occurred reported in Somalia in 1977. After several years with no reported cases of the disease, the WHO declared smallpox eradicated in 1980.

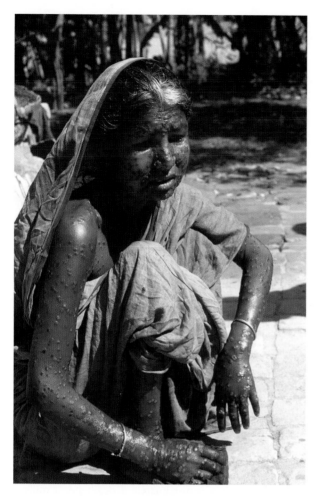

This 1974 image depicts an adult female Bangladeshi villager who contracted smallpox. She displays the classic maculopapular rash covering her arms, legs, and face with pustules. The symptoms of smallpox begin with high fever, head and body aches, and sometimes vomiting. A rash follows, which spreads and progresses to raised bumps and pus-filled blisters that crust, scab, and fall off after about three weeks, leaving pitted scars. The majority of patients with smallpox recover, but death may occur in up to 30 percent of cases. Many smallpox survivors have permanent scars over large areas of their body, especially their faces. Some are left blind. *Jean Roy/U.S. Centers for Disease Control and Prevention.*

The only smallpox vaccine that is in use today—a preparation called Dryvax—is made from vaccinia, a poxvirus that is very similar to the smallpox virus. The reaction of the immune system to vaccinia confers protection to the smallpox virus. The vaccinia virus that is administered is alive and causes a mild infection, which is inconsequential in most people. However, in a small minority of people, the use of the live virus does carry a risk that the virus will spread from the site of injection, and that side effects will result.

The side effects are typically minor (e.g., sore arm at the injection site, a fever, and generalized body aches). However, rare severe side effects are possible, which can even be life threatening. These include encephalitis (a swelling of the brain and spinal cord), gangrene, extreme eczema, and blindness. People whose immune systems are not functioning properly are especially at risk, as are those people who have had skin ailments such as eczema or atopic dermatitis. The fatality rate due to the vaccine is estimated to be 1 in 8 million.

Despite the risk, smallpox vaccine is worthwhile if exposure to smallpox is possible. A single injection of vaccinia vaccine preparation provides up to five years of immunity to smallpox. A subsequent injection extends this protection. Studies have demonstrated that up to 95 percent of vaccinated people are protected from smallpox infection. Protection results after just a few days. If exposure to smallpox is anticipated—such as in a military campaign—vaccination a short time before can be a wise precaution.

In late 2009 and early 2010, media and Internet reports circulated of a potential outbreak of smallpox centered around the Ugandan village of Mityana. The reports were proven false after emergency investigations by the WHO and Ugandan Ministry of Health officials correctly attributed the disease outbreak to chicken pox rather than smallpox.

⊕ Impacts and Issues

Following the declared global eradication of smallpox, the WHO initially set 1999 as the deadline for the destruction of all smallpox-causing variola virus stocks (viable samples of the disease held in laboratories). However, both the United States and Russia failed to carry out the WHO directive, citing the need for further research on the virus. In 2010, a review by a WHO advisory team concluded that smallpox samples should be allowed to remain stored in designated research facilities in order to develop new antiviral medications, as well as a vaccine against smallpox that has fewer side effects than the current vaccine.

Since the 1990s, there has been ongoing debate about whether or not remaining stocks of smallpox should be destroyed. Issues include the morality of deliberately causing the extinction of a species; whether continued possession of the virus might someday result in its escape, potentially causing millions of deaths; whether the virus might be used to develop biological weapons; and whether keeping the virus intact is necessary as a precaution against the possible use of smallpox as a biowar or bioterror weapon or its accidental or natural rerelease into human populations.

Population Vulnerability

The eradication of smallpox saw the end of routine smallpox vaccination programs. Individuals in the United States under the age of 40 have not received the vaccine as part of their normal, recommended course of

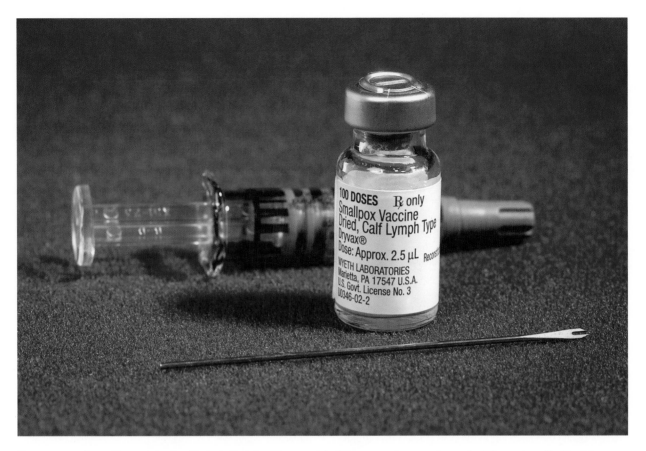

Components of a smallpox vaccination kit, including the diluent, a vial of Dryvax smallpox vaccine, and a bifurcated needle. Vaccinia (smallpox) vaccine, derived from calf lymph and licensed in the United States, is a lyophilized, live-virus preparation of infectious vaccinia virus. It does not contain smallpox (variola) virus.   *James Gathany/U.S. Centers for Disease Control and Prevention.*

vaccinations. Smallpox vaccine was discontinued as part of the recommend vaccine protocol in the United States in the early 1970s. Even in older Americans, immunity has likely faded. After the bioterrorist anthrax attacks on U.S. citizens in the latter months of 2001, concern heightened that smallpox could be used as a terrorist weapon on a population that is once again susceptible to infection.

Beginning January 2003, health-care workers at strategic hospitals and research centers across the United States received the smallpox vaccine in order to provide a population of immune responders in case of a smallpox outbreak or mass exposure due to bioterrorism. Mass vaccination programs are again under study by researchers. As of 2013, approximately 300 million doses of standard smallpox vaccine and 40 million new-version smallpox vaccine are stockpiled for use in the event of a bioterrorist-mediated smallpox outbreak.

Bioengineering Perils

After approving limited and specific genetic engineering experiments in 2004, in 2005, a WHO advisory committee also voted to allow the transfer of variola DNA fragments up to 55 base pairs long between laboratories,

the manufacture of gene chips containing smallpox DNA, and the splicing of smallpox genes into other viruses.

In 2005, a bill passed by the U.S. Congress made it illegal to "produce, engineer, [or] synthesize" the variola virus from scratch. The possibility of from-scratch (also called de novo) manufacture of smallpox virus is not far-fetched. Poliovirus was first synthesized from scratch in 2001, starting solely with a record of its genome and without the aid of preexisting RNA, DNA, or living cells. In 2006, Sandia National Laboratory, an arm of the U.S. government, began experiments that involved inserting synthetic (de novo) variola genes into other organisms. Some critics of the continued existence of variola stocks say that since Sandia's historical mission has been the production of nuclear weapons and the laboratory has no biomedical mission, its research with variola virus genes is inappropriate and signifies deteriorating WHO control over smallpox research. In January 2007, the WHO Executive Board called for a United Nations resolution to forbid genetic engineering of the variola virus.

Safe Facilities

By U.S. law, smallpox virus can be stored and handled only at Biosafety Level 4 (BSL-4) facilities. Such a facility

SMALLPOX AS BIOTERRORISM AGENT

Bioterrorism refers to the use of lethal biological agents to wage terror against a civilian population. It differs from biological warfare in that it also thrives on public fear, which can demoralize a population. An example of bioterrorism is provided by the anthrax outbreak that occurred from September to November 2001 in the United States. Anthrax spores intentionally spread in the mail distribution system caused five deaths and a total of 22 infections. The U.S. Centers for Disease Control classifies bioterror agents into three categories.

Category A Diseases/Agents can be easily disseminated or transmitted from person to person, which can result in high mortality rates while causing public panic and social disruption. Although declared eradicated as a disease, smallpox virus still exists in high-security laboratories in the United States and Russia. Smallpox joins anthrax, botulism, plague, tularemia, and viral hemorrhagic fever viruses as a Category A disease agent.

Category B Diseases/Agents are moderately easy to disseminate and can result in low mortality rates. Brucellosis, food and water safety threats, melioidosis, psittacosis, staphylococcal enterotoxin B, and typhus belong to this category.

Category C Diseases/Agents include emerging pathogens that could be engineered for mass dissemination in the future because of availability or ease of production and dissemination.

The variola (smallpox) virus has been used as an agent of warfare. During the French and Indian Wars (1754–1767), British colonial commanders distributed blankets that were used by smallpox victims in order to initiate an epidemic among Native Americans. The mortality rate associated with these outbreaks was as high as 50 percent in certain tribes. More recently, in the years leading up to World War II (1939–1945), the Japanese military explored smallpox weaponization during operations of Unit 731 in Mongolia and China.

There are a number of characteristics that make the variola virus an excellent candidate for use as a biological weapon. An aerosol suspension of variola can spread widely and have a very low infectious dosage. In general, the dissemination of a pathogen by aerosol droplets is the preferred deployment method for biological weapons. Smallpox is highly contagious and is spread through droplet inhalation or ingestion. As there are no civilian or military smallpox vaccination requirements at this time, a large susceptible population is at risk from the infection. The incubation period in naturally occurring cases averages seven to fourteen days. However, the period could be shortened to three to seven days, especially in the cases of aerosol application. People who have contracted the disease are contagious during the late stages of the incubation period, even though they remain asymptomatic. Thus, transmission of the disease can occur as early as two days after exposure to the virus. Depending on the climate, corpses of smallpox victims remain infectious for days to months. The duration of the disease is long, and coupled with the complex isolation and protection requirements of smallpox treatment, each infected person would require the efforts of several medical support personnel.

consists of a separate building or architecturally isolated section of a building specially equipped for biological isolation. Persons entering and leaving the facility must take sterilizing showers; air and sewage leaving the building must pass through special filters to remove any possible disease-carrying particles; and separate air supply and exhaust must be arranged for workers inside the laboratory space. The building must be ventilated so that air flows into the building and toward the part of the building where the most hazardous materials are kept. The building must also remain sealed in the event of a power failure.

⊕ Future Implications

Scientists at the CDC published findings in November 2009 that shed light on the mechanisms by which smallpox infection rapidly spreads. Research showed that cells infected with the smallpox-causing variola virus create a blocking protein that binds to human interferon molecules that normally suppress variola virus reproduction at the molecular level.

Despite ongoing research and discoveries utilizing the variola virus, debate concerning the fate of smallpox maintained in government laboratories resumed with vigor in 2011. International policy statements call for setting a definitive date for the destruction of variola virus stocks, but officials in both the United States and Russia continue to oppose their elimination. Although some experts argue that no life-form, however virulent, should be destroyed (in part because of potential future usefulness), other experts counter that accidents are inevitable should the virus remain in storage and subject to experimentation. The WHO maintains that smallpox stores in the United States and Russia serve "no essential public health purpose."

Viruses, including the SARS virus, have previously escaped high-security laboratories—often on the clothes of lab workers—and critics argued that risk analysis requirements for Bio Security Level 3 (BSL-3) or BSL-4, the most secure labs, often are insufficient to ensure public safety.

The WHO has authorized some research with existing variola stocks but faces continued controversy. Research using the surviving smallpox virus stocks will remain controversial especially because developing countries would be much more vulnerable to a new smallpox outbreak. Accordingly, developing nations are typically strong proponents of the complete and final destruction of existing smallpox virus stocks.

PRIMARY SOURCE

FDA Statement on Vials of Smallpox Found on July 1, 2014

SOURCE *"Update on Findings in the FDA Cold Storage Area on the NIH Campus," FDA Statement. U.S. Food and Drug Administration, July 16, 2014. http://www.fda.gov/newsevents/ newsroom/pressannouncements/ucm405434.htm (accessed January 25, 2015).*

INTRODUCTION *This primary source is a statement from the U.S. Food and Drug Administration (FDA) in response to the discovery of vials containing biological samples of infectious agents at the FDA laboratories on the campus of the National Institutes of Health (NIH).*

UPDATE ON FINDINGS IN THE FDA COLD STORAGE AREA ON THE NIH CAMPUS

For Immediate Release

July 16, 2014

Statement

As previously reported, on July 1, 2014, biological samples were found in the cold storage area of U.S. Food and Drug Administration laboratories on the National Institutes of Health campus. The FDA has since acquired additional information from the federal investigative agencies regarding inventories of the materials.

The investigation found 12 boxes containing a total of 327 carefully packaged vials labeled with names of various biological agents such as dengue, influenza, Q fever, and rickettsia. Upon the discovery of these vials on July 1, 2014, FDA employees followed standard protocol and turned them all over to the appropriate NIH safety program officials, who in turn transferred them to the appropriate investigative agencies, as per standard protocols.

As announced on July 8, 2014, six vials labeled "*variola*" (the causative agent of smallpox) along with ten other samples with unclear labeling were transported safely and securely with the assistance of federal and local law enforcement agencies in a government aircraft to CDC's high-containment facility in Atlanta. In addition, 32 samples were destroyed following inventory at the NIH facility, including 28 labeled as normal tissue and four labeled as "*vaccinia*," the virus used to make the smallpox vaccine. To be clear, *vaccinia* does not cause smallpox. These vials represented no value to forensic sciences and were destroyed according to standard protocols.

The remaining 279 biological samples were then transferred by the investigating agencies to the U.S. Department of Homeland Security's National Bioforensic Analysis Center for safeguarding. There were no smallpox samples included in this transfer. The FDA received confirmatory information about the samples yesterday, thus permitting public disclosure of this additional information.

While an investigation continues regarding the origin of these samples, this collection was most likely assembled between 1946 and 1964 when standards for work with and storage of biological specimens were very different from those used today. All of the items labeled as infectious agents found in the collection of samples were stored in glass, heat-sealed vials that were well-packed, intact, and free of any leakage, and there is no evidence that anyone was exposed to these agents.

Overlooking such a sample collection is clearly unacceptable. The FDA has already taken steps to ensure that similar material is not present in its other cold storage areas by initiating a thorough review of all common cold storage spaces. The agency is in the process of reviewing its policies and procedures in order to implement a corrective action plan so that potentially hazardous samples are never overlooked in the future.

SEE ALSO *Conflict, Violence, and Terrorism: Health Impacts; Vaccine-Preventable Diseases; Viral Diseases*

BIBLIOGRAPHY

Books

Arita, Isao. *The Smallpox Eradication Saga: An Insider's View*. Edited by Alan Schnur and Masanobu Sugimoto. New Delhi: Orient Blackswan, 2010.

Boom, Julie A., and Rachel M. Cunningham. *Understanding and Managing Vaccine Concerns*. New York: Springer, 2014.

Crisp, Nigel. *Turning the World Upside Down: The Search for Global Health in the Twenty-First Century*. London: Royal Society of Medicine Press, 2010.

Foege, William H. *House on Fire: The Fight to Eradicate Smallpox*. Berkeley: University of California Press, 2011.

Furgang, Adam. *Smallpox*. New York: Rosen, 2011.

Henderson, Donald A. *Smallpox: The Death of a Disease*. Amherst, NY: Prometheus Books, 2014.

Lakoff, Andrew, and Stephen J. Collier, eds. *Biosecurity Interventions: Global Health and Security in Question*. New York: Columbia University Press, 2012.

Roy, Jonathan. *Smallpox Zero: An Illustrated History of Smallpox and Its Eradication*. Johannesburg, South Africa: Umlando Wezithombe, 2010.

Stepan, Nancy. *Eradication: Ridding the World of Diseases Forever?* Ithaca, NY: Cornell University Press, 2011.

Williams, Gareth. *Angel of Death: The Story of Smallpox.* Basingstoke, UK: Palgrave Macmillan, 2010.

Periodicals

Arita, I. "Smallpox: Should We Destroy the Last Stockpile?" *Expert Review of Anti-infective Therapy* 9, no. 10 (2011): 837–839.

Lane, J. M., and G. A. Poland. "Why Not Destroy the Remaining Smallpox Virus Stocks?" *Vaccine* 29, no. 16 (2011): 2823–2824.

Meseda, C. A., and J. P. Weir. "Third-Generation Smallpox Vaccines: Challenges in the Absence of Clinical Smallpox." *Future Microbiology* 5, no. 9 (2010): 1367–1382.

Mombouli, J. V., and S. M. Ostroff. "The Remaining Smallpox Stocks: the Healthiest Outcome." *The Lancet* 379, no. 9810 (2012): 10–12.

Shchelkunov, S. N. "Emergence and Reemergence of Smallpox: The Need for Development of a New Generation Smallpox Vaccine." *Vaccine* 29 (2011): 49–53.

Tucker, Jonathan B. "Destruction of the Smallpox Virus Stocks: Negotiating for Consensus in the World Health Organization." *Negotiating and Navigating Global Health: Case Studies in Global Health Diplomacy* (2011): 221–247.

Wickett, J., and P. Carrasco. "Logistics in Smallpox: The Legacy." *Vaccine* 29 (2011): 131–134.

Websites

"Smallpox." *U.S. Centers for Disease Control and Prevention (CDC).* http://emergency.cdc.gov/agent/smallpox/index.asp (accessed March 1, 2015).

"Smallpox." *World Health Organization (WHO).* http://www.who.int/topics/smallpox/en (accessed March 1, 2015).

"Smallpox: Conquered Killer." *National Geographic Society.* http://science.nationalgeographic.com/science/health-and-human-body/human-diseases/smallpox-article.html (accessed March 1, 2015).

"Smallpox Vaccine." *U.S. Centers for Disease Control and Prevention (CDC).* http://emergency.cdc.gov/agent/smallpox/vaccination/index.asp (accessed March 1, 2015).

"Vaccine Safety: Smallpox." *U.S. Centers for Disease Control and Prevention (CDC).* http://www.cdc.gov/vaccinesafety/emergency/smallpox.htm (accessed March 1, 2015).

K. Lee Lerner

Social Theory and Global Health

🌐 Introduction

Global health is a collection of challenges that span a wide breadth of cultural, scientific, political, economic, and practical disciplines. As these challenges often require knowledge and sensitivity about how both biological and social factors relate to health problems, many actors in global health now use a biosocial approach in solving them. Although most medical literature still focuses on the biological aspects of disease, the biosocial approach takes a wider view to causality and factors in local conditions of community, economy, and the lifeways of the population experiencing sickness and health.

As the human immunodeficiency virus/acquired immune deficiency syndrome (HIV/AIDS) epidemic erupted throughout the world in the 1980s, for example, previously reticent cultural attitudes gave way to frank and open discussion about safe sex practices and how HIV transmission could be reduced. When effective antiviral medicines and other treatments for HIV became available in the developed world, larger questions of how to make them affordable and available to the world's poor and those in medically underserved areas occupied health and governmental experts. Addressing inequities, especially in access and delivery of medical care, is a cornerstone in the biosocial approach to global health challenges.

Rarely does biology alone fully explain disease, and conversely, rarely do social factors explain the full picture of health. These two factors interact with each other to influence health and disease and to provide the best view of the health status of a person and his community.

🌐 Historical Background

Early concepts of global health began with European colonizers who sought opportunity in mostly tropical lands in which malaria and other diseases were endemic. Emphasis on reducing disease in lands far from the homeland was initially considered for the benefit of the colonizers rather than the local populations. The advent of quinine allowed the 19th-century European conquest of most of Africa, which in turn brought about the arrival of global health as a medical specialty. The concurrent development of germ theory and Koch's postulates of the agents of infectious disease encouraged social considerations of global health because attention could then be focused on the microbial cause of disease, rather than the previous assumption of tropical heat and native populations as disease threats.

The Iron Cage

German sociologist Max Weber (1864–1920) provided a framework for different types of authority, which was soon integrated into health systems both at home and in colonies abroad. Rather than emphasizing the art of medicine, it became a system of bureaucratic authority ingrained with new technical rationality, paradigms, and standards, and was a system seen as capable of export anywhere in the world, regardless of the prevailing culture. Advantages of Weberian bureaucracy in health included efficient systems for treating more patients and the advent of modern standards. Disadvantages include diminished roles for traditional aspects of medicine that were effective, and more difficulty in employing innovative solutions for betterment or to solve problems (escaping the iron cage of bureaucracy).

Biopower

Biopower is a concept shaped by the 20th-century French philosopher Michel Foucault (1926–1984), with its origins in 18th-century Europe, a time just after the Enlightenment and just before the first French Revolution, when the power of the monarchy in France was (temporarily) eliminated and a centralized state resulted. At this time, the French government began to utilize statistics and apply them to their populations, for troop movement purposes, for example. Foucault's biopower concept includes the controls exerted over humans for regulation, discipline, welfare, or other control.

HAITI AND THE 2010 EARTHQUAKE: REBUILDING HEALTH CARE

After a catastrophic earthquake, measuring 7.0 on the Richter scale, struck Haiti on January 12, 2010, leveling its capital city along with many of its health-care facilities, and killing or injuring hundreds of thousands of people, American medical anthropologist Paul Farmer made his way quickly to the island nation to offer assistance in treating the injured. He was no stranger to the island, having first traveled to the island's central plateau almost 30 years prior.

In the midst of the chaos, Farmer writes in his book *Haiti after the Earthquake*, of "frustration among many volunteers and disaster relief experts rooted in their inability to find a system capable of effectively using their resources and good will." Before the earthquake, Haiti's institutional health-care system was long underfunded and dysfunctional, and so numerous were the nongovernmental organizations (NGOs) that responded to the many needs of the vulnerable population, that Haiti was often known in international aid circles as "the republic of NGOs." For many reasons, both political and practical, most governments and organizations chose to bypass the existing Haitian public health infrastructure and to operate independent systems

for providing health care and other assistance to the people of Haiti. This lack of investment further weakened the public sector and, together with facilities collapsed by the earthquake, left it incapable of an effective response in the aftermath of the disaster.

Farmer argued that building a strong public health infrastructure in Haiti would be a better investment, one that would better meet the needs of the people. If both private and governmental humanitarian aid agencies showed confidence in the public sector by helping them build an efficient health-care system with adequate equipment and supplies, assisting with the ability to pay a well-trained staff regularly, and most importantly, providing accessibility to all the population without regard to the ability to pay, then Haiti's public health system would become the first-considered and most-desired option for both the Haitian people and for contributors. Partners in Health, an organization founded by Farmer, set about building the University Hospital in Mirebalais, which in 2014 was one of the largest providers of health services in Haiti and was training a new generation of Haitian physicians and nurses to care for Haiti's people.

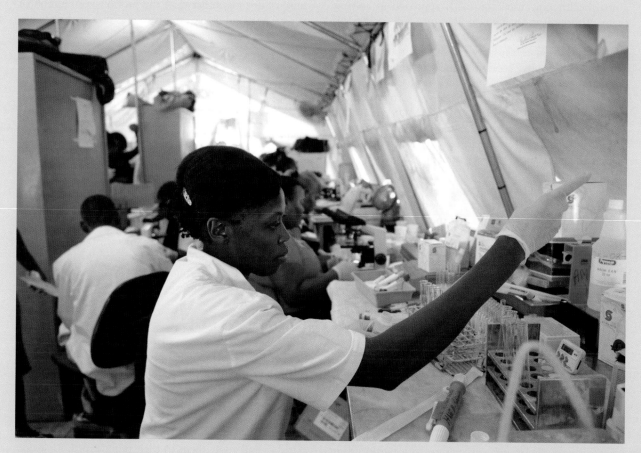

A Haitian health worker does tests in a temporary tent laboratory on August 26, 2010, in Port-au-Prince, Haiti. © *arindambanerjee/ Shutterstock.com.*

An expanded definition that is more relevant to global health views biopower as governmentality, the surveillance or control of populations by the state in the development of health policy.

Biopower can work at both the level of the individual or family, as in China's one-child policy, or at the level of a population, as in prohibiting the sale of alcohol to children. The exertion of biopower can be either voluntary, as in the National Health and Nutrition Examination Survey (NHANES), a health survey of Americans conducted periodically by the U.S. government, or compulsory, as in vaccination requirements or no-smoking zone laws. Another example of biopower is found in the American medical anthropologist Arthur Kleinman's "Four Social Theories for Global Health," which details a "biological citizenship" among a large group of citizens in Ukraine after the Chernobyl nuclear accident in 1986. These citizens were not certified as exposed to radiation, but claimed disability from the trauma of the event and expected "compensation from a caring state that exerts the power of governance via the welfare rolls."

Social Suffering

Kleinman also helped to define the concept of social suffering (pain and suffering caused by social forces) that is key to understanding the necessity of resolving inequities as a moral imperative in achieving global health. Structural violence, the routine or daily present difficulties in life that conspire to constrain a person's potential, is often the cause of social suffering. For many people, racism, political violence, sexism, and grinding poverty limit both everyday and important life choices, especially those that can impact health and wellness. One example is poverty as a risk factor for increased maternal mortality. Kleinman argues that medicine cannot be separated from moral and political concerns, and that disparities across economic status, gender, ethnic group, and age cohort mean that inequality is at the heart of global health policy.

Unintended Consequences of Purposive Social Action

The American sociologist Robert K. Merton (1910–2003) theorized that for every action that has a purpose there are usually unanticipated, unintended consequences. In global health, Merton's theory has multiple illustrations; the pesticide DDT (dichlorodiphenyltrichloroethane) reduced malaria deaths in the 1950s and 1960s by killing vast numbers of the mosquitoes that harbor the malaria parasite but also reduced many bird species' populations by thinning their eggshells. When the Canadian government relocated the Grassy Knoll Indians of Ontario in the 1980s to a suburb where the men could not fish due to high mercury levels in the water, rates of depression and violence against women skyrocketed. Additionally, the advent of magnetic

resonance imaging brought about clear and detailed diagnostic images, but has contributed to escalating health-care costs and excessive radiation exposure with overuse in the United States.

⊕ Impacts and Issues

Water, sanitation, and hygiene (WASH) remain the most pressing and basic needs to improve health for the world's poor, along with basic health-care infrastructure and access, food security, housing, electricity, and education. Providing jobs is the next key point in breaking the cycle of poverty, which is inevitably linked to both improving social mobility and good health. Social sciences, especially anthropological and political strategies, are expected to figure heavily in both short-term and future global health initiatives.

India, for example, is a rapidly developing lower-middle-income country that has a considerable network of policies in place, many enacted into law, that are intended to provide access to health care for all Indian citizens. Yet, according to the World Bank in 2012, of India's 1.24 billion people, almost one-third or about 400 million people fall below India's national poverty line and cannot afford health services, and 48 percent of children under five years of age are chronically malnourished.

During the 1980s and 1990s, India was the recipient of health-care aid and interest from multiple countries with different ideologies, including the Soviet Union's centralized methods, and the Western neoliberal approaches that included the mandating of loans, structural adjustments, and implementing user fees in exchange for aid. Additionally, the presence of nongovernmental organizations (NGOs), whether faith-based or secular, political or apolitical, or simply humanitarian in motivation, blossomed in India during these years. Most of these programs also featured vertical approaches designed to meet a specific health challenge rather than to shore up the existing state health infrastructure. Today, India continues to rely on much of this structurally and ideologically disparate aid as it builds its own health-care system.

Developing countries like India are now encouraged politically to commit more of their own resources toward health-care infrastructure and medical personnel, regardless of the input of peripheral resources from the world community. India expends only 1 percent of its gross domestic product (GDP) on public health systems, contrasting with other lower-middle-income countries such as Ukraine (3.5 percent) and Honduras (3.8 percent), according to the World Bank in 2012. India also fell short of its modest goal to commit an amount equal to 2 percent of GDP expenditure on public health by 2010, as proposed in its revised 2002 national health policy.

One result of this lack of internal investment has been the proliferation of an abundance of similar well-meaning national or state-level health policies that are not realized, a situation that is referred to by some social theorists as negative governmentality. Weber's legal bureaucratic hierarchy is in place; the public health policies and objectives are clearly defined, but especially in the rural areas of India and in the urban slums, the policies do not reach the people they were intended to serve. NGOs are increasingly encouraged to cooperate and integrate with Indian systems in order to strengthen them and broaden their reach, rather than to operate independently.

Ethnography (an anthropological tool for documenting a culture and its practices) is also playing an increasingly important role in building health systems around the world. By learning what a particular culture values, as well as how health and wellness are approached, health strategies can be formed that have a better chance of acceptance and long-term success. In India, for example, faced with a lack of trust in or access to state medical facilities, along with the inability to pay for private health care, many people turn to traditional healers. The training of traditional AYUSH healers (practitioners of

Ayurveda, yoga and naturopathy, Unani, Siddha, and homoeopathy) overlaps with evidence-based medicine to a sufficient degree that by Indian law, AYUSH healers can practice medicine under some restrictions and with supervision. AYUSH healers who also invest their confidence in evidence-based medicine programs are often effective in delivering modern health care to their community, especially as the local population already consults them. AYUSH healers serve as trusted physician extenders and as a link between tradition and the governmental health service.

Cultural considerations also played a key role in the response to the 2014–2015 Ebola outbreak in western Africa, where the traditional practice of washing and laying hands on bodies of deceased family members before burial was amplifying the spread of the disease. In Guinea alone, the World Health Organization estimated that 60 percent of Ebola cases were acquired through these pre-burial rituals. Health officials and local citizens worked together to combine the rituals with safe practices, such as wrapping the deceased in a protective plastic covering, leaving the head exposed during farewell prayers, and ceremonial washing of the deceased within the protective covering by a skilled

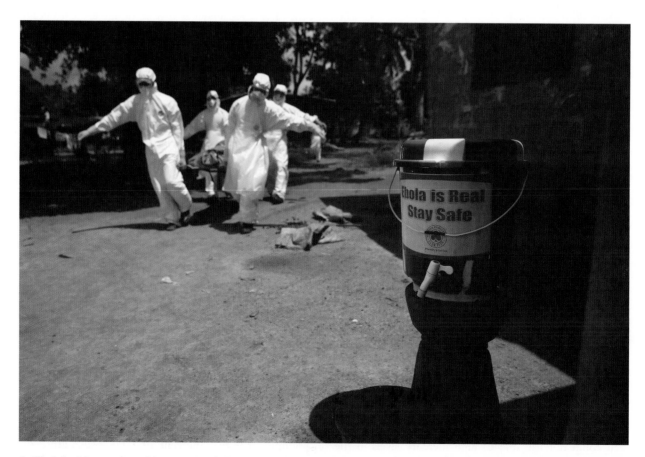

An Ebola burial team, dressed in protective clothing, carries the body of a woman while passing a bucket of chlorinated water for hand washing in the New Kru Town suburb of Monrovia, Liberia.   *© John Moore/Getty Images.*

worker using disinfectant spray in the presence of the family. Trained burial teams then helped with a traditional procession and burial. This intervention is credited with dramatically slowing the epidemic in Liberia and Guinea, where officials estimate 80 percent of Ebola victims family members eventually requested safe burials.

⊕ Future Implications

Biopower will likely surface, either as an conflicting issue or as a useful tool for health policy development, as Haiti rebuilds from its 2010 earthquake, along with postcolonial nation-states in Africa and Asia that are forming centralized governments and building health-care systems. Efficient use of governmentality to build health infrastructure and policy will also play an important role in developing countries, and those who accept foreign aid are likely to insist that aid entities work with existing governments to build lasting health-care systems, instead of working independently. Where intended health benefits are not reaching the people, removing negative governmentality will be a key focus for reducing inequities in health care. Equitable access to health care is a major human rights challenge of modern medicine in the 21st century.

When responding to disease and disability, whether it is a chronic condition or especially amid a disaster situation, both social and biological factors are important considerations in mounting the most effective response. A biosocial approach to problem solving provides a more complete picture of the causes of human suffering than either biology or social factors alone. When social factors are considered, medical interventions are often more effective in the long term, and clinicians, researchers, and decision makers can embrace a united framework for understanding.

SEE ALSO   *Conflict, Violence, and Terrorism: Health Impacts; Cultural and Traditional Medicine; Food Security and Hunger; Gender and Health; Global Health Initiatives; Health as a Human Right and Health-Care Access; Health-Related Education and Information Access; International Health Regulation, Surveillance, and Enforcement; Médicins Sans Frontières; NGOs and Health Care: Deliverance or Dependence; Population Issues; Stigma; Universal Health Coverage; Vulnerable Populations*

BIBLIOGRAPHY

Books

Biehl, João, and Adriana Petryna, eds. *When People Come First: Critical Studies in Global Health.* Princeton, NJ: Princeton University Press, 2013.

Crisp, Nigel. *Turning the World Upside Down: The Search for Global Health in the Twenty-First Century.* London: Royal Society of Medicine Press, 2010.

De Maio, Fernando. *Global Health Inequities: A Sociological Perspective.* Houndmills, UK: Palgrave Macmillan, 2014.

Farmer, Paul. *Partner to the Poor: A Paul Farmer Reader.* Edited by Haun Saussy. Berkeley: University of California Press, 2010.

Farmer, Paul, Jim Yong Kim, Arthur Kleinman, and Matthew Basilico. *Reimagining Global Health.* Berkeley: University of California Press, 2013.

Hall, Peter A., and Michèle Lamont, eds. *Successful Societies: How Institutions and Culture Affect Health.* New York: Cambridge University Press, 2009.

Keshavjee, Salmaan. *Blind Spot: How Neoliberalism Infiltrated Global Health.* Berkeley: University of California Press, 2014.

Kleinman, Arthur. *The Illness Narratives: Suffering, Healing, and the Human Condition.* New York: Basic Books, 1988.

Nichter, Mark. *Global Health: Why Cultural Perceptions, Social Representations, and Biopolitics Matter.* Tucson: University of Arizona Press, 2008.

Singer, Merrill, and Pamela I. Erickson. *Global Health: An Anthropological Perspective.* Long Grove, IL: Waveland Press, 2013.

Periodicals

Gelmanova, I., et al. "'Sputnik': A Programmatic Approach to Improve Tuberculosis Treatment Adherence and Outcome among Defaulters." *International Journal of Tuberculosis and Lung Disease* 93, no. 10 (2011): 1373–1379.

Kleinman, Arthur. "Four Social Theories for Global Health." *The Lancet* 375, no. 9725 (2010): 1518–1519.

Ruger, J. P. "Ethics and Governance of Global Health Inequalities." *Journal of Epidemiology & Community Health* 60, no. 11 (2006): 998–1002.

Websites

"Achieving the Global Public Health Agenda: Dialogues at the Economic and Social Council." *United Nations.* http://www.un.org/en/ecosoc/docs/pdfs/achieving_global_public_health_agenda.pdf (accessed March 1, 2015).

Blas, E., J. Sommerfeld, and A. S. Kurup, eds. "Social Determinants Approaches to Public Health: From Concept to Practice." *World Health Organization (WHO)*, 2011. http://www.who.int/social_determinants/tools/SD_Publichealth_eng.pdf (accessed March 1, 2015).

"Closing the Gap in a Generation: Health Equality through Action on the Social Determinants of Health." *World Health Organization (WHO)*, 2008. http://whqlibdoc.who.int/publications/2008/9789241563703_eng.pdf (accessed March 1, 2015).

Partners in Health. http://www.pih.org (accessed March 1, 2015).

"PEPFAR and the Global Context of HIV (December 2009)." *U.S. President's Emergency Plan for AIDS Relief (PEPFAR)*, December 2009. http://www.pepfar.gov/about/strategy/global_context/index.htm (accessed March 1, 2015).

Brenda Wilmoth Lerner

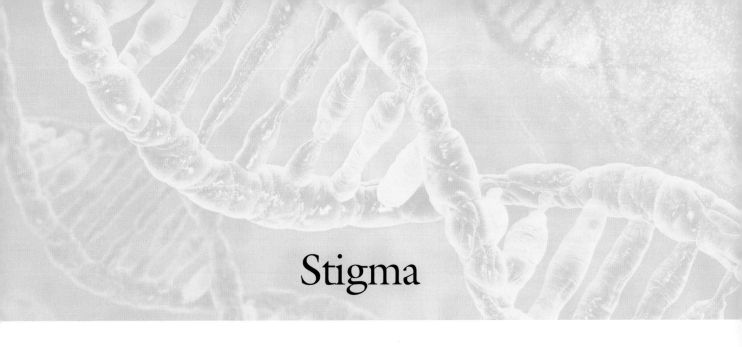

Stigma

⊕ Introduction

Stigma is defined as a mark of shame or discredit, or an identifying mark of disease. The word derives from the Latin term for a "mark" or "brand," and from the Greek meaning "to tattoo." The phrase "stigma of disease" refers to negative perceptions of people with certain diseases, who become part of a stereotyped group that faces discrimination and prejudice.

Being stigmatized because of an illness can lead to a wide range of social, economic, and health problems such as difficulties finding a home or alienation from friends and family, as well as discrimination in schooling, employment, and health care. People who are stigmatized often suffer from problems with self-esteem and self-worth.

⊕ Historical Background

The stigma of illness is deeply rooted in history. Leprosy, also known as Hansen's disease, is closely associated with stigma. Leprosy is caused by the bacterium *Mycobacterium leprae*; it is characterized by skin lesions that become insensate (they have no physical sensation), leading to more serious infections. Damage to the nerves, eyes, and limbs may occur. Leprosy has a long incubation period and symptoms can take up to 30 years to appear.

Leprosy is mentioned frequently in the Bible; in Leviticus, it is commanded to shun lepers and separate from them. At that time, however, the term may have encompassed a wide range of skin infections and diseases. The earliest written report of a disease appearing to be leprosy was found in an Egyptian papyrus written around 1550 BCE. It was also described in writings from India dating to 600 BCE.

In Greece, leprosy spread after Alexander the Great returned from India, around 327 BCE. It appeared in Rome about 62 BCE, with the return of Roman troops

from campaigns and was endemic (regularly found in the region) during the Middle Ages (1000 CE–1500 CE). Early reports of the disease in the United States are from the 1800s, when specific areas were established in order to banish those with the disease.

The history of leprosy in the United States illustrates the stigma of disease and the discrimination that victims suffer. In 1866, a colony was established on the U.S. island of Molokai, Hawaii, to which victims were banished for life with neither medical care nor provisions. Westerners in charge enacted the quarantine law but 97 percent of victims were Hawaiian natives, illustrating how the political atmosphere and racial overtones of those policies influenced health decisions. More than disability, it was the "loathesome appearance" of patients and concept of "moral filth" that led to this law. It was not until Father Damien arrived in Molokai in 1873 that routine care was established. He contracted the disease, died in 1889, and was canonized for his work in 2009. It was not until 1969 that the Hawaiian law regarding leprosy was retracted.

Also in the United States in the late 1800s, leprosy sufferers were exiled to a plantation in Carville, Louisiana (see sidebar). An 1881 law in Chicago, Illinois, stated that anyone with a disease that was deemed "unsightly or disgusting" could not expose themselves to public view. Interestingly, at about the same time, Norwegians adopted a policy to treat these patents in local hospitals. They were neither arrested nor exiled. It was a Norwegian doctor, Gerhard Armauer Hansen (1841–1912), who discovered the disease-causing bacterium in 1873; the disease now bears his name.

Leprosy is still prevalent in many countries today. It is estimated that at least 1 million people are affected in India. In the southern United States, 213 new cases were reported in 2009 with an estimate of 6,500 cases throughout the country.

Mental illness is another disease whose victims suffer from social stigma and discrimination. Early beliefs that mental illness was the result of sorcery or demonic

CARVILLE

From the ruins of an old plantation on the banks of the Mississippi River, just south of Baton Rouge, Louisiana, rose the world's leading hospital, rehabilitation center, and research facility on Hansen's disease, or leprosy.

The Gillis W. Long Hansen's Disease Center, otherwise known as Carville, was founded in 1894 in order to quarantine patients with leprosy. The first eight patients were exiled there by law. They arrived by river barge, as no wagon driver would take them. Conditions were terrible. The plantation building was dilapidated and the area was hot and swampy, but there were old slave cottages that were used as shelter. The resident doctor left within a year, leaving the patients alone to live and care for themselves for nearly two years.

In 1896, the nuns of the Daughters of Charity order were asked to care for the patients. Only four volunteered, but eventually at least 120 nuns would serve at Carville. Dr. Isadore Dyer (1865–1920) of Tulane University was the doctor responsible for establishing Carville and overseeing care.

Louisiana purchased the hospital in 1905, began massive renovations and construction, and became the first state to fund custodial care for patients. In 1921, the U.S. Public Health Service took over the facility. Over the years, improvements were made, adding amenities such as a newspaper run by patients, a lake with boating, and opportunities for socializing.

However, this was not just a hospital. Quarantine was permanent, and the conditions were cruel. Patients were called inmates. They were separated by sex; the law forbade them to marry, and if a baby was born, it was taken away. Patient names were changed to protect families from the stigma of the disease. It was not until the 1920s that families could visit, and even then no touching was allowed. Patients were subjected to experimental treatments. They could not vote.

Then, one day in 1941, everything changed. Two patients were given injections of Promin, a new sulfone drug. They improved, and others soon followed. Leprosy sufferers were cured for the first time in history. Spouses were now allowed to come and live with their loved ones. When discharged, however, many patients still faced the stigma of the disease, and had not known life outside of the hospital for most of their lives. They returned to Carville and stayed on, living in cottages and provided for even after the hospital closed in 1998. The facility is now on the National Park Service Historic Registry; the research branch relocated to the Louisiana State University Veterinary School in Baton Rouge.

physical pain to drive out the impure. The ancient Egyptians were apparently more enlightened. In early papyrus writings, the brain is identified as the site of mental dysfunction, and recommendations for those with mental disorders included pleasant activities such as dance and art.

Hippocrates (c. 460–c. 377 BCE) proposed that mental illness had natural causes, particularly pathology in the brain. He and later Galen (129–c. 199 CE) championed the idea of the four bodily fluids, or humors: blood, phlegm, yellow bile, and black bile. Combinations of these fluids were believed to create individual personalities. A disturbance in the balance could cause disease. During the Middle Ages, belief in humors persisted, and treatments were aimed at restoring the balance. These treatments included blood letting, laxatives, inducing vomiting, and concoctions of various types.

In the Middle Ages, the mentally ill were often punished, arrested, and thrown in jail, sometimes for life. Care of patients was left to families, and they were often hidden from society, chained, caged, or abandoned. Social stigma was tied to family. In cultures where marriages were arranged, the mentally ill family member could cause the entire family to experience discrimination.

In a 2006 survey conducted in Australia, one in four respondents considered mental illness the result of personal weakness and said they would not employ someone with a mental disorder. Forty-two percent said that people with depression are unreliable, 25 percent thought people with schizophrenia are dangerous, and 20 percent said they would not disclose depression if affected. Of those with a mental disorder, 75 percent reported experiencing stigma.

Research has shown that the activity with the sense of highest self-worth is the ability to work, but 61 percent of people with mental health problems are out of the workforce. Unemployment rates for those with serious problems such as schizophrenia range from 80 to 90 percent. A survey of U.S. employers reveals that half are reluctant to hire people with current or past mental disorders.

Untreated mental illness can result in suicide. Historically, people who survive suicide attempts and the families who have lost members to suicide also have been stigmatized. In the Middle Ages, the corpses of suicides were mutilated to prevent the release of evil spirits and could not be buried in church cemeteries. Today, the stigma associated with suicidal thinking continues to prevent people throughout the world from seeking help. The World Health Organization (WHO) map of suicide rates per 100,000 population reveals that in many parts of the world the suicide rate is greater than 15 percent. Reducing the stigma of suicide can improve the effectiveness of suicide prevention programs.

possession led to brutal treatment of affected people. Mesopotamians, Persians, and the Hebrews thought mental illness indicated demonic possession or punishment from God; treatment took the form of threats and

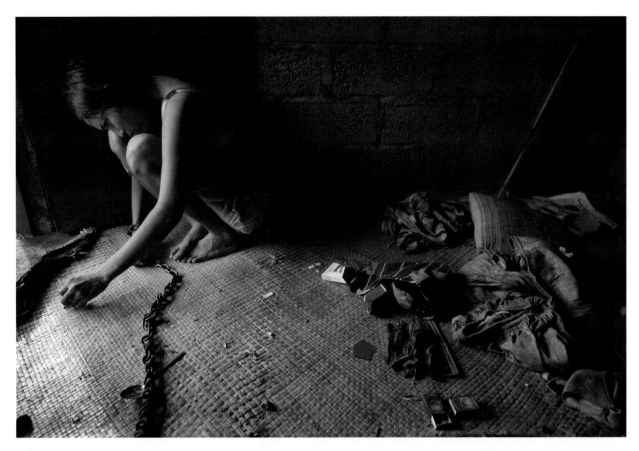

An Indonesian woman diagnosed with schizophrenia sits in her room, where she is shackled by her own family. They say it is to control her so she does not run away and disturb the community. She comes from a poor family with six siblings and has been chained off and on for years while taking medication for her illness. Many poor families do not have money to pay for hospitalization or go to doctors. In addition, inside the Balinese society there is often a stigma and misinformation about mental illness. Some people feel that it is the work of the supernatural and their hope of solving the mental disorder is to let traditional healers do the work. The Indonesian health ministry has a shortage of psychiatrists and only one government-run mental hospital in Bali. *© Paula Bronstein/Getty Images.*

Throughout history, patients with sexually transmitted diseases (STDs) also have been stigmatized. They have often been viewed as bringing the illness upon themselves. An American Medical Association (AMA) article describes a woman in 1728 who went to the church for aid, admitting she had the "pox," or an STD; she was sent to a workhouse and given mercury treatments. During that time, men with an STD were usually hospitalized, but women were treated differently. Wealthy patients could be discreetly treated at home. The stigma of STD had political, cultural, and moral implications: the Italians called it the French disease and the French called it the Spanish disease.

Perhaps the most stigmatized STD in recent history has been human immunodeficiency virus/acquired immune deficiency syndrome (HIV/AIDS). The first cases, in five homosexual men, were described in 1981 in the United States. Case numbers rose, and the disease was initially called gay-related immune deficiency (GRID). This led to widespread discrimination and fear of homosexuals. People with HIV/AIDS

lost jobs and were denied housing. In 1985, Ryan White (1971–1990), a teen who contracted the disease through a blood transfusion, was denied entrance to school. This provoked a highly publicized court fight resulting in his return to school. White's family also suffered the stigma of AIDS when their property was vandalized and they were ostracized in their community. Lack of a cure fueled the hysteria, as people feared this new fatal disease.

Other infectious diseases continue to cause panic and are associated with stigma. Plague, cholera, and yellow fever still occur today and provoke fear, although influenza epidemics kill more people worldwide than these diseases. Ebola is a recent example of a viral infectious disease that causes fear and misunderstanding. While Ebola is deadly in most cases, there are survivors. Despite this, those infected still face the stigma of their disease, even after they are cured.

There also is stigma associated with noncommunicable, chronic conditions such as overweight and obesity. According to the WHO, in 2014, more than one-third of

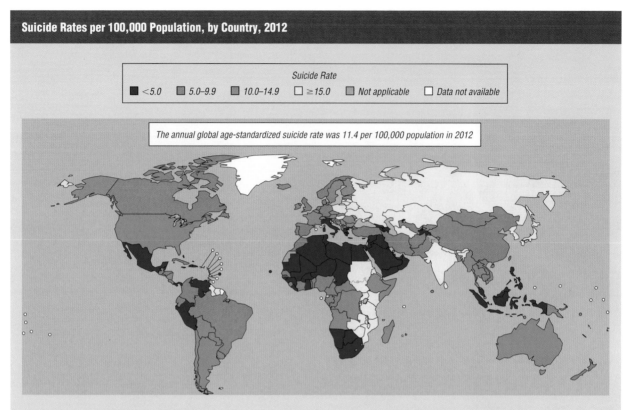

Suicide Rates per 100,000 Population, by Country, 2012

Suicide Rate

■ <5.0 ■ 5.0–9.9 ■ 10.0–14.9 □ ≥15.0 ■ Not applicable □ Data not available

The annual global age-standardized suicide rate was 11.4 per 100,000 population in 2012

SOURCE: Adapted from "Map 1. Age-standardized suicide rates (per 100,000 population), both sexes, 2012," in *Preventing Suicide: A Global Imperative*, World Health Organization (WHO), 2014, p. 16, http://apps.who.int/iris/bitstream/10665/131056/1/9789241564779_eng .pdf?ua=1&ua=1 (accessed January 14, 2015).

adults (39 percent) worldwide were overweight and 13 percent were obese. In the United States, more than one-third (35 percent) of adults are obese. Despite the widespread prevalence of obesity, negative attitudes toward people who are obese has resulted in stigmatization and discrimination. Along with discrimination in the areas of education, employment, and health care, people who are obese have faced discrimination in adoption proceedings, jury selection, and housing.

⊕ Impacts and Issues

Because of fear, stigma, and discrimination associated with some diseases, governments have had to intervene to ensure the well-being of those affected. However, not all official intervention has been humane or appropriate.

In the United States, laws have been passed to address many of these issues. Section 504 of the 1973 Rehabilitation Act states that people with illnesses and disabilities may not be excluded from or be denied benefits from certain programs, but the law did not address private entities. In 1990, the Americans with Disabilities Act was passed, making it illegal to discriminate based on

disability. To address fears of privacy invasion, the Health Insurance Portability and Accountability Act was passed in 1996; it protects patient privacy with regard to medical records and health information. The Office for Civil Rights ensures compliance with this legislation.

In the United Kingdom, the Disability Discrimination Act (1995) prohibits discrimination in employment, education, access to services, and housing. In the same year, Hong Kong and India passed similar laws. However, in some cases laws do not provide for legal procedures to deal with complaints and violations of the law.

Cultural aspects affect adherence and enforcement of laws. The AMA reports that villagers in India are shunned even after triple drug therapy for leprosy has rendered them cured. A new bill introduced there in 2014 aims to give those with disabilities equal rights in areas such as education, employment, and legal redress, according to the article "India's Disabilities Bill Raises Hopes of an End to Discrimination" in the *Guardian*. However, some fear it will make no difference when existing laws are not enforced. The *Guardian* reports that negative attitudes toward disabled people in India are entrenched, with the result that forced sterilization, sexual abuse, and sexual assaults on women with disabilities are often ignored by police.

are such topics as compassion and respect for human rights, betterment of public health, and access to medical care for all.

🌐 Future Implications

There is still much work to be done in helping people who suffer from the stigma of disease. Stigma affects all aspects of life, bringing shame, distress, blame, and hopelessness. The social, personal, and financial costs are high. While some countries have dealt with stigma legally, many have not yet passed protective legislation or do not enforce existing laws.

Certain diseases such as leprosy and HIV/AIDS become associated with certain groups within the population, causing group members to experience prejudice and discrimination even though they are not ill. Patients may fear losing their jobs, friends, or families and becoming social outcasts. This fear of discrimination often deters patients from seeking help for treatable conditions. Today, mental illness and obesity are preeminent examples of the negative effects of stigma. Once labeled, a diagnosis can jeopardize an individual's educational attainment, career, or social life.

Race has often been used as an excuse for prejudicial treatment. Both HIV/AIDS and Ebola originated in Africa, resulting in discrimination against those of African descent, even those who are not ill. Native Hawaiians with leprosy were sent to Molokai, but residents of Western descent were not dispatched there, even though they too were affected by the illness. They were treated at home or quietly allowed to leave Hawaii. Immigrants are frequently feared and blamed for outbreaks of disease. It was not until 2009 that the United States lifted the ban against travel to the United States by people with AIDS.

Overcoming cultural bias is difficult. Antidiscrimination laws must be enacted and enforced, and countries without legal recourse for victims need to reevaluate their laws. Education on the causes, treatment, and spread of disease is one of the best ways to help with stigma. First and foremost, health-care workers must respond to these diseases with positive attitudes. Treating each patient with respect, regardless of disease, not only will encourage those affected to seek treatment but also models appropriate behavior to the community at large.

Reducing and, ideally, eliminating stigma will enable people to access education and care for themselves, rather than depending on government aid for survival. It will also enable early detection and treatment, which in turn will decrease the costs associated with caring for patients. Nations must continue to discuss stigma and discrimination openly. For example, after much discussion in 2009, the Office of the United Nations High Commissioner for Human Rights established guidelines for eliminating the stigma of leprosy. Finally, it is important to realize that

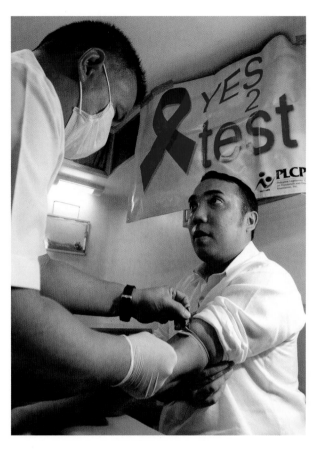

A medical worker extracts blood from Congressman Ibarra Gutierrez for an HIV/AIDS test in Manila, Philippines, on December 2, 2013, as legislators and advocates, during the launching of "YES 2 TEST," called for the elimination of stigma and discrimination against populations most at risk for HIV infection. The Department of Health in the Philippines recorded a total of almost 500 HIV/AIDS cases in October 2013, or 66 percent higher than the 295 cases in October 2012, making it the highest ever recorded in a month in the country. © *Jay Directo/AFP/Getty Images.*

The U.S. Emergency Medical Treatment and Labor Act was passed in 1986, stating that no one can be denied treatment on arrival at an emergency room. Patients must at a minimum be examined and stabilized within that hospital's capability; only then can they be transferred. Hospital licensing requirements in certain states specify that refusal to provide care for cases of infectious disease can result in disciplinary action. Nurses or doctors employed by the hospital that refuse to treat patients with specific diseases or conditions may also may face dismissal or licensing actions. However, in some states there is no provision to force a physician in private practice to treat patients with certain conditions, unless refusal is based on race, sex, or religion. A doctor has the legal right to refuse new patients, but cannot abandon a current patient.

The AMA has a code of nine ethical principles for physicians, several of which concern stigma. Included

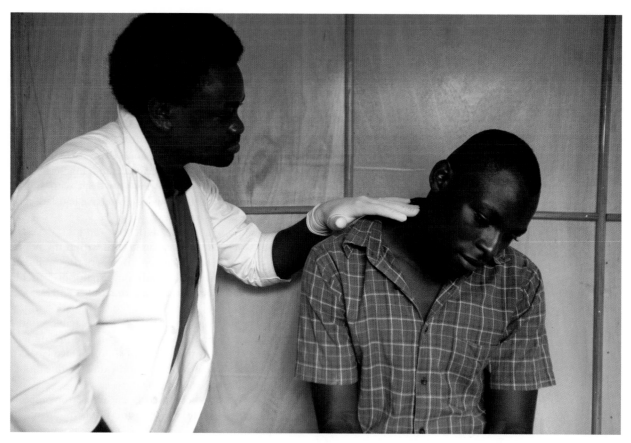

Auf Usaam Mukwaya, a Ugandan homosexual man, gets a checkup from a doctor who has many gay and lesbian patients. Homosexual acts are illegal in Uganda (and several other African nations) and were punishable by up to 14 years in prison before a tougher law was proposed in 2009. David Bahati's Anti-homosexuality Bill was passed in 2013 and includes a punishment of life imprisonment for homosexuals and penalties for individuals or organizations that know gay people or support lesbian, gay, bisexual, transgender, and questioning (LGBTQ) rights. Mukwaya believes the country's antigay bill will lead to "supercriminalization" of HIV, making it difficult for the LGBTQ community to gain access to health care. AIDS is a "disaster for public health—not just for queers," he says. A constitutional court ruled the law invalid in August 2014, however, this ruling was being appealed as of late 2014.   *© Benedicte Desrus/ Sipa Press/AP Images.*

throughout history there have been diseases that strike fear in people spark stigma and discrimination. Education about health and disease and enforcing legislation banning discrimination based on health status can help to reduce the long-term consequences of stigmatization on population health and quality of life.

PRIMARY SOURCE

Positive Women in Ukraine: Living with Denial, Discrimination and HIV/AIDS

SOURCE *Namjilsuren, Tunga. "Positive Women in Ukraine: Living with Denial, Discrimination and HIV/AIDS."* The 3 by 5 Initiative. *World Health Organization (WHO). http://www.who.int/3by5/news19/en/ (accessed January 25, 2015).*

INTRODUCTION *This primary source is an article on women in Ukraine and their children who are living with HIV. It focuses on the discrimination that the women and their children face on a daily basis.*

POSITIVE WOMEN IN UKRAINE: LIVING WITH DENIAL, DISCRIMINATION AND HIV/AIDS

World AIDS Campaign 2004: Women, Girls and HIV/AIDS

A large republic in the east of Europe, Ukraine is the country hardest hit by HIV/AIDS in the region. An estimated 360,000 people—nearly 1% of country's population—are currently living with HIV. More than 70% of them are injecting drug users (IDU) who became infected through sharing used syringe needles.

But drugs are not the only thing driving the AIDS epidemic in the Ukraine. HIV infection is rising sharply among the general population. "HIV is not just drug users' problem anymore. It's everywhere now," said Svetlana Antonyak, an experienced HIV/AIDS physician at Kiev's Lavra clinic. In April 2004, half of the new HIV cases in her clinic were not drugs users at all. "This shows HIV/AIDS is now a broader social problem that concerns everyone in the country," she said.

According to the UNAIDS 2004 global epidemiological report, women and young people are the most vulnerable groups to HIV infection. In Ukraine, 120 000 people—some 30 per cent—of all people living with HIV are women. Lack of awareness of the right information regarding HIV infection is a major contributing factor.

"I got HIV, because I did foolish things without reflecting how much devastation it can bring to my life," says Valeria, from Odessa.

Valeria contracted HIV when she was 18, injecting drugs with friends. Like many others she didn't know that she might become infected with HIV by sharing used needles.

Since then she had to live with the devastating consequences. One of the first people in the country to be diagnosed with HIV/AIDS, Valeria says she has faced extreme discrimination. She was rejected by those around her, she lost her sports career as a member of the national women's volleyball team and was forced to give up her university studies. Faced with such rejection and discrimination, Valeria says she lost her self confidence and plunged deeper into drug addiction.

Ten years on and Valeria has turned her life around. She works as a treatment counsellor for Life+, an NGO providing self-help and counselling services to people living with HIV/AIDS.

She is also in charge of the day-care centre for HIV positive children and is fierce in fighting against stigma and discrimination towards children living with AIDS. She's faced this first hand, as her daughter was born with HIV. "Many nurses and doctors are scared of providing services to people and even children living with HIV," she said, describing how a nurse refused to take a blood sample from her daughter for her first HIV test.

"I had to take the blood myself", confirms Valeria. "Safety conditions are not always perfect in our clinics but they shouldn't bear actions to violate our human rights."

Further discrimination followed Valeria's daughter. With "HIV" featured in her health records, no kindergarten or school would admit her. "Children are at no fault, they have a right to schooling and treatment, just like other children," said Valeria.

SEE ALSO *Ebola Virus Disease; Genetic Testing and Privacy Issues; Health as a Human Right and Health-Care Access; HIV/AIDS; Isolation and Quarantine; Mental Health Treatment Access; Obesity; Parasitic Diseases; Poliomyelitis (Polio); Pregnancy Termination; Tobacco Use; Tuberculosis (TB); Viral Diseases*

BIBLIOGRAPHY

Books

Doka, Kenneth J. *Aids, Fear, and Society: Challenging the Dreaded Disease*. New York: Taylor and Francis, 1997.

Flynn, James, Paul Slovic, and Howard Kunreuther, eds. *Risk, Media, and Stigma: Understanding Public Challenges to Modern Science and Technology*. London: Earthscan, 2001.

Lee, Jon D. *An Epidemic of Rumors: How Stories Shape Our Perception of Disease*. Boulder, CO: Utah State University Press, 2014.

Liamputtong, Pranee. *Stigma, Discrimination and Living with HIV/AIDS: A Cross-Cultural Perspective*. Dordrecht, Netherlands: Springer, 2013.

Mmana, Clement. *Stigma and HIV/AIDS: A Case Study*. Zomba, Malawi: Kachere Series, 2011.

Websites

"India's Disabilities Bill Raises Hopes of an End to Discrimination." *Guardian*, February 26, 2014. http://www.theguardian.com/global-development/2014/feb/27/india-disabilities-bill-end-discrimination (accessed May 31, 2015).

"Stigma and Disease: Changing Paradigms." *The Lancet*. http://www.thelancet.com/pdfs/journals/lancet/PIIS0140-6736(98)08068-4.pdf (accessed March 14, 2015).

"Stigma and Illness." *U.S. Centers for Disease Control and Prevention (CDC)*. http://www.cdc.gov/mentalhealth/about_us/stigma-illness.htm (accessed March 14, 2015).

"Stigmatization Complicates Infectious Disease Management." *American Medical Association*. http://journalofethics.ama-assn.org/2010/03/mhst1-1003.html (accessed March 14, 2015).

"Stigmatized Illnesses and Health Care." *National Institutes of Health*. http://www.ncbi.nlm.nih.gov/pmc/articles/PMC2080544/ (accessed March 14, 2015).

Virginia Herbert McDougall

Tobacco Use

⊕ Introduction

Tobacco use long has been a recreational activity worldwide. The nicotine in tobacco works on receptors in the brain, creating relaxing and pleasurable sensations, which is why using tobacco, usually in the form of smoking cigarettes, tends to be addictive. However, the smoke and tar from tobacco is known to be harmful to health, and smoking is responsible for around 6 million deaths per year, mainly from heart disease, chronic obstructive pulmonary disease, and lung cancer.

By far the most common form of tobacco use is cigarette and pipe smoking. However, a minority use smokeless tobacco, in the form of chewing tobacco or snuff. A 2012 survey showed that 5.5 percent of those in the 18–25 age group in the United States used smokeless tobacco. Some people use smokeless tobacco as a substitute for cigarettes in environments where smoking is not permitted. Smokeless tobacco increases the risk of oral and esophageal cancer, as well as causing dental problems. Since the introduction of smoking bans, tobacco companies have promoted smokeless tobacco, particularly to young people, by adding flavorings to make them seem more attractive.

There are around 1 billion smokers in the world, and around 80 percent of them live in low- and middle-income countries. A survey by the World Lung Foundation and the American Cancer Society found that rates of smoking are highest in Eastern Europe. Serbia has the highest smoking rate in the world, with a consumption of 2,841 cigarettes per person per year. Outside of Eastern Europe, the highest rates of smokers are in South Korea, Kazakhstan, and Japan. China is not far behind and, because of the size of its population, is the biggest consumer of cigarettes in the world.

The United States is 34th in the world ranking for smoking prevalence, similar to Israel, Australia, and Ireland. The lowest rates of smoking are in sub-Saharan Africa and South Asia. Annual cigarette consumption in India is 96 cigarettes per person per year and in Ethiopia the figure is only 46.

Rates of smoking have declined in the United States, the United Kingdom, and many other countries in the years since the 1980s. According to a study by the University of Washington, smoking rates in the United States were down to 18 percent in 2012, compared with 42 percent in 1980. Overall, smoking rates worldwide have decreased from an overall average of 26 percent in 1980 to 18.7 percent in 2012. However, smoking is increasing in developing countries and among women. Faced with tightening controls on their activities in many parts of the world, the tobacco industry is targeting lower-income countries, where regulations tend to be weaker. Women are being targeted as their social and financial independence increases.

If nothing is done to curb smoking, the annual death toll could rise to more than 8 million by 2030. The impact of smoking will be not just on those who already smoke, but upon those who will take up the habit, if efforts to dissuade them fail. Fortunately, there are many proven methods to reduce tobacco use, from imposing controls upon the tobacco industry to public health campaigns aimed at helping people quit.

⊕ Historical Background

The tobacco plant was grown and widely used in the Americas for 2,000 to 3,000 years before it was introduced into Europe by the explorer Francis Drake (c.1540–1596). It was used for both recreational and medicinal purposes, with cigarettes mainly replacing cigars and pipes by the end of the 19th century. By the conclusion of World War I (1914–1918), the majority of men in the United Kingdom and the United States were smokers, and the habit began to grow among women during the 1920s. The physical harm that tobacco caused would not, however, become apparent for many years.

During the early years of the 20th century, physicians began to note an increase in the rate of myocardial infarction, commonly known as heart attack. This condition

Smokers in Ten Countries Accounted for More Than 65 Percent of All Smokers Globally in 2008

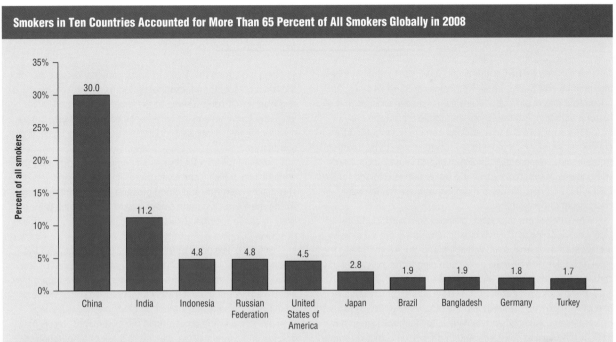

SOURCE: Adapted from "Nearly Two Thirds of the World's Smokers Live in 10 Countries," in *WHO Report on the Global Tobacco Epidemic, 2008*, World Health Organization (WHO), 2008.

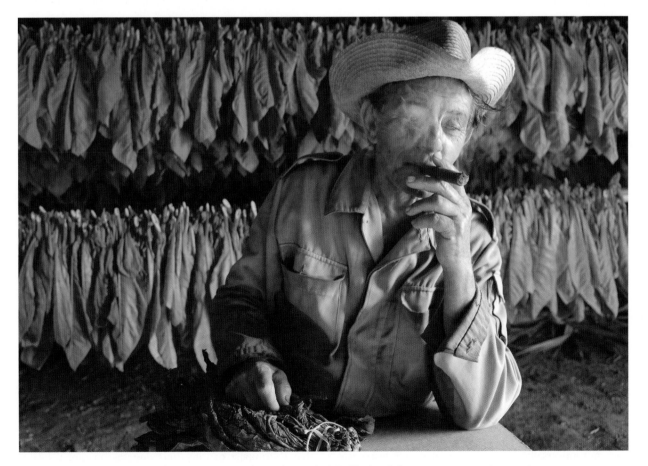

A tobacco farmer smokes a homemade cigar in his tobacco drying shed, in Viñales, Cuba. © *Klemen Misic/Shutterstock.com.*

HOW TOBACCO KILLS

Tobacco kills around half of those who use it. One in four smokers dies prematurely, that is, between the ages of 35 to 74 years, and one in four dies in old age. It is not the nicotine in tobacco that is harmful to health, but the smoke that tobacco produces.

Tobacco smoke is a toxic cocktail of more than 7,000 different chemicals, of which more than 250 are known to be harmful to the body, and more than 50 are known to cause cancer. Many components of tobacco smoke have not even been studied for their effects on cells, tissue, and organs, so these figures well could be an underestimate.

The carcinogens that tobacco smoke contains include formaldehyde, benzene, and vinyl chloride. Then there are toxic heavy metals, such as arsenic, lead, cadmium, and chromium. Finally, the smoke contains several toxic gases, including hydrogen cyanide, carbon monoxide, butane, and ammonia.

The chemicals in tobacco smoke are inhaled and reach every part of the body via the lungs and the bloodstream. Cells and tissues become inflamed and damaged. The immune system has to fight this damage constantly and, if the person carries on smoking, the body never really gets a chance to heal the damage that smoking inflicts on every part of it. Inhaling cigarette smoke inflicts both short and long-term damage. Blood clots, heart attacks, and strokes can be triggered by cigarettes at any time. Meanwhile, years of smoking gradually damage tissue, resulting in a number of health problems, including lung disease and cancer.

Every cigarette a person smokes increases his or her risk of developing cancer. The carcinogens in tobacco smoke are known to damage DNA in cells in a way that may cause the cells to multiply out of control, eventually forming a tumor. This is a process that may take many years, which is why increases in cancer in a population often occur many years after smoking rates peak. The good news is that once smoking rates decline, cancer rates also will fall eventually. Under normal circumstances, the immune system protects the body from cancer. But, as stated above, smoking weakens the immune system. Thus, not only can smoking cause cancer, it can also block the body's natural defenses against it.

The link between smoking and lung cancer is well known. Nearly 9 out of 10 men who die from lung cancer are smokers. Moreover, around 3,000 nonsmokers die from inhaling secondhand smoke every year. In addition, it has become known that

smoking is a strong risk factor in many other cancers: cancer of the mouth, nose, throat, esophagus, kidneys, stomach, cervix, and bladder. Of course, some of these parts of the body are a long way from the lungs, where smoke enters the body, but as mentioned, the chemicals in cigarette smoke readily reach all cells and tissues.

Inhaling tobacco smoke has an immediate effect upon the endothelium, which is the layer of cells lining the blood vessels. This makes heart rate and blood pressure increase immediately. At the same time, cigarette smoke makes blood platelets more likely to clump together, which increases the risk of heart attack or stroke.

Smoking also contributes to the buildup of plaque in the blood vessels serving the heart. Plaque is a fatty deposit of scar tissue and cholesterol. It narrows the arteries and eventually may block them, causing a potentially fatal heart attack or stroke. In addition, the plaque may narrow or block arteries in the legs, thereby impeding the circulation in the lower limbs. Ulcers may develop and tissue may die, leading to a risk of amputation of toes, feet, or even the leg itself.

Smoking is a risk factor for developing type 2 diabetes. People who already have type 1 diabetes will tend to need more insulin to control their condition if they smoke. Smokers with diabetes also have higher risks of complications such as heart and kidney disease, retinopathy, and peripheral neuropathy.

Tobacco smoke harms the tissue in the upper and lower respiratory tract, from the mouth to the lungs. It damages the cilia, which are the tiny hairs that line the airways. Normally, these keep the airways clear by a sweeping motion. Once they are damaged, the lungs do not clear as easily, and the smoker develops a chronic cough.

Over time, smoking causes the lungs to lose their elasticity and their function declines. Scar tissue replaces healthy elastic tissue, and it becomes harder to breathe. Smoking causes chronic obstructive pulmonary disease, which is a condition comprising both emphysema and chronic bronchitis. In emphysema, lung tissue is destroyed progressively, and it becomes harder to breathe in and out. Chronic bronchitis involves swelling of the lining of the bronchial tubes, leading to chronic cough and reduced airflow.

previously had been virtually unknown. Researchers soon began to suspect a link between heart disease and cigarette smoking. Cancer of the lung also had been a rare disease. Again, many doctors noted that patients with lung cancer were often also heavy smokers.

In 1950, a number of groundbreaking case-control studies published by British and American researchers led to the conclusion that smoking is an important factor in lung cancer. These results were publicized widely but were not universally accepted. The tobacco industry was quick to try to disprove the link between smoking and

cancer, but the research findings triggered new studies and forced governments to look into the implications of smoking on public health.

⊕ Impacts and Issues

The advent of antibiotics and vaccination, improved sanitation, and increasing life expectancy worldwide meant that the impact of infectious diseases on global health began to recede. Therefore, the focus of efforts by the

World Health Organization (WHO) and other health policy makers has begun to shift toward noncommunicable diseases such as cancer, cardiovascular disease, and diabetes. Because tobacco use is known to harm both individuals who smoke and those around them, everyone stands to benefit from effective tobacco control measures.

The Smoking Epidemic

The Royal College of Physicians in England and the U.S. surgeon general issued reports on smoking in 1962 and 1964, respectively, that revealed that the impact of smoking on health was greater than previously realized. An increasing number of diseases were linked to smoking in addition to myocardial infarction and lung cancer. It is believed that 35 diseases, some of them admittedly rare, are smoking related. Of these, 22 emerged from a large study on British doctors and in the landmark study of 1 million men and women undertaken by the American Cancer Society.

It generally takes 30 to 40 years for lung cancer caused by smoking cigarettes to develop. Because this cancer has a poor survival rate, research has been able to link levels of smoking in the 1920s in different countries with lung cancer mortality in 1955. Although correlation is not exact—because many other factors affect rates of lung cancer—in general, where smoking rates were high (in Finland, Greece, and the United Kingdom), lung cancer cases also were high, compared with those occurring in countries where smoking rates in the 1920s were lower (Sweden, Norway, and Portugal).

Data on the health impact of smoking in developing countries are scarcer. However, it is known that in China, cigarette consumption increased from around one cigarette per person per day in 1952 to 10 per day in 1992. A case-control study of a million deaths in 98 parts of China, both urban and rural, and another of a quarter of a million Chinese men provided information on smoking habits and cause of death. The finding showed quite clearly that 12 percent of male deaths were attributed to smoking. However, the pattern of deaths was different from that found in the more developed world, with an emphasis on stroke, chronic obstructive pulmonary disease, and cancer of the esophagus, liver, and stomach, rather than on heart disease and lung cancer.

Secondhand Smoke

Secondhand smoke, also known as environmental tobacco smoke, is the smoke that fills the space around those who smoke cigarettes and other tobacco products. It is inhaled by those nearby and is known to cause a number of health problems. In adults, secondhand smoke is linked to heart disease and lung cancer, and in pregnant women it is linked to low birth weights of babies. Around 600,000 deaths per year around the world result from secondhand smoke exposure.

Children in particular are vulnerable to the effects of secondhand smoke. Nearly half of children worldwide inhale smoke from a parent who smokes. Secondhand smoke exacerbates asthma in both children and adults. Many of the people who have health problems from secondhand smoke have never smoked themselves. According to the WHO, there is no safe level of exposure to secondhand smoke.

Tobacco Control

Growing awareness of the health impact of tobacco led to pressure for public policy on tobacco control in the 1990s. A resolution calling for action was passed in May 1996, initiating the WHO Framework Convention on Tobacco Control (FCTC). For the first time in the history of the WHO, its power to conclude treaties was applied when an intergovernmental body, comprising all the WHO member states, was established in 1999. The treaty itself was adopted in 2003 and entered into force in February 2005. The FCTC generally is acknowledged as a success in global health diplomacy. It is, indeed, one of the most widely adopted treaties in United Nations history, with 178 parties, covering 89 percent of the world's population. It is the WHO's prime tool for tobacco control and is seen as an important milestone in public health.

The FCTC is evidence-based and provides a legal dimension to global health cooperation and sets high standards for compliance. In 2008, the WHO gave a push to the implementation of the FCTC, with the introduction of the 6 MPOWER measures, which are designed to educate people about tobacco and also combat the activities of the tobacco industry. These focus on demand reduction and comprise: monitoring tobacco use and prevention policies; protecting people from tobacco smoke; offering help to quit tobacco use; warning people about the dangers of tobacco use; enforcing bans on tobacco advertising, promotion and sponsorship; and raising taxes on tobacco. Currently around 2.3 billion people, which is around one-third of the world's population, are covered by at least one effective tobacco control measure and nearly 1 billion are covered by two or more measures. It is not just the comprehensive content of the FCTC that is important but the solidarity and commitment that has developed around the shared goal of tackling the harm caused by tobacco use.

Demand Reduction

Persuading people away from tobacco is an important part of tobacco control. It may involve trying to prevent people from starting to smoke or helping those who smoke to stop, or, if this cannot be achieved, then at least to cut down. There are many approaches to demand reduction. Price and tax measures cause smoking to become an expensive habit, which may mean that the cigarettes become increasingly unaffordable. This is the

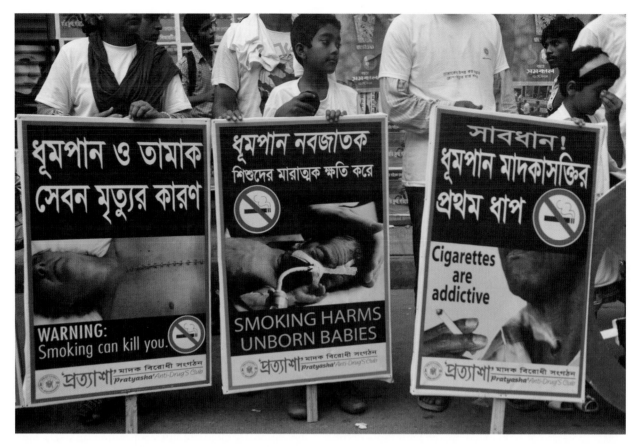

A human chain forms in front of the Press Club in Dhaka, Bangladesh, to promote the World No Tobacco Day campaign on May 31, 2014. The global tobacco epidemic kills nearly 6 million people each year, of which more than 600,000 are nonsmokers dying from breathing secondhand smoke, according to the World Health Organization. *© Mohammad Asad/Pacific Press/LightRocket via Getty Images.*

most cost-effective way of reducing tobacco use, for a 10 percent increase reduces consumption by 4 to 5 percent. However, the potential of taxation is far from fully exploited. Only 32 countries, representing less than 8 percent of the world's population, have tobacco tax rates that are greater than 75 percent of the retail price index.

Education and awareness also may help reduce the demand for tobacco. If, for instance, an individual sees a prominent advertisement showing a graphic description of what tobacco tar does to the lungs, that person may be less inclined to smoke. There also is value in putting health warnings on cigarettes, which may give people pause for thought. Research conducted after the introduction of such warnings in Brazil, Canada, Singapore, and Thailand showed how the warnings significantly increase awareness of the harms of tobacco use.

Health-care professionals also have a role to play in demand reduction. They can ask their patients about their smoking habits. While they cannot force their patients to quit, they can talk to them about the dangers of smoking. If a patient is motivated, that person can be supported through a cessation program. Here, psychological support in the form of group therapy, or motivational interviewing, can be combined with medication such as

bupropion or nicotine replacement therapy. Most health authorities assert that the best way to quit smoking is to give up immediately, completely and permanently. However, there is another approach, known as harm reduction, which uses nicotine replacement therapy, including the use of nicotine gum, patches, or electronic cigarettes. These nicotine products acts as a bridge to permanent cessation by satisfying a smoker's cravings without the smoke of cigarettes. Thus, the smoker and those around them are at least not exposed to the harmful health effects of tobacco smoke.

However, electronic cigarettes are controversial. Their marketing is extensive and growing, but it is too soon to know what, if any, adverse health effects are associated with their use. Some critics argue that electronic cigarettes normalize smoking behavior. They also prolong the time taken for smokers to quit their dependence on nicotine. However, there is some evidence that electronic cigarettes may be as good as nicotine patches in helping someone to quit. It remains to be seen whether it is mainly current or ex-smokers who use electronic cigarettes or if they are being used as a gateway to conventional smoking by never smokers. Findings from the 2014 National Youth Tobacco Survey conducted by the U.S. Centers

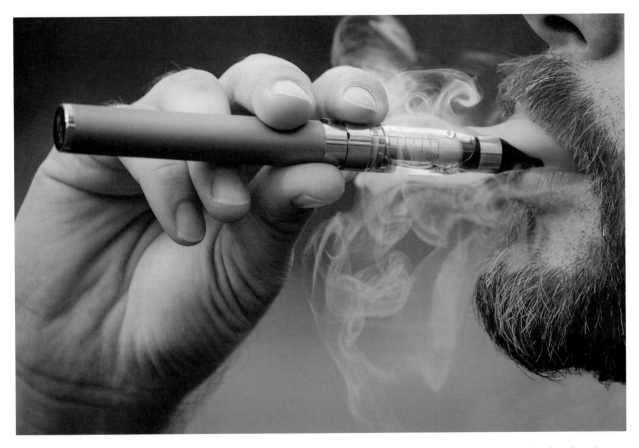

A man smokes an electronic cigarette. In discussing electronic cigarettes and their increased use by middle and high school students in a press release from 2015, U.S. Centers for Disease Control director Tom Friedan warned that nicotine is dangerous in any form, whether it is from traditional cigarettes or electronic cigarettes. This is especially true for those whose brains are still developing.
© *Marc Bruxelle/Shutterstock.com.*

for Disease Control and Prevention's Office on Smoking and Health (OSH) and the U.S. Food and Drug Administration, Center for Tobacco Products (CTP) found that e-cigarette use by high school students tripled from 4.5 to 13.4 percent from 2013 to 2014. There is also controversy over whether electronic cigarettes should be allowed in places where conventional smoking is not. Currently, the WHO is carrying out an investigation into the health issues around electronic cigarettes.

Whereas smoking cessation programs do not have a high success rate on the first attempts, many more people will quit if they make multiple attempts. There is a need to expand these programs, for they are available (and are not always free to participate in) in only 21 countries, representing 15 percent of the world's population.

Taking on the Tobacco Industry

The tobacco industry is adept at advertising and other promotional activities to maintain demand for its products, for it must replace those smokers who either die or quit. In the language of tobacco control, these activities are known as TAPS (tobacco advertising, promotion, and sponsorship). It is known that exposure to TAPS is associated with higher smoking rates, particularly where initiation and continuation of smoking by young people is concerned. A comprehensive TAPS ban drastically reduces exposure to smoking. Around one-third of youthful experimentation with smoking arises from TAPS, which portrays an attractive image of the smoking habit either through advertising or some less direct means. Protecting people from TAPS through a comprehensive ban has been shown to reduce cigarette consumption in all countries where this was implemented, regardless of their income.

Research by the WHO shows that partial TAPS bans merely cause the tobacco industry to divert its budget into permitted activities instead. If television advertising is banned, for instance, then spending on billboard and magazine advertising will be increased. A total ban on advertising merely increases spending on sponsoring events that are attractive to young people such as sports or music, which gets the message across indirectly. In one example, Singapore restricted cigarette advertising, so companies instead increased spending on advertising on television in neighboring Malaysia, which could still be seen by viewers in Singapore.

The packaging of cigarettes is another form of promotion that can greatly increase the attractiveness of smoking. Therefore, as well as requiring a health warning, banning the branding, and thus the message, on the packet is equally important. This goes hand in hand with banning store signage and point-of-sale displays. Currently, very few countries ban point-of-sale displays. In Ireland, such displays were banned in 2009 and worked to reduce smoking initiation by causing young people to be less likely to believe that their peers were smoking. In other words, smoking began to seem less like a normal activity. Similar effects have been reported in other countries that have introduced a point-of-sale ban on tobacco products.

⊕ Future Implications

Reduction of tobacco use is a key element of the WHO global action plan for the prevention and control of non-communicable disease. The plan, which runs from 2013 to 2020, aims to reduce premature mortality from such diseases by 25 percent in 2025 and to generate a 30 percent relative reduction in prevalence of tobacco use in those aged 15 or older. It is likely that the trend toward banning smoking in public places will spread. There is, for instance, discussion about banning smoking in cars. Whether this, or the more ambitious goal of banning smoking altogether, will be achievable in the future is debatable. What can be predicted is that the war between the tobacco industry and tobacco control organizations will increase.

Against this must be set an increasing trend in tobacco use in some places. Richard Doll (1912–2005), the pioneering tobacco researcher, noted in 1993 that the prevalence of smoking and smoking-related mortality in China resembled what had been happening in the United States 40 years prior. For Chinese men who began smoking in adolescence, the risk of death from smoking was one in four in 2005 and predicted to become one in two by 2025. Two-thirds of Chinese men currently become smokers before the age of 25. Should this continue, around 100 million of the 300 million Chinese men under the age of 30 as of 2015 will die from a tobacco-related cause.

PRIMARY SOURCE

WHO Report on the Global Tobacco Epidemic, 2013

SOURCE *"Summary," in* WHO Report on the Global Tobacco Epidemic, 2013: Enforcing Bans on Tobacco Advertising, Promotion and Sponsorship. *Geneva: World Health Organization (WHO), 2013, 13–14. http://apps.who.int/iris/bitstream/10665/85380/1/9789241505871_eng.pdf?ua=1 (accessed January 25, 2015).*

INTRODUCTION *This primary source is taken from the 2013* WHO Report on the Global Tobacco Epidemic. *It is "the fourth in a series of WHO reports that tracks the status of the tobacco epidemic and the impact of interventions implemented to stop it."*

SUMMARY

The WHO Framework Convention on Tobacco Control (WHO FCTC) recognizes the substantial harm caused by tobacco use and the critical need to prevent it. Tobacco kills approximately 6 million people and causes more than half a trillion dollars of economic damage each year. Tobacco will kill as many as 1 billion people this century if the WHO FCTC is not implemented rapidly.

Although tobacco use continues to be the leading global cause of preventable death, there are proven, cost-effective means to combat this deadly epidemic. In 2008, WHO identified six evidence-based tobacco control measures that are the most effective in reducing tobacco use. Known as "MPOWER", these measures correspond to one or more of the demand reduction provisions included in the WHO FCTC: Monitor tobacco use and prevention policies, Protect people from tobacco smoke, Offer help to quit tobacco use, Warn people about the dangers of tobacco, Enforce bans on tobacco advertising, promotion and sponsorship, and Raise taxes on tobacco. These measures provide countries with practical assistance to reduce demand for tobacco in line with the WHO FCTC, thereby reducing related illness, disability and death....

There continues to be substantial progress in many countries. More than 2.3 billion people living in 92 countries—a third of the world's population—are now covered by at least one measure at the highest level of achievement (not including Monitoring, which is assessed separately). This represents an increase of nearly 1.3 billion people (and 48 countries) in the past five years since the first report was released, with gains in all areas. Nearly 1 billion people living in 39 countries are now covered by two or more measures at the highest level, an increase of about 480 million people (and 26 countries) since 2007.

In 2007, no country protected its population with all five or even four of the measures. Today, one country, Turkey, now protects its entire population of 75 million people with all MPOWER measures at the highest level. Three countries with 278 million people have put in place four measures at the highest level. All four of these countries are low- or middle-income.

Most of the progress in establishing the MPOWER measures over the past five years since the first report was launched, has been achieved in low- and middle-income countries and in countries with relatively small populations. More high-income and high-population countries need to take similar actions to fully cover their people by completely establishing these measures at the highest achievement level.

…

The WHO FCTC demonstrates sustained global political will to strengthen tobacco control and save lives. As countries continue to make progress in tobacco control, more people are being protected from the harms of second-hand tobacco smoke, provided with help to quit tobacco use, exposed to effective health warnings through tobacco package labelling and mass media campaigns, protected against tobacco industry marketing tactics, and covered by taxation policies designed to decrease tobacco use and fund tobacco control and other health programmes.

SEE ALSO   *Cancer; Noncommunicable Diseases (Lifestyle Diseases); World Health Organization: Organization, Funding, and Enforcement Powers*

BIBLIOGRAPHY

Books

Boyle, Peter, et al., eds. *Tobacco: Science, Policy, and Public Health*, 2nd ed. New York: Oxford University Press, 2010.

Moyer, David. *The Tobacco Book: A Reference Guide of Facts, Figures, and Quotations about Tobacco*. Santa Fe, NM: Sunstone Press, 2005.

Rabinoff, Michael. *Ending the Tobacco Holocaust: How Big Tobacco Affects Our Health, Pocketbook, and Political Freedom—and What We Can Do about It*. Santa Rosa, CA: Elite Books, 2010.

U.S. Department of Health and Human Services. *A Report of the Surgeon General: How Tobacco Smoke Causes Disease: What It Means to You*. U.S. Department of Health and Human Services, Centers for Disease Control and Prevention, National Center for Chronic Disease Prevention and Health Promotion, Office on Smoking and Health, 2010. Available online at http://www.cdc.gov/tobacco/data_statistics/sgr/2010/consumer_booklet/index.htm (accessed May 31, 2015).

Periodicals

Stellman, Steven, and Lawrence Garfinkel. "Smoking Habits and Tar Levels in a New American Cancer Society Prospective Study of 1.2 Million Men and Women." *Journal of the American Cancer Society* 76, no. 6 (June 1986): 1057–1063.

Websites

"E-Cigarette Use Triples among Middle and High School Students in Just One Year." Press Release. *U.S. Centers for Diseases Control and Prevention (CDC)*, April 16, 2015. http://www.cdc.gov/media/releases/2015/p0416-e-cigarette-use.html (accessed May 31, 2015).

Fisher, Max. "Who Smokes Most: A Surprising Map of Smoking Rates by Country." *Washington Post*, October 19, 2012. http://www.washingtonpost.com/blogs/worldviews/wp/2012/10/19/who-smokes-most-a-surprising-map-of-smoking-rates-by-country (accessed January 16, 2015).

Partnership for Public Service. "Putting the Science behind FDA's Tobacco Regulation." *Washington Post*, May 1, 2012. http://www.washingtonpost.com/politics/putting-the-science-behind-fdas-tobacco-regulation/2012/04/29/gIQAHorgpT_story.html (accessed January 16, 2015).

"Tobacco." *World Health Organization*. http://www.who.int/topics/tobacco/en/ (accessed November 23, 2014).

"Tobacco Industry." *Action on Smoking and Health*. http://www.ash.org.uk/information/tobacco (accessed November 23, 2014).

Susan Aldridge

Tuberculosis (TB)

⊕ Introduction

Tuberculosis (TB) is an infectious disease caused by the bacterium *Mycobacterium tuberculosis*. It affects around one-third of the world's population.

TB can affect any part of the body, but in around 80 percent of cases it is the lungs that are infected. In most people, TB remains latent, and they do not have symptoms or infect others. Around 2 billion people around the world are infected with TB, and there are around 9 million active cases. TB claims around 2 million lives each year. The disease tends to take hold when immunity is compromised, which is why there has been a resurgence of TB coincident with the spread of human immunodeficiency virus/acquired immune deficiency syndrome (HIV/AIDS) and the breakdown of post-Soviet health systems. However, with effective programs of awareness, diagnosis, and treatment in place, TB is both preventable and curable.

TB is spread in aerosol droplets that are emitted from the lungs and throat when an actively infected person coughs or sneezes. When people breathe in these droplets, they become infected too. An untreated person with active pulmonary TB can infect 10 to 15 people each year. Thus, there are around 30 million new TB infections annually. Crowded circumstances, malnutrition, the presence of HIV, and inadequate health care increase the risk of contracting infection. Certain groups, including migrants, miners, prisoners, and drug users, are more at risk. The symptoms of active TB are a persistent cough, night sweats, weakness, and loss of appetite. However, symptoms may be mild for many months, which leads to delays in diagnosis.

There are two different forms of TB: smear positive and smear negative, according to the results seen at diagnosis. If left untreated, one-third of those with active smear-negative TB will die, one-third will recover, and the rest will remain ill and capable of infecting others. In smear-positive TB, which is both more infectious and more deadly, up to 70 percent will die within 10 years. Added to the morbidity and mortality of the disease, people with TB often suffer from discrimination and social isolation, as well as the problems of poverty, which make the disease more likely in the first place.

The diagnosis of TB in resource-poor settings relies on the classic microscopic examination of a smear of the person's sputum. These tests can distinguish between smear-negative and smear-positive TB. However, the use of more precise and rapid molecular tests for TB is spreading. The treatment of TB involves two months administration of a combination of the drugs isoniazid, rifampin (also known as rifampicin), ethambutol, and pyrazinamide, followed by another four months with isonazid and rifampin only.

Most people with TB can be cured if they take the complete course of drugs. However, the relatively long course of treatment brings its own problems. People who are at work may be reluctant to take time out for treatment, particularly if their symptoms are mild. Furthermore, access to a continuing supply of high-quality drugs is necessary, which can be challenging where health systems are weak. If a person does not take the full course of treatment, however, the disease will linger, or return, and probably in a drug-resistant form that will be harder and more expensive to treat.

The World Health Organization (WHO) has recognized TB as a major public health problem and has taken action accordingly. The Stop TB Strategy is aligned with Millennium Development Goal (MDG) 6, which is to combat HIV/AIDS, malaria, and other diseases. The MDGs were formulated in 2000 at the United Nations (UN) Millennium Summit. There are eight MDGs, all related directly or indirectly to global health. The TB-specific target within MDG 6 is to have reversed the incidence of TB by the end of 2015. The world is on track to achieve this, although incidence is falling very slowly. Furthermore, all WHO regions except Africa and Europe are on track to reach the Stop TB target of 50 percent decline in mortality.

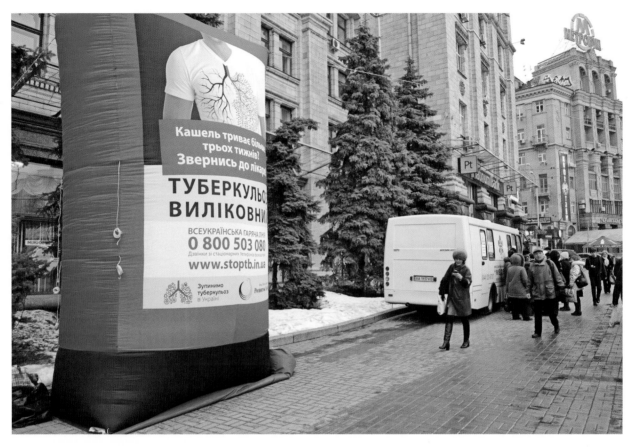

A Stop TB in Ukraine sign is set up near a mobile x-ray lab in Kiev, Ukraine. According to the World Health Organization, "Ukraine is among the 27 high multidrug-resistant tuberculosis (MDR-TB) burden countries in the world." © *fmua/Shutterstock.com.*

⊕ Historical Background

TB was known as consumption or phthisis, from the Greek word for "wasting," before the 20th century. These terms arise from the tendency of the disease to appear to consume its victims. It is probably as old as humanity, but began to reach epidemic proportions in the United States and Europe in early industrial society. It was the biggest killer of young adults and was feared greatly. The English romantic poet John Keats (1795–1821) was one victim. Perhaps because the disease targeted the young, it began to acquire a romantic and mysterious image in Victorian society. Heroines with TB, with their pale, tragic faces and wasted features, star in many famous works from the 1800s, including the novel *La Dame aux Caméllias* by Alexandre Dumas (1824–1895) and the opera *La Traviata* by Giuseppe Verdi (1813–1901). From the late 19th century, however, TB began to recede in many places, probably because of improvements in hygiene and housing.

TB causes lesions in the lungs known as tubercles. In 1882, German microbiologist Robert Koch (1843–1910) identified *Mycobacterium tuberculosis* in tubercles

in both humans and animals and went on to establish this bacterium as the cause of the disease. *Mycobacterium tuberculosis* is smaller than many other bacteria, it divides slowly, and has a lipid cell wall that allows it to survive in drier conditions, all factors that contribute to its efficient ability to cause chronic infections.

In the 20th century, TB shed its romantic image, and it was more common for victims to be stigmatized. Treatment consisted of moving patients to a special hospital known as a sanatorium, where they would be prescribed a regime of rest, fresh air, nutritious food, and sunshine under constant medical supervision. Physicians widely believed that high altitude was beneficial in TB, so many sanatoriums were located in Switzerland and other mountainous countries. With the development of mass use of x-ray technology following World War II (1939–1945), diagnosis became easier via the detection of tubercles in the lungs. Indeed, the chest x ray became part of a routine medical examination. Nevertheless, there was still no cure for TB, and the disease claimed some famous victims, including British author George Orwell (1903–1950), New Zealand writer Katherine Mansfield (1888–1923), and British actress Vivien Leigh (1913–1967).

STOP TB, END TB

The World Health Assembly endorsed the creation of Stop TB in 2001, following the Amsterdam Declaration to Stop TB in 2000, which called for new action to combat the disease. Stop TB has evolved into a global health initiative, run by the World Health Organization (WHO) with seven working groups. The Stop TB Partnership, the people putting the campaign into action, consists of more than 1,200 partners across 100 countries. The main goal of Stop TB is aligned with Millennium Development Goal 6, that the global burden of tuberculosis (TB) be reduced by 2015 by halving prevalence and incidence levels compared with 1990 levels. The long-term vision of Stop TB is a TB-free world, where the next generation will see the disease eliminated in its lifetime. The mission of Stop TB is to stop transmission of TB and to ensure that every TB patient has access to effective diagnosis, treatment, and cure. It also aims to develop and implement new preventive diagnostic tools and strategies to stop TB and finally to reduce the social and economic toll of the disease.

Stop TB relies upon a program called TB REACH, which aims to get effective diagnosis and treatment to more people who have TB, because one-third of all cases are not detected or treated properly. The program funds and supports innovative techniques, interventions, and approaches. It awards grants of up to $1 million to institutions with research proposals that support the objectives of TB REACH. The program also provides the Global Fund to Fight AIDS, Tuberculosis and Malaria with successful research models that can be scaled up to a national level.

Also essential to the Stop TB is the Global Drug Facility, which was created in 2001. Its role is to increase access to high-quality and affordable TB diagnostics and treatments. The facility also provides support to countries, donors, and programs on procurement of drugs and diagnostics. It makes sure supplies are there where and when needed and provides any technical assistance required to those managing TB on the ground.

Besides the technical programs outlined above, Stop TB must engage all stakeholders in the fight against the disease, from patients and health-care professionals to governments and wider society. To this end, the campaign uses its Challenge Facility for Civil Society, which is an instrument to promote the role of communities in TB programs operating at a national level, particularly targeting locations supported by the Global Fund. The facility has supported various community-based organizations engaged in advocacy and social mobilization to ensure that they have a voice in the fight against TB.

DOTS stands for directly observed therapy, short course, which is central to the Stop TB Strategy. It aims to support patients through a long course of TB treatment and make sure they complete it. This helps prevent the development of multidrug-resistant TB and also ensures the best outcome for the patient. The regimen itself consists of isoniazid, rifampin, pyrazinamide, and ethambutol for two months, then isoniazid and rifampin for the next four months. The key to DOTS is that a local care provider dispenses the medication and observes it being taken by the patient.

The DOTS strategy has a number of components. A political commitment to a national TB program is necessary in the first place. Then access to a quality-assured diagnostic service is needed. Once an active case is identified, then a supply of the drugs needed for the six-month treatment is required. The direct observation component is required to ensure the patient takes the entire course of medication. The observers can be health-care workers, nongovernmental organization staff, teachers, religious leaders, or other respected community figures. The drugs needed for DOTS are cheap. However, for the program to achieve and be cost effective, a regular supply of quality-assured medication is needed, which is where the Global Drug Facility has a key role to play.

In 2015, the global initiative against TB escalates to an end-game strategy called End TB by the WHO, and includes a target date of 2035 for reducing TB deaths worldwide by 95 percent.

Treatment for TB

Ukrainian American biochemist Selman Waksman (1888–1973) studied the bacteria that live in the soil and synthesize many compounds that can fight infection. Waksman coined the term *antibiotic* for these compounds and discovered streptomycin, the first effective drug against TB, in 1943. Streptomycin was isolated from the soil bacterium *Streptomyces griseus.* Waksman was awarded the Nobel Prize for his discovery in 1952.

Unfortunately, streptomycin began to lose its power against TB after only a few months, owing to the development of resistance. However, Waksman's discovery had stimulated the search for drugs to counter TB. Several more drugs, including isoniazid, kanamycin, rifampin, and pyrazinamide, were discovered in the 1950s. All these drugs attack the TB bacterium in a different way, and it was soon realized that the best approach to TB treatment was to use a combination of drugs because resistance is then less likely to develop. Since the 1960s, the pharmaceutical industry has shown less interest in developing new drugs against infection, including TB, focusing more upon noncommunicable diseases such as cancer and heart disease. Thus, TB treatments in the 2010s rely on drugs discovered 50 or more years ago.

⊕ Impacts and Issues

A Worldwide Public Health Problem

TB is the fifth-most-important cause of death worldwide, and the second-leading cause of death from infectious disease, after HIV/AIDS. It is overwhelmingly a disease of poverty and primarily affects people between the ages of 15 to 64, robbing them of their most productive years. Most cases of TB and deaths occur among men, but women also are affected. Out of 1.5 million total TB deaths in 2013, around half a million women died from the disease (about a third of whom also had HIV). TB is not generally a disease of children, but there were 80,000 deaths among HIV-negative children from the disease in 2013.

TB is present in all regions of the world. In 2013, the South-East Asia and Western Pacific WHO Regions accounted for 56 percent of the world's cases of TB.

The African region had around 25 percent of cases and the highest rates of cases and deaths relative to the population. India and China had the highest absolute number of cases, because of their large populations, and accounted for 24 percent and 11 percent of the global total, respectively. There are also high numbers of TB cases in Nigeria, Pakistan, Indonesia, and South Africa. The rates of incident TB vary widely among countries. The lowest rates are found in high-income countries, including most countries in western Europe, Canada, the United States, Japan, Australia, and New Zealand.

Globally, the UN MDG 6 target of stopping and reversing TB incidence by 2015 has been achieved, as the incidence rate has fallen by 1.5 percent, on average, each year since 2000. Since 1990, the TB mortality rate has declined by 45 percent, and the prevalence rate by 41 percent. Although TB is on the decline, and effective

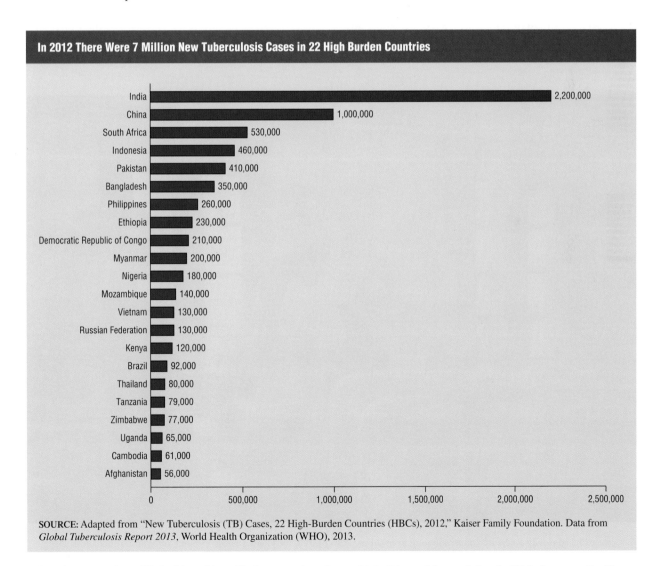

In 2012 There Were 7 Million New Tuberculosis Cases in 22 High Burden Countries

India	2,200,000
China	1,000,000
South Africa	530,000
Indonesia	460,000
Pakistan	410,000
Bangladesh	350,000
Philippines	260,000
Ethiopia	230,000
Democratic Republic of Congo	210,000
Myanmar	200,000
Nigeria	180,000
Mozambique	140,000
Vietnam	130,000
Russian Federation	130,000
Kenya	120,000
Brazil	92,000
Thailand	80,000
Tanzania	79,000
Zimbabwe	77,000
Uganda	65,000
Cambodia	61,000
Afghanistan	56,000

SOURCE: Adapted from "New Tuberculosis (TB) Cases, 22 High-Burden Countries (HBCs), 2012," Kaiser Family Foundation. Data from *Global Tuberculosis Report 2013*, World Health Organization (WHO), 2013.

Tuberculosis is a major public health problem affecting approximately one-third of the world's population. In 2012, there were 7 million new cases of tuberculosis in 22 high-burden countries alone.

diagnosis and treatment have saved an estimated 37 million people between 2000 and 2013, the death toll remains high, given that this is a largely preventable and curable disease. Indeed, to achieve the Stop TB Partnership target of halving the TB mortality and prevalence rate by 2015, compared to a 1990 baseline, an acceleration in current rates of decline is required.

TB and HIV Coinfection

HIV infection renders a person susceptible to active TB because it undermines the immune system. Thus, part of the resurgence of TB since the late 1990s can be attributed to the spread of HIV. Around 1.1 million of the 9 million people who developed TB in 2013 were HIV positive. The WHO African Region accounts for 80 percent of HIV-positive TB cases and TB deaths among those who are HIV positive. In part of southern Africa, more than half of TB cases also have HIV. At least one-third of the 35 million people living with HIV worldwide are infected with latent TB. If active TB develops, and diagnosis and treatment are delayed, HIV patients are at high risk of dying from drug-resistant TB.

TB accounts for 30 to 40 percent of mortality from AIDS. The interaction between TB and HIV is an urgent public health issue because it influences both the transmission of TB and the morbidity and mortality from both TB and HIV. The lifetime risk of an HIV-negative person developing TB is just 10 percent, but when the person is HIV-positive, this increases to 10 percent per year. Moreover, TB may affect areas other than the lungs in the HIV-positive patient, and it tends to be more difficult to diagnose. Between 2005 and 2011, collaborative WHO TB/HIV activities have saved an estimated 1.3 million lives. However, more needs to be done in terms of ensuring universal access to life-saving diagnosis and treatment in this vulnerable group.

Drug-Resistant TB

There has been an increase in TB that is resistant to the drugs normally used to treat it. These infections are either resistant to one drug or to more than one. The latter are known as multidrug-resistant TB (MDR TB) or extensively drug resistant TB (XDR TB). The main

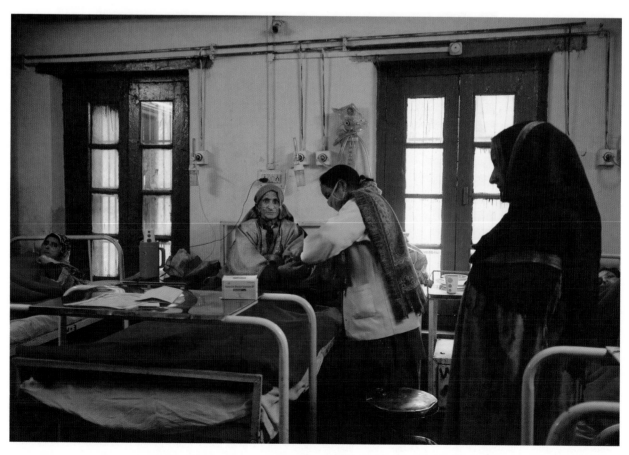

A doctor treats an elderly Kashmiri woman suffering from tuberculosis (TB) at the Chest Disease Hospital on World Tuberculosis Day in Srinagar, India. India has the highest incidence of TB in the world, according to the World Health Organization's *Global Tuberculosis Report 2013*, with as many as 2.4 million cases. The disease kills about 300,000 people every year in the country. India also saw the greatest increase in multidrug-resistant TB between 2011 and 2012. © *Mukhtar Khan/AP Images.*

reason for drug-resistant TB is failure to complete a course of treatment. The mechanism is similar to that for antibiotic resistance in other infections: the drug kills the weaker bacteria first, and the whole course must be taken to kill the whole bacterial population. If treatment stops early, the stronger bacteria, which are more resistant to the drug, remain.

Drug-resistant strains of TB are found in many countries and are, as the name suggests, hard to treat, which adds to the cost of treatment. The lengthier treatment required for drug-resistant TB can be up to 200 times as expensive as standard treatment. MDR TB is a particular problem where health systems are weak or in disarray because of conflict or poverty. It is also found where there are high rates of HIV infection. Thus, the locations where drug-resistant TB are more likely to exist are precisely those least able to afford the added difficulty and costs of treatment.

In 2013, 5 percent of all TB was estimated to be MDR TB. An estimated 480,000 people developed MDR TB of whom 210,000 died. Meanwhile, 100 countries reported XDR TB in 2013 and around 9 percent of those with drug-resistant TB have XDR TB. If all TB patients had been tested for drug resistance in 2013, an estimated 300,000 cases of MDR TB would have been identified. More patients with drug-resistant TB are being treated: around 97,000 patients began treatment in 2013, which is a threefold increase compared with 2009. There are two new drugs, bedaquiline and delamanid, for the treatment of drug-resistant TB. Also, there are novel and shortened treatments currently under investigation.

Action on TB

The WHO declared TB to be a global emergency in 1993 following its sudden resurgence. This has led to significant progress in the fight against the disease. The mortality rate has fallen by 45 percent since 1990, and TB incidence rates are decreasing in most parts of the world.

In the global health context, AIDS, TB, and malaria are seen as the key threats to countries and communities. Therefore, the Global Fund to Fight AIDS, Tuberculosis and Malaria was formed in 2002. The role of the fund is to provide the financial support to put plans in place to fight these diseases into action. The fund is a partnership between public and private sectors with the WHO, the Joint United Nations Programme on HIV/AIDS (UNAIDS), and the World Bank. It is financed by governments, the public and private sector, and charitable foundations, such as the Bill & Melinda Gates Foundation. Although the fund does carry out some advocacy work, its main role is to finance programs in its three diseases, with a particular focus upon AIDS and Africa. The fund provides 80 percent of funding for TB globally.

⊕ Future Implications

The year 2015 marks the beginning of the post-MDG era. The WHO has set up a post-2015 global strategy for TB known as End TB Strategy (as opposed to the Stop TB Strategy). This was approved by all member states at the WHO May 2014 World Health Assembly. The overall goal of End TB is to eradicate the global TB epidemic. This means aiming for a 95 percent reduction in TB deaths and a 90 percent reduction in TB incidence by 2035, compared with levels in 2015.

Within the End TB Strategy, there are some important five-year milestones to keep the plans on track. For instance, by 2020 no TB patients or their families should be experiencing a heavy financial burden because of their TB disease. By 2025, there should be a 75 percent reduction in TB deaths, compared with 2015. The WHO has set out three strands to its post-2015 TB strategy: patient-centered care and prevention, bold policies and supportive systems, and intensified research and innovation.

TB Research and Innovation

Current technology for prevention, care, and control will not be sufficient to eliminate TB by 2050. However, investment by the Global Fund already is producing new tools that will strengthen the fight against the disease. In diagnostics, there is the Xpert MTB/RIF test, a DNA-based molecular assay that can diagnose both TB and rifampin resistance rapidly. As of late 2014, this had been introduced in more than 108 countries, and there were many new diagnostic tests under development.

There are also 10 new or repurposed drugs in late clinical development and new drug combinations that allow shorter treatment of all forms of TB. Meanwhile, there are 15 new vaccines in clinical trial as of late 2014. However, there are still some significant gaps in TB research. The WHO is calling for research across a broad spectrum, from basic science to socio-behavioral research, to improve health-related practices of TB patients, caregivers, and health-care workers. There also is a need to innovate in the larger policy and health system environment. In short, there needs to be a multidimensional approach, with creation of a research-enabling environment at both the national and international levels.

PRIMARY SOURCE

Reaching People with MDR-TB

SOURCE The Expand-TB Project: Progress and Impact Brief: Reaching People with MDR-TB: Progress in Diagnosis: A Key Step in Overcoming the MDR-TB Crisis. *The Expand-TB Project, World Health Organization (WHO)*, 2014, 1–2. http://www.who.int/campaigns/tb-day/2014/tb-brochure.pdf?ua=1 (accessed January 25, 2015).

INTRODUCTION *This primary source is excerpted from a 2014 brief produced by the EXPAND-TB Project of the World Health Organization. The project "was initiated in 2009 to accelerate access to diagnostics for patients at risk of MDR-TB in 27 low- and middle-income countries."*

THE MDR-TB CRISIS

BACKGROUND

In 2013, the World Health Organization (WHO) called for multidrug-resistant tuberculosis (MDR-TB) to be addressed as a public health crisis. MDR-TB is a global health security risk and carries grave consequences for those affected.

Globally in 2012, WHO estimates that 450 000 people fell ill with MDR-TB and there were 170 000 MDR-TB deaths.

The public health crisis of MDR-TB has three main elements which need to be addressed urgently.

1. Access to diagnostic services:

In 2012, only as few as 94 000 people (one in four) who were estimated to have MDR-TB were detected. This includes 84 000 people with confirmed MDR-TB plus 10 000 with rifampicin resistance. While this number represents nearly a 50% increase in MDR-TB detection as compared to 2011, progress towards reaching all people with MDR-TB remains far off-track.

2. Treatment coverage:

Beyond expanding access to diagnostic services, a key challenge is treatment coverage for people with MDR-TB. Just over 77 000 people with MDR-TB were started on second-line treatment in 2012, leaving at least 16 000 detected patients without treatment. Treatment coverage gaps for detected cases were much larger in some countries, especially in the African Region (51% enrolled in treatment), and widened in China, Pakistan and South Africa.

3. Quality of care:

Intensified efforts are also needed to improve quality of care for drug-resistant TB. The treatment success rate for MDR-TB patients is currently low at 48%. This suggests that most countries are not achieving high treatment success due to high mortality rates and a large number of patients being lost to follow up.

DIAGNOSING DRUG-RESISTANT TB: WHY IT MATTERS

Worldwide, less than one in four of the people estimated to have fallen ill with MDR-TB were detected in 2012.

Overcoming the MDR-TB crisis hinges on the scaling up of diagnostic capacity in countries to detect drug-resistant TB. Matching this with improved access to quality treatment and care completes the chain to enable people with MDR-TB to get the care they need.

BOTTLENECKS IN REACHING PEOPLE WITH MDR-TB

Limited access

Diagnostic services for MDR-TB are generally not easily accessible to patients.... The high prices of some new diagnostic tests also pose financial barriers for access.

Lack of functional laboratories capable of providing quality assured TB diagnostic services

Modern diagnostics available through a network of appropriate and quality-assured laboratories will have a sustainable impact on MDR-TB control. However, laboratory capacity currently varies widely among resource-constrained countries, with generally few having reference laboratories capable of performing the recommended tests for MDR-TB including TB culture and drug susceptibility testing (DST).

Most countries still use outdated techniques which miss many people with TB and MDR-TB. The high price of new diagnostic equipment, together with the costs of training of staff and establishing new procedures inhibits countries from taking first steps towards modernizing their laboratories.

Shortage of well-trained staff

The tests for diagnosis of MDR-TB require skilled operators. Human resources at country level often don't have the skills required.

SEE ALSO *Antibiotic/Antimicrobial Resistance; Bacterial Diseases; Global Health Initiatives; HIV/AIDS*

BIBLIOGRAPHY

Books

Bynum, Helen. *Spitting Blood: The History of Tuberculosis.* Oxford: Oxford University Press, 2012.

Dubos, René, and Jean Dubos. *The White Plague: Tuberculosis, Man, and Society.* New Brunswick, NJ: Rutgers University Press, 1987.

Murphy, Jim, and Alison Blank. *Invincible Microbe: Tuberculosis and the Never-Ending Search for a Cure.* Boston: Clarion Books, 2012.

Skolnik, Richard. *Essentials of Global Health.* Sudbury, MA: Jones and Bartlett, 2008.

Periodicals

Babaria, Palav. "Threatened Hope: PEPFAR and Health in Africa." *New England Journal of Medicine* 369, no. 15 (October 10, 2013): 1388–1389.

Barry, Clifton, and Maija Cheung. "New Tactics in the Fight against Tuberculosis." *Scientific American* (March 2009): 62.

Websites

"Global Tuberculosis Report 2014." *World Health Organization*, 2014. http://www.who.int/tb/publications/global_report/en/ (accessed January 16, 2015).

Stop TB Partnership. http://www.stoptb.org/ (accessed January 16, 2015).

"Tuberculosis," Fact Sheet no. 104. *World Health Organization (WHO)*, October 2014. http://www.who.int/mediacentre/factsheets/fs104/en/ (accessed January 16, 2015).

Susan Aldridge

Universal Health Coverage

⊕ Introduction

Universal health coverage (UHC) means that all people within a country or region will have access to the categories of health services that they require, defined by the World Health Organization (WHO) as "prevention, promotion, treatment, rehabilitation, and palliative care, of sufficient quality to be effective," without potentially experiencing financial devastation in order to obtain necessary care.

Obtaining needed care does not imply that every possible desired service will be provided by a UHC scheme. There will nearly always be services that exist outside the system and are available on an as-desired basis, often requiring direct, or out-of-pocket, payment. An example of an à la carte service might be desired cosmetic surgery to reverse the appearance of aging. Needed care would be the menu of services that ensure ongoing health, such as annual well-checks and periodic health screenings, sick care to include diagnostics, treatment protocols and medications, surgical and intensive medical interventions when called for, and palliative care at the end of life to ensure a comfortable death. Palliative care is the range of services and medications necessary to ensure comfort and to eliminate or manage pain, but not aimed at curing a disease or reversing a terminal process.

There are three core principles underlying the provision of UHC. The first is that the coverage must be delivered equitably to all who need it; that is, quality and access to care are not dependent on socioeconomic status. The second is that the services must be of good quality and should be aimed not just at treatment of illness, but also at prevention, wellness, and health improvement. The third core value is that costs of care should be sufficiently low as to prevent financial hardship. Out-of-pocket costs should be kept as low as possible, to minimize the burden on the patient and family. When costs are high, individuals do not seek out preventive care and often remain either undertreated or entirely untreated in times of illness, injury, or chronic condition.

⊕ Historical Background

The concept of UHC is not new. In the late 19th century, German Chancellor Otto von Bismarck sought to make widespread health coverage available to blue-collar workers. In 1883, he introduced legislation called the Health Insurance Bill, which was an effective means of ensuring quality and affordable health care for the working class.

After World War II (1939–1945) and the vast medical and economic challenges in its aftermath, many countries began to consider new ways of providing care for widespread populations. Many industrialized nations, democracies and socialist countries alike, sought to provide universal access to quality health care regardless of ability to pay for services and created sweeping health care reforms.

According to data published by the WHO, the first region to set up a national health-care system was the United Kingdom, in 1948. The National Health Service was financed by taxation of the general population, and all citizens were equally entitled to care. Japan was next in 1961, with reforms that provided UHC across the nation. The underlying rationale had to do with a philosophy of providing the people with needed and desired benefits. South Korea's national health insurance was promoted by President Park Chung-hee in 1977. In 1988, Brazil launched universal health services, financed by taxation revenues and spurred on by a new government. South Africa was next, in 1994. The African National Congress government put tax-financed services in place for children below the age of six years, as well as pregnant women. The newly installed populist government of Thailand extended universal coverage in 2001. In 2006, Zambia launched free health care for people in rural areas and extended the program to urban areas in 2009. Free health care for pregnant women and their children was initiated in Burundi in 2006, in Ghana in 2008, and in Sierra Leone in 2010. Nepal adopted universal free health care up to the hospital level in 2008.

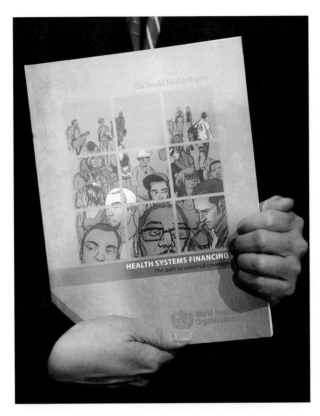

The director-general of the World Health Organization (WHO) Margaret Chan holds a copy of *The World Health Report 2010*, its presentation at the German health ministry in Berlin on November 22, 2010. More than 100 million people are plunged into poverty every year by illness or "catastrophic" medical bills, the WHO said, as it launched a global drive for universal health care.
© *Odd Andersen/AFP/Getty Images.*

By the end of 2008, it was reported that approximately 50 countries had instituted some form of UHC.

In response to unrest in the populace, China significantly expanded public spending programs to enhance service coverage and to cover financial protections (lowering out-of-pocket costs for those seeking care) in 2009. In 2012, the country of Georgia expanded health coverage to all citizens. The United States is the only developed country without a universal health-care system as of the mid-2010s. The Patient Protection and Affordable Care Act is a national health-care system reform instituted by President Barack Obama's administration as a means of ensuring affordable health care in a manner that is designed to dramatically decrease the number of uninsured or underinsured citizens, however, it does not cover everyone under one national plan. That a nation or region has UHC does not necessarily mean that health care is free. Nearly every UHC system involves some direct payment, or out-of-pocket costs. (See graphic.)

According to the WHO, the next block of countries focused on for universal health-care provision are those with developing and emerging economies. India is

a prime example, having launched in 2008 a health insurance system designed to provide systematically increasing health care access to its most impoverished areas. The program is called Rashtriya Swasthya Bima Yojana (National Health Insurance Program); by 2012 it was providing free and easily accessible health care to about 100 million people being served in more than 8,000 public and private medical centers, health-care facilities, and hospitals across the country. The nation's goal is to provide health care that is affordable and accessible to the entire population of India by 2022.

⊕ Impacts and Issues

In many areas of the world, medical care has historically been largely financed by out-of-pocket, or direct, payments for services. This has often had one of two outcomes. First, people choose not to seek necessary preventive, restorative, or required care because they are unable to afford it, leading to negative and often far more costly health outcomes. Or second, they expend all personal resources, take out loans, divest themselves of personal property such as homes and vehicles, lose employment, or borrow money in order to obtain necessary care, as in the case of devastating illness or the aftermath of an accident. This can push people, even those of middle income and relative financial security, into financial ruin. In developed or high-income countries, the direct payment cost of catastrophic illness has been a primary cause of financial collapse and has led to a significant percentage of personal bankruptcies.

In order for UHC to be possible, there must exist a health delivery system that is efficient, effective, financially sound, and accessible to virtually the entire population. It must offer a broad-based package of consistent, good-quality services delivered by well-trained, competent health-care workers. It must offer ready access to a continuum of medications and pharmaceutical products and have available the technologies necessary for diagnosis and treatment, such as x rays, scanners, and surgical systems.

The finance mechanisms for a system of UHC must be sound, efficient (offering good to excellent value for the cost), and equitable (offering necessary services to all without preferential treatment given to those who can afford to pay high direct costs). In addition, they must offer a program that protects people from extreme financial hardship when contributing to the cost of their health care. No person or group should be pushed into poverty to pay for needed care and services in a system of UHC.

There are two primary funding schemes for UHC systems: the Beveridge model and the Bismarck model. The Beveridge model funds services through a government organized health-care system and pays for them through tax revenues. Some countries using variations of

THE UNITED STATES AND "OBAMACARE"

The United States is unique in many ways, not the least of which is its diversity. It has a very heterogeneous population, with many cultures, sets of values, and attitudes toward public health care. In the developed world of middle- and high-income countries, the United States stands alone, as of 2015, in its lack of implementation of a universal-health-care system. A significant proportion of the populace has been arguing in favor of universal health coverage for decades and has been quite vocal in expressing the need for affordable health care for all.

The Obama administration made affordable health-care insurance for all Americans a central part of its campaign platforms. The correct name for what is colloquially referred to as "Obamacare" is the Patient Protection and Affordable Care Act (PPACA), and it was enacted on March 23, 2010. Since its inception, it has been at the epicenter of significant bipartisan debate and the subject of federal lawsuits. It was alleged that requiring all people in the United States to obtain some form of health-care coverage was a violation of constitutional rights. The U.S. Supreme Court, in a ruling published on June 28, 2012, deemed that all provisions but one of the PPACA were within the law. The one segment that was deemed unconstitutional had to do with requiring all states to expand their Medicaid coverage to all otherwise-eligible individuals living at up to 133 percent of the federal poverty level.

The U.S. Census Bureau reported that the percentage of individuals in the United States without health insurance in 2010 was 16.3, which translates to 49.9 million uninsured. During the first quarter of 2015, the uninsured percentage was estimated to be approximately 12 percent, down from a high of 20 percent in 2013. It has been reported that, by the end of the 2014 open enrollment period, in excess of 15 million people who were uninsured prior to 2010 when the PPACA was enacted had ongoing, affordable (based on continuing payment of health-care premiums) health insurance coverage.

PPACA requires that all people residing in the United States obtain and maintain health-care coverage. In order to make it affordable, the legislation increased subsidies for middle-income families, while increasing taxes for those at the highest incomes as well as a continuum of health-care providers who are also high wage earners. It is considered the most comprehensive health-care reform in the United States since 1935's Social Security Act.

Some of the guiding principles of the PPACA are: (1) parents may now keep their children on their health insurance plans until the offspring are 26 years of age; and (2) there was an issue called a donut hole in prescription benefits for those on Medicare, in which beneficiaries might be required to pay a large portion of prescription costs after utilizing specific benefit amounts; PPACA subsidizes those costs and proposes to eliminate them by 2020; and (3) Those with preexisting conditions may no longer be excluded from obtaining health insurance coverage or dropped from coverage because of development of a catastrophic illness.

PPACA has initiated the use of health-care exchanges, which are typically either federal- or state-run cooperatives where individuals can go, either in person or online, to view a menu of health insurers and choose the provider and service menu that best suits their needs. This is believed to be especially useful for individuals who are self-employed or whose employers do not offer health insurance plans.

The overarching goal of PPACA is to encourage prevention, health promotion, and increased wellness by ensuring low-cost or free wellness and preventive care, while providing affordable health care to all and lowering health-care costs over time. The theory is that costs will go down when people are paying more attention to remaining healthy, thereby avoiding many of the chronic noncommunicable diseases such as diabetes,

this model are Thailand, Brazil, Sri Lanka, Malaysia, and Indonesia. The Bismarck model utilizes a mixed funding model with mandatory insurance coverage paid for with contributions from employers and workers through the use of direct deductions from the employee's payroll. Most countries use a mixed funding scheme combining aspects of both models.

When people have access to quality and affordable health care, they are far more likely to seek preventive and maintenance services. Rather than waiting until an illness or injury has reached a critical phase and will require hospitalization, surgery, or extensive treatment, people are more likely to engage in a program wherein they manage low-level, ongoing care, such as an exercise or therapy program to rehabilitate an injury rather than having it worsen and require aggressive intervention; a daily course of maintenance medications for a

chronic health condition rather than becoming very ill and requiring an extended hospital stay; or a program for systematic, outpatient treatment of a potentially life-threatening illness or condition rather than critical, acute inpatient care or potential loss of life.

Often, UHC systems offer programs for preventive care, such as smoking cessation, respiratory and cardiac disease management programs, nutritional counseling, family planning, prenatal care and education, and diabetes and kidney disease management programs, encouraging members to make positive health decisions that minimize the need for more intensive interventions over time. In sum, people tend to be healthier and to make more positive lifestyle choices when afforded UHC.

There is no single algorithm or formula to help countries determine how much capital they should be able to allocate for health care. According to the WHO, hypertension, and many forms of cancer, and needing to use fewer high-end services. Many of those currently uninsured avoid routine well visits, and do not engage with the health-care system until they are seriously ill and require urgent or emergency services, leading to preventable hospitalizations and costly treatment.

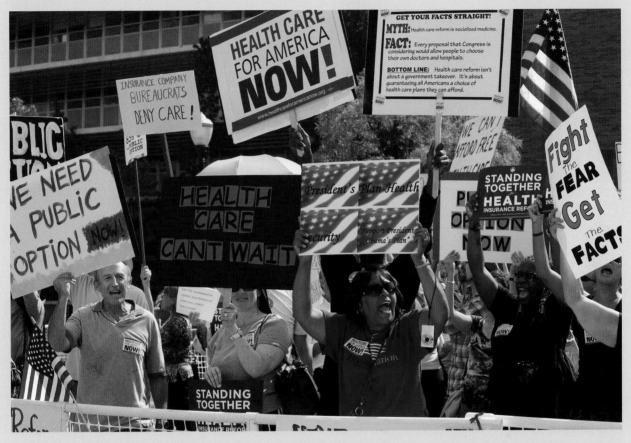

Universal-health-care proponents demonstrate at the University of California, Los Angeles, on August 21, 2009, prior to the implementation of the Patient Protection and Affordable Care Act in the United States, which offered health-care insurance to millions more Americans, but not without controversy that continued into 2015. © *Jose Gil/Shutterstock.com.*

the biggest determinant of a successfully funded system lies in broadening the scope of public entitlement systems and shifting the population base from privately funded health care to public health programming. At the same time, it is necessary to create a package of services that addresses the needs of the entire population, regardless of ability to pay out-of-pocket fees. Historically, health care has been privatized, meaning that it was only accessible to those who could afford to pay substantial premiums.

An ongoing challenge for all health-care systems, particularly those utilizing public funding, is the constantly increasing cost of diagnostic and treatment technology, as well as extremely expensive pharmaceuticals (solvable by increasing competition or preferentially using generic rather than name-brand medications when available). As the global population ages and lives longer, the need for health services increases as well. The type, number, and quantity of services must be determined by each country and region, as the disease burden varies by climate, environment, and, to a significant extent, by lifestyle. Developing countries might be more likely to have endemic diseases such as malaria, diarrheal diseases, and tuberculosis, with higher maternal and infant mortality rates. Their health-care needs will be quite different from those of a developed, middle- to high-income country with a higher incidence of lifestyle-related diseases such as obesity, substance abuse, and diabetes.

Although the estimates per person per country for annual health-care needs will vary widely by economy, the WHO suggests that each nation must be able to allocate a minimum of US$60 dollars per person per year in order to address a basic set of noncommunicable and communicable diseases. For some impoverished and

In 2013 Different Countries Had Varying Levels of Out-of-Pocket Expenditures as a Percent of Total Expenditures on Health

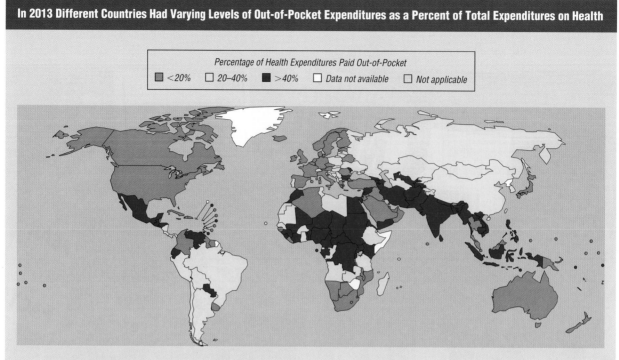

Percentage of Health Expenditures Paid Out-of-Pocket

◼ <20% ☐ 20–40% ◼ >40% ☐ Data not available ☐ Not applicable

SOURCE: Adapted from "Fig. 1.3. Out-of-pocket expenditures on health as a percentage of total expenditure on health, 2013," *The World Health Report 2013*, World Health Organization (WHO), 2013, p. 14, http://apps.who.int/iris/bitstream/10665/85761/2/9789240690837_eng .pdf?ua=1 (accessed January 14, 2015).

developing economies, this is cost-prohibitive, leading the nation to require novel sources of sustainable funding in order to create universal health care. One means of broadening funding is called pooling, in which prepaid contributions in the form of taxes or payroll deductions are combined and then used as a mechanism to pay for services for all, regardless of ability to pay out-of-pocket fees.

Overall, however funded, UHC must be fair and equal for all (equitable); must keep administrative and extraneous costs to a minimum so that the funds go to services provided rather than to highly paid specialty service providers (efficient); and must meet the needs of the population to be served (effective).

⊕ Future Implications

In order for the global community to continue to thrive and grow, for individuals to live healthy and productive lives, and for epidemic and endemic diseases to be managed and in many cases eradicated, there must be a viable means of providing health care to the masses. UHC has been shown to be a solid answer, but there are many issues that must be managed in order for the plans to succeed. As the WHO has repeatedly pointed out, universal health care is a paradigm that is as much politically driven as social and medical. Governments must first support

the idea of UHC, then work to find creative and appropriately sustainable means of funding.

The government must actively support capacity building, including the creation of an infrastructure for developing and maintaining clinics, hospitals, and diverse health-care delivery systems throughout the country. This is often a strain on fragile economies, made more challenging by a lack of available or trained care providers. One way of supporting staffing needs is to hire local community members and offer on-the-ground training and support for them to provide paraprofessional and community-based care for non-emergency issues.

It is also critical for the prevailing government to embrace the idea of UHC as a means of advancing wellness and making the workforce more robust. If there are more healthy workers, there is higher productivity, which stimulates the economy. The investment in creating a large-scale, sustainable, affordable health-care system is sizable. It is not a static process; as technology rapidly advances and diagnostic and other health-care treatment and prevention tools become more sophisticated, the system becomes more expensive to maintain and grow. The costs of providing care continually rise, and it is imperative to build into the system ways of addressing this. The WHO has developed a compendium designed to both illustrate what is currently working and what is evolving in the global movement toward UHC.

When viewed in the context of large-scale epidemics such as SARS, human immunodeficiency virus/acquired immune deficiency syndrome (HIV/AIDS), and Ebola, the financial and human costs of which have been enormous, the investment in preventive care has a rational appeal. There are also human rights issues to be considered in the evolution of UHC systems, particularly in the provision of accessible, affordable care to pregnant women, children, the elderly, and those who are chronically ill or differently abled.

Another formidable challenge, once funding has been implemented, is making certain that the services are targeted to all population segments and that those who most need services receive them in the necessary proportions. That provides special challenges to developing and low-income countries with significant rural communities. Part of the answer lies in the judicious use of highly paid professionals such as doctors, nurses, and pharmacists, and the widespread deployment of paraprofessionals, in order to make the funds go as far as possible. Efficiency and economy of staffing is critically important.

SEE ALSO *Global Health Initiatives; Health as a Human Right and Health-Care Access; Social Theory and Global Health; Vulnerable Populations*

BIBLIOGRAPHY

Books

Altman, Stuart H., and David Shactman. *Power, Politics, and Universal Health Care: The Inside Story of a Century-Long Battle.* Amherst, NY: Prometheus Books, 2011.

Bristol, Nellie. *Global Action toward Universal Health Coverage: A Report of the CSIS Global Health Policy Center.* Washington, DC: Center for Strategic & International Studies, 2014.

Bump, Jesse B. *The Long Road to Universal Health Coverage: A Century of Lessons for Development Strategy.* Seattle, WA: PATH—A Catalyst for Global Health, 2010.

Giedion, Ursula, Eduardo Andres Alfonso, and Yadira Diaz. *The Impact of Universal Coverage Schemes in the Developing World: A Review of the Existing Evidence.* Washington, DC: World Bank, 2013.

Maeda, Akiko, et al. *Universal Health Coverage for Inclusive and Sustainable Development: A Synthesis of 11 Country Case Studies.* Washington, DC: World Bank, 2014.

Redwood, Heinz. *Why Ration Health Care?: An International Study of the United Kingdom, France, Germany and Public Sector Health Care in the USA.* London: Institute for the Study of Civil Society, 2000.

Shimazaki, Kenji. *The Path to Universal Health Coverage—Experiences and Lessons from Japan for Policy Actions.* Tokyo: Japan International Cooperation Agency, 2013.

World Health Organization. *Arguing for Universal Health Coverage.* Geneva: WHO Press, 2013.

Periodicals

White, Franklin. "Primary Health Care and Public Health: Foundations of Universal Health Systems." *Medical Principles and Practice* 24, no. 2 (2015): 103–116.

Websites

Banthin, Jessica, and Sarah Masi. "CBO's Estimate of the Net Budgetary Impact of the Affordable Care Act's Health Insurance Coverage Provisions Has Not Changed Much Over Time." *Congressional Budget Office (U.S.)*, May 14, 2013. http://www.cbo.gov/publication/44176 (accessed March 26, 2015).

Cook, Lindsey. "Percentage of Uninsured Americans Now Lowest on Record." *U.S. News & World Report*, July 10, 2014. http://www.usnews.com/news/blogs/data-mine/2014/07/10/percentage-of-uninsured-americans-now-lowest-on-record (accessed March 26, 2015).

"Health Insurance: Highlights 2010." *U.S. Census Bureau.* http://www.census.gov/hhes/www/hlthins/data/incpovhlth/2010/highlights.html (accessed March 23, 2015).

Mendes, Elizabeth. "Fewer Americans Getting Health Insurance from Employer." *Gallup*, February 22, 2013. http://www.gallup.com/poll/160676/fewer-americans-getting-health-insurance-employer.aspx (accessed March 26, 2015).

Mukherjee, Anit. "India's New Health Policy: A Work in Progress." *Center for Global Development*, March 16, 2015. http://www.cgdev.org/blog/indias-new-health-policy-work-progress (accessed March 23, 2015).

"Universal Health Coverage (UHC)," Fact Sheet No. 395. *World Health Organization (WHO)*, September 2014. http://www.who.int/mediacentre/factsheets/fs395/en/ (accessed March 26, 2015).

"What Is Universal Coverage?" *World Health Organization (WHO).* http://www.who.int/health_financing/universal_coverage_definition/en/ (accessed March 23, 2015).

Pamela V. Michaels

Vaccine-Preventable Diseases

🌐 Introduction

Vaccine-preventable diseases are communicable afflictions that currently have an available and effective immunization method. In 2013, the World Health Organization (WHO) estimated approximately 1.5 million deaths among children under the age of five were caused by vaccine-preventable diseases. Ninety-six percent of these deaths were caused by only five diseases (pneumococcal diseases, rotavirus, *Haemophilus influenzae* type b [Hib], pertussis, and measles). More than one-third of all deaths in children under age five are preventable through vaccination.

Vaccines, or immunizations, are currently listed by the WHO for 24 different infectious agents or illnesses; 15 of these are recommended as routine, while others are recommended for those traveling to areas where certain agents or illnesses are endemic. Vaccine-preventable diseases are caused by invading bacteria or their toxins, viruses, and parasites. Younger children and the elderly and immunocompromised are at greater risk for these infections due to their immature immune systems. However, this susceptibility is compounded in developing countries where limited health services and environmental conditions allow these pathogens to spread relatively uncontested. Overpopulation, pollution, and scarcity of food are all conditions that increase the likeliness that vaccine-preventable diseases will result in serious illness or death.

The human immune system protects itself through two methods: innate and acquired immunity. Innate immunity includes a variety of primordial mechanisms to prevent pathogens from invading the body. In the event of an infection, the innate immune system can also dispatch specific cells, referred to as phagocytic cells, to kill and digest the pathogen. Intruding microorganisms are also destroyed by substances in the skin, blood, saliva, and tears. Acquired immunity, a relatively more recent human adaptation to combating diseases, involves the recognition of specific pathogens and producing a tailor-made immune response. Each pathogen carries a distinct substance called an antigen, which triggers the creation of antibodies. Antibodies then attach to the antigens and begin inactivating or removing the pathogen.

Vaccines rely on an important characteristic of the acquired immune response. The acquired immune response has the ability to recall every previous encounter it has had with an antigen. With each following exposure, the immune response becomes faster and more effective at signaling a defense. This "immunological memory" is the underlying mechanism that makes vaccination so effective. By exposing the human body's immune system to inert forms of different pathogens, antibodies are produced that serve as primers for an effective defense against future infections.

🌐 Historical Background

As of 2013, the WHO recommends 21 vaccines for preventable diseases in the 18th WHO Model List of Essential Medicines. Vaccine-preventable diseases are generally caused by either viral or bacterial infections. Bacterial microorganisms, one form of infectious microbes, cause diseases such as cholera, diphtheria, and pertussis. Viruses, another form of infectious pathogen, are responsible for illnesses like measles and poliomyelitis (polio).

Bacterial Vaccine-Preventable Diseases

The *Haemophilus influenzae* type b (Hib) bacteria is one of the primary causes of death in children under age 5 around the world. Originally thought to be the pathogen responsible for influenza, this bacteria was recognized as its own separate entity in 1918. Contrary to what its name implies, Hib is actually a bacterial infection that is spread through direct contact with respiratory secretions. Children living in crowded households with poor sanitation are particularly susceptible to this disease. Following infection, the Hib bacteria weakens the host's immune system as it spreads through the bloodstream, causing a variety

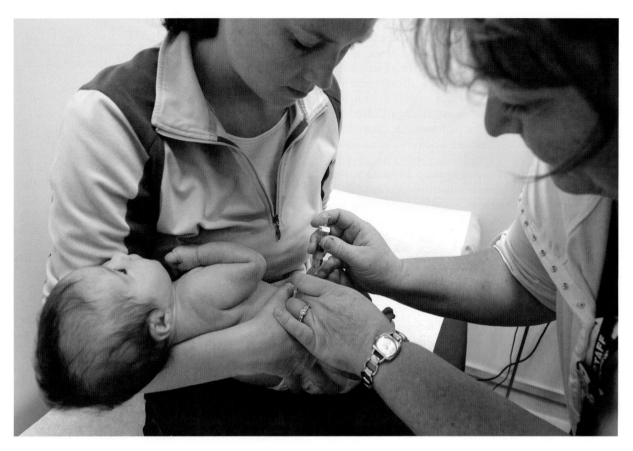

A newborn receives the first of what will be a series of more than 20 vaccinations recommended in the first two years of life for all children to help minimize the risk of vaccine-preventable diseases such as tetanus, diphtheria, pertussis, chicken pox, and other infectious diseases. © *ChameleonsEye/Shutterstock.com.*

of different diseases. The most common conditions associated with Hib are meningitis (infection of the membranes protecting the brain and nervous system) and pneumonia (infection of the lungs). As of 2006, the Hib vaccination has been included on the WHO's list of essential medicines.

Pertussis or "whooping cough" is caused by the *Bordetella pertussis* bacterium. The bacteria infects the respiratory tract and causes damage to the cilia, which are small hair like structures that work to remove particulate matter from the lungs. When the cilia are impaired, mucus begins to build up, triggering a coughing response. The term whooping comes from the unabated fits of violent coughing attacks, which often result in sudden gasping for air (the term pertussis is derived from the Latin per, meaning "thoroughly," and tussis, which means "to cough"). Infants are less capable of forceful coughing in order to maintain an open airway. Any prolonged oxygen deprivation can result in brain damage. Primarily a childhood disease, adults and adolescents can serve as a potential reservoir for the pertussis pathogen, thereby spreading it to younger populations. Recent epidemiological evidence shows 95 percent of the pertussis cases worldwide occurred in developing countries, resulting in about 200,000 deaths. In 2012, the WHO estimated

22.8 million children did not receive the pertussis vaccination before their first birthday.

Pneumococcal disease is caused by the *Streptococcus pneumonia* bacterium. This pathogen lives in the upper portion of the respiratory system, located just below the nasal cavity. As the name suggests, this bacterial infection can result in pneumonia if it spreads to the lungs. The pathogen can also spread to other locations and bodily tissues, resulting in middle ear infections (otitis media), sinus infections (sinusitis), and in rare cases, infections can spread to the joints, bones, and the bloodstream. The disease usually presents with a fever, difficulty breathing, and chest pain. As with the other respiratory illnesses discussed, risk of contracting the disease is increased by crowded living spaces and poor hygienic conditions. A variety of risk factors can also increase a person's susceptibility to pneumococcal diseases, such as HIV infections, diabetes, chronic lung disorders, alcohol abuse, smoking, or asthma. In 2009, a newly developed vaccination against pneumococcal disease was added to the WHO vaccination schedule for children as early as six weeks of age. The WHO strongly encourages vaccination programs for countries with mortality rates for children under five years of age over 50 per 1,000 births.

The causative agent for tetanus is the bacterium *Clostridium tetani*. Unlike the previously described vaccine-preventable diseases, tetanus infections do not spread from person to person. The bacterium, in its very stable spore form, is pervasive throughout the environment and is introduced to the body through injuries or puncture wounds (old, rusty nails serve as prime candidates for tetanus infections). Once the pathogen has entered the body, it reproduces and releases a powerful neurotoxin. This toxin interferes with the human body's muscle contractile functions, resulting in spasms. Individuals that have contracted the disease often initially experience these muscle spasms in the face and neck, resulting in a condition referred to as lockjaw (or medically as trismus). As the illness progresses, patients may experience additional spasms of the back muscles, an ailment called opisthotonos posturing. Pregnant women and newborns are especially susceptible to tetanus infections, particularly during unhygienic birthing practices. Due to worldwide vaccination efforts, the WHO estimated tetanus infections resulted in the deaths of 49,000 newborns in 2013, down 94 percent from the 1988 estimate of 787,000 newborn deaths.

The WHO also recommends vaccinations for bacterial infections that cause cholera, diphtheria, meningococcal meningitis, tuberculosis, and typhoid. Cholera outbreaks typically occur as a result of unsanitary drinking water. Cholera was generally on the decline from 1991 to 2004, however, outbreaks began to increase in 2005, especially in Africa (representing more than 90 percent of all cases from 2001 to 2009) until 2010, when an outbreak in Haiti began. By 2013, cholera levels had decreased again, with Haiti representing 47 percent of all cases and Africa 44 percent.

Diphtheria infections cause sore throat and breathing difficulties, which can be fatal if untreated. As of 2012, fewer than 5,000 diphtheria cases were reported, and the global coverage for the diphtheria vaccine among infants is 84 percent.

Meningococcal meningitis has a high fatality rate (more than half of those infected die), and commonly arises in sub-Saharan Africa. Transmission of the disease takes place through coughing, sneezing, or contact with infected saliva. In 2010, the WHO developed an effective meningococcal vaccine that was able to reach over 150 million people by 2013, although one serogroup, type B, did not have a vaccine for it until the following year.

Tuberculosis is a respiratory infection that can be fatal if left untreated. Although as much as one-third of the global population is infected with this bacterium, most people do not exhibit symptoms. However, a positive skin test can show previous exposure. The current tuberculosis vaccine (bacille Calmette-Guérin, or BCG) provides partial protection in children against the pathogen but is not used in many parts of the developed world and is contraindicated in children infected with HIV.

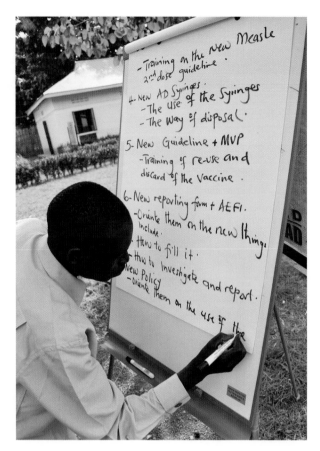

A participant gives instructions in a training session in South Sudan, as part of the East Africa Training Project (EATP). The endeavor aims to improve the routine immunization systems and protect the inhabitants of Uganda, Ethiopia, and South Sudan from vaccine-preventable diseases. According to the U.S. Centers for Disease Control and Prevention, "Due to its success, EATP, originally planned for 18 months, received funding so it could continue for another year (through mid-2014). The extension means even more officers will develop the skills necessary to protect the children in their country from deadly but vaccine-preventable diseases." *Steve Stewart/U.S Centers for Disease Control and Prevention.*

Typhoid is spread via contaminated food or water. Typhoid fever is a more severe disease caused by the *Salmonella typhi* bacteria, while paratyphoid is less severe and caused by a subspecies of the same pathogen. Currently the WHO estimates between 200,000 and 600,000 deaths from typhoid worldwide, with concentrations of the disease in the developing world. Two different vaccinations are available for typhoid; one is recommended for children under two years of age, the other is for children over five years of age. The vaccines do not prevent paratyphoid or other forms of salmonellosis.

Viral Vaccine-Preventable Diseases Rotavirus infections are caused by a virus that enters the body through the mouth. Under extreme magnification, the virus is circular and appears wheel-like. Along its surface, the virus has protruding spokes that attach to human intestinal cells. After attaching, the virus causes a variety of absorption abnormalities. Absorption dysfunction causes an inability to properly take in electrolytes and vital minerals, often resulting in watery diarrhea. Additional signs and symptoms can include fever, abdominal pain, or vomiting. The virus is spread through contact with the stool of infected individuals, either through sharing children's toys or consuming food that was contaminated with infected feces. Approximately 800,000 to 1 million deaths of children under five years of age can be attributed to rotavirus in developing countries. The WHO recommends administering rotavirus vaccines to all children following six weeks of age. Use of rotavirus vaccines in Mexico led to a 50 percent reduction in deaths from diarrhea.

Measles is caused by a single-stranded RNA virus belonging to the genus *Morbillivirus*. The virus enters the body through the droplets and airborne transmission. The pathogen incubates in the upper respiratory tract and in the lymph nodes, which play an important role in the body's immune system. Within a few days following the infection, measles typically presents with a high fever, followed by a distinctive rash. Additional complications resulting from a measles infection include middle ear infections (otitis media), pneumonia, and diarrhea. These complications tend to arise in children under the age of 5 and adults over 20 years of age. Occasionally, measles results in a condition that causes the brain to swell, referred to as acute encephalitis. According to the WHO, vaccination efforts have lowered the number of

worldwide deaths from this pathogen from 562,000 deaths in 2000 to 122,000 deaths in 2012. Currently, most of the deaths occurring from measles infections are the result of poor access to health resources.

Vaccine-preventable diseases caused by viral infections that currently have effective immunizations available also include dengue, hepatitis A/B/E, human papillomavirus (HPV), influenza, Japanese encephalitis, mumps, polio, rabies, rubella, tick-borne encephalitis, varicella (chicken pox and shingles), and yellow fever.

⊕ Impacts and Issues

Populations have increased protection from infectious disease through a process referred to as herd immunity. Herd immunity is the resistance provided to a susceptible group of individuals by a larger proportion of immune individuals. How does this work? Diseases spread through human populations when an infected person comes in contact with a susceptible person (i.e., individuals not immune to the pathogen). By having a large proportion of the population immunized against diseases, the chances of an infected person coming into contact with a vulnerable person is reduced, thereby slowing or even stopping the spread of disease.

Unfortunately, herd immunity does not work against all types of pathogens. If the pathogen can exist in a reservoir (like the tetanus-causing bacteria, *Clostridium*

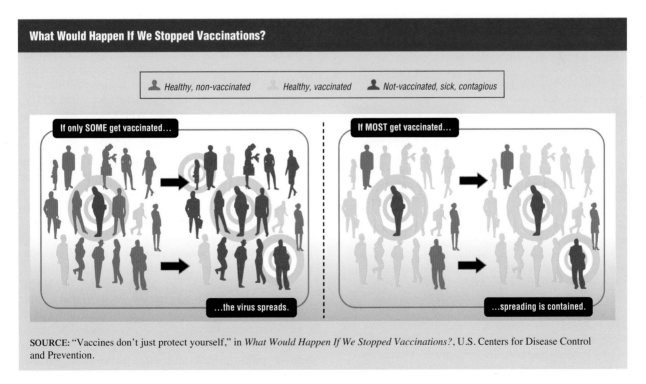

SOURCE: "Vaccines don't just protect yourself," in *What Would Happen If We Stopped Vaccinations?*, U.S. Centers for Disease Control and Prevention.

Herd immunity only works when a majority of people are vaccinated against diseases.

MMR FRAUD AND ANTI-VACCINE MOVEMENTS

In February 1998, an article was published by Andrew Wakefield, a physician from the United Kingdom, in *The Lancet*, one of the United Kingdom's premier medical journals. The paper described a possible link between the measles, mumps, and rubella (MMR) vaccination and autism, a neurodevelopmental disorder, in a small set of children. The findings in the paper asserted, "onset of behavioral symptoms was associated by the parents with measles, mumps, and rubella vaccination in eight of the 12 children." The results went on to declare that the children's symptoms of autism had started within a few weeks after receiving the MMR vaccination.

Rates of autism had been rising for some time when the article was published. Researchers had been unable to answer even the most basic questions on the origin of autism or its causes. When research was published in a respected journal that raised suspicions about the MMR vaccination, what ensued was a "perfect storm" of poor journalism, hysteria, scientific illiteracy, and scandal.

Despite the small sample size in the study, the lack of controls, and no explanation of biological plausibility, many parents in the United Kingdom and United States refused to vaccinate their children with the MMR vaccination. In order for herd immunity to remain in effect for a highly communicable disease like measles, vaccination rates have to stay around 95 percent. In 1995, MMR vaccination rates in the United Kingdom had reached 94 percent. Following the publication of the article, MMR vaccination rates plummeted to 78 percent by 2003. The UK physician Trevor Jones, director of the Association of British Pharmaceutical Industry, issued this public statement: "The development of modern vaccines has been one of the greatest successes of medical science, with many diseases effectively eradicated in Britain. It is vital that we do not squander the position we have reached."

In 2008, a measles endemic was declared in England and Wales. In 2010, *The Lancet* paper was retracted, and Wakefield's medical license was revoked for fraud and medical misconduct. Evidence eventually surfaced that revealed the diagnosis and immunization dates were falsified. Unfortunately, the damage from this calamity has been long lasting and severe. In 2013, a measles outbreak occurred in Swansea, a coastal city in Wales. Before it was declared over, health officials diagnosed more than 1,000 cases and one person was killed as a result of the disease. In the United States, a multistate outbreak occurred beginning in December 2014 at Disneyland in California. By March 20, 2015, 146 people in seven states had been reported as having contracted measles.

In the United States, concerns about vaccination safety centered around the preservative thimerosal. This mercury-containing substance was used in small amounts until it was removed from most vaccinations in 1999. Despite numerous reviews, meta-analyses, and scientific reports published between 2004 and 2014 that demonstrate the lack of evidence for the claim that autism is linked to vaccinations, vaccine concerns persist. Many of these unsubstantiated claims are propagated by entertainment celebrities without expertise in vaccines or public health.

tetani), other means of disease transmission make it impossible for the disease to spread outside of person-to-person contact. Herd immunity can be hindered if infections do not produce complete protection from the disease; partially immune populations do not safeguard susceptible individuals.

Herd immunity also requires that human contact within a population is constantly mixing. In other words, if infected individuals only come into contact with vulnerable individuals, the disease will continue to spread. Obviously, the degree to which people associate with complete strangers varies between populations and cultures. For a highly contagious disease like measles, scientists have projected as much as 95 percent of the population must be immune before herd immunity can occur.

The greatest advantage to successful vaccination programs is that many nonimmune people can be protected from disease because vaccinated individuals serve as a protective barrier against infectious agents. Immune individuals are also less likely to transmit vaccine-preventable disease to susceptible individuals. Between 1958 and 1961, the effect of herd immunity from polio vaccinations in the United States substantially reduced the number of observed cases, saving children from paralysis or death.

⊕ Future Implications

Vaccine sales have historically represented a paltry contribution to the global pharmaceutical market, averaging between 2 to 3 percent. Yet the vaccine market value has quadrupled between 2000–2013. According to a 2012 report from the International Federation of Pharmaceutical Manufacturers and Associations, research is currently underway to develop vaccinations for over 30 diseases, ranging from human immunodeficiency virus (HIV) to malaria to hookworm. The WHO has predicted the arrival of these new immunizations could drive the vaccine market value to US$100 billion by 2025. The other factors that influence the market value of vaccinations include higher prices for new vaccines, greater demand for vaccines in developing countries, global eradication of some vaccine-preventable diseases, and additional potential markets (adults and adolescents).

Unlike standard pharmaceutical substances, the procurement of vaccines poses additional complications that require foresight, planning, collaboration, and transparency. Vaccines are usually funded by governments, intergovernmental organizations like WHO or the United Nations Children's Fund (UNICEF), or nongovernmental organizations. In developing nations, vaccines can also be procured with the help of public-private and nongovernmental partnerships like Gavi, the Vaccine Alliance, Médecins Sans Frontières Campaign for Access to Essential Medicines, the Clinton Global Initiative, and the Bill & Melinda Gates Foundation.

Vaccine supply is largely provided by a limited number of pharmaceutical multinational corporations. GlaxoSmithKline (GSK), Sanofi Pasteur, Pfizer, Merck, and Novartis produce nearly 80 percent of the global vaccination supply. Emerging market manufacturers play an increasingly important role in vaccine supply by directing production efforts to the needs of developing countries. These new manufacturers introduce competition and drive down the cost of vaccinations by expanding the production abilities of essential immunizations. Overall, this change has had a positive effect on pooled procurement organizations like UNICEF, who have begun purchasing more of their vaccination supply from these emerging market manufacturers.

Vaccine demand is controlled by the governments of developed countries, pooled procurement initiatives like UNICEF and the Pan American Health Organization, and private-sector corporations. The majority of vaccination sales come from high-income countries (HICs). Newer and more expensive immunizations are frequently purchased by HICs, which represent an estimated 82 percent of annual worldwide vaccination sales. Despite this high proportion of global sales, this figure represents only one-fifth of the annual volume of vaccine sales. In low-income countries and middle-income countries (LICs and MICs, respectively) where vaccine need is highest, the ratios are exactly opposite. Approximately 80 percent of the global volume of vaccine purchases are from LICs and MICs, yet this accounts for only 18 percent of the annual vaccination sales.

The issue of equitable access to vaccinations came under scrutiny in 2009 when developed countries purchased advanced orders of the 2009-H1N1 vaccine. Even after the WHO and United Nations requested monetary donations to help supply developing countries with the 2009-H1N1 vaccine, there was a limited supply available to combat the disease. The Canadian and Australian governments refused to donate any of their country's vaccines until local needs were fulfilled. The United States had offered 10 percent of their H1N1 supply to the WHO, then rescinded this donation until they could provide all at-risk citizens with the immunization.

In the 2010s the WHO launched the Vaccine Product, Price, and Procurement (V3P) Project. The project's goal is to "identify, develop and establish the most appropriate and comprehensive method(s), mechanism(s) and/or tools to provide countries with accurate, reliable and useful data on vaccine product, price and procurement." Funded by the Bill & Melinda Gates Foundation,

the V3P platform will consist of an open price database, information repository, and resource gateway. This project began in 2011 and is expected to be fully operational in 2015. When completed, this tool should provide data for evidence-based international policies and guidelines for vaccine price-setting and procurement.

SEE ALSO *Vaccines*

BIBLIOGRAPHY

Books

Abbas, Abul, Andrew Lichtman, and Shiv Pillai. *Cellular and Molecular Immunology*, 8th ed. Philadelphia: Elsevier Saunders, 2015.

Centers for Disease Control and Prevention. *Epidemiology and Prevention of Vaccine-Preventable Diseases*, 13th ed. Edited by J. Hamborsky, A. Kroger, and S. Wolfe. Washington, DC: Public Health Foundation, 2015.

Cunningham, Rachel M., et al. *Vaccine-Preventable Disease: The Forgotten Story*. Houston: Texas Children's Hospital, 2009.

Offit, Paul. *Autism's False Prophets: Bad Science, Risky Medicine, and the Search for a Cure*. New York: Columbia University Press, 2008.

Plotkin, Stanley, Walter Orenstein, and Paul Offit, eds. *Vaccines*, 6th ed. Philadelphia: Elsevier Saunders, 2013.

Periodicals

Deer, Brian. "How the Case against the MMR Vaccine Was Fixed." *British Medical Journal* 342, no. 7788 (January 8, 2011): 77–82.

Websites

"Immunizations, Vaccines, and Biologicals." *World Health Organization (WHO)*. http://www.who.int/ immunization/en/ (accessed March 4, 2015).

Specter, Michael. "Jenny McCarthy's Dangerous Views." *New Yorker*, July 16, 2013. http://www .newyorker.com/tech/elements/jenny-mccarthys-dangerous-views (accessed March 4, 2015).

"Swansea Measles Epidemic Officially Over." *BBC News*. July 3, 2013. http://www.bbc.com/news/uk-wales-23168519 (accessed March 4, 2015).

"Vaccines and Diseases." *World Health Organization (WHO)*. http://www.who.int/immunization/dis eases/en/ (accessed March 4, 2015).

Martin James Frigaard

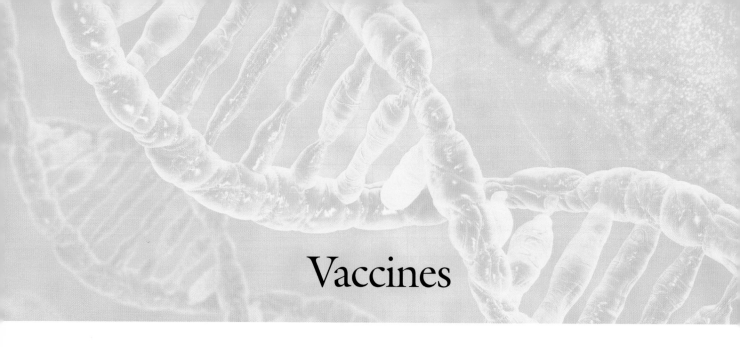

⊕ Introduction

Vaccinations are considered one of the single greatest disease prevention achievements in medical history, along with clean water and good sanitation. Usually administered in the form of injectable serums containing weakened or altered pathogens, vaccinations are designed to stimulate an immune response in individuals. This response prompts the sensitization of certain lymphocytes and the formation of antibodies, which then target specific structures in the pathogen, called antigens. The human immune system protects the body against future infections by retaining the distinct information from each communicable disease antigen it has encountered.

Vaccines rely on the biological mechanism of immunity. Immunity is the ability of an organism to resist infections and disease. In humans, the immune response is the body's protective defense against an invasion by a bacterial or viral pathogen. For example, human skin provides a physical barrier to infection and has antimicrobial properties to ward off harmful microorganisms. Additional protection comes from the mucosal tissues in the lungs, gut, eyes, nose, mouth, throat, uterus, and reproductive organs, all of which play an important role in the immune system. The mucosal tissues in the gut have evolved to absorb useful foodstuffs while identifying and destroying dangerous pathogens. The hallmark of a healthy immune system is the capacity to recognize and eliminate infectious agents. Other bodily systems and organs involved in immune defense include bone marrow, the thymus, lymph and lymph nodes, the spleen, and the bloodstream.

Vaccinations, or immunizations, are considered a form of primary prevention against contagions. Primary prevention strategies are deliberate actions taken to thwart the development of diseases among healthy, at-risk individuals. Vaccinations exist for smallpox, anthrax, measles, rubella, chicken pox, cholera, meningococcal disease, influenza, diphtheria, mumps, tetanus, hepatitis A, pertussis, tuberculosis, hepatitis B, pneumococcal disease, typhoid fever, hepatitis E (though not always easily available), poliomyelitis, tick-borne encephalitis, *Haemophilus influenzae* type b, rabies, shingles, human papillomavirus (HPV), rotavirus, yellow fever, and Japanese encephalitis. The U.S. Centers for Disease Control and Prevention (CDC) recommends that children receive more than 20 vaccinations between birth and age 6 to combat many of the most common childhood diseases. Despite attempts to remove these afflictions entirely, smallpox remains the only disease to be eradicated completely (and thus children no longer receive a smallpox vaccination).

Scientists have estimated that worldwide vaccinations and immunization programs save 2.5 million lives every year. Specifically, these efforts have reduced deaths dramatically of children under five years of age between 2000 and 2010, despite an increase in the number of children born. Children can be particularly susceptible to pneumonia and diarrhea, often resulting in death if not treated properly. Advancements in technology and health equity have made vaccines for these ailments (specifically the pneumococcal and rotavirus vaccinations) available to millions of children worldwide.

The World Health Organization (WHO) considers access to immunizations and vaccines to be a basic human right to health and a governmental responsibility. Its report titled *Global Vaccine Action Plan: 2011–2020* was published in 2013 and states that one of the WHO's missions is to provide access to immunizations to "all people, regardless of where they are born, who they are, or where they live" by 2020. One success has been in vaccinations for diphtheria, pertussis, and tetanus, which are usually combined in one vaccine, which had increased from 20 percent coverage in 1980 to 85 percent in 2010. According to WHO statistics in the mid-2010s, there has been a 78 percent drop in global deaths from measles. Unfortunately, 21.8 million children under 12 months of age remain incompletely vaccinated.

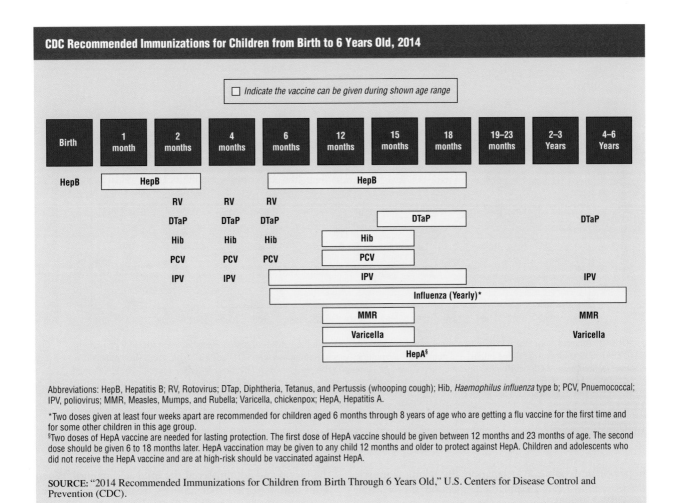

CDC Recommended Immunizations for Children from Birth to 6 Years Old, 2014

☐ *Indicate the vaccine can be given during shown age range*

Abbreviations: HepB, Hepatitis B; RV, Rotovirus; DTap, Diphtheria, Tetanus, and Pertussis (whooping cough); Hib, *Haemophilus influenza* type b; PCV, Pnuemococcal; IPV, poliovirus; MMR, Measles, Mumps, and Rubella; Varicella, chickenpox; HepA, Hepatitis A.

*Two doses given at least four weeks apart are recommended for children aged 6 months through 8 years of age who are getting a flu vaccine for the first time and for some other children in this age group.

§Two doses of HepA vaccine are needed for lasting protection. The first dose of HepA vaccine should be given between 12 months and 23 months of age. The second dose should be given 6 to 18 months later. HepA vaccination may be given to any child 12 months and older to protect against HepA. Children and adolescents who did not receive the HepA vaccine and are at high-risk should be vaccinated against HepA.

SOURCE: "2014 Recommended Immunizations for Children from Birth Through 6 Years Old," U.S. Centers for Disease Control and Prevention (CDC).

⊕ Historical Background

Discovering the Conceptual Framework for Vaccinations

English physician and scientist Edward Jenner (1749–1823) became interested in smallpox prevention in the late 1700s. The common preventive practice for smallpox during this time was a process called variolation, which involved administering tissues or discharges from smallpox-infected patients to healthy patients. Jenner noticed this process often resulted in death from the smallpox or from additional infections, so he began searching for a safer alternative. Having heard claims that dairymaids were immune to smallpox after having contracted a milder disease referred to as cowpox, Jenner surmised that a similar mechanism could be used to pass immunity between individuals.

In 1796, Jenner attempted a smallpox vaccination by administering material from a cowpox pustule to a young boy named James Phipps (1788–1853). Six weeks later, young Phipps remained immune from smallpox. After two years of research and replications of this process, Jenner published his findings. His book, *Inquiry*

into the Causes and Effects of the Variolae Vaccinae, issued in 1798, demonstrated how cowpox can be passed among individuals, transferring widespread immunity from smallpox. This publication and procedure set the groundwork for using preparations containing a killed or weakened pathogen to stimulate an immune response, referred to as inoculation.

Although Jenner usually receives the credit for discovering the cowpox/smallpox inoculation technique, English farmer Benjamin Jesty had successfully vaccinated his wife and two sons in 1774, more than two decades prior to Jenner's initial experiment. Jesty had grown up hearing anecdotes of dairymaids being immune to smallpox, and inoculated his family after becoming aware of a local smallpox outbreak. Evidence of Jesty's contributions to the vaccination discovery include his portrait in the Original Vaccine Pock Institution and the etching on his tombstone that reads, "the first person (known) who introduced the cowpox inoculation."

The next major advance in vaccinations came from the work of French chemist Louis Pasteur (1822–1895) on the chicken cholera bacterium. Pasteur began experimenting with a strain of chicken cholera in 1878 in the

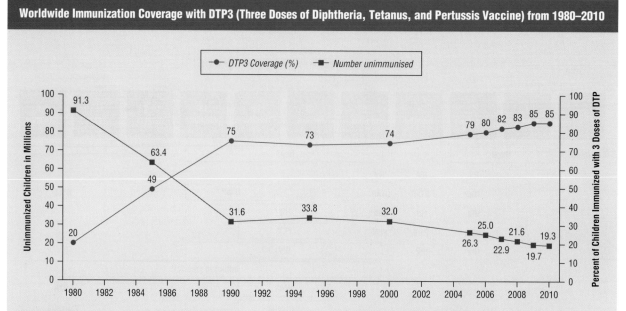

Worldwide Immunization Coverage with DTP3 (Three Doses of Diphtheria, Tetanus, and Pertussis Vaccine) from 1980–2010

SOURCE: Adapted from "Fig. (1). Global routine immunization coverage with three doses of diphtheria and tetanus toxoid with pertussis (DTP3) vaccine among surviving infants and number of surviving infants unimmunised with DTP3, 1980–2010," from Brown, David W., et al, "A Summary of Global Routine Immunization Coverage Through 2010," in *The Open Infectious Diseases Journal*, 2011, Volume 5. Data from United Nations Children's Fund (UNICEF), United Nations, Department of Economic and Social Affairs, Population Division, and World Health Organization (WHO), 2011.

Worldwide immunization against diphtheria, tetanus, and pertussis has increased to nearly 90 percent as of 2010.

hopes of developing a vaccination. By taking a muscle tissue sample from an inflamed injection site, Pasteur discovered that cultures from this tissue became acidic. Chickens previously inoculated with acidic cultures that were exposed to chicken cholera survived the disease. Through a series of experiments, Pasteur again demonstrated the principle that laboratory substances derived from a weakened or killed form of a pathogen can be used to elicit an immune response.

Vaccinations Meet the Scientific Method   Anthrax is an ancient disease that dates back to the literary works of Virgil (70–19 BCE) and Homer (c. 850 BCE). *Bacillus anthracis*, the bacterium that causes anthrax, had been discovered by German scientist Robert Koch (1843–1910) in 1876. Koch used this bacterium to develop his famous postulates—a checklist used for illustrating the causal relationship between specific microbes and diseases. Pasteur began working on a vaccination for anthrax in 1877, coinciding with his research on the chicken cholera vaccination.

Veterinarian Henry Toussaint (1847–1890) had learned of Pasteur's experiment and hoped to create an inoculation using blood from cattle that had died from anthrax. Toussaint attempted to develop his vaccination using a variety of experimental conditions. He first attempted to filter the *Bacillus anthracis* from the blood, which was unsuccessful. Toussaint later heated

the blood and administered the mild acid phenol. When Toussaint reported that animals treated with all three vaccinations had developed immunity, Pasteur and other members in the medical community questioned the validity of Toussaint's vaccine. In a follow-up experiment, Toussaint successfully inoculated 22 sheep with the blood and phenol solution. In 1890, Toussaint died at the young age of 43 from a neurological disease. Although Touissaint received recognition for his efforts (including the Legion of Honor), Pasteur often is credited as the sole researcher to develop the anthrax vaccine successfully.

Pasteur gained additional prestige following his widely publicized vaccination experiment in 1881. Over the course of one month, witnesses observed inoculated livestock (24 sheep and 1 goat) survive exposure to anthrax, whereas the same number of uninoculated control animals succumbed to the disease. Unlike the smallpox vaccination technique, this was the first time a vaccination was tested using the scientific method of controlled experimentation. Pasteur would later receive notoriety for his involvement in the unorthodox and controversial administration of the rabies vaccine to two young boys in 1885.

Joseph Meister (age 9) and Jean-Baptiste Jupille (age 14) were given a weakened form of the rabies virus after being bitten by a rabid dog. Pasteur had discovered that dried-out spinal columns contained a less deadly form of the pathogen. Many researchers and members of the general public were appalled to hear that a deadly disease had been used as a form of treatment. Up to this point, the administration of disease-containing materials to treat illnesses was seen as a relic of the past. Jenner's smallpox vaccination method of using similar but nondeadly pathogens for inoculation had become the current standard. Fortunately, both boys survived their inoculations and injuries. And despite the initial public outcry, Pasteur eventually was seen as an innovative medical genius.

Due to the safety concerns of administering pacified forms of pathogens, researchers continued searching for a more innocuous means of providing immunization. In 1886 American researchers Daniel Salmon (1850–1914) and Theobald Smith (1859–1934) discovered that by exposing the microbes to heat, it rendered them inert. This was an attractive alternative to giving abated versions of pathogens. In 1887, German physician Paul Ehrlich (1854–1915) coined the term antibodies and used it to describe the antigen receptor theory of immunity. This groundwork later would be used to distinguish between active and passive immunity. By the early 1900s, researchers also had discovered that tetanus and diphtheria were bacterial infections, caused by toxoids. Soon vaccines were developed for typhoid, cholera, and *Yersinia pestis* (plague).

As described by Ehrlich, active and passive immunity refer to how an individual has acquired resistance to an infection. Active immunity involves the creation of particular antibodies after either being exposed to a disease or following an inoculation. Conversely, passive immunity is the direct transfer or administration of antibodies. Passive immunity provides a quick, temporary form of protection whereas active immunity takes longer to develop but remains part of the body's permanent immunological memory. Each human also possesses a certain degree of innate immunity. Innate immunity is the resistance to a disease prior to any exposure or contact to its specific antigen. This is the result from the selective pressures of thousands of years of evolution shaping the human immune system.

In 1927, a live, attenuated vaccination for tuberculosis was made available. The next major scientific advancement that paved the way for a vast expansion in vaccine development was the invention of the stable monolayer cell culture. This new method for growing human pathogens safely outside of their normal biological environment was created in 1949 by John Enders (1897–1985), Thomas Weller (1915–2008), and Fred Robbins (1916–2003) from Boston Children's Hospital. The researchers would go on to receive the Nobel Prize for Physiology or Medicine in 1954 for their contribution. The first virus successfully grown on a cell culture was the *poliovirus*, the causative agent for poliomyelitis.

⊕ Impacts and Issues

Live, Attenuated vs. Inactive Vaccinations

A live, attenuated vaccine is a pathogen that has been altered or weakened to reduce the disease's virulence, or ability to cause harm. Unlike Pasteur's live, attenuated rabies vaccine, which relied on exposure to air and time to diminish its strength, the common process used to weaken pathogens is to pass it through a series of animal cell cultures. In each successive culture, the pathogen must adapt to successfully replicate in the animal cells. These adaptations result in the pathogen becoming less effective at replicating in human cells. However, this altered pathogen still can be recognized by the human body's immune system.

After receiving a live, attenuated vaccination, the immune system produces specific antibodies against the disease. The antibodies created also serve as future instructions for the body's immunological response. This mechanism is why live, attenuated vaccines tend to produce strong, long-lasting immune responses with a single dose. In rare cases, pathogens can mutate and become virulent again, causing disease. Although these events are extremely uncommon, as a precaution, most live, attenuated vaccines are not given to people with compromised immune systems. Live vaccines currently exist for measles, mumps, rubella, varicella, adenovirus, shingles, polio, and rotavirus.

Killed vaccines are pathogens that are unable to replicate, but are otherwise intact. By exposing the virus antigens (or toxoid if the disease is caused by bacteria) to either heat or toxic chemicals such as formaldehyde, the pathogen is rendered inactive. These inactive strains are unable to cause the disease, but the immune system still will recognize the infection and begin to protect itself. Unfortunately, killed or inactive vaccines provide a shorter duration of immunity and often require several doses, or "boosters." Examples of killed or inactivated vaccinations include hepatitis A, rabies, and one form of polio vaccine.

Polio Rates Decline after Vaccines Introduced

Poliomyelitis, commonly referred to as polio, is a viral infection that often results in muscle weakness and eventually paralysis. Throughout the first half of the 20th century, paralytic polio wreaked havoc on children in Western Europe and North America. U.S. President Franklin Roosevelt (1882–1945) established the National Foundation for Infantile Paralysis (which later became the March of Dimes) in 1938 in response to the outbreaks and his own struggles with the disease, which he acquired in 1921. Despite many efforts, the attempts to develop a vaccination against polio were largely unsuccessful in the first half of the century. The one exception was a successful live, attenuated strain developed by Polish American immunologist Hilary Koprowski (1916–2013) and tested in 1950.

EXPERIMENTAL VACCINE USE IN EBOLA OUTBREAK

The World Health Organization (WHO) published the first formal notification of an Ebola outbreak in Guinea in early 2014. Six months later, the organization declared that the Ebola virus had become a health emergency of "international concern." Ebola outbreaks soon spread across Sierra Leone, Liberia, and other African countries, and cases were exported out of Africa into the United States and Spain. The rapid transmission of this disease was due in part to the difficulty involved in properly identifying the Ebola pathogen as the causative agent. This region of West Africa had become accustomed to fighting off malaria and cholera outbreaks, whereas the Ebola virus previously had been limited to the Central African coast.

Scientists from INSERM and the Institut Pasteur in Paris subsequently confirmed that the disease was Zaire ebolavirus. The first case of the Ebola virus was traced to a two-year-old child in the Meliandou village, located in southern Guinea. Within three months, there were more than 100 suspected cases and 79 deaths. By May 2015, the WHO estimated that there had been more than 27,000 cases and more than 11,100 deaths from the outbreak.

Ebola was discovered in 1976 as a highly contagious pathogen that presented with fever, headaches, diarrhea, and hemorrhaging. The disease was referred to as "Ebola hemorrhagic fever," although the current outbreaks from the pathogen do not necessarily present with hemorrhages. For this reason, the name has been changed to Ebola virus disease to aid in early diagnosis.

In the mid-2010s, there are limited treatment options for individuals infected with the Ebola virus. Symptoms tend to appear between 8 to 10 days after exposure to the disease. If diagnosed early, patients receiving adequate supportive care (including intravenous fluids and supplemental oxygen) have significantly higher chances of survival. Unfortunately, between 30 and 90 percent of individuals contracting the Ebola virus die as a result of the disease, with higher rates in those not receiving immediate care.

Not long after the 2014 Ebola virus outbreaks, two pharmaceutical companies emerged as front-runners for vaccine candidates. One set of experiments involved a genetically modified vaccination created by the pharmaceutical company GlaxoSmithKline (GSK) and the U.S. National Institute of Allergy and Infectious Diseases. This vaccination contains a benign chimpanzee adenovirus containing genes for an Ebola virus surface protein. Ideally, the immune system would begin making antibodies in response to the surface protein. Human dosage and safety trials for this vaccination began in November 2014. As of early 2015, an application for phase II trials was being reviewed by national authorities in Cameroon, Ghana, Mali, Nigeria, and Senegal.

A second vaccine was developed by the smaller U.S. biotech company NewLink and licensed by the Canadian government. Similar to the GSK vaccination, this vaccination is based on inserting the genes from an Ebola surface protein into an attenuated, livestock version of the vesicular stomatitis virus. Large-scale, worldwide production of this vaccination was seen as a daunting prospect for this relatively modest corporation. Fortunately, NewLink entered a licensing agreement with the pharmaceutical giant Merck following phase II and III trials.

Additional experimental treatment methods utilizing specific antibodies produced in tobacco plants also have shown preliminary promise against Ebola infections. One treatment, termed ZMapp, provides passive immunity in the form of a dose of neutralizing antibodies. Another experimental treatment, TKM-Ebola, interferes with the ability of the Ebola virus ability to replicate. A third experimental therapeutic method involves recovering the antibodies from Ebola patients' blood or plasma—a process referred to as convalescent therapy.

Jonas Salk (1914–1995) was the first researcher to develop an inactivated polio vaccine. In 1954, Salk's vaccine was tested in the largest clinical trial ever conducted in the United States. More than 1 million children participated in this massive, nationwide experiment. After one year, the Salk vaccination was approved for distribution and use. Yet even with this Herculean achievement of medical science, researchers continued searching for a live, attenuated virus that would provide longer lasting immunity. Albert Sabin (1906–1993), a U.S. physician working at Cincinnati Children's Hospital, successfully created the first live, attenuated polio vaccine.

The newly developed live, attenuated vaccine prompted the formulation and design of a second monumental human trial, this time in the Soviet Union. Although the Soviet scientists reported positive results, the international political climate was suspicious of information out of the Soviet bloc. The WHO enlisted the help of epidemiologist and virologist Dorothy Horstmann (1911–2001). After independently reviewing the results of the Soviet trials, Horstmann concluded the findings were positive and the vaccination was approved for worldwide use. Both Sabin's live, attenuated vaccine and Salk's inactivated vaccine remain in use, and have led to a 99 percent decrease in the disease from 1988 to 2014. In 1988 polio was endemic in 128 countries, however, by 2014, it was endemic in only three (Afghanistan, Pakistan, and Nigeria). The WHO has predicted that polio will be eradicated completely by 2018.

⊕ Future Implications

Genetics Advancements and Vaccinations

Vaccine development continues to progress. Advancements in genetic modification technologies now allow researchers to use a process called genetic reassortment. The influenza vaccination is created using reassortment technology. By mixing a disease-causing form of influenza with an innocuous form in fertilized chicken eggs,

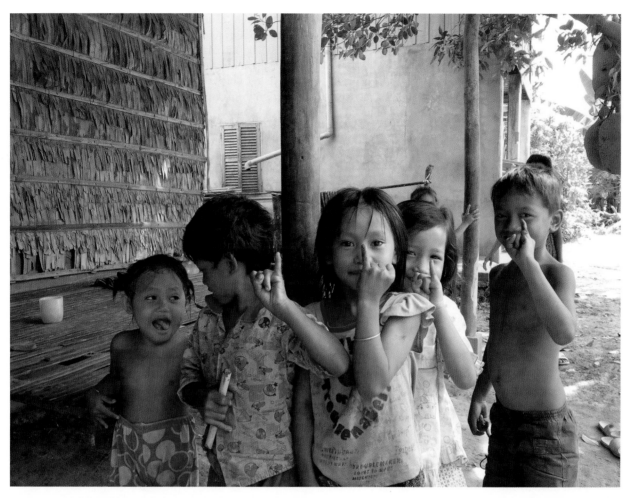

Cambodian children show off their purple-marked pinkie fingers, indicating they have been vaccinated against measles and rubella during a 2013 mass measles-rubella vaccination campaign in Cambodia. Measles is one of the most contagious diseases in the world and is a leading cause of vaccine-preventable death among children. Rubella infection during pregnancy can cause congenital rubella syndrome (CRS), the leading vaccine-preventable infectious disease cause of birth defects, which can also be fatal. Although the two have similar symptoms, they are different but can be easily prevented with combined vaccines. The Measles & Rubella Initiative is a global partnership committed to ensuring no child dies from measles or rubella, or is born with CRS.   *Sue Chu/U.S. Centers for Disease Control and Prevention.*

scientists can select a newly blended strain that has the ability to replicate in the eggs but does not cause the disease. This "assorted" influenza strain then is administered as the vaccination.

Recombinant subunit vaccines, such as for hepatitis B, are created by locating genes that code for specific antigens. Scientist select the subunit antigens that stimulate a strong immune response, and insert them into a cell culture containing yeast. As the yeast cells grow, the pathogen genes replicate, and scientists can use the recombined antigens in vaccinations. A recombinant vaccine also was developed for HPV in 2006.

Bacterial Vaccinations

Most bacterial pathogens have an outer coating that conceals the antigens, making it invisible to the body's immune system. This protective shield is made of sugar molecules, called polysaccharides. When initially

developing polysaccharide vaccines, scientists discovered the immune response was inconsistent in children under two years old. Additional doses were unsuccessful at producing an improved response.

Researchers later found they could provoke a stronger immune response by attaching antigens or toxoids in the form of "carrier proteins." This process, referred to as conjugation, essentially primes the immune system to recognize the bacterial coating. Conjugate, polysaccharide vaccines have been created for *Haemophilus influenzae* type B, pneumococcal disease, and meningococcal disease.

The initial bacterial pertussis vaccination was developed in 1926 and contained a "whole-cell" form of the pathogen. In 1971, the Japanese Ministry of Health suspended use of the vaccination due to adverse reactions. Soon after, the immunization rates began to plummet in the United Kingdom from 77 percent in 1974 to only 10

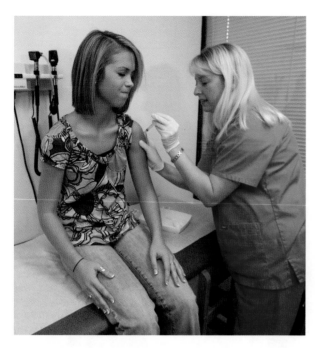

A patient winces as she has her third and final application of the HPV vaccine administered by a nurse at a doctor's office. The groundbreaking vaccine prevents cervical cancer, which is caused by HPV. © *John Amis/AP Images.*

Research also is being performed on so-called naked DNA vaccines. DNA fragments can be inserted into small, circular pieces of DNA called plasmids. These plasmids can be injected into the body with a syringe or delivered by microscopic particles ejected from a high-pressure gas device. Introducing the genes for a pathogen's antigens into human cells causes the cells to begin making antigen molecules. The antigens are displayed on the cells' surfaces, instigating an immune response. Researchers are conducting tests on this type of vaccine in the mid-2010s for the West Nile virus.

PRIMARY SOURCE

Principles of Vaccination

SOURCE *"Chapter 1: Principles of Vaccination," in* Epidemiology and Prevention of Vaccine-Preventable Diseases: The Pink Book: Course Textbook, *12th ed., 2nd printing. U.S. Centers for Disease Control and Prevention, Atkinson, William, Charles (Skip) Wolfe, and Jennifer Hamborsky, eds. Washington, DC: Public Health Foundation, 2012, 1–7. Available online at http://www.cdc.gov/vaccines/pubs/pinkbook/downloads/prinvac.pdf (accessed January 25, 2015).*

INTRODUCTION *This primary source is from a publication of the U.S. Centers for Disease Control and Prevention. It gives a brief overview of immunology and introduces the types and characteristics of vaccines.*

PRINCIPLES OF VACCINATION

Immunology and Vaccine-Preventable Diseases

Immunology is a complicated subject, and a detailed discussion of it is beyond the scope of this text. However, an understanding of the basic function of the immune system is useful in order to understand both how vaccines work and the basis of recommendations for their use. The description that follows is simplified. Many excellent immunology textbooks are available to provide additional detail. Immunity is the ability of the human body to tolerate the presence of material indigenous to the body ("self"), and to eliminate foreign ("nonself") material. This discriminatory ability provides protection from infectious disease, since most microbes are identified as foreign by the immune system. Immunity to a microbe is usually indicated by the presence of antibody to that organism. Immunity is generally specific to a single organism or group of closely related organisms. There are two basic mechanisms for acquiring immunity, active and passive.

percent in 1979. By the time vaccination rates rose again to 45 percent in 1981, the lapse had caused more than 100,000 cases and three deaths from pertussis.

In response to the outbreaks, an acellular pertussis vaccination was developed in 1981 by Japanese researchers Yuji Sato and Hiroko Sato. By 1996, the United States and other countries licensed the use of the acellular pertussis vaccination that often is given in combination with diphtheria and tetanus. Unfortunately, pertussis continues to be a major problem in many developing countries—the WHO reported nearly 90,000 deaths from this disease in 2012.

Experimental Vaccination Techniques

Scientists are experimenting with the use of recombinant vector vaccinations. During infection, viruses attach to cells and manipulate the cell's metabolism to generate copies of themselves, thereby spreading their genetic material. Scientists have seized this ability and can use this mechanism to transport weakened or attenuated genetic information into cells to stimulate an immune response.

A similar recombinant vector process is being developed using bacteria as the vehicle for delivery. As stated earlier, bacterial microbes have an outer coating that can be used to carry antigens. By inserting genetic material of disease-causing antigens into the bacteria, the immune system assumes the bacterium is a harmful microbe and produces antibodies to defend itself.

Active immunity is protection that is produced by the person's own immune system. This type of immunity is usually permanent. Passive immunity is protection by products produced by an animal or human and transferred to another human, usually by injection. Passive immunity often provides effective protection, but this protection wanes (disappears) with time, usually within a few weeks or months.

The immune system is a complex system of interacting cells whose primary purpose is to identify foreign ("nonself") substances referred to as antigens. Antigens can be either live (such as viruses and bacteria) or inactivated. The immune system develops a defense against the antigen. This defense is known as the immune response and usually involves the production of protein molecules by B lymphocytes, called antibodies (or immunoglobulins), and of specific cells (also known as cell-mediated immunity) whose purpose is to facilitate the elimination of foreign substances.

The most effective immune responses are generally produced in response to a live antigen. However, an antigen does not necessarily have to be alive, as occurs with infection with a virus or bacterium, to produce an immune response. Some proteins, such as hepatitis B surface antigen, are easily recognized by the immune system. Other material, such as polysaccharide (long chains of sugar molecules that make up the cell wall of certain bacteria) are less effective antigens, and the immune response may not provide as good protection.

...

Classification of Vaccines

There are two basic types of vaccines: live attenuated and inactivated. The characteristics of live and inactivated vaccines are different, and these characteristics determine how the vaccine is used.

Live attenuated vaccines are produced by modifying a disease-producing ("wild") virus or bacterium in a laboratory. The resulting vaccine organism retains the ability to replicate (grow) and produce immunity, but usually does not cause illness. The majority of live attenuated vaccines available in the United States contain live viruses. However, one live attenuated bacterial vaccine is available.

Inactivated vaccines can be composed of either whole viruses or bacteria, or fractions of either. Fractional vaccines are either protein-based or polysaccharide-based. Protein-based vaccines include toxoids (inactivated bacterial toxin) and subunit or subvirion products. Most polysaccharide-based vaccines are composed of pure cell wall polysaccharide from bacteria. Conjugate polysaccharide vaccines contain polysaccharide that is chemically linked to a protein. This linkage makes the polysaccharide a more potent vaccine.

Live Attenuated Vaccines

Live vaccines are derived from "wild," or disease-causing, viruses or bacteria. These wild viruses or bacteria are attenuated, or weakened, in a laboratory, usually by repeated culturing. For example, the measles virus used as a vaccine today was isolated from a child with measles disease in 1954. Almost 10 years of serial passage using tissue culture media was required to transform the wild virus into attenuated vaccine virus.

To produce an immune response, live attenuated vaccines must replicate (grow) in the vaccinated person. A relatively small dose of virus or bacteria is administered, which replicates in the body and creates enough of the organism to stimulate an immune response. Anything that either damages the live organism in the vial (e.g., heat, light) or interferes with replication of the organism in the body (circulating antibody) can cause the vaccine to be ineffective.

Although live attenuated vaccines replicate, they usually do not cause disease such as may occur with the "wild" form of the organism. When a live attenuated vaccine does cause "disease," it is usually much milder than the natural disease and is referred to as an adverse reaction.

The immune response to a live attenuated vaccine is virtually identical to that produced by a natural infection. The immune system does not differentiate between an infection with a weakened vaccine virus and an infection with a wild virus. Live attenuated vaccines produce immunity in most recipients with one dose, except those administered orally. However, a small percentage of recipients do not respond to the first dose of an injected live vaccine (such as MMR or varicella) and a second dose is recommended to provide a very high level of immunity in the population.

Live attenuated vaccines may cause severe or fatal reactions as a result of uncontrolled replication (growth) of the vaccine virus. This only occurs in persons with immunodeficiency (e.g., from leukemia, treatment with certain drugs, or human immunodeficiency virus (HIV) infection).

A live attenuated vaccine virus could theoretically revert to its original pathogenic (disease-causing) form. This is known to happen only with live (oral) polio vaccine.

Active immunity from a live attenuated vaccine may not develop because of interference from circulating antibody to the vaccine virus. Antibody from any source (e.g., transplacental, transfusion) can interfere with replication of the vaccine organism and lead to poor response or no response to the vaccine (also known as vaccine failure). Measles vaccine virus seems to be most sensitive to circulating antibody. Polio and rotavirus vaccine viruses are least affected.

Live attenuated vaccines are fragile and can be damaged or destroyed by heat and light. They must be handled and stored carefully.

Currently available live attenuated viral vaccines are measles, mumps, rubella, vaccinia, varicella, zoster (which contains the same virus as varicella vaccine but in much higher amount), yellow fever, rotavirus, and influenza (intranasal). Oral polio vaccine is a live viral vaccine but is no longer available in the United States. Live attenuated bacterial vaccines are bacille Calmette-Guérin (BCG—not currently available in the U.S.) and oral typhoid vaccine.

Inactivated Vaccines

Inactivated vaccines are produced by growing the bacterium or virus in culture media, then inactivating it with heat and/or chemicals (usually formalin). In the case of fractional vaccines, the organism is further treated to purify only those components to be included in the vaccine (e.g., the polysaccharide capsule of pneumococcus.)

Inactivated vaccines are not alive and cannot replicate. The entire dose of antigen is administered in the injection. These vaccines cannot cause disease from infection, even in an immunodeficient person. Inactivated antigens are less affected by circulating antibody than are live agents, so they may be given when antibody is present in the blood (e.g., in infancy or following receipt of antibody-containing blood products.)

Inactivated vaccines always require multiple doses. In general, the first dose does not produce protective immunity, but "primes" the immune system. A protective immune response develops after the second or third dose. In contrast to live vaccines, in which the immune response closely resembles natural infection, the immune response to an inactivated vaccine is mostly humoral. Little or no cellular immunity results. Antibody titers against inactivated antigens diminish with time. As a result, some inactivated vaccines may require periodic supplemental doses to increase, or "boost," antibody titers.

Currently available whole-cell inactivated vaccines are limited to inactivated whole viral vaccines (polio, hepatitis A, and rabies). Inactivated whole virus influenza vaccine and whole inactivated bacterial vaccines (pertussis, typhoid, cholera, and plague) are no longer available in the United States. Fractional vaccines include subunits (hepatitis B, influenza, acellular pertussis, human papillomavirus, anthrax) and toxoids (diphtheria, tetanus.) A subunit vaccine for Lyme disease is no longer available in the United States.

Polysaccharide Vaccines

Polysaccharide vaccines are a unique type of inactivated subunit vaccine composed of long chains of sugar molecules that make up the surface capsule of certain bacteria. Pure polysaccharide vaccines are available for three diseases: pneumococcal disease, meningococcal disease, and *Salmonella* Typhi. A pure polysaccharide vaccine for *Haemophilus influenzae* type b (Hib) is no longer available in the United States.

The immune response to a pure polysaccharide vaccine is typically T-cell independent, which means that these vaccines are able to stimulate B cells without the assistance of T-helper cells. T-cell independent antigens, including polysaccharide vaccines, are not consistently immunogenic in children younger than 2 years of age. Young children do not respond consistently to polysaccharide antigens, probably because of immaturity of the immune system.

Repeated doses of most inactivated protein vaccines cause the antibody titer to go progressively higher, or "boost." This does not occur with polysaccharide antigens; repeat doses of polysaccharide vaccines usually do not cause a booster response. Antibody induced with polysaccharide vaccines has less functional activity than that induced by protein antigens. This is because the predominant antibody produced in response to most polysaccharide vaccines is IgM, and little IgG is produced.

In the late 1980s, it was discovered that the problems noted above could be overcome through a process called conjugation, in which the polysaccharide is chemically combined with a protein molecule. Conjugation changes the immune response from T-cell independent to T-cell dependent, leading to increased immunogenicity in infants and antibody booster response to multiple doses of vaccine.

The first conjugated polysaccharide vaccine was for Hib. A conjugate vaccine for pneumococcal disease was licensed in 2000. A meningococcal conjugate vaccine was licensed in 2005.

Recombinant Vaccines

Vaccine antigens may also be produced by genetic engineering technology. These products are sometimes referred to as recombinant vaccines. Four genetically engineered vaccines are currently available in the United States. Hepatitis B and human papillomavirus (HPV) vaccines are produced by insertion of a segment of the respective viral gene into the gene of a yeast cell or virus. The modified yeast cell produces pure hepatitis B surface antigen or HPV capsid protein when it grows. Live typhoid vaccine (Ty21a) is *Salmonella* Typhi bacteria that have been genetically modified to not cause illness. Live attenuated influenza vaccine has been engineered to replicate effectively in the mucosa of the nasopharynx but not in the lungs.

SEE ALSO *Bacterial Diseases; Ebola Virus Disease; Poliomyelitis (Polio); Smallpox Eradication and Storage of Infectious Agents; Vaccine-Preventable Diseases; Viral Diseases*

BIBLIOGRAPHY

Books

Abbas, Abul, Andrew Lichtman, and Shiv Pillai. *Cellular and Molecular Immunology*, 8th ed. Philadelphia: Elsevier Saunders, 2015.

Plotkin, Stanley A., ed. *History of Vaccine Development.* New York: Springer, 2011.

Weisberg, Susan Shoshana. *Factcines: Facts on Vaccines.* Charleston, SC: BookSurge, 2008.

Periodicals

Carleton, Heather A. "Putting Together the Pieces of Polio: How Dorothy Horstmann Helped Solve the Puzzle." *Yale Journal of Biology and Medicine* 84, no. 2 (June 2011): 83–89.

Marks, Harry. "The 1954 Salk Poliomyelitis Vaccine Field Trial." *Clinical Trials* 8, no. 2 (April 2011): 224–234.

Websites

"Global Vaccination Action Plan 2011–2020." *World Health Organization (WHO)*, 2013. http://www.who.int/immunization/global_vaccine_action_plan/en/ (accessed January 30, 2015).

"Immunizations, Vaccines, and Biologicals." *World Health Organization (WHO)*. http://www.who.int/immunization/en/ (accessed January 30, 2015).

"Vaccine Information Statements." *Vaccines.gov*. http://www.vaccines.gov/more_info/vis/index.html (accessed January 30, 2015).

Martin James Frigaard

Viral Diseases

🌐 Introduction

Viral diseases are infections caused by viruses, and they are commonly called viral infections. The National Institute of Allergy and Infectious Diseases describes viruses as "capsules with genetic material inside." Viruses are tiny, much smaller than bacteria, and they are easily transmitted from person to person. The viruses themselves, or their deoxyribonucleic acid (DNA) or ribonucleic acid (RNA), invade healthy cells and quickly multiply by using these normal cells as vehicles to make more viruses. As a group, viral diseases are widespread infections and are highly contagious. Viral diseases are found throughout the world.

Some viral diseases are not as serious, such as the common cold, but others may be deadly, such as hepatitis, Ebola virus disease, and human immunodeficiency virus (HIV). For instance, an estimated 1.5 million people died globally due to HIV-related illnesses in 2013. In another example, during the outbreak of Ebola virus that began in 2014 in West Africa, in just a few of the most affected countries (Guinea, Sierra Leone, and Liberia), it is estimated by the U.S. Centers for Disease Control and Prevention (CDC) that the virus had infected more than 25,000 and almost 10,500 had died by March 2015.

🌐 Historical Background

When the medical community began to identify viruses they named them in an informal, unplanned manner. Some viruses were named for the associated diseases they caused. For example, in 1908 Austrian biologist Karl Landsteiner (1868–1943) and Austrian physician Erwin Popper (1879–1955) discovered that the disease known as poliomyelitis (commonly called polio) was caused by something other than bacteria; it was determined to be a virus. The virus was named poliovirus after the disease.

Other viruses were named for the body parts they were affected. For example, rhinoviruses predominantly cause the common cold in humans. There are three species: *Rhinovirus A*, *Rhinovirus B*, and *Rhinovirus C*. Because they largely affect the nose, and *rhino-* is the Greek word for "nose," they were dubbed nose viruses.

Other viruses are named for the geographic locations where they were first isolated. American scientist Gilbert Dalldorf (1900–1979) and his colleague Grace Sickles discovered the Coxsackie virus in the late 1940s. Dalldorf was investigating viruses in the feces of polio patients when he found the group of viruses that were eventually given the name Coxsackie. They were named after Coxsackie, New York, the town in which Dalldorf first recognized that some of its residents carried these viruses.

Still other viruses are named after the scientists who discovered them. Epstein-Barr virus (EBV), also called EB virus and human herpesvirus 4, is one of eight viruses in the family of *Herpesviridae*. It was named after its discoverers, English pathologist Michael Anthony Epstein (1921–) and English virologist Yvonne Barr (1932–), who discovered it in 1964. The EB virus causes infectious mononucleosis, commonly known as mono.

In the 1960s, a classification system was developed as new viruses were studied using powerful electron microscopes. Electron microscopy allowed miniscule-sized viruses to be divided into groups based on composition, shape, and size. Using the traditional system of classification developed by Swedish botanist Carolus Linnaeus (1707–1778), French microbiologist André M. Lwoff (1902–1994) and colleagues suggested that all viruses be grouped according to their properties. Many of their principles were accepted for use in an international format to classify viruses.

Viruses are now grouped with respect to common characteristics: (1) nature of the nucleic acid (DNA or RNA) in the virion (a whole virus consisting of an outer protein shell, or capsid, and an inner core of nucleic acid, (2) symmetry of the capsid, (3) presence or absence of an envelope (lipid membrane), and (4) dimensions of the virion and capsid. In the 21st century, the International Committee on Taxonomy of Viruses is responsible for the global classification scheme for viruses.

The viruses that most commonly produce disease include those that result in chicken pox, shingles, and other herpes infections; chikungunya (transmitted by mosquitoes, the symptoms of which include fever and joint pain); the common cold; Ebola hemorrhagic fever; infectious mononucleosis; influenza (flu); mumps; measles; rubella; viral gastroenteritis; viral hepatitis; viral meningitis; and viral pneumonia. HIV and the human papillomavirus (HPV) are other common viruses.

Chicken Pox

Chicken pox (also called varicella), caused by the varicella-zoster virus (VZV), is usually diagnosed in children under age 15; however, older children and adults also can acquire the infection. Like many other viruses, it is airborne and is spread by exposure to the coughing and sneezing of an infected person. The CDC describes its initial symptom as a rash that appears on the face and trunk that eventually spreads over the entire body.

The CDC reports that about 4 million people in the United States contracted chicken pox annually before the chicken pox vaccine was available. Of those, about 10,600 people were hospitalized, and 100 to 150 died. By the mid-2010s, the number of chicken pox cases and hospitalizations has been dramatically reduced from these pre-vaccine numbers. Although chicken pox is not entirely preventable, the vaccine (Varivax) provides nearly a 90 percent protection from the virus for young children and prevents the most severe cases of the disease so that those infected will have milder symptoms and fewer blisters.

Shingles

Shingles is caused by the VZV, the same virus that causes chicken pox. It causes a painful rash that can occur anywhere on the body but usually appears on either side of the torso or on the thigh or leg as a single stripe of blisters. Anyone who has had chicken pox carries the virus in nerve tissues near the spinal cord and brain.

The virus may become active years or decades after having chicken pox. Although not a deadly condition, shingles can be very painful. The CDC recommends that adults age 60 and older be vaccinated to prevent shingles.

Chikungunya

Chikungunya is a viral infection caused by the chikungunya virus that is passed to humans by the two species of mosquitoes, the *Aedes albopictus* and *Aedes aegypti*. Joint pain and fever are its two main symptoms. Fever usually lasts from two to seven days, which is normally followed by joint pain that can continue for weeks or even months.

The virus is commonly found in the countries of Africa, Asia, Europe, and the Indian and Pacific Oceans. There is no cure for the infection. The best way to prevent the disease is to practice mosquito control.

Common Cold

The common cold is an infection of the upper respiratory tract involving the nose and throat. It is usually harmless but highly contagious and generally only involves a stuffy nose, sore throat, and cough. The virus enters through the eyes or nose after the person touches a surface or breathes in air impregnated with cold viruses. It takes the virus about two or three days to multiply enough to produce the first symptoms. According to the U.S. National Institutes of Health (NIH), about 1 billion cases of the cold occur in the United States annually.

More than 100 different viruses cause the common cold. Rhinoviruses (among the smallest viruses) are the most common cause and account for 10 to 40 percent of all colds. Adenoviruses (family *Adenoviridae*) can also cause the common cold, as can coronaviruses (family *Coronaviridae*).

Ebola Hemorrhagic Fever

Ebola hemorrhagic fever, also called Ebola virus disease (EVD), is a rare but deadly viral disease caused by one of the Ebola virus strains in the *Filoviridae* family and genus *Ebolavirus*. It primarily affects humans and primates such as chimpanzees, gorillas, and monkeys.

The CDC identifies five Ebola virus species. Four of them cause disease in humans: Ebola virus (*Zaire ebolavirus*); Sudan virus (*Sudan ebolavirus*); Taï Forest virus (*Taï Forest ebolavirus*, formerly *Côte d'Ivoire ebolavirus*); and Bundibugyo virus (*Bundibugyo ebolavirus*). The fifth species causes disease only in nonhuman primates: Reston virus (*Reston ebolavirus*).

Herpes

Herpes is the general medical term for oral herpes and genital herpes. Oral herpes generally causes cold sores or fever blisters on the body above the waist (usually on the mouth), while genital herpes generally causes genital sores (on the external sexual organs) or sores anywhere below the waist. A large family of viruses, called *Herpesviridae*, comprises the viruses that cause herpes. The virus that usually causes oral herpes is herpes simplex type 1 (HSV-1), while the one that usually causes genital herpes is herpes simplex type 2 (HSV-2), however both viruses can occur in either oral and genital sites.

Either form of herpes is transmitted by direct contact with a bodily lesion or from body fluid of a herpes-infected person. Sexual contact is a common way to contract herpes, which is why it is classified as a sexually transmitted disease (STD). According to Planned Parenthood, a provider of reproductive health care, about half of all adults in the country have oral herpes, and just over 16 percent have genital herpes.

Human Immunodeficiency Virus (HIV)

HIV is a lentivirus, which is a retrovirus that produces illness sometime after infection. HIV, which is

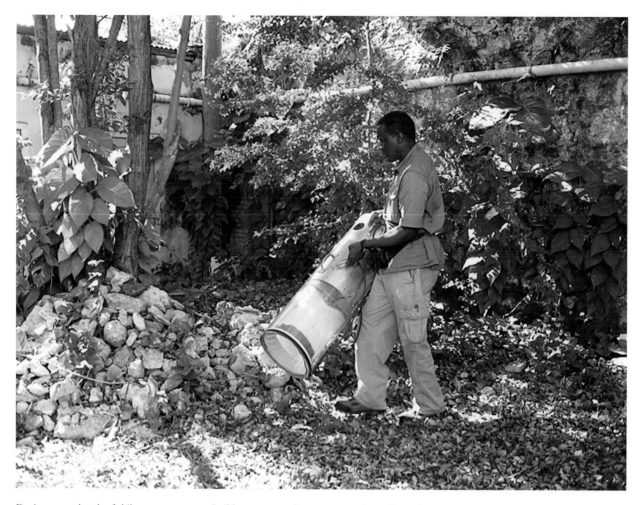

During an outbreak of chikungunya among Caribbean nontravelers, an entomologist from the Centers for Disease Control and Prevention (CDC), John-Paul Mutebi, uses a Nasci aspirator in order to collect mosquitoes for testing on the island of St. Croix, U.S. Virgin Islands. Health officials at the CDC and across the Americas were tracking the spread of the chikungunya virus since December 2013, when it was first discovered in the Caribbean on Saint Martin. While outbreaks of the virus have previously been reported in some parts of Africa, Europe, Asia, and the Pacific, this was the first time the virus was found among nontravelers in the Western Hemisphere. Chikungunya virus is transmitted to people through mosquito bites. Mosquitoes become infected when they feed on a person with the virus. Infected mosquitoes then spread the virus to other people. *U.S. Centers for Disease Control and Prevention.*

transmitted from bodily fluids, can lead to acquired immune deficiency syndrome (AIDS), which can progressively deteriorate the immune system. An HIV-infected person is more prone to infections, cancers, and other medical problems. Without proper treatment, the average survival time (from the time of infection) is from 9 to 11 years.

The CDC reports that about 50,000 people in the United States are infected with HIV each year. At the end of 2011, about 1.2 million Americans were living with HIV, and about 14 percent of them were unaware of their infection. Globally, Joint United Nations Programme on HIV/AIDS (UNAIDS) data from the publication *Global Report: UNAIDS Report on the Global AIDS Epidemic 2013* shows that though rates of new infections have been on the decline since 2000, in 2012

an estimated 1.9 million people acquired the virus. About 35 million were living with HIV that year, but it was estimated that about 55 percent did not know they had the virus.

Human Papillomavirus

HPV is a viral infection from viruses in the *Papillomaviridae* family and are commonly known as papillomaviruses. They are small, double-stranded DNA viruses that infect the epithelium (a type of tissue lining the cavities and surfaces of humans). HPV refers to the more than 150 different viruses that produce infections on the keratinocytes (epidermal cells) of the skin or mucous membranes. Of the different viruses associated with HPV, each is assigned a number that is called its HPF type.

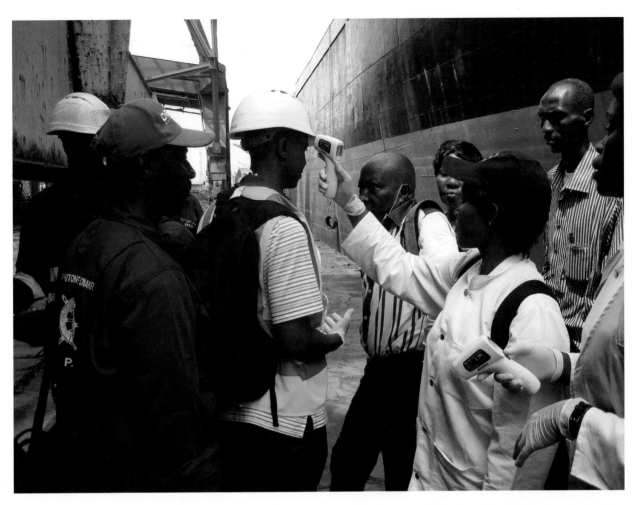

In the West African port city of Conakry, the capital of Guinea, during the 2014 Ebola hemorrhagic fever (Ebola HF) outbreak, a health screening procedure is conducted on a port worker. The health-care screener takes a thermal reading on a worker's head using a Thermo-Flash infrared thermometer, which monitors the temperature of a person's skin surface, enabling a trained investigator to determine if an individual is exhibiting a fever. Those exhibiting a fever are then monitored for 21 days, so that they can be isolated, and treated as soon as possible if they develop additional symptoms of Ebola HF. *U.S. Centers for Disease Control and Prevention.*

As the most common STD, HPV can be transmitted through skin contact with an infected person, or by having anal, oral, or vaginal sex with such a person. The CDC explains that HPV is so common that "nearly all sexually active men and women get it at some point in their lives." Two vaccines (Cervarix, by GlaxoSmithKline, and Gardasil, from Merck & Company) protect against infection with HPV. The CDC recommends that the vaccine be given to adolescents and teens prior to beginning sexual relations, preferably at age 11 or 12.

Infectious Mononucleosis

Commonly referred to as mono or "the kissing disease," infectious mononucleosis is caused by EBV. The virus is spread through saliva, which is frequently transmitted when people kiss. The disease can be acquired at any age but it is more common in teenagers and young adults.

A blood test detects the presence of EBV antibodies and helps to diagnose infectious mononucleosis. The

test can distinguish between past and current infections based on the presence of antibodies against three specific antigens.

There is no treatment for infectious mononucleosis, however, symptoms usually subside on their own in one or two months.

Influenza

The illness commonly called the flu is a viral infection that invades the respiratory system (lungs, nose, and throat). Although some gastrointestinal problems are often mistakenly termed stomach flu, influenza does not cause diarrhea and vomiting. Instead, it causes aching muscles, chills and sweats, dry cough, fatigue and weakness, headache, fever, and nasal congestion.

Most cases of the flu are effectively treated with supportive care—bed rest, sleep, and plenty of fluids. Complications are rare in healthy children and young adults. Pneumonia is the most frequently occurring serious

THE DECLINE OF HIV/AIDS

Research suggests that HIV infection and AIDS probably originated in west-central Africa early in the 20th century. It then spread throughout the world. The United Nations (UN) reports that in 2013, about 35.3 million people worldwide were infected with HIV. The same year the UN reported a decrease in both the number of persons infected with HIV and AIDS-related deaths over the previous few years. As the number of people receiving treatment increases, infection rates decrease.

The Joint United Nations Programme on HIV/AIDS (UNAIDS) 2013 annual report observes that there were 2.3 million AIDS-related deaths in 2005. Since then, the number of deaths attributable to AIDS has steadily decreased, from 1.7 million in 2011 to 1.6 million in 2012.

By the end of 2012, about 9.7 million people in the lower- to middle-income countries of the world had access to treatment for HIV/AIDS. By 2015, the UN was aiming to provide 15 million people worldwide with treatments. In fact, Michel Sidibé, the executive director of UNAIDS, declared, "Not only can we meet the 2015 target of 15 million people on HIV treatment, we must also go beyond and have the vision and commitment to ensure no one is left behind."

The WHO confirms that in 2013 the estimated number of deaths from HIV-related causes was 1.5 million, which was 22 percent less than the number of deaths in 2009 and 35 percent less than in 2005. When considering only children, the statistics were even better. For children younger than 15 years of age, 31 percent fewer HIV-related deaths were reported in 2013 than in 2009 and 40 percent fewer deaths than in 2005.

The declining trend of HIV-related deaths was especially evident in Africa. In the WHO African Region (western, southern, and central Africa), 1.1 million people died in 2013, a 24 percent decrease from 1.5 million deaths in 2009.

The UNAIDS report concluded that increased availability of medical care, including antiretroviral treatment, throughout the world has contributed to the decline of the disease. Total funding for HIV/AIDS was US$18.9 billion in 2012. By 2015, UNAIDS estimates that total funding must reach $22 billion to $24 billion to continue to effectively combat the epidemic.

complication, and for older adults and people with a chronic illness, pneumonia can be deadly.

Mumps, Measles, and Rubella

Mumps, also called epidemic parotisis, is a viral disease that is caused by the mumps virus, which is a member of the *Paramyxovirus* family and genus *Rubulavirus*. A childhood disease, it produces swelling of the parotid glands and salivary glands. Mumps can cause serious complications, such as deafness, encephalitis (inflammation of the brain), and even death. About 1 in 5,000 cases of mumps will result in encephalitis. The mumps vaccine effectively prevents the disease and is included in the combination measles-mumps-rubella (MMR) and measles-mumps-rubella-varicella (MMRV) vaccines.

Measles is caused by the measles virus (MeV), which is a virus in the *Paramyxoviridae* family and the genus *Morbillivirus*. It is also called rubeola. Although it initially causes a runny nose, red eyes, and a cough, its most visible symptoms occur about two or three days later, when small white spots appear on the inside of the mouth, and a rash spreads over the body. Although most cases resolve without any complications, 25 percent of people who contract measles are hospitalized. One in 1,000 will develop encephalitis, and 1 or 2 out of every 1,000 people with measles will die as a result of the disease. The measles vaccine prevents the disease and is included in the combination MMR and MMRV vaccines.

The CDC reports that in 2011, only 220 cases of measles occurred in the United States. Most children (91 percent, as of 2012) in the United States are vaccinated for measles, mumps, and rubella between the ages of 19 and 35 months. However, in 2015, a multistate outbreak of the disease occurred that was traced back to the Disneyland amusement park in California. The CDC reported that during the first three months of 2015, at least 178 people were diagnosed with measles in 17 states. Globally, measles is a top cause of death for children under age five. An estimated 145,700 deaths were caused by measles in 2013, according to the WHO. This is down from more than half a million deaths from measles in 2000, due to effective vaccination campaigns.

Rubella, also called German measles, is generally a milder viral infection when compared to measles and mumps. It is caused by togaviruses (*Togaviridae* family). It affects children the most, causing joint pain, a face and neck rash, and swollen glands. These symptoms usually subside within two to three days. Like mumps and measles, the combination MMR and MMRV vaccines effectively prevent rubella.

The MMR vaccine is recommended by the CDC to be given to all children from 12 months to 12 years of age.

Viral Gastroenteritis

Viral gastroenteritis, commonly called stomach flu (though unrelated to the influenza virus), is a viral infection of the intestines. Viruses known to cause gastroenteritis include those viruses within the genus *Rotavirus* and the genus *Sapovirus*, along with the families of *Adenovirus* and *Astrovirus*. Symptoms of viral gastroenteritis include abdominal cramps, watery diarrhea, nausea that often includes vomiting, and sometimes fever. Viral gastroenteritis may be contracted from contact with someone infected with the virus or contact with contaminated water or food.

Treatment for gastroenteritis in healthy persons consists of resting until the symptoms subside. The best way to prevent viral gastroenteritis is to avoid foods and fluids that may be likely sources of contamination.

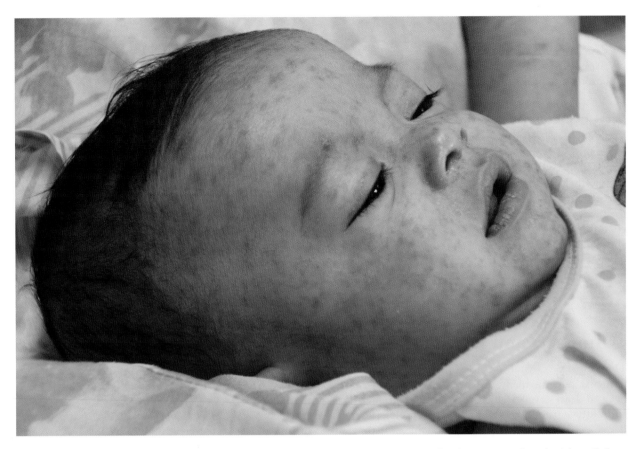

A baby in a hospital in Manila, Philippines, exhibits the maculopapular rash that is one of the hallmark symptoms of measles (also called rubeola). After Typhoon Haiyan (Yolanda) in 2013, the Philippines, especially metropolitan Manila, experienced a large measles outbreak. Measles is a highly contagious respiratory disease caused by the measles virus. Measles causes fever, runny nose, cough, and a rash all over the body. According to the U.S. Centers for Disease Control and Prevention, about 1 out of every 20 children who gets the measles also gets pneumonia and out of 1,000 children who get measles, 1 or 2 will die. *Jim Goodson/U.S. Centers for Disease Control and Prevention.*

Viral Hepatitis

Viral hepatitis is an inflammation of the liver attributable to one of five viruses. Hepatitis A, or infectious jaundice, is caused by the hepatitis A virus (HAV). A vaccine for HAV became available in the United States in 1995, and according to the CDC, infection rates have decreased 95 percent since then. Hepatitis B is caused by the hepatitis B virus (HBV), and hepatitis C is caused by the hepatitis C virus (HCV). In 2012, 2,895 cases of acute HBV were reported to the CDC. However, many more cases are unreported. Males from 25 to 44 years of age are most likely to acquire HBV. In 2011, the CDC reported 1,229 cases of HCV, and the next year 1,778 cases were reported. HCV also is under reported because between 60 to 70 percent of those infected have no symptoms. These are the three most common types of viral hepatitis that occur in the United States. Globally, about 240 million are infected with hepatitis B and 150 million are infected with hepatitis C, according to the WHO. More than 1 million people die each year from hepatitis B- and C-related illnesses.

HBV is transmitted through blood and body fluids. HCV is commonly transmitted via exposure to infected blood, which is why injection drug users who share needles are at high risk of developing the disease. Less frequently, HCV may be transmitted during sexual contact.

HAV is an acute disease, while HBV and HCV can also be chronic diseases. Those with chronic cases of viral hepatitis can develop cirrhosis of the liver and liver cancer. Other viral hepatitis types include hepatitis D virus and hepatitis E virus.

Viral Meningitis

Viral meningitis is an inflammation of the meninges (tissue-like membrane) that surround the brain and spinal column. Most cases of viral meningitis are caused by enteroviruses, a genus of viruses from the *Picornaviridae* family. Other viruses that can cause viral meningitis include those involving influenza, mumps, and measles, along with West Nile virus and various others in the *Hepadnaviridae* family.

The CDC warns that those at greatest risk are babies younger than one month of age and anyone with a compromised immune system. Although most people who contract viral meningitis recover completely in 7 to 10 days, some of the more serious cases, such as those cases caused by herpesviruses and the influenza virus, require treatment with antiviral medications.

Viral Pneumonia

Viral pneumonia is inflammation of the lungs commonly caused by the influenza virus and respiratory syncytial virus, along with human parainfluenza viruses in children. Other viruses also can cause the disease.

Most people with viral pneumonia recover in one to three weeks. However, those at higher risks for the condition, such as those with serious medical problems and older adults, may require a hospital stay to prevent complications from setting in. Serious cases of viral pneumonia can lead to heart failure, liver failure, or respiratory failure.

⊕ Impacts and Issues

The impact of viral diseases around the world is immense and, in many instances, deadly. There have been at least seven influenza pandemics in the 19th and 20th centuries, killing millions of people. The pandemic of 1918–1919 alone resulted in an estimated 21 million deaths. In the 21st century, the first influenza pandemic occurred in 2009–2010. The influenza A-H1N1 virus quickly spread throughout the world, after starting in North America. The CDC estimates that it sickened more than 60 million Americans, caused more than 270,000 to be hospitalized, and resulted in 12,500 deaths.

Historically, viral diseases have disproportionately affected the poorer, less developed countries of the world, where health care and living conditions are lacking. For example, the CDC reports that of the 35 million people throughout the world living with HIV/AIDS in 2012, more than two-thirds live in sub-Saharan Africa. Furthermore, of the nearly 2 million new cases of HIV infection that occurred globally in 2012, approximately 75 percent were in this African region.

Depending primarily on the type of virus that has invaded the body and the resulting, viral diseases are treated differently. Beginning in the early decades of the 20th century, vaccines were developed to prevent many viral diseases. For example, chicken pox and measles are two viral infections that have been drastically reduced in numbers because of widespread vaccination. Hepatitis A and hepatitis B, along with HPV, are other viral infections that are effectively prevented with vaccines.

Most antiviral drugs work by interfering with the infection process. If viruses are unable to enter the cells, then they will be unable to reproduce and infect other cells of the host. Some antiviral agents act by blocking the virus from attaching to healthy cells. Others target the modification of the viral components after they enter the host cell, making them ineffective in spreading infection.

⊕ Future Implications

Several viral diseases have emerged as major public health problems and are projected to persist as problematic in the future. For example, EVD is frequently fatal. The first fatal cases of EVD occurred in remote areas of Central Africa (primarily in Sudan and the Democratic Republic of the Congo) during the 1970s. One case in a village along the Ebola River gave the disease its name. These cases occurred sporadically.

In 2014, however, cases were reported in urban and rural areas of western Africa. These were some of the largest, most deadly outbreaks of Ebola since its discovery. It spread to several countries, including Guinea, Liberia, Nigeria, Senegal, and Sierra Leone, and a few cases were exported to countries outside of Africa. According to the WHO, as of April 2015, there are no licensed Ebola vaccines but testing is underway of two candidate vaccines.

The WHO reported in March 2015 that the number of Ebola cases had stopped increasing in some regions, including the "hot spot," which is the common borders of Guinea, Liberia, and Sierra Leone. In May 2015 Liberia was declared free of Ebola for the first time since the 2014 outbreak began, and the cases in Guinea and Sierra Leone were dwindling. However, the WHO warned that "with only partial success, Ebola could become a permanent presence in this part of the world. In other words, it could become endemic in the human population." The WHO further cautioned, "Even with a successful outcome this time around, we must never forget: the genie will continue to lurk in the bottle, waiting for an opportunity to emerge again."

Influenza is a viral disease that has caused serious problems worldwide in the past and will continue to be an international threat in the future. The influenza virus claims about 36,000 lives annually in the United States, and about 250,000 to 500,000 annually worldwide.

In the 2010s, there has been concern about avian (bird) strains of influenza from the H5N1 subtype, which has caused deadly disease in domestic poultry in Asia and the Middle East. Should H5N1 mutate in a way that enables airborne transmission, it would have the potential to cause a pandemic (global epidemic). Vaccines have been developed and are available for such an event. According to Flu.gov (as of March 2015), an online service of the U.S. Department of Health and Human Services, the WHO reported that 650 people had contracted H5N1 (through direct or close contact with poultry) in 15 countries since 2003.

In the foreseeable future, viral diseases will continue to threaten the health of humans and animals. They will pose challenges for public health agencies, health-care systems, and clinical research centers worldwide.

SEE ALSO *Avian (Bird) and Swine Influenzas; Ebola Virus Disease; Hemorrhagic Diseases; HIV/AIDS; Influenza; Pneumonia and Pneumococcal Diseases; Poliomyelitis (Polio); Vaccines; Viral Hepatitis*

BIBLIOGRAPHY

Books

Cook, Nigel, ed. *Viruses in Food and Water: Risks, Surveillance and Control.* Cambridge, UK: Woodhead, 2013.

Domingo, Esteban, Colin Ross Parrish, and John J. Holland, eds. *Origin and Evolution of Viruses.* Amsterdam: Elsevier Academic Press, 2008.

Feng, Zhi, and Ming Long, eds. *Viral Genomes: Diversity, Properties, and Parameters.* Hauppauge, NY: Nova Science, 2009.

Flint, S. Jane, et al. *Principles of Virology: Molecular Biology, Pathogenesis and Control of Animal Viruses,* 3rd ed. Washington, DC: ASM, 2009.

Global Report: UNAIDS Report on the AIDS Epidemic. Joint United Nations Programme on HIV/AIDS (UNAIDS), 2013. Available online at http://www.unaids.org/sites/default/files/en/media/unaids/contentassets/documents/epidemiology/2013/gr2013/UNAIDS_Global_Report_2013_en.pdf (accessed March 31, 2015).

Jerome, Keith R., and Edwin H. Lennette, eds. *Lennette's Laboratory Diagnosis of Viral Infections,* 4th ed. New York: Informa Healthcare USA, 2010.

Johnson, Nicholas, ed. *The Role of Animals in Emerging Viral Diseases.* San Diego, CA: Academic Press, 2014.

Madigan, Michael T., et al. *Brock Biology of Microorganisms,* 14th ed. Boston: Pearson, 2015.

M'ikanatha, Nkuchia M., and John K. Iskander, eds. *Concepts and Methods in Infectious Disease Surveillance.* Hoboken, NJ: Wiley, 2015.

Novel and Re-emerging Respiratory Viral Diseases. London: Wiley, 2008.

Oldstone, Michael B. A. *Viruses, Plagues, and History: Past, Present, and Future,* rev. ed. Oxford: Oxford University Press, 2010.

Zimmer, Carl. *A Planet of Viruses.* Chicago: University of Chicago Press, 2012.

Periodicals

Esposito, Joseph J., et al. "Genome Sequence Diversity and Clues to the Evolution of Variola (Smallpox) Virus." *Science* 313 (2006): 807–812.

Websites

"Diseases and Conditions." *Mayo Clinic.* http://www.mayoclinic.org/diseases-conditions/ (accessed March 19, 2015).

"Ebola in West Africa: Heading for Catastrophe?" *World Health Organization (WHO).* http://www.who.int/csr/disease/ebola/ebola-6-months/west-africa/en/ (accessed March 19, 2015).

"Ebola Virus Disease." *World Health Organization (WHO).* http://www.who.int/mediacentre/factsheets/fs103/en/ (accessed March 19, 2015).

"Facts about the Common Cold." *American Lung Association.* http://www.lung.org/lung-disease/influenza/in-depth-resources/facts-about-the-common-cold.html (accessed March 19, 2015).

"Herpes." *Planned Parenthood.* http://www.plannedparenthood.org/health-info/stds-hiv-safer-sex/herpes (accessed March 19, 2015).

"HIV/AIDS." *Global Fund.* http://www.theglobalfund.org/en/about/diseases/hivaids/ (accessed March 20, 2015).

"Measles Cases and Outbreaks." *U.S. Centers for Disease Control and Prevention (CDC).* http://www.cdc.gov/measles/cases-outbreaks.html (accessed March 31, 2015).

"M-M-R II (Measles, Mumps, and Rubella Virus Vaccine Live)." *U.S. Food and Drug Administration (FDA).* http://www.fda.gov/downloads/BiologicsBloodVaccines/Vaccines/ApprovedProducts/UCM123789.pdf (accessed March 19, 2015).

"Number of Deaths Due to HIV/AIDS." *World Health Organization (WHO).* http://www.who.int/gho/hiv/epidemic_status/deaths_text/en/ (accessed March 19, 2015).

"Shingles Vaccination: What You Need to Know." *U.S. Centers for Disease Control and Prevention (CDC).* http://www.mayoclinic.org/diseases-conditions/ (accessed April 1, 2015).

"Vaccines and Immunizations: Influenza." *U.S. Centers for Disease Control and Prevention (CDC).* http://www.cdc.gov/vaccines/pubs/pinkbook/flu.html (accessed March 19, 2015).

"Viral Hemorrhagic Fevers (VHFs)." *U.S. Centers for Disease Control and Prevention (CDC).* http://www.cdc.gov/vhf/virus-families/index.html (accessed March 20, 2015).

"Viral Hepatitis." *U.S. Centers for Disease Control and Prevention (CDC).* http://www.cdc.gov/vhf/virus-families/index.html (accessed April 1, 2015).

"Viral Pneumonia." *U.S. National Institutes of Health.* http://www.nlm.nih.gov/medlineplus/ency/article/000073.htm (accessed March 19, 2015).

William Atkins

Viral Hepatitis

⊕ Introduction

Hepatitis is inflammation of the liver, a potentially life-threatening disease most frequently caused by viral infections but which may also result from liver damage caused by toxic substances such as alcohol and certain drugs.

Hepatitis A virus (HAV) is one of five major hepatitis viruses. HAV infection is one of the identified causes of the disease hepatitis. HAV infection also is known as infectious hepatitis. Hepatitis B virus (HBV), formerly known as post transfusion or serum hepatitis, is transmitted through infected blood and other body fluids, rather than by food or casual contact. Formerly known as non-A non-B hepatitis, hepatitis C (HCV) was discovered in 1989. HCV accounts for the majority of cases acquired through infected blood transfusions that cannot be attributed to hepatitis B virus. Hepatitis D (HDV) is an unusual virus in that it cannot infect people on its own. It requires the presence of hepatitis B. Anyone who is at risk of hepatitis B infection may also be at risk of hepatitis D if they live an area where the virus is common. Being infected with both viruses leads to a poorer prognosis than being infected with HBV alone.

Hepatitis E virus (HEV) was shown to be a separate form of hepatitis in 1980. Reports of a hepatitis F virus remain unconfirmed, although there appear to be some rare viruses that cause unexplained cases of hepatitis. All types are potentially serious and, because clinical symptoms are similar, positive identification of the infecting strain is possible only through laboratory testing. Symptoms often include a generalized feeling of listlessness and fatigue, perhaps including mental depression, nausea, vomiting, lack of appetite, dark urine and pale feces, jaundice (yellowing of the skin), pain in the upper right portion of the abdomen (where the liver is located), and enlargement of both the liver and the spleen. Severe cases of some types of hepatitis can lead to scarring and fibrosis of the liver (cirrhosis), and even to cancer of the liver.

⊕ Historical Background

The Greek physician Hippocrates (c.460–c.377 BCE) recorded an outbreak of liver disease. Hippocrates described an epidemic of jaundice and fulminant hepatitis in patients who died in less than two weeks. Patients with jaundice were isolated because they were considered impure and treated with a diet of honey and water. Although it was not prescribed for the scientifically correct reason, because hepatitis is highly contagious, isolation was a reasonable approach for containing hepatitis epidemics.

Hepatitis epidemics were rampant during the military campaigns of the 18th century. During the American Civil War (1861–1865) there were 52,000 reported cases of hepatitis. During World War II (1939–1945), hepatitis accounted for an estimated 16 million deaths. Of these, an estimated 150,000 were U.S. military and the balance were German military and civilians throughout Europe.

Although researchers described the different forms of hepatitis during the early 1940s, the landmark experiments performed by Saul Krugman (1911–1995) in the mid-1960s confirmed that there were distinct forms of viral hepatitis (at that time described as a short incubation period (30–45 days) virus and the other a long incubation period virus (60–90 days). Hepatitis viruses identified to date occur in five types: HAV, HBV, HCV, HDV, and HEV.

Despite major advances in diagnosis, treatment, and prevention methods over past decades, viral hepatitis remains one of the most serious global health problems facing humans today.

The Hepatitis A Virus

Discovered in the early 1970s, HAV is a single-stranded RNA virus (with nuclear genetic material composed of RNA, not DNA), unrelated to the other hepatitis viruses. HAV is transmitted through the fecal-oral route, generally transmission of fecal material from one organism

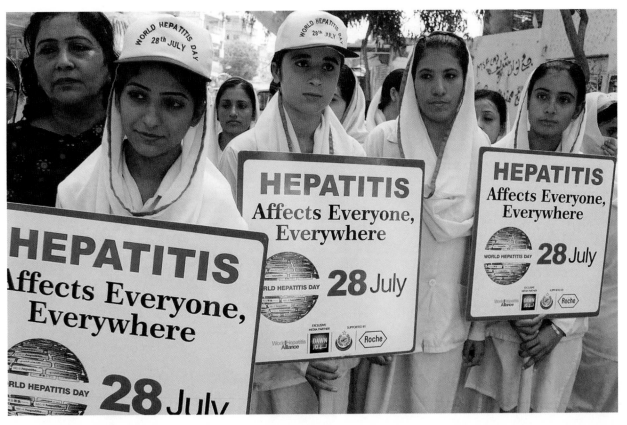

Demonstrators participate in Walk against Hepatitis organized by the Hepatitis Control Program on the occasion of World Hepatitis Day on July 28 in Hyderabad, Pakistan. © *Asianet-Pakistan/Shutterstock.com.*

(human or animal) to the mouth of another organism, via contaminated seafood, vegetables, or fruit. Contamination is often via contact with virus-bearing sewage.

After infection with HAV, and during an average incubation time of 28 days, HAV migrates into the liver where it ultimately produces an acute disease, with symptoms that include nausea, malaise, diarrhea, and enlarged liver. Although some infected people, particularly children, are asymptomatic (lacking symptoms), the onset of disease is often marked with nausea, loss of appetite, diarrhea, and fever. A person with hepatitis A may experience pain and tenderness in the upper right abdomen. Many cases develop secondary jaundice, a yellowing of the skin and eyes, that results from liver inflammation. The majority of HAV cases are self-limiting (disappearing or resolving without treatment). About 15 percent of infections last longer than a week or relapse after seeming recovery.

The Hepatitis B Virus

HBV is unrelated to any known human virus, although similar liver viruses are found in other animal species. It exists as spherical particles with double-stranded DNA as the genetic material. Transmission does not occur through casual contact. Transmission of HBV occurs through infected blood and other body fluids. Sexual contact with an infected person, or injection drug use with the sharing of needles and other items, is associated strongly with HBV transmission. The virus is highly infectious, but for most people the HBV infection clears up within a few weeks. However, those with chronic disease remain infectious, even if they do not have symptoms. HBV infection also can pass from mother to child through contact with infected blood during childbirth.

HBV infection can cause acute disease, with symptoms that include nausea, malaise, diarrhea, joint pain, and abdominal pain. About 12 weeks after exposure, around 70 percent of those infected with HBV develop disease symptoms. These symptoms include nausea, diarrhea, joint pain, abdominal discomfort, fatigue, and loss of appetite. Jaundice may also occur, with symptoms lasting for several months. In around 10 percent of cases, the HBV infection results in chronic viral hepatitis with potentially fatal damage to the liver (cirrhosis) and/or liver cancer. Adequate nutrition and rest are most often recommended to ease symptoms. Chronic infection can be treated with interferon, an immune system protein, and antiviral drugs such as lamivudine. The hepatitis B vaccine is genetically engineered, in part by inserting the HBV genetic material into yeast cells. It was introduced in 1982, and is highly effective protecting against mother-to-child transmission and accidental exposure.

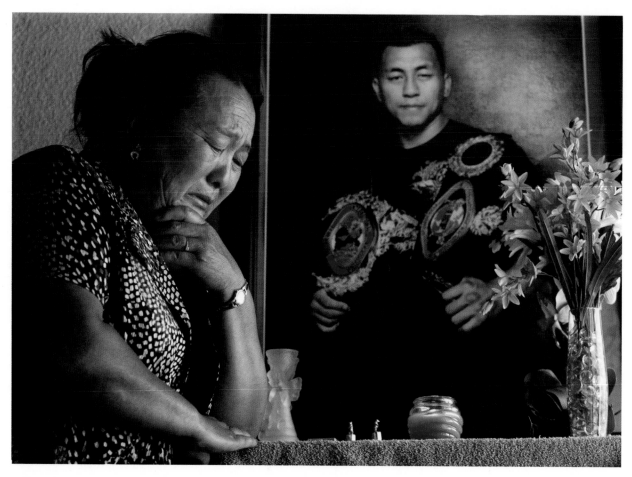

Yeng Mua grieves the loss of her only son, 34-year-old Yia Mua, a champion kickboxer. He had hepatitis B, which caused liver cancer. She encourages those in the Hmong community in the San Joaquin Valley of California where she lives to be tested for the hepatitis B virus and get treatment early, as the rate of infection among Hmong immigrants is exceptionally high compared to the general population. Hepatitis B can lead to cirrhosis of the liver and liver cancer, but often there are no symptoms until the person is very ill. © *John Walker/ The Fresno Bee/ZUMApress.com/Alamy.*

The Hepatitis C Virus

HCV is a ribonucleic acid (RNA) virus (that is, its genetic material consists of RNA rather than DNA). It is also a flavivirus and thus related to the viruses causing yellow fever and dengue. It exists in six different genotypes that have varying distributions around the world; each responds differently to treatment.

HCV is a blood-borne pathogen. In humans, the incubation period for HCV is 6 to 12 weeks, and most acute infections do not cause any symptoms. Transmission of HCV by blood transfusion or receipt of blood-clotting factors has become rare in Western countries. This leaves injection drug use as the main route of HCV infection in North America and Europe. To a lesser extent, hepatitis C is transmitted through body fluids during sexual contact. Occupational exposure, through needlestick injuries by health-care workers, also may transmit HCV. In addition, hepatitis C can pass from an infected mother to her baby during childbirth, although the risk is relatively low.

Hepatitis C is not spread through coughing, sneezing, kissing, or casual contact between people.

In 55 to 85 percent of cases, HCV becomes chronic over a period of several years, during which time the liver becomes progressively inflamed and damaged. Around 70 percent of those who are chronically infected with HCV subsequently develop significant liver disease, including cirrhosis (scarring) and/or liver cancer. Hepatitis C is a major indication for liver transplantation. Antiviral treatment is available for hepatitis C, but there is, as yet, no vaccine to protect against the disease. Hepatitis C is often a silent killer because many people do not realize they are infected and pass the virus on to others. Moreover, the infection causes progressive damage to the liver but may not produce any symptoms for many years.

Traditional treatment for hepatitis C has consisted of injections of the immune system protein interferon, often combined with ribavirin over several months. Treatment response varies by the genotype (the genetic makeup) of

HCV. The objective of treatment is to lower levels and remove HCV from a patient's blood via a process called sustained virological response.

The Hepatitis D Virus

HDV is a single-stranded RNA virus that exists as one of seven genotypes (genetic identities). Transmission of HDV is similar to that of HBV, that is, through infected blood and other body fluids. Sexual contact with an infected person or injecting drugs with shared needles is strongly associated with HDV transmission. Rarely, HDV infection can pass from mother to child through contact with infected blood during childbirth.

There are two types of HDV infection. Hepatitis D may occur as a coinfection, that is, simultaneously with HBV, or it may be seen as a superinfection in someone who already has chronic HBV infection. The symptoms of acute HDV infection are difficult to distinguish from those of hepatitis A and hepatitis B. A condition called fulminant hepatitis, which is a sudden, severe form of the disease with rapid onset, is more likely to develop from acute HDV infection than with hepatitis A or hepatitis B. Around 2 to 20 percent of those with coinfection will develop acute liver failure, which is often fatal. Superinfection causes a worsening in the severity and progression of hepatitis B; those affected are likely to develop chronic cirrhosis of the liver or liver cancer.

Limited surveillance data exist for hepatitis D, but the disease is found mainly in southern Europe, Africa, and South America and is less prominent in the United States, northern Europe, and Japan. WHO estimates put the number of people infected with hepatitis D at about 15 million people worldwide. Chronic infection can be treated with interferon, although response is less effective than if the person is infected only with hepatitis B. Higher doses of interferon may be necessary with coinfection. Liver failure can be treated with liver transplant. Transmission of HDV is prevented in the same way as HBV, preventing contact with infected blood.

The Hepatitis E Virus

HEV is a single-stranded RNA virus, with no outer envelope. It is distinguished by the appearance of spikelike structures on its surface. HEV is transmitted by the fecal-oral route, via contaminated water and foods such as shellfish and raw fruits and vegetables. Unlike hepatitis B and hepatitis C, hepatitis E is not transmitted sexually or through blood.

The incubation time of HEV is three to eight weeks. Infection may give rise to no symptoms or just very mild illness. Symptoms of HEV infection can include jaundice, a yellowing of the skin and whites of the eyes, nausea, vomiting, diarrhea, fatigue, fever, dark urine, and pale stools. In 0.5 to 4 percent of cases, HEV infection is fulminant, that is, severe and rapid in onset. Fulminant hepatitis E is fatal to mother and fetus in about 20 percent

of cases if it occurs during late pregnancy. It is difficult to distinguish HEV from HAV infection and other forms of acute viral hepatitis. It does not progress to chronic disease, unlike hepatitis B and hepatitis C.

Hepatitis E infection is always acute, like HAV infection. It causes symptoms such as nausea, malaise, diarrhea, and enlarged liver.

Hepatitis E infection is usually self-limiting, and there is no specific treatment for it, other than rest and adequate nutrition. There is no globally commercially available vaccine against HEV, but China has produced and licensed the first vaccine to prevent HEV infection. In the absence of a widely available vaccine, prevention of HEV infection depends upon maintaining a good standard of personal hygiene, including hand washing after using the bathroom and before eating or preparing food.

Testing for antibodies against HEV has suggested that strains of the virus occur around the world. However, HEV infection is more of a problem in developing countries; epidemics occur in Central and Southeast Asia, North and West Africa, and Mexico. The risk is highest where access to clean water is restricted and where sanitation is poor. Travelers to such areas are at risk of HEV infection, as they are to infection with HAV. Symptomatic infection with HEV is most common in the 15 to 40 age group. Children get infected also, but are more likely to be asymptomatic.

⊕ Impacts and Issues

Unlike other forms of hepatitis, hepatitis A generally does not progress to chronic disease. According to the U.S. Centers for Disease Control and Prevention (CDC), less than one-half of 1 percent of cases prove fatal, with a marked rise in mortality with age. Reported HAV cases have generally declined in developed countries since the 1970s. HAV infections continue to be most common under conditions of overcrowding and poor hygiene. Epidemics of hepatitis A are also most frequently observed institutionally in prisons and nursing homes. The U.S. National Center for HIV/AIDs, Viral Hepatitis, STD and TB Prevention estimates that approximately one-third of Americans show evidence of past HAV infection and thus some level of immunity to subsequent infection. Adults who live closely with or are sexual partners of people infected with hepatitis A and both injecting and non-injecting drug users have an elevated risk for the disease.

According to the CDC, as of 2012 the incidence rate of HBV in the United States was 0.9 cases per 100,000 population. Hepatitis A is a risk for travelers to areas with poor sanitation. Basic protection is offered by proper hand washing with soap and water after defecation, after changing a diaper with fecal material, and before preparing or eating food. There are also two hepatitis A

HEPATITIS A EXPOSURE DURING TRAVEL

People travel more widely now than ever before, which means they may be exposed to novel diseases for which they lack immunity (usually conferred by prior exposure or proper vaccination). For travelers, hepatitis A is the most common preventable infection. The extent of the risk depends upon the length of stay, the living conditions in the place visited, and the level of hepatitis A in the country visited. In general, the risk of contracting hepatitis A is low in North America (except Mexico), New Zealand, Australia, and developed European countries. However, epidemics still occur even on standard tourist itineraries. Before traveling, it is advisable to check out the latest information on proposed destinations through public health departments and the U.S. Centers for Disease Control and Prevention.

In destinations where high standards of hygiene and sanitation may be lacking, it is recommended to stick to bottled water and avoid ice, seafood, raw fruit and vegetables, and foods sold by street vendors. Personal hygiene is also essential—thorough handwashing after using lavatories and bathrooms and before eating or preparing food will help avoid transmission of hepatitis A virus.

Despite food safety measures, outbreaks of hepatitis A sometimes occur. Health authorities and epidemiologists generally attempt to track down and contact people potentially exposed to the disease by, for example, an infected kitchen worker or server. The standard precaution is for potentially exposed individuals to undergo immune globulin injections to prevent hepatitis A infection.

vaccines that offer immunity. Both are made of inactivated virus. (Inactivated virus is incapable of causing disease but still stimulates the immune system to respond by forming antibodies to subsequent exposure.) One vaccine protects against hepatitis A only, whereas the other is a combined hepatitis A and hepatitis B vaccine.

Blood is not screened specifically for HBV and HDV in all countries, so this is a possible route of infection, particularly when traveling abroad, for someone who already has hepatitis B. If someone is protected against HBV, then he or she is automatically protected from HDV as well. Therefore, the HBV vaccine is an effective method of preventing HDV transmission. Researchers are working on a vaccine specific for HDV.

In countries where HBV infection is common, liver cancer rates are relatively high. Since the advent of screening of blood for HBV in developed countries, rates of infection have gone down, although people are still at risk through injecting drug use and sexual contact. According to the World Health Organization (WHO) report "Global Immunization 1989–2012,"

global public health efforts resulted in 79 percent of infants receiving third-dose coverage against hepatitis B by 2012. (See graphic.) An effective vaccine helps to protect babies from mother-to-child transmission and to stop those who work with blood from being infected with HBV through accidental exposure. Infants are most at risk of developing chronic HBV infection even though they are unlikely to have symptoms of acute disease. Others at high risk include those living closely with or sexual partners of those with chronic HBV, intravenous drug users, and those with routine exposure to blood (e.g., health-care workers).

The social and economic effects of populations with high rates of HBV infections are substantial. Care of patients with chronic HBV is costly. HBV is one of the few viruses that can lead to cancer, although the way in which it does so is not well understood. HBV-related liver cancer and cirrhosis increase demand for liver transplants in an environment already strained by a lack of suitable donor organs. If the HBV vaccine could be made more readily available in those countries where infection is common, it could reduce the number of cases of liver cancer among the population. Around 10 percent of those with the human immunodeficiency virus (HIV) are also chronic carriers of HBV. Rates of HBV in part of Africa and Asia are high and liver cancer accounts for 20 to 30 percent of all cancer cases in these areas.

HCV is about four times as easy to transmit as HIV/AIDS. The WHO estimates that worldwide, many asymptomatic infected persons will progress to the end stages of the disease, and the incidence of cirrhosis, liver cancer, and liver failure will rise dramatically. This impending HCV epidemic has spurred a significant and apparently successful effort to find effective new treatments. According to the National Center for HIV/AIDs, Viral Hepatitis, STD and TB Prevention, the number of new hepatitis C infections per year has declined dramatically since the 1980s. Most hepatitis C infections are due to illegal injection drug use. Transfusion-associated cases occurred prior to blood donor screening; they now occur in fewer than 1 per 2 million transfused units of blood. The CDC estimates that by 2014 approximately three and a half million people in the United States suffered from chronic hepatitis C virus infection. Globally, the WHO estimates that worldwide, for every one person infected with the virus that causes AIDS, four people are infected with HCV. By 2035, many of these persons currently displaying relatively few symptoms will progress to the end stages of the disease. Researchers expect the number of cases of cirrhosis, hepatocellular carcinoma (liver cancer), and liver failure to increase dramatically, placing a major burden on health-care resources. The need for donor livers for transplantation is projected to increase more than fivefold.

Many persons with tattoos and body piercings obtained from unlicensed sources may be at higher risk

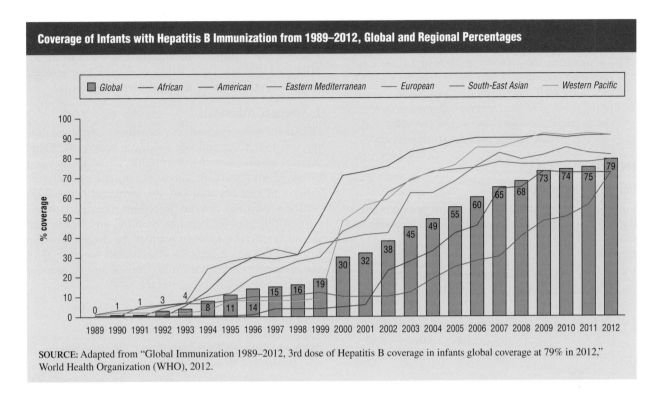

Coverage of Infants with Hepatitis B Immunization from 1989–2012, Global and Regional Percentages

■ Global — African — American — Eastern Mediterranean — European — South-East Asian — Western Pacific

SOURCE: Adapted from "Global Immunization 1989–2012, 3rd dose of Hepatitis B coverage in infants global coverage at 79% in 2012," World Health Organization (WHO), 2012.

of harboring HCV than previously thought. Research at the University of Texas Southwestern Medical Center has shown that commercially acquired tattoos among persons in one study group accounted for more than twice as many hepatitis C infections as injection-drug use. Data from the CDC does not support this conclusion because only a small percentage of hepatitis C cases reported to the CDC involve people with a documented history of receiving tattoos. CDC officials have found, however, that outbreaks of hepatitis C can be traced to tattoo and piercing establishments, and that often oversight of sterilization techniques at such establishments is lacking and not adequately monitored by health authorities. The CDC is conducting studies that could provide definitive scientific evidence of any links that exist between tattooing, body piercing, and HCV infection.

Hepatitis E is rare in the United States, but common in Asia and Africa, where epidemics may occur. Like HAV, HEV is spread through contaminated water and food. It is, therefore, a risk for travelers to areas where sanitation standards are poor, and those who live or travel to developing countries may be at risk of exposure. While the disease is generally not serious, it occasionally develops into a potentially fatal form called fulminant hepatitis that can be especially dangerous in pregnant women. Therefore, travelers to areas where HEV is endemic are advised to take precautions. In destinations where high standards of hygiene and sanitation may be lacking, it is best to drink bottled water and avoid ice, seafood, and raw fruit and vegetables.

⊕ Future Implications

According to the WHO, by 2014 annual deaths from viral hepatitis routinely surpassed deaths from HIV/AIDS, in part due to the success of efforts to combat AIDS, but also because efforts to lessen the burden of disease from viral hepatitis remain underfunded and often unknown.

Since receiving an endorsement by the WHO in 2010, the World Hepatitis Alliance has sponsored an annual World Hepatitis Day coordinating awareness and activist events in approximately 150 countries. All 194 governments belonging to the United Nations have formally pledged to increase efforts to stem viral hepatitis and mitigate its personal, economic, and social impacts. In 2014, the World Health Assembly adopted a resolution calling on all countries to develop comprehensive strategies to combat viral hepatitis, including developing educational programs to raise awareness, increase testing, and promote participation in prevention efforts.

PRIMARY SOURCE

Prevention & Control of Viral Hepatitis Infection: Framework for Global Action

SOURCE *"Introduction," from* Prevention & Control of Viral Hepatitis Infection: Framework for Global Action. *Geneva: World Health Organization (WHO), 2012, 2–3. http://www.*

who.int/csr/disease/hepatitis/GHP_Framework_En.pdf?ua=1 (accessed January 25, 2015).

INTRODUCTION *This primary source is part of the introduction section from a World Health Organization (WHO) report on the global public health problem of viral hepatitis. It summarizes the disease, reasons for concern, and potential solutions for controlling viral hepatitis infection.*

INTRODUCTION

What is the problem?

Viral hepatitis is a global public health problem affecting millions of people every year, causing disability and death.
Overall:

- Around 500 000 000 people are chronically infected with hepatitis B virus (HBV) or hepatitis C virus (HCV).

- Approximately 1 000 000 people die each year (~2.7% of all deaths) from causes related to viral hepatitis, most commonly liver disease, including liver cancer.

- An estimated 57% of cases of liver cirrhosis and 78% of cases of primary liver cancer result from HBV or HCV infection.

Why should we be concerned?

Millions of people are living with viral hepatitis and millions more are at risk. Most people who were infected long ago with HBV or HCV are unaware of their chronic infection. They are at high risk of developing severe chronic liver disease and can unknowingly transmit the infection to other people.

Viral hepatitis places a heavy burden on the health care system because of the costs of treatment of liver failure and chronic liver disease. In many countries, viral hepatitis is the leading cause of liver transplants. Such end-stage treatments are expensive, easily reaching up to hundreds of thousands of dollars per person. Chronic viral hepatitis also results in loss of productivity.

Some groups are at more risk of contracting viral hepatitis than others. In communities where food and sanitation services are not optimal, hepatitis A and E tend to be more common. New hepatitis B and C infections are seen more often in recipients of organs, blood, and tissue, along with persons working or receiving care in health settings, and in vulnerable groups.

In recent decades, viral hepatitis has not received the attention it deserves from the global community. Although the burden of disease is very high, the problem has not been addressed in a serious way for many reasons, including the relatively recent discovery of the causative viruses, the mostly silent or benign nature of the disease in its early stages, and the insidious way in which it causes chronic liver disease. Decades-long delay between infection and the expression of chronic liver disease or liver cancer made it difficult to link these diseases to earlier HBV or HCV infections. All these factors have resulted in "the silent epidemic" we are experiencing today.

Is there a solution?

Affordable measures, such as vaccination, safe blood supply, safe injections, and safe food, can reduce the transmission of viral hepatitis infections. These are detailed below. Most of these measures not only reduce the transmission of viral hepatitis but also have spill over effects on the prevention of other infectious diseases. Further, current therapies for hepatitis B and C give health care providers effective tools to combat the disease. For the first time in history, hepatitis C is curable. New therapies are also being developed for hepatitis B and C, and the future is more promising than ever.

SEE ALSO *Epidemiology: Surveillance for Emerging Infectious Diseases; Food Preparation and Food Safety; Sanitation and Hygiene; Vaccine-Preventable Diseases; Viral Diseases; Waterborne Diseases*

BIBLIOGRAPHY

Books

Bartenschlager, Ralf, ed. *Hepatitis C Virus: From Molecular Virology to Antiviral Therapy.* Berlin: Springer, 2013.

Ruggeri, Franco Maria, Ilaria Di Bartolo, Fabio Ostanello, and Marcello Trevisani. *Hepatitis E Virus: An Emerging Zoonotic and Foodborne Pathogen.* New York: Springer, 2013.

Shetty, Kirti, and George Y. Wu, eds. *Chronic Viral Hepatitis: Diagnosis and Therapeutics*, 2nd ed. New York: Humana Press, 2012.

Thomas, H. C., et al. eds. *Viral Hepatitis*, 4th ed. Chichester, UK: Wiley, 2014.

Viral Hepatitis: The Secret Epidemic: Hearing before the Committee on Oversight and Government Reform, House of Representatives, One Hundred Eleventh Congress, Second Session, June 17, 2010. Washington, DC: U.S. G.P.O., 2011.

World Health Organization. *Guidance on Prevention of Viral Hepatitis B and C among People Who Inject Drugs.* Geneva: World Health Organization, 2012.

Periodicals

Shimokura, Gayle H., and Paul R. Gully. "Risk of Hepatitis C Virus Infection from Tattooing and Other Skin Piercing Services." *Canadian Journal of Infectious Diseases* 6, no. 5 (September/October 1995): 235–238.

Trepo, Christian. "A Brief History of Hepatitis Milestones." *Liver International* 34, suppl. 1 (February 2014): 29–37.

Websites

"The Future of HCV." *Axium Healthcare.* http://www.axiumhealthcare.com/hepatitis-c-guide-book-practices-part-3/ (accessed April 7, 2015).

"Hepatitis." *World Health Organization (WHO).* http://who.int/topics/hepatitis/en/ (accessed April 7, 2015).

"Surveillance for Viral Hepatitis—United States, 2012." *U.S. Centers for Disease Control and Prevention (CDC).* http://www.cdc.gov/hepatitis/Statistics/2012Surveillance/index.htm (accessed April 7, 2015).

"Viral Hepatitis." *U.S. Centers for Disease Control and Prevention (CDC).* http://www.cdc.gov/hepatitis/index.htm (accessed April 7, 2015).

"WHO to Launch Guidelines on Hepatitis C Treatment." *World Health Organization (WHO).* http://www.who.int/hiv/events/2014/hepctreatmentguidelines/en/ (accessed April 7, 2015).

K. Lee Lerner

Vulnerable Populations

⊕ Introduction

Population groups that have limited access to health care, food, housing, employment, and other basic life necessities are considered vulnerable. These vulnerable populations are less equipped to cope with the risks of poverty and disease due to their lower social status. Vulnerable populations include women, children, the elderly, members of religious and ethnic minority groups, indigenous people, individuals with physical or mental disabilities, refugees, people living in remote rural areas, and those living in urban slums.

Vulnerable populations are typically on the periphery of mainstream health systems, leading to poor access to medical care and disease prevention. These populations face a higher incidence of disease and illness and increased disease mortality. For instance, children from poor and rural communities in developing countries are two times more likely to die under the age of five when compared to their richer counterparts in the developed world. In the United States, African Americans and Hispanics have a much higher rate of human immunodeficiency virus (HIV) infection and acquired immune deficiency syndrome (AIDS) than the white population.

Social determinants of health for vulnerable populations put them at a higher risk of negative health outcomes. Determinants include the social, economic, and physical conditions where people live and work. The distribution of resources, power, and wealth impact these conditions. The World Health Organization (WHO) identifies poor social determinants as a primary cause of health inequality within and between countries.

Organizations such as Médicins Sans Frontières (MSF; Doctors Without Borders) have programs aimed at meeting the basic health needs of vulnerable members of society, including reaching victims of war, natural disasters, and other calamities. The United Nations (UN) World Food Program supplements the nutritional needs of vulnerable children through its school-feeding program. The WHO highlights the plight of indigenous people who have the highest rates of suicide, diabetes, infant mortality, and other health-related issues. Educating policy makers and leaders about the realities facing vulnerable populations is considered an important strategy for improving health outcomes.

⊕ Historical Background

Attention to the health issues facing vulnerable populations can be traced back to the Lalonde Report published in Canada in 1974. Prior to the report, health care followed the medical model of researching and treating diseases. This seminal work proposed looking at other determinants of health including lifestyle choices, human biology, and social and physical environments where people live. Additionally, the report suggested interventions to improve public health should focus on those population groups with the highest level of risk for certain diseases as determined by large-scale studies. These included focus on those who smoke, drink alcohol, or have high blood pressure. The report considered these risk factors to be due to choices made by individuals. This populations-at-risk model was successful in bringing awareness to the health risks associated with certain behaviors and lifestyles.

Critiques of the populations-at-risk model maintained that this approach would lead to victims being blamed for the health conditions they experienced, which would lead to stigmatizing certain population groups. Secondly, there was a critique that intervention aimed at these population groups would not address the root problems and societal forces that lead members to participate in high-risk behaviors. An alternative to the populations-at-risk model was the population model discussed in the *Strategy of Preventive Medicine* by Geoffrey Rose, first published in 1992. The strategy population model was to focus public health interventions toward the entire population instead of focusing on high-risk individuals.

Population level interventions are weak because they lack focus on those with the highest risk of developing

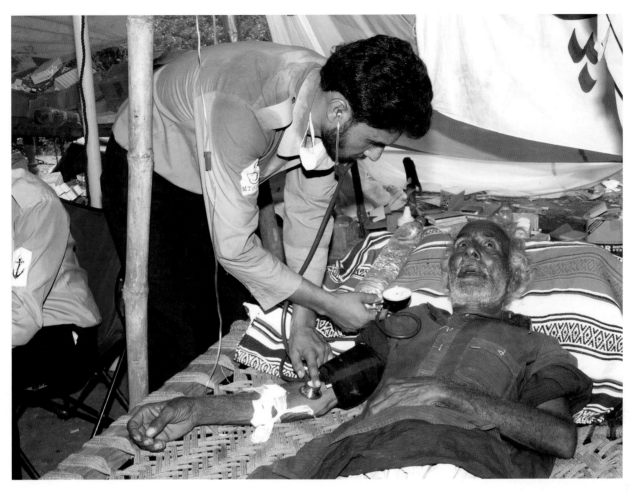

An elderly man is treated at a relief camp established by the Pakistani navy for flood-displaced victims after a flood hit Sind Province in Pakistan. The elderly are one group considered vulnerable, and they may be at increased risk during events such as natural disasters. *© Asianet-Pakistan/Shutterstock.com.*

negative health outcomes. A population model approach may increase health inequities, particularly if those who are most at risk of suffering health problems do not receive the interventions they need. Katherine Frohlich and Louise Potvin argued in 2008 that vulnerable groups within a population face shared social characteristics, increasing their risk of experiencing negative impacts from environmental, biological, or other health threats. This vulnerable populations approach called for a focus of public health intervention toward root causes of health problems. These include increasing socioeconomic status and improving education.

⊕ Impacts and Issues

Economic inequality is one of the primary drivers keeping vulnerable populations from accessing the medical and social services they need to decrease health risks. Those in poverty and on the fringes of society are often desperate to find the resources to survive each day. The

desperation caused by poverty may further put people in harm's way. Poverty can exacerbate domestic problems and violence. Children are often not in school, instead they help the family increase income or food production, making cycles of poverty difficult to break.

Government policies and programs must recognize the needs of the most vulnerable and improve access to vital services. Interventions are needed to improve access to health-care services, education and job skills training, and community support and awareness of the plight of vulnerable people. A number of nongovernmental organizations, including international organizations, recognize the difficulties vulnerable groups face. The UN Population Fund identifies a life of health and equal opportunity as a right for every woman, man, and child.

Vulnerable population groups face physical, psychological, and social disabilities. Those with physical concerns include the chronically ill, disabled, people living with HIV/AIDS, and mothers and infants. Psychological concerns include those with chronic mental conditions, such as schizophrenia, depression, suicidal tendencies,

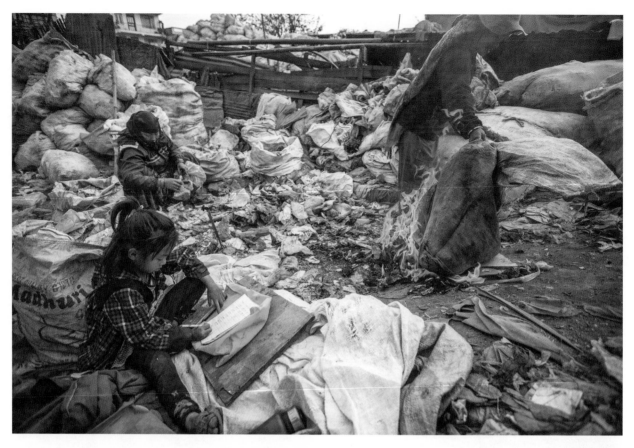

A child does her homework while her family works at a landfill in Kathmandu, Nepal. Nepal is one of the poorest countries in the world, with more than one-third of children living below the national poverty level in 2010, according to the United Nations Children's Fund. © De Visu/Shutterstock.com.

and substance abuse. Social related difficulties encompass those experiencing abuse in the family, the homeless, immigrants, and refugees. Vulnerable groups often face issues in each of these categories, which further complicates the health concerns they face.

Women and Maternal Health

Women are a vulnerable group throughout the world due to gender-based discrimination that results in social and economic barriers that may limit their ability to access goods and services necessary to maintain their health and well-being. Approximately half of the women in developing regions receive the recommended amount of health care they need. Treatable complications from pregnancy and childbirth kill more than one woman every two minutes in the developing world. For each woman that dies, another 20 to 30 women have serious or long-lasting complications. Surviving children are also at risk for increased poverty and poor health outcomes when they lose a mother or a mother is disabled.

The Millennium Development Goals (MDGs), a coordinated effort begun in 2000 by the UN to focus on identified priorities, set the goal of reducing maternal mortality 75 percent from 1990 levels by 2015. While the reduction has been significant, at 45 percent in 2015,

the goal was not reached. To further improve maternal health, improvements need to be made to increase access to skilled nursing personnel during delivery. Also, all women need access to reproductive health services and prenatal services. There is a lack of resources available to provide the specialized care women need.

There are a number of international organizations and programs working to advocate for women and the health-care challenges they face. One nongovernmental organization, Partners In Health (PIH), considers health care a human right for both men and women. PIH works to meet the specific health and cultural requirements of women in the communities where they are present. They provide trained health workers in the remote mountains of Lesotho, in southern Africa, to give the health care women need before, during, and after pregnancy and birth. PIH also addresses the root causes of poverty and provides financial assistance to women for transportation to and from health clinics. They advocate for the needs of women and those in poverty.

The UN chartered an organization, UN Women, to draw attention to and improve the plight of women throughout the world. They support a more equitable distribution of resources, particularly credit, seeds, and information technology in agricultural areas around the world.

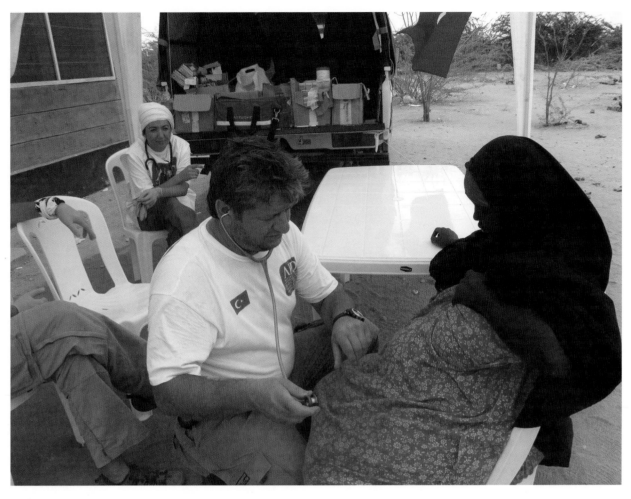

A woman is examined at one of the refugee camps in Dadaab, Kenya, where thousands of Somalis have lived since the 1990s. © *Sadik Gulec/Shutterstock.com.*

Women are vulnerable to abuse but are not empowered to speak out. UN Women assists in expanding economic opportunities for women, with a goal of improving women's sense of self-worth and societal respect for women.

Refugees and Internally Displaced People

Refugees have typically been displaced from their home country to escape conflict or human rights violations. Although they may have escaped immediate conflict or violence, they are very vulnerable because the country in which they seek refuge may not protect their basic rights and security. They are particularly vulnerable, as there is a risk that the source of the violence, which could be their country's military, might still reach them. Displaced people often live in densely populated camps for extended periods in a state of instability, not knowing if and when they will return to their homes.

Providing for the health needs of displaced people is one of the primary focus areas for the UN Refugee Agency (UNHCR). The 1951 Refugee Convention says that refugees should have access to the same health services available to the citizens of the country of refuge. The top five causes of mortality for displaced children under the age of five are malaria, malnutrition, measles, diarrhea, and respiratory infections. The UNHCR works with partner organizations to provide nutritional support, immunizations, reproductive services, and monitoring of public health among refugee populations.

There are often particular vulnerabilities among displaced people, including victims of trafficking, people with disabilities, the elderly, and women and children, and those facing sexual violence. The protection of women and children includes providing safe access to basic needs such as food, water, and latrines. It is the responsibility of the UNHCR and other agencies to ensure vulnerable refugees receive the services and protection they need.

There were 1.7 million Syrian refugees in Turkey in March 2015 due to violent insurgents in the region. Many of the refugees arriving in Turkey were women, children, and the elderly, who had to walk over rough roads with luggage. The elderly and disabled unable to walk had to be carried.

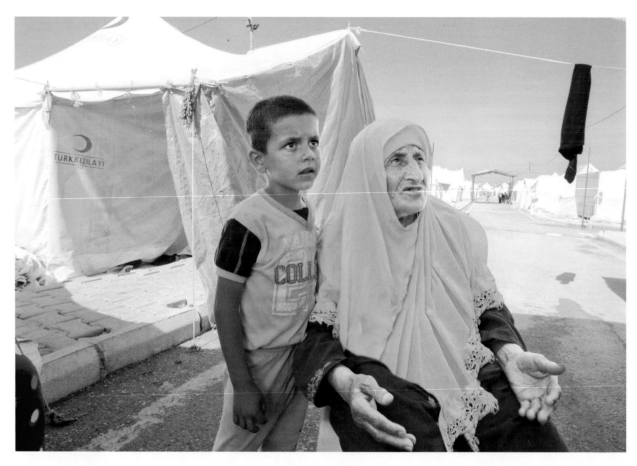

A Syrian woman and child sit outside a tent at a refugee camp on the Turkish-Syrian border. The United Nations High Commissioner for Refugees (UNHCR) estimates that of the 1.7 million Syrian refugees in Turkey in March 2015 about half are children. © *Dona_Bozzi/ Shutterstock.com.*

Street Children

There are approximately 100 million children living in the streets of urban areas throughout the world. Children may spend their days on the streets begging for food or money to help their families survive. Other children have no families, and call the streets their home. It is not uncommon for girls on the street to become pregnant and give birth to additional street children. Street children often band together in large groups for support and means of survival. Street children engage in begging, shoe shining, collecting trash, and prostitution, increasing their risk of sexually transmitted diseases, to find the resources to survive.

Poverty is the primary reason children are on the streets. In some cases a child's parents may have died due to conflict or disease, such as HIV/AIDS. Natural disaster and civil unrest are also reasons families separate. Other times, sexual abuse, or other social stigma, may force children away from their homes.

Children face many risks when living and work in the streets. Street children are vulnerable to physical health problems, violence, depression, and social discrimination. Police forces victimize street children. Substance abuse is common among street children. The WHO

reports that the rates of disease morbidity, mortality, and disability are high among street children. Many street children receive little or no formal education.

The WHO has a street education program to improve the well-being of children on the streets. Education includes reading programs, counseling about substance abuse, teaching how to prevent sexually transmitted diseases, and guiding children to seek assistance for health and social problems. Other programs focus on teaching children life skills so they can better earn an income. Depending on the circumstance through which a child ended up on the streets, it may not be in the best interest of the child to return.

Mental Health Disabilities

Individuals with mental health disabilities are particularly stigmatized and discriminated against in societies throughout the world. These individuals experience high rates of physical and sexual abuse. It is not uncommon for mentally ill people to be restricted from accessing social and medical services, including emergency care. It is also difficult for people with such disabilities to attend school, and they have limited employment opportunities.

HUMAN RIGHTS OF PEOPLE WITH DISABILITIES

People with physical and mental disabilities in many societies are very vulnerable as a result of being excluded from the social, health, and protective services enjoyed by the majority of the population. The Convention on the Rights of Persons with Disabilities is a United Nations treaty that came into force in 2008. The treaty's primary purpose is to protect the fundamental human rights and freedoms of people who have long-term physical, mental, intellectual, or other disabilities.

The principles of the Convention include: a. Respect for inherent dignity, independence, and freedom to make one's decisions; b. Non-discrimination; c. Full and effective participation and belonging in society; d. Acceptance of the human diversity and humanity of disabled people; e. equal opportunities; f. accessibility to the built world, transportation, information technology, and services; g. equality for men and women; and h. respect for the changing capacities of disabled children and ensuring their ideas and voices are considered.

Countries who have ratified the Convention agree to ensure and promote the human rights and freedoms of all people with disabilities free of discrimination. Countries agree to a. adopt appropriate legislative and administrative actions; b. modify or remove existing laws and customs that violate rights; c. promote the rights of the disabled in all programs and policies; d. ensure that authorities and institutions conform to the convention; e. take measures to eliminated discrimination of the disabled in all organizations and businesses; f. implement and promote research for the development of goods, services, equipment, and facilities to be universally used by all people with minimal need for adaptation for the disabled; g. promote the development of mobility technology, information technology, and other assistive technology to meet the needs of the disabled at an affordable cost; h. provide information to the disabled about available mobility aids, assistive technology, and support services and technology; and i. promote the training of those working with the disabled of the rights recognized in this Convention.

Countries also agree to take measures to devote economic resources to achieving the economic, social, and cultural rights of the disabled. They also agree to collaborate internationally to meet the goals of the Convention. Countries agree to involve those with disabilities and representative organizations, including children, to participate in developing and implementing policies to meet the goals of the Convention.

The Convention recognizes that women and girls with disabilities are particularly vulnerable to discrimination. States who sign the Convention agree to take measures to ensure the protection of rights and freedoms of women and girls. The Convention highlights the need to protect the disabled in times of risk and humanitarian emergencies. It also indicates that countries should ensure the disabled are not subject to inhuman treatment or punishments.

The Convention highlights the right to education for the disabled. Countries must facilitate the disabled receive a quality education with special needs being met, such as instruction in braille for the visually impaired. Easily accessible health services must also be provided to disabled individuals under the Convention, including access to reproductive health and other public health programs.

The Convention has 153 party countries as of 2015. The European Union ratified the Convention in 2010. The United States, while a signatory, has been unable to ratify the Convention.

These complex factors lead to higher rates of disease, and shorter life spans compared to rates in the larger population.

The WHO points out that many vulnerable groups targeted for intervention programs often suffer from mental disabilities. For example, many refugees fleeing violence in a country are likely to suffer from post-traumatic stress. Up to 67 percent of HIV/AIDS patients also suffer from depression. More than 50 percent of homeless people suffer from a mental health disability. Mental health issues are typically not addressed in intervention programs, and it is not uncommon for those with mental health problems to be excluded from programs.

The UN Convention on the Rights of People with Disabilities entered into force in 2008 to address the serious concerns facing this vulnerable group. The WHO has identified a number of evidenced-based strategies that should be integrated into development and assistance programs to address the needs of people specifically with mental disabilities. The goal of these measures is to improve outcomes for patients, families, and their communities.

First, services for mental health must be integrated into all health services, including at the level of primary care. Second, mental health issues must be considered at the broader health policy level. Third, in times of emergencies and crises, mental health services should be provided. Fourth, social services and housing development should consider mental health problems, so people receive the support services they need. Fifth, schools need to integrate mental health issues, and provide support to people with mental disabilities, helping them to access education. Sixth, the mentally ill must receive support to find employment opportunities. Seventh, laws and policies to protect the human rights of people with mental disabilities need to be developed. Eighth, those with mental issues should be enabled to engage in community and public affairs. Finally, development organizations should design programs to bring those with mental illness into decision-making processes.

Health Inequities in the United States

Vulnerable populations exist in both developing and developed countries. According to the 2010 U.S. Census, approximately 36 percent of the U.S. population identified with a racial or ethnic minority group. Minorities in the United States experience a higher rate of preventable disease, death, and disabilities than do whites. The U.S. Centers for Disease Control and Prevention (CDC) explains that health disparities exist in the United States based on gender, sexual identity, age, disability, income level, and geographic location.

The CDC says influences on health include access and availability of quality education, healthful food, adequate housing, reliable and safe transportation, health-care providers who are culturally sensitive, health insurance, and clean water and air. The CDC facilitates the creation of policies and programs to reduce health inequities. It regularly chooses new public health topics on which to focus its resources. Focus areas are chosen only if they are highly related to premature death and disease burden, are distributed unequally to vulnerable groups, and have feasible interventions. Current topics include increasing access to more healthful food retailers, decreasing HIV transmission, and reducing work-related injuries.

⊕ Future Implications

The WHO member states adopted the Rio Political Declaration at the 2011 World Conference. First, the declaration calls countries to adopt improved governance for health and development, particularly recognizing the needs of vulnerable population groups. Second, it recognizes the need for community participation in health-related policy making. Third, it highlights a commitment for reorienting the health-care sector toward reducing inequity. Fourth, it calls for strengthened global attention and collaboration toward the social determinants of health. Finally, the declaration calls for improved monitoring and accountability of health inequities.

The MDGs and the UN Development Group have a strong influence on the development priorities addressed by governments and development organizations throughout the world. They recognize that development improvements achieved from 1990 to 2015 did not reach the most vulnerable groups. Through the development of new goals and strategies, it is recognized that governments need the capacity to recognize and address the health and poverty concerns of the most vulnerable groups.

The Robert Wood Johnson Foundation (RWJF), a large think tank on public health issues in the United States, includes the role of the social determinants of health when considering the health outcomes of vulnerable populations. RWJF promotes research to improve public health outcomes for vulnerable groups, including minorities, victims of abuse, and immigrants. RWJF engages stakeholders, policy makers, business leaders, and community groups while researching solutions to U.S. health issues.

SEE ALSO *Centers for Disease Control and Prevention (CDC); Child Health; Conflict, Violence, and Terrorism: Health Impacts; Drug/Substance Abuse; Food Security and Hunger; Global Health Initiatives; Health as a Human Right and Health-Care Access; Health-Related Education and Information Access; HIV/AIDS; Life Expectancy and Aging Populations; Malnutrition; NGOs and Health Care: Deliverance or Dependence; Nutrition; Population Issues; Sanitation and Hygiene; Stigma; Water Supplies and Access to Clean Water*

BIBLIOGRAPHY

Books

Aday, Lu Ann. *At Risk in America: The Health and Health Care Needs of Vulnerable Populations in the United States*, 2nd ed. San Francisco, CA: Jossey-Bass, 2001.

Awotona, Adenrele A. *Rebuilding Sustainable Communities with Vulnerable Populations after the Cameras Have Gone: A Worldwide Study*. Newcastle upon Tyne, UK: Cambridge Scholars, 2012.

Estrine, Steven, et al., eds. *Service Delivery for Vulnerable Populations: New Directions in Behavioral Health*. New York: Springer, 2011.

Frohlich, Katherine L. "Learning from the Social Sciences in Chronic Diseases Health Promotion: Structure, Agency, and Distributive Justice," in *Global Handbook on Noncommunicable Diseases and Health Promotion*, edited by David V. McQueen, 73–82. New York: Springer, 2013.

Greif, Geoffrey L., and Paul H. Ephross, eds. *Group Work with Populations at Risk*, 3rd ed. Oxford: Oxford University Press, 2011.

Lalonde, Marc. *A New Perspective on the Health of Canadians*. Ottawa, Canada: Minister of Supply and Services, 1981. Available online at http://www.phac-aspc.gc.ca/ph-sp/pdf/perspect-eng.pdf (accessed March 20, 2015).

Link, Bruce G., and Jo C. Phelan. "Fundamental Sources of Health Inequalities," in *Policy Challenges in Modern Health Care*, edited by David Mechanic, L. B. Rogut, D. C. Colby, and J. R. Knickman. New Brunswick, NJ: Rutgers University Press, 2004, 71–84. Available online at http://www.rwjf.org/content/dam/farm/books/books/2004/rwjf11410 (accessed March 5, 2015).

Matherly, Deborah, Jane Mobley, and Beverly G. Ward. *Communication with Vulnerable Populations: A Transportation and Emergency Management Toolkit*. Washington, DC: Transportation Research Board, 2011.

Rose, Geoffrey. *The Strategy of Preventive Medicine*. Oxford: Oxford University Press, 1992.

Shi, Leiyu, and Gregory D. Stevens. *Vulnerable Populations in the United States*, 2nd ed. San Francisco, CA: Jossey-Bass, 2010.

Society of American Law Teachers, and Golden Gate University, eds. *Vulnerable Populations and Transformative Law Teaching: A Critical Reader*. Durham, NC: Carolina Academic Press, 2011.

Periodicals

Centers for Disease Control and Prevention. "The CDC Health Disparities and Inequalities Report— United States, 2013." *Morbidity and Mortality Weekly Report* 62, Suppl. 3 (November 22, 2013): 1–187. Available online at http://www.cdc.gov/mmwr/preview/ind2013_su.html (accessed March 5, 2015).

Frohlich, Katherine L., and Louise Potvin. "Transcending the Known in Public Health Practice: The inequality Paradox: The Population Approach and Vulnerable Populations." *American Journal of Public Health* 98, no. 2 (February 2008): 216–221.

Sugarman, Jonathan R., et al. "The Safety Net Medical Home Initiative: Transforming Care for Vulnerable Populations." *Medical Care* 52, Suppl. 4 (November 2014): S1–S10.

Uddin, Jasmim, et al. "Vulnerability of Bangladeshi Street-Children to HIV/AIDS: A Qualitative Study." *BMC Public Health* 14 (2014): 151.

Websites

"2015 UNHCR Country Operations Profile - Turkey." *United Nations High Commissioner for Refugees*. http://www.unhcr.org/pages/49e48e0fa7f.html (accessed May 31, 2015).

"Convention on the Rights of Persons with Disabilities." *United Nations (UN)*. http://www.un.org/disabilities/convention/conventionfull.shtml (accessed February 14, 2015).

"Delivering the Post-2015 Development Agenda." *United Nations Development Group*, 2014. https://www.worldwewant2015.org/diglogues2015 (accessed March 20, 2015).

"Minority Health." *U.S. Centers for Disease Control and Prevention (CDC)*. http://www.cdc.gov/minorityhealth/populations/atrisk.html (accessed February 14, 2015).

"Vulnerable Populations." *U.S. Department of Health and Human Services*. http://www.hhs.gov/ohrp/policy/populations/ (accessed February 14, 2015).

"Vulnerable Populations." *Urban Institute*. http://www.urban.org/health_policy/vulnerable_populations/index.cfm?gclid=CKDm67Ld4sMCFXJp7Aod01QARw (accessed February 14, 2015).

"Managing Vulnerable Populations." *World Health Organization (WHO)*. http://www.who.int/substance_abuse/publications/vulnerable_pop/en/ (accessed January 14, 2015).

Steven Joseph Archambault

Water Supplies and Access to Clean Water

⊕ Introduction

There are approximately 748 million people worldwide who do not have access to sources of clean drinking water, according to the World Health Organization (WHO). The majority of these people live in developing countries in Africa, Asia, and Latin America. Over 2.5 billion people do not have access to basic sanitation facilities. Nearly 3.5 million people die each year as a result of unsafe drinking water and poor water sanitation. Waterborne illnesses include diarrhea, cholera, intestinal worms, and malaria.

Water covers about 70 percent of Earth's surface, but only 2.5 percent of this water is drinkable. Much of the world's freshwater is in the form of ice caps in Antarctica and Greenland, or it is in the form of soil moisture. Less than 1 percent of freshwater is easily accessible for human consumption in the form of surface water (rivers, lakes, and human-made reservoirs) and groundwater. Snow and rain renew these sources, however, in some of the more arid parts of the world, water is consumed faster than the replenishment rate.

The distribution of water supplies and the ability for people to access freshwater varies throughout the world. North Africa, the Middle East, other parts of Central and southern Asia, southwestern North America, and southern Africa face existing and growing scarcity of physical water. Sub-Saharan Africa, south Asia, and parts of South America are burdened by economic water scarcity, lacking the physical infrastructure to harvest river water and groundwater.

Agriculture production is responsible for 70 percent of the water used worldwide. Remaining water uses include household (domestic) human consumption, manufacturing, and electricity production. Water that evaporates or is used up by crops and plants through transpiration is called consumptive water. A large percentage of the surface water used by humans is nonconsumptive, where it returns to groundwater or surface water sources for later use. Groundwater is an increasingly relied upon source of freshwater.

Drinking water sources naturally protected from contamination, or constructed to keep out contamination, are improved drinking water sources. The primary contamination of concern is fecal matter. Many people in the Western world have clean drinking water piped directly into their homes. Improved sources of drinking water for poor individuals and communities in developing countries are likely to come from a public tap or a community well from which households collect water to use in their homes. Water sources are also at risk from runoff and contamination from contact with animals. Improved water sources include dug wells, springs, and the collection and storage of rainwater.

⊕ Historical Background

Access to ample supplies of water has driven human behavior and settlements throughout human history. Early hunter-gatherers often returned to lakes and fertile river valleys where they were likely to find more food. To survive they were forced to understand climatic variation and the seasonality of temperature and rainfall. The size of these communities was limited to the scarcity of resources, including water.

The development of the first agricultural communities 10,000–13,500 years ago required the development of irrigation technologies. Raising animals also required a reliable source of water. People in communities in China and North Africa carried water to their homes in clay pots as early as 9,000 years ago. Early settlements developed nearby springs and reliable streams to mitigate the problem of a lack of water.

Ancient cultures, including the Mayans and Egyptians, recognized water as important for survival. Early Egyptian farmers were taxed in years when the Nile River spring flows were high, as the waters carried extra nutrient rich silt that increased farm production. Ancient Egyptians developed some of the first plumbing systems to carry water from the Nile to their fields. Egyptians

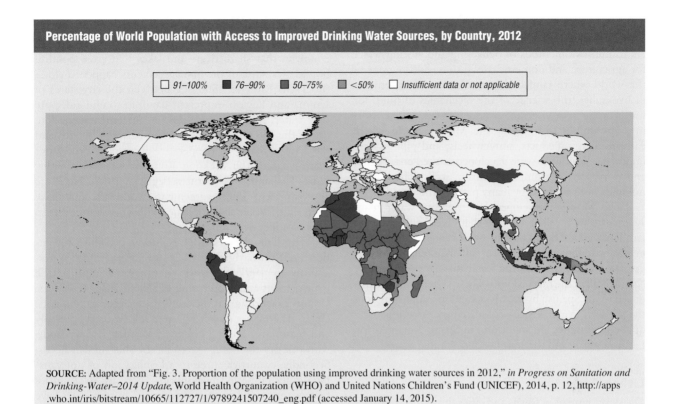

Percentage of World Population with Access to Improved Drinking Water Sources, by Country, 2012

□ 91–100%　■ 76–90%　■ 50–75%　■ <50%　□ Insufficient data or not applicable

SOURCE: Adapted from "Fig. 3. Proportion of the population using improved drinking water sources in 2012," *in Progress on Sanitation and Drinking-Water–2014 Update*, World Health Organization (WHO) and United Nations Children's Fund (UNICEF), 2014, p. 12, http://apps .who.int/iris/bitstream/10665/112727/1/9789241507240_eng.pdf (accessed January 14, 2015).

Approximately 748 million people worldwide do not have access to clean drinking water. The majority live in developing countries in Africa, Asia, and Latin America.

also built one of the first waste collection systems. The Palace of Knossos, built in 1900 BCE, had a system of flushable latrines that brought waste to underground holding facilities.

There is evidence that the Mayans had sophisticated systems for bringing water from its source to where it could be used for domestic and agricultural purposes. Water was carried to cisterns, where it was stored until it was needed by households or in agricultural fields. There is evidence of Mayan settlements relocating following periods of drought. The collapse of Mayan communities occurred in part due to changes in climate, including an extended period of drought.

Aqueducts

The development of the aqueduct and other technologies to move water allowed ancient Roman and Greek communities to live farther from freshwater sources. The early Roman aqueducts would carry water to urban developments in brick or stone conduits after being siphoned from springs, lakes, or reservoirs. The conduits often ran underground, using the power of gravity over a slight gradient. Viaducts or bridges would enable water to cross large valleys. The conduits would often feed water tanks that would distribute the water supply as needed.

The city of Rome is surrounded by freshwater springs, which supplied water fountains and public baths

via aqueducts. Eleven aqueducts provided water to a population of 1 million by 200 CE. Rome built hundreds of other aqueducts throughout its empire. The aqueduct systems required regular maintenance and repair. Most of the aqueducts were not maintained as the Roman Empire collapsed; however there are portions of aqueducts still in existence today.

Issues of water quality and sanitation were very important for the health of early cities. Technology for measuring water quality was limited to smell and visual inspections. Water with the poorest quality was used for irrigation. There were some attempts to clean water in settling tanks, particularly after rain events, which would carry debris into the aqueduct system. The Romans controlled water conditions by warming water for baths using underground furnaces.

The Romans collected sewage and other wastewater, and deposited it into nearby bodies of water. There was some risk to the population, who was exposed to sewage flowing in semi-open channels near residential areas. The constant movement of water from the aqueducts allowed wastes to be washed away quickly, which likely improved sanitation conditions.

Muslim Influence

Muslim communities throughout North Africa, the Middle East, and Central Asia advanced water technology and management after the fall of Rome. Muslims integrated techniques developed by Romans, the Chinese, and others to improve methods of delivering and storing water for agriculture and domestic use in these arid regions of the world where rainfall was unreliable. Advancements in hydraulics, the science of the mechanics of fluid, for use in industry and power production have their roots in communities throughout the Muslim world where early Roman aqueducts, waterwheels, and piping were improved. Windmills were developed in the Persia region and were used to pump water from wells. These technologies were adopted by many parts of the world.

The Muslims developed an irrigation water management system called *acequias* that divert river water to farmlands via a series of human-made canals. The acequias involve communal governance and maintenance of the irrigation channels, with the water manager of a specific channel called the mayordomo. These systems were introduced to the Spanish by the Moors and spread throughout the Western world as Spain colonized the Americas. Acequia communities are still found in Spain, North Africa, Latin America, and the southwestern United States.

Urban Areas

The development of towns and cities throughout Europe in the Middle Ages (c. 500–c. 1500 CE) required advancements in water management and technology to be used by city residents. In addition to drinking and bathing, water was used for trades including milling, slaughtering, tanning, brewing, and papermaking. Water was also used for defense. Issues of sewage disposal, water pollution, sanitation, the spread of disease, and fire control became important concerns for medieval towns as they grew. Feudal lords and town councils had to encourage community members to maintain pipes and sewage systems, and to put in regulations to discourage pollution and damaging waste disposal practices.

The growth of cities such as Paris and London in the 17th, 18th, and 19th centuries introduced important water supply and sanitation problems. London was extracting water from shallow wells and by waterwheels from the River Thames. The Thames was also the place where sewage was piped. This led to numerous health concerns, including outbreaks of cholera, as polluted water was distributed back to factories and households. The 1800s and 1900s saw the advancement of underground sewage systems and water treatment facilities.

The septic tank, an on-site system that stores and treats wastes, was developed in France by John Mouras in the late 1800s. Septic tanks break down solids and allow liquids to leach into the ground where they are purified by soil. Septic systems diminished the problem of sewage polluting freshwater supplies. The septic tanks were patented and brought to other parts of the world in the late 1800s. The first septic systems were installed in the United States in Boston in 1883.

International Water Agreements

There have been numerous historical agreements between countries that share rivers and lakes that cross political boundaries. One of the first agreements happened along the Tigris River in 2500 BCE between the city-states of Umma and Lagash in present-day Iraq to end a dispute over water. In the early 1900s, an agreement regarding use of the Rio Grande was reached between Mexico and the United States. A cooperative agreement over water sharing along the Mekong River between Cambodia, Laos, Thailand, and Vietnam began in 1957. There are approximately 3,600 agreements worldwide that have been signed to enable countries with mutual interests to avoid conflict over water.

The United Nations (UN) developed the Convention on Non-navigational Uses of International Watercourses in 1997 to assist countries to improve the management and monitoring of shared water resources. Countries who signed the convention agree to two principles. The first is that freshwater will be used equitably and reasonably among countries sharing a water body, with priority for water use to be for vital human needs. Secondly, countries agree to an obligation of not causing significant harm to neighbors. There are 36 countries that are included in the convention, but only 16 have signed it as of 2015.

⊕ Impacts and Issues

Governments, development agencies, nonprofit organizations, and private companies recognize the importance of improving the access and use of water throughout the world. The UN created an administrative body, UN-Water, to coordinate efforts to address water and sanitation issues, particularly in developing countries. Through the Millennium Development Goals (MDGs) the international community made a commitment to reduce by half the number of people who did not have access to safe drinking water and basic sanitation between 1990 and 2015. The access to safe drinking water goal was met in 2010; however, 11 percent of the world's population continued to use unsafe sources of water. It was projected that by 2015, about 8 percent of the world's population would have access to safe water sources. The goal to improve sanitation (75 percent of the population with improved sanitation) has not been reached, particularly due to rapid growth in urban areas, with only 63 percent of the world's population with access to improved sanitation in 2010, projected to be 67 percent in 2015.

Water as a Human Right

In 2010, the UN passed a resolution to acknowledge that water is a human right, and that all human rights cannot be realized if people do not have access to clean drinking water and sanitation. The motivation was, in part, to encourage the international community to do more to

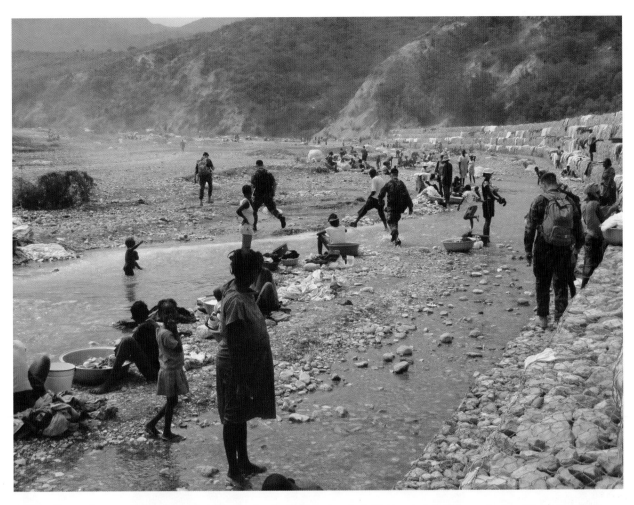

Haitian villagers who were displaced from their houses after the 2010 earthquake in Haiti wash their clothes and eating utensils in a stream, while U.S. Public Health Service officers inspect the source of drinking water. *Lt. Cmdr. Gary Brunette/U.S. Centers for Disease Control and Prevention.*

provide the resources countries need to improve water and sanitation facilities. Many developing countries do not have the financial resources to build and maintain modern water distribution and treatment centers. The resolution says water should be in sufficient quantities, safe for consumption, acceptable based on needs and culture, within reasonable physical proximity, and affordable for all people.

The World Health Organization (WHO) says that individuals need between 13 to 26 gallons (50 and 100 liters) of water per day to ensure their basic needs are met. This is considered sufficient water for drinking, personal sanitation, washing clothes, preparing food, and maintaining personal and household hygiene. The UN Development Programme (UNDP) reports that people who do not have access to sufficient drinking water use approximately 1.32 gallons (5 liters) of unsafe water per day, in stark contrast to water use in the United States and Europe where about 53 to 80 gallons (200 to 300 liters) per day of safe water use is common. Women who are lactating and involved in physical activity need approximately 7.5 liters per day.

To be considered safe, water must be free of chemicals, radiological hazards, and microorganisms that could threaten a person's health. The WHO provides guidelines for drinking water standards that can be used by authorities to create local and national water management policy. Sanitation facilities should be hygienic, with wastewater and excrement disposed of safely. Public toilet facilities, the only available facilities for many people in developing countries, should be in locations where their security can be ensured. Safe sanitation also means toilets should be constructed to prevent collapse, and should be available at all times, including both day and night.

Acceptable water and sanitation facilities ensure water is of an acceptable color, odor, and taste for personal use. To be acceptable also includes ensuring all male and females have equal access to water and to sanitation facilities in a way that ensures privacy and dignity. In rural areas of developing countries, it is not uncommon that schools do not have facilities that are separate for boys and girls. This causes girls to try and avoid using the facilities by not drinking water and potentially becoming dehydrated. Without separate facilities, girls are more likely to miss school when they are menstruating.

The collection of water is primarily the responsibility of women and children in developing countries. On average, women in Africa and Asia walk 3.73 miles (6 kilometers) to collect water, which takes away from other activities including education, agriculture, and wage earning. In sub-Saharan Africa, women spend nearly 40 billion hours per year carrying water to their homes, which is equivalent to the annual working hours of the French labor force. The WHO says people have good access to water and sanitation when those services are located within a distance of 0.62 miles (1 kilometer) of a household, workplace, school, or health facility, and when water collection takes less than 30 minutes. In addition to women and children, the needs of the disabled and elderly should not be overlooked when considering access to water and sanitation.

Water and sanitation services in Latin America, Asia, and Africa often require a higher percentage of household income than services in the world's richest cities. The cost of water and sanitation services for median income households is approximately 1.1 percent of income. In Nicaragua and El Salvador, the poorest 20 percent of households pay nearly 10 percent of their income on water and sanitation services, and those services are generally of lower quality. Unaffordable water and sanitation require households to sacrifice purchases of other basic needs, such as food, housing, health care, and education. The right of affordable water and sanitation services does not indicate that these services should be free of charge, but the cost should not exceed 5 percent of a household's income.

Economic Impacts and Considerations

The lack of access to water and sanitation services impacts economic advancement for household, communities, and countries. Children in villages and cities with minimal access to clean water suffer from higher rates of illness, causing them to miss over 440 million school days each year. This is equivalent to all of the seven-year-old children in Ethiopia missing a year of school. Decreased attendance and performance in school negatively impacts the long-term ability for students to break out of poverty cycles.

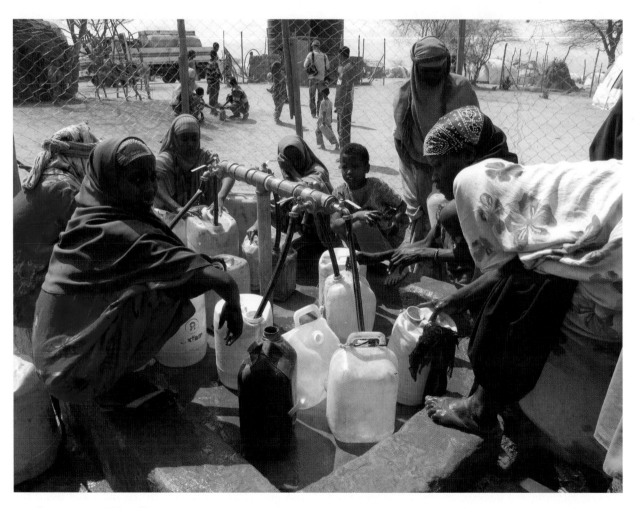

Somali women and children fill up water containers at the refugee camp in Dadaab, Kenya. © *Sadik Gulec/Shutterstock.com.*

WATER SECURITY

The rate of water use has grown twice as fast as the rate of population growth throughout the last century. Anthropogenic (human) water use in developing countries is expected to increase by 50 percent from the levels used in 2013. Developed countries will see an increase of 18 percent over the same period. This places stress on both surface water and underground aquifers. It is estimated that 1.8 billion people will be living in countries with water scarcity by 2025. Two-thirds of the world's population could be under water stress conditions by 2025. Water stress occurs when available water supplies are less than the water demanded during certain times of the year or when poor quality restricts water use.

Global climate change adds increased uncertainty to the world's water supplies. Increases in the world's temperature will likely lead to less reliable snow packs and early and more rapid snow melt. This adds difficulties for agricultural users and water managers who rely on predictable water flows. Higher temperatures also increase the evaporation rate, drying out soils. Lower precipitation in some areas, including the Sahel in Africa, have led to more persistent drought. Other areas have experienced more extreme storms and rainfall events leading to increases in flooding disasters.

One in nine people does not have access to drinking water that has been improved to make it safe from pollution and waterborne illnesses. One in three people does not have access to improved sanitation, including toilets, which properly dispose of wastewater and sewage. Eighty percent of the world's sewage in developing countries is directly discharged untreated into water bodies. Industry is another large polluter of the world's fresh-water bodies.

Freshwater ecosystems including rivers, lakes, streams, and wetlands have been degraded and threatened more than other ecosystems, with the population of freshwater species declining by more than 70 percent in the 40 years prior to a 2014 report by the World Wildlife Fund. The services provided by freshwater ecosystems, including supplies of clean water, production of food, soil formation, habitat, flood control, and recreation have often been overlooked as these ecosystems are damaged. Water officials and policy makers must consider the value of these services when developing conservation and water management strategies.

Countries and development organizations around the globe have recognized the need to protect water security as part of meeting sustainable development goals. The UN's interagency coordinating body of water issues, UN-Water, defined water security as "The capacity of a population to safeguard sustainable access to adequate quantities of and acceptable quality water for sustaining livelihoods, human well-being, and socioeconomic development, for ensuring protection against water-borne pollution and water-related disasters, and for preserving ecosystems in a climate of peace and political stability."

UN-Water identified several key aspects for improving and maintaining water security for the world's poor and vulnerable populations. 1) Ensure access to affordable drinking water that is safe and sufficient to meet basic needs and maintain good health. 2) Protect human rights, livelihoods, cultural values, and recreational values of water. 3) Allocate water to preserve and protect ecosystems that provide critical ecosystem services. 4) Maintain water for economic development activities including energy production, transportation, industry, and tourism. 5) Properly treat wastewater to protect against disease and environmental pollution. 6) Develop collaborative and cooperative approaches to cross border water resource management within and between countries. 7) Increase the capacity to manage the risks and uncertainty from natural and human-made disasters including floods, drought, and pollution. 8) Good governance and accountability through the consideration of all interests and stakeholders, appropriate policy, transparency; planning and maintenance of infrastructure; and building capacity.

The Water and Sanitation Program has investigated the economic impact of poor sanitation, saying high health-care costs, lost time and productivity, decreased water quality, and decreased tourism cost the world US$260 billion a year. This amounts to an average of 1.5 percent of each country's gross domestic product. The economic costs in India alone are US$54 billion per year. Health-care costs are the largest component of the economic burden of poor sanitation.

Studies by the WHO indicate that for each US$1 invested in improving sanitation, there is an average economic return of US$5.50. For investments in improved water supplies, the rate of return is US$2 for each US$1 invested. These numbers vary across regions, with the highest returns seen in Latin America, East Asia, and South Asia. In all regions, the costs of needed investment are greater in urban areas when compared to rural areas. The capital costs, or initial investments, of improving water and sanitation services are 1.7 times higher in urban areas than they are in rural areas.

To improve water and sanitation there is a need for new reservoirs, wells, water delivery systems, toilets, sewage systems, and other infrastructure projects. Additionally, there is a need to maintain water and sanitation systems and to replace aged systems. These recurring costs are important for government planning and the creation of budgets. Investments are also needed for improving human capacity in areas of hygiene education, policy planning, monitoring, and regulation.

⊕ Future Implications

Water takes on aspects of a community or common resource, where a particular individual or household does not own it. This leads to a case of the tragedy of the commons, in which individuals acting in their own self-interest do not have an incentive to ensure resources are protected, while it is in the best interest of all users that the resource is protected. In the case of water, this can lead to problems including overuse and excessive pollution. To avoid these negative effects that can lead to disagreement and violence, it is necessary to have good policy that incorporates all of the needs and interests of communities members to share and regulate water use so it is used sustainably.

There is a growing understanding of the role that ecosystems play in protecting water supplies. Healthy forests regulate water flows for urban, agricultural, and industrial water users. In Costa Rica, upstream landowners are paid by hydroelectric producers to restore and maintain forests to ensure downstream flows. Wetland ecosystems are natural water purifiers and are particularly important for reducing the costs of water purification. Water management plans and strategies must consider the role of healthy ecosystems to meet production and conservation objectives.

Global climate change is causing changes in weather conditions that are projected to impact rainfall, snowmelt, river flows, and groundwater. Increases in natural disasters related to extreme storms and other weather events are attributed in part to global climate change. As temperatures rise, higher rates of evaporation decrease freshwater supplies. It is likely that climate change will deteriorate water quality, putting continued pressure on poor communities throughout the world. The likelihood of climate change increases the need for protecting water resources that are already under stress.

UN-Water highlights the need to adapt land and water management strategies to increase the ability to adapt to climate change, and improve water security. Taking these measures has the potential to improve economic development. Implementation of innovative technological strategies in agriculture, land use management, and water conservation need to be implemented at appropriate scales to assist communities in adapting to climate change.

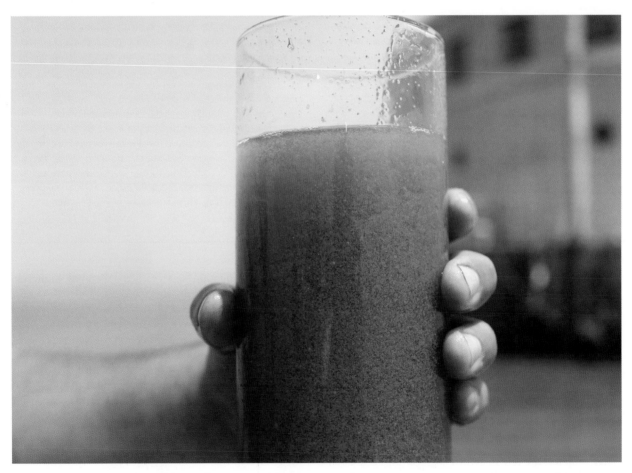

A sample glass of Lake Erie water is shown near the city of Toledo, Ohio, water intake plant, August 3, 2014, about 2.5 miles (4 kilometers) off the shore of Curtice, Ohio. The mayor of Toledo warned 400,000 people in the region to avoid drinking tap water for a second day while tests were conducted to ensure toxins were out of Toledo's water supply. Toledo officials had issued the warning early the previous day after tests at one treatment plant showed two sample readings for microcystin (a liver toxin) above the standard for consumption, possibly because of algae on Lake Erie.   © Haraz N. Ghanbari/AP Images.

Water, Energy, and Agriculture

The 2014 UN *World Water Development Report* highlights the strong interconnections between water and energy. Most energy sources, particularly those derived from oil, natural gas, coal, nuclear, hydropower, and biofuel, require some input of water for production, transportation, and use. The water available for energy production is highly dependent on how water resources are used, conserved, and managed. Energy is also needed for the extraction, treatment, and distribution of water.

As population grows, energy production must compete for water with agriculture, manufacturing, human consumption, and maintaining healthy ecosystems. There is a need for policy makers to manage and consider the different needs for water that communities have. Water utilities find energy costs to be their number one expense. It is necessary to invest in urban water management technologies and strategies that conserve energy. One approach is to treat water to the quality that is needed. Water used for agriculture and certain industries does not require purification to drinking water standards.

The growth in population requires more efficient methods for food production that protect water resources. The UN Food and Agriculture Organization highlights the important connection between water management and food security. Agricultural practices that better use and conserve water resources include small-scale water storage projects, agroforestry, methods to improve soil quality, precision irrigation, and systems allowing for reuse of water. Building human capacity to implement water conservation technologies and cropping strategies is also important. International research organizations such as the International Crop Research Institute for the Semi-arid Tropics are also involved with projects to make irrigation in agriculture more efficient and sustainable.

Growing crops for bioenergy has resulted in one of the largest increases in demand for agriculture products. Bioenergy can have a bigger water consumption rate than fossil fuel use, as water is needed for the production of crops and for the conversion to energy. Many bioenergy crops are subsidized, given an incentive for farmers to deplete groundwater to produce the crops. It is necessary to consider impacts on water sustainability when analyzing the long-term benefit of bioenergy.

SEE ALSO *Child Health; Cholera and Dysentery; Global Health Initiatives; High Blood Pressure; Noncommunicable Diseases; Nutrition; Population Issues; Vulnerable Populations; Waterborne Diseases*

BIBLIOGRAPHY

Books

Fagan, Brian. *Elixir: A History of Water and Humankind.* New York: Bloomsbury, 2011.

Gleick, Peter. *The World's Water.* Vol. 8: *The Biennial Report on Freshwater Resources.* Washington, DC: Island Press, 2014.

United Nations World Water Assessment Programme. *United Nations World Water Development Report 2014: Water and Energy.* Paris: UNESCO, 2014. Available online at http://www.unwater.org/publications/publications-detail/en/c/218614/ (accessed March 9, 2015).

World Health Organization. *Global Costs and Benefits of Drinking-Water Supply and Sanitation Interventions to Reach the MDG Target and Universal Coverage.* Geneva: World Health Organization, 2012. Available online at http://www.who.int/water_sanitation_health/publications/2012/global_costs/en/ (accessed March 9, 2015).

World Health Organization. *UN-Water Global Analysis and Assessment of Sanitation and Drinking-Water (GLAAS) 2014 Report: Investing in Water and Sanitation: Increasing Access, Reducing Inequalities.* Geneva: World Health Organization, 2014. Available online at http://www.who.int/water_sanitation_health/glaas/en/ (accessed March 9, 2015).

World Health Organization and United Nations Children's Fund. *Progress on Drinking Water and Sanitation, 2014 Update.* Geneva: World Health Organization and UNICEF, 2014. Available online at http://www.who.int/water_sanitation_health/publications/2014/jmp-report/en/ (accessed March 9, 2015).

Periodicals

Dodds, Walter K., Joshuah S. Perkin, and Joseph E. Gerken. "Human Impact on Freshwater Ecosystem Services: A Global Perspective." *Environmental Science and Technology* 47, no. 16 (August 20, 2013): 9061–9068.

Flörke, M., et al. "Domestic and Industrial Water Uses of the Past 60 Years as a Mirror of Socio-economic Development: A Global Simulation Study." *Global Environmental Change* 23, no. 1 (February 2013): 144–156.

Yoshihide, Wada, and Marc F. P. Bierkens. "Sustainability of Global Water Use: Past Reconstruction and Future Projections." *Environmental Research Letters* 9, no. 10 (October 2014). Available online at http://iopscience.iop.org/1748-9326/9/10/104003 (accessed March 9, 2015).

Websites

International Crop Research Institute for the Semi-arid Tropics. http://www.icrisat.org (accessed March 5, 2015).

UN-Water. http://www.unwater.org (accessed March 5, 2015).

"Water." *World Health Organization (WHO).* http://www.who.int/topics/water/en/ (accessed March 5, 2015).

"Water and Sanitation." *United Nations Children's Fund (UNICEF).* http://www.unicefusa.org/mission/survival/water (accessed March 5, 2015).

"Water & Sanitation Specialists." *Médicins Sans Frontières/Doctors Without Borders.* http://www.msf.ca/en/water-sanitation-specialists (accessed March 5, 2015).

"Water Projects & Programs." *The World Bank.* http://www.worldbank.org/en/topic/water/projects (accessed March 5, 2015).

Water.org. http://water.org/water-crisis/water-facts/water/ (accessed March 5, 2015).

Steven Joseph Archambault

Waterborne Diseases

⊕ Introduction

Waterborne diseases are caused by pathogenic bacteria, parasites, and viruses spread primarily from ingesting or washing in contaminated water or from poor storage of treated water. Organisms that cause these diseases may be introduced to the water supply through human or animal feces or by way of organisms that naturally spend part of their life cycle in water.

Symptoms of these diseases vary, but diarrhea and vomiting are the most commonly reported and often do the most damage. About 88 percent of the 4 billion diarrhea cases reported worldwide are linked to unsafe water, inadequate sanitation, or insufficient hygiene. The waterborne diseases that do not cause diarrhea cause a host of other ailments including malnutrition, skin infections, and organ damage.

Some of these diseases, once contracted, resolve themselves on their own. However, others may require medical interventions with antimicrobials or salt tablets that help restore fluids lost due to dehydration. The World Health Organization (WHO) estimates that 94 percent of diarrheal cases are preventable through modifications to the environment, including interventions that increase the availability of clean water, improved sanitation, and hygiene.

Of the more than 6.5 billion people living in the world, an estimated 748 million lack access to safe drinking water and 2.5 billion, or 38 percent, do not have access to basic sanitation, according to WHO. Furthermore, hundreds of millions lack soap and clean water necessary for basic hand washing, a practice that prevents the spread of diarrheal and respiratory illness. Roughly 2 million people die each year from diarrheal diseases directly attributable to unsafe water, sanitation, and hygiene; of those, more than 600,000 are children. These diseases are particularly common and virulent in poor and rural areas of the world where underlying health problems such as malnutrition and HIV/AIDS make the effects worse. Lack of education and resources for clean water further exacerbate the problem.

⊕ Historical Background

It is likely that waterborne diseases have always existed. It is also likely that they gave the earliest humans considerable trouble, and that early humans discerned good water from bad through trial and error.

Over the centuries, humans developed sophisticated ways of bringing in clean water and taking away waste. Some archaeological evidence suggests that the Mayans may have had pressurized water as early as 6500 BCE. Early Romans had an elaborate series of aqueducts and irrigation channels to bring in clean water and get rid of their wastewater; the Greeks, as well as many other civilizations, boiled their rainwater before they drank it.

Still, there have been outbreaks of waterborne disease with catastrophic consequences. Typhoid fever, a disease caused by the bacteria *Salmonella enterica* (serotpye Typhi), is believed by some scholars to have been one of the diseases that killed many of the first settlers who came to Jamestown, Virginia, in 1607. Scholars also believe typhoid and dysentery, another waterborne illness that causes severe diarrhea, killed more than 86,000 Union soldiers in the American Civil War. Dysentery is caused by the bacterium *Shigella* and by some types of amoebae.

Another example of waterborne disease is cholera. Cholera, caused by the bacteria *Vibrio cholerae*, was responsible for several recurring pandemics throughout the 1800s and may have been causing outbreaks in India since the 16th century. The ultimate death toll of cholera during those pandemics is not known, but scholars with the U.S. National Institutes of Health cite the deaths of as many as 7,000 people in Paris over the course of 18 days in 1832 as an example of cholera's devastation.

By the mid-1800s, scientists began advancing the notion that disease was caused by microorganisms. At that time, miasmata—believed to be particles of disease-causing, foul-smelling decaying matter suspended in the air—were thought to be responsible. The idea that disease is caused by the presence and actions of microorganisms

JOHN SNOW, CHOLERA AND THE BROAD STREET PUMP HANDLE

John Snow, a British physician, was one of the first to discover that cholera was spread through contaminated water and food. Born in 1813 in York, England, to a coal laborer, Snow was an exceptionally bright student. After attending school, he was apprenticed at the age of 14 to a local physician named Dr. William Hardcastle. Four years later, Snow was working for Hardcastle when a cholera pandemic hit London.

Cholera, which is caused by the bacteria *Vibrio cholerae*, is believed to have been endemic in India and caused outbreaks as early as the 16th century. In some of those infected, the disease causes severe diarrhea within hours of contracting it, and it can cause death from dehydration if not treated. In 1817, a fierce outbreak struck the East Indian state of Bengal. After spreading through India, it made its way to Persia, the Middle East, and Southeast Asia. By 1823 it had reached the Mediterranean before slowing down. Just four years later, in 1827, cholera once again struck in India and by 1829 showed up in Russia, Europe, and the Middle East. By 1832, it reached North America by way of Quebec and New York.

When the pandemic hit London in 1831, Hardcastle found himself with more patients than he could treat. He sent his young apprentice out to tend to a group of coal miners who had fallen ill. At age 18, equipped only with the treatment tools available to him at the time (bleeding, brandy, laxatives, opium, and peppermint), he found himself unable to help the men.

By 1832, the outbreak in London was over, and Snow went on to earn his degree. He became a practicing physician and spent years studying the effects of anesthetics. He was also interested in causes of contagious disease, and he came to believe that instead of being caused by miasmata, or malodorous air arising from the decay of organic matter (a popular theory at the time), disease might be caused by microorganisms.

This idea, which would become known as germ theory, had been around in one form or another since the 1600s when Dutch scientist Antonie van Leeuwenhoek (1632–1723) first discovered organisms while looking through his microscope. Until Snow, however, no one had given it any credence.

A second cholera pandemic hit London in 1848, and Snow began studying and tracking the disease and speaking with its victims. Through his medical detective work, he reasoned that cholera was spread by contaminated water and espoused this belief for several years to much criticism. When an outbreak hit the Soho area of London in 1854, Snow had gathered enough evidence to pinpoint locations of cholera cases on a map. Many of the cases clustered around a communal water pump on Broad Street. Officials still were not convinced, but when the pump handle was removed, the cases of cholera in that area dropped off dramatically.

Though Snow's germ theory still would not be widely accepted until the 1860s, he is now considered the founder of modern epidemiology.

---

is known as germ theory, and once accepted, radically changed the science of medicine.

Communities around the world have now developed various ways of treating water to remove microorganisms that cause disease. Despite this, the largest outbreak of a waterborne illness in the United States happened in 1993, when a treatment plant in Milwaukee, Wisconsin, became contaminated with *Cryptosporidium*, a parasite that causes the diarrheal disease cryptosporidiosis, the symptoms of which are fever, stomach cramps, diarrhea, and dehydration. The disease sickened 403,000 people and killed 100 (though most of the severe cases were in persons with diminished immunity, such as those infected with human immunodeficiency virus [HIV].)

⊕ Impacts and Issues

Though waterborne diseases have been all but eradicated in the developed world, they remain a problem in many developing countries. Lack of access to clean water and proper sanitation as well as poor storage of treated water are among the biggest barriers to eradicating waterborne diseases. Risk of these diseases is highest among poor and rural populations. Some of the most prevalent waterborne diseases found in these areas are diarrhea, cholera, dysentery, shigellosis, guinea worm disease, schistosomiasis, and typhoid fever.

Diarrhea

Diarrhea due to gastrointestinal infection is widespread throughout the world and kills 2.2 million people each year. It is the cause of 4 percent of all deaths and 5 percent of health loss to disability, according to the WHO. In Southeast Asia and Africa alone, diarrhea is responsible for as much as 8.5 percent and 7.7 percent of all deaths respectively. The U.S. Centers for Disease Control and Prevention (CDC) reports that, globally in 2012, it caused 11 percent of all deaths in children under age five for which cause of death was known (see graphic).

Diarrhea is caused by a variety of microorganisms including viruses, bacteria, and protozoans, and is most common in places where there is a shortage of adequate sanitation, hygiene, and safe water for drinking, cleaning, and cooking. Rotavirus, a genus of double-stranded RNA virus in the family Reoviridae, and *Escherichia coli* (also known as *E. coli*), rod-shaped bacterium of the genus *Escherichia* commonly found in the lower intestine of warm-blooded organisms, are the two most common etiological agents, or originators, of diarrhea in developing countries.

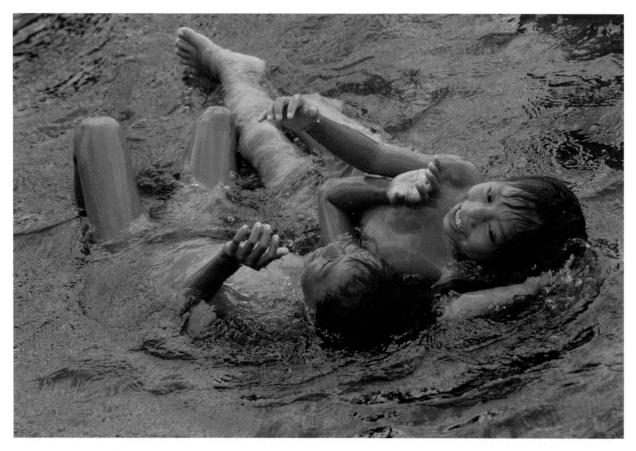

Children from impoverished areas escape the summer heat by swimming in the waters of Manila Bay, Philippines, on April 2, 2013, despite warnings issued by city and national authorities prohibiting swimming due to pollution in the bay. The health department has warned that those who swim in the bay are putting themselves in danger from diarrhea, cholera, typhoid fever, hepatitis, encephalitis, and various infections. © *Jay Directo/AFP/Getty Images.*

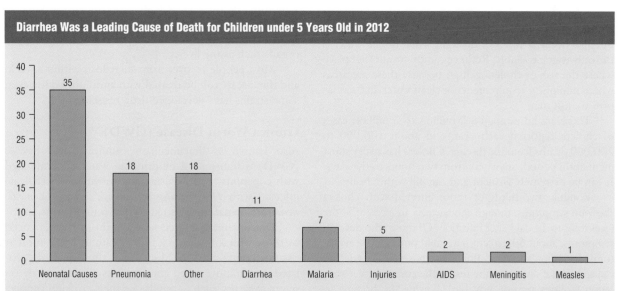

Diarrhea Was a Leading Cause of Death for Children under 5 Years Old in 2012

SOURCE: Adapted from data in *The Safe Water System: Disease & SWS Impact*, U.S. Centers for Disease Control and Prevention (CDC). Data from Liu, L., et al., "Global, Regional, and National Causes of Child Mortality: An Updated Systematic Analysis for 2010 with Time Trends since 2000," *Lancet* 379, no. 9832 (2012): 2151–2161.

Symptoms can include episodes of acute watery or bloody stools lasting several hours or days; persistent diarrhea may last 14 days or longer. A person suffering from diarrhea loses water and electrolytes, which can lead to dehydration and in extreme cases death. According to the United Nations Children's Fund (UNICEF), children account for 90 percent of the deaths from diarrhea each year. Those who survive are more vulnerable to other diseases and malnutrition.

As an example of how deadly diarrhea can be, UNICEF points to Rwandan refugees who fled the country in 1994 to areas around Goma, now the Democratic Republic of the Congo. After just one month, 50,000 refugees had died; of those deaths, 85 percent were attributed to diarrhea.

Along with access to adequate sanitation facilities, UNICEF estimates that simple hand washing with soap and water could cut diarrheal disease by one-third. Treatment usually includes administration of a solution of clean water, sugar, and salt, and sometimes zinc tablets. Access to vaccines such as that for rotavirus can greatly reduce incidence and death from diarrheal diseases.

Cholera

According to the WHO's fact sheet on water-related diseases, cholera is an acute diarrheal infection caused by ingestion of food or water contaminated with the bacterium *Vibrio cholera*. The bacterium thrives in salty water such as that in estuaries, and can be associated with algal blooms (a rapid increase or accumulation of algae).

Cholera is still reported in 58 countries and is present on every continent but Antarctica. It is most prominent in slums located in peri-urban areas (those located on land between rural and urban areas), where safe drinking water is limited and proper sanitation is scarce. Cases of cholera often spike during rainy seasons with flooding but also occur at times of drought when unsafe water is the only water available. Refugee camps are another place where the risk of cholera is high because these are areas where minimum requirements of clean water and sanitation are not met.

There are an estimated 3 million to 5 million cases of cholera reported each year, and about 100,000 to 200,000 deaths from the disease. Cholera has a very short incubation period, anywhere from two hours to five days. It can be extremely virulent and can kill within hours.

Roughly two-thirds of those infected with cholera show no symptoms, though the bacteria are present in the feces for 7 to 14 days after infection. Of those who develop symptoms, about 80 percent have mild or moderate symptoms, including diarrhea. But even those mildly affected can spread the disease to the rest of the community if sanitation facilities are not available, allowing the bacteria to shed back into the environment. The remaining 20 percent who experience severe cases of cholera develop acute watery diarrhea with severe dehydration, according to the WHO.

There are two serogroups, or variations, of *V. cholerae* linked to outbreaks; they are identified as *V. cholerae* O1 and *V. cholerae* O139. *V.cholerae* O1 is responsible for the majority of outbreaks while *V. cholerae* O139, which was first identified in Bangladesh in 1992, is largely confined to Southeast Asia. Other variations of *V. cholerae* can cause illness but generally do not produce outbreaks. New variations have been detected in recent years in Asia and Africa. These strains seem to cause more severe cholera and have higher fatality rates.

The vast majority of cases, as much as 80 percent, can be treated with oral rehydration salts, which is clean water mixed with sugar and salt, as well as supplemental zinc. If the case is severe, however, intravenous fluids and antibiotics are necessary.

Dysentery

Dysentery is bloody diarrhea that is loose and watery. Symptoms also include fever, abdominal cramps, and rectal pain. Dysentery is most often caused by the *Shigella* species of bacteria, known as bacillary dysentery, but it can also be caused by *Entamoeba histolytica*, known as amoebic dysentery.

Shigellosis occurs throughout the world and is transmitted by food or water contaminated with the *Shigella* bacteria, or through person-to-person contact. It only requires a few organisms of *Shigella* to transmit infection, so person-to-person transmission is frequent. Once in the body, the *Shigella* bacteria destroy the cells lining the large intestine, causing mucosal ulceration and bloody diarrhea.

Amoebic dysentery is caused by the amoeba *Entamoeba histolytica*, which forms cysts in fecal matter that can be transmitted through contaminated water. The symptoms of amoebic dysentery are much the same as shigellosis, except that if left untreated, the amoeba can spread outside the intestine and form abscesses on other organs such as the liver.

Most people recover from shigellosis within a week, and the disease can be treated with antibiotics. However, some strains have developed drug resistance.

Guinea Worm Disease (GWD)

Also known as dracunculiasis, guinea worm disease (GWD) is transmitted by drinking water contaminated with copepods (small crustaceans known as water fleas) infected with *Dracunculus medinensis* larvae. *D. medinensis* are nematodes, also known as roundworms.

Dracunculiasis is rarely fatal, but the pain experienced by those who suffer from it is debilitating. Those most at risk for contracting the disease are those in rural, isolated, and impoverished communities who must rely on stagnant water, such as ponds, for their drinking supply.

After a person drinks contaminated water, ingesting the fleas, the fleas die and release their larvae. The larvae then make their way through the stomach and intestinal

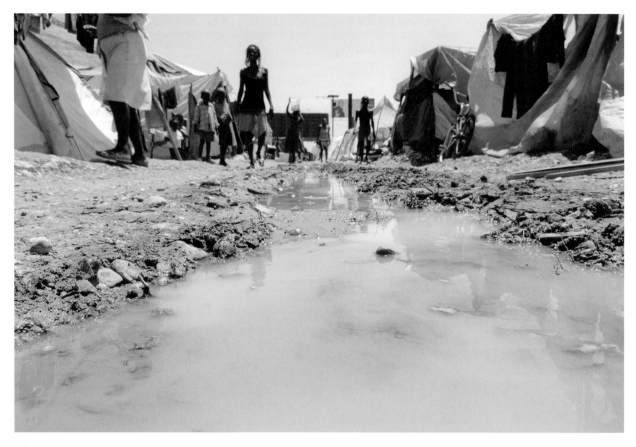

After the 2010 earthquake in Haiti, many Haitians were forced to live in internally displaced person camps, many of which had unclean water that became breeding grounds for waterborne and insect-borne diseases, including cholera. © *arindambanerjee/Shutterstock.com.*

wall into the abdominal cavity. Here they mature and mate, after which the males die. Meanwhile, the females, which can grow to a length of between 2 and 4 feet (70 to 120 centimeters), migrate to the skin surface.

After a year, the female worm breaks through the skin (usually in the foot or leg) via a blister it has created. When the person infected with the worm next puts his or her foot into water, the worm comes out of the blister, releases larvae, and the cycle starts again.

GWD has been on a steady decline since the 1980s; at that time the disease was endemic in 20 countries, and more than 3.5 million cases were reported per year. As of 2014, the disease is endemic in Chad, Ethiopia, Mali, and South Sudan, and according to WHO, between January and October 2014 there were only 115 reported cases of GWD.

Currently there is no vaccine to prevent the disease and no known medication for treatment. Instead, the disease is on the verge of eradication through a variety of strategies that include an increase in surveillance to detect every case within 24 hours of the worm emerging. Once the worm emerges, transmission can be prevented by treating, cleaning, and bandaging the affected area until the worm is completely out of the body, according to the WHO.

Other strategies include keeping the affected person from wading into water sources, providing access to improved drinking water supplies, filtering water from open water bodies before drinking, using the larvicide temephos, and promoting health education and behavior change.

Schistosomiasis

Trematode flatworms of the genus *Schistosoma* are the cause of schistosomiasis, also known as bilharzia (after the man who discovered schistosomes, Theodor Bilharz). Intestinal schistosomiasis is caused by *S. mansoni* and found primarily in Africa, the Middle East, and some parts of South America. *S. haematobium*, which causes urinary or urogenital schistosomiasis, is limited to Africa and the Middle East. *S. japonicum* and *S. mekongi* also cause intestinal schistosomiasis but only in the Far East, and *S. intercalatum* causes the disease in small pockets of Central Africa.

At various stages of the life cycle, these worms and their eggs live in freshwater snails; in water, where they can survive for 48 hours; and in humans. The worms invade a human host through the skin while the person is swimming or washing in contaminated water.

Once in the body, the larvae reach maturity inside the host's blood vessels. For as many as five years, the female flatworms release an estimated 300 eggs per day, which break out of the blood vessels and migrate into the bladder and intestine. These eggs can also pass out of the body in urine or feces or can get stuck in body tissues, such as the liver and urinary bladder, resulting in an immune reaction with scarring.

Urinary schistosomiasis causes progressive damage to the bladder, ureters, and kidneys, while intestinal schistosomiasis causes progressive enlargement of the liver and spleen, intestinal damage, and hypertension of the abdominal blood vessels. *S. mansoni* eggs collect in the liver, where they are trapped. When they die, they cause fibrosis, which is the thickening and scarring of connective tissue, over time. *S. haematobium* eggs cause genital lesions and bladder wall fibrosis.

About 240 million people are infected with schistosomiasis; of those, 20 million suffer severe consequences, according to UNICEF. Another 700 million are at risk of infection. Control of schistosomiasis is based on drug treatment, snail control, improved sanitation, and health education, say WHO researchers. According to UNICEF, studies have shown that adequate water supply and sanitation, which reduces contact with contaminated surface water, could reduce infection rates by 77 percent.

Typhoid Fever

Typhoid fever is a bacterial disease caused by *Salmonella enterica typhi*, which is transmitted through ingesting food or water contaminated by the feces of people with the bacteria. *Salmonella paratyphi* bacteria cause a similar but less severe disease.

Symptoms can be mild or severe, develop one to three weeks after exposure, and include high fever, malaise, headache, constipation or diarrhea, rose-colored spots on the chest, and enlarged spleen and liver. The most severe cases can cause death. The CDC estimates that there are 21 million typhoid cases worldwide, with 200,000 typhoid-related deaths annually.

There are two vaccines for typhoid that have been used with some success, according to the WHO. Once infected, a person can be treated for typhoid fever with antibiotics. However, resistance to common antimicrobials is widespread.

⊕ Future Implications

The biggest impediment to the eradication of waterborne diseases is the lack of potable water, proper sanitation, and hygiene. In 2000, the United Nations created eight Millennium Development Goals (MDGs) to be accomplished by 2015. These included measurable progress in reducing income poverty, hunger, disease, and lack of adequate shelter. Also among the MDGs was the directive to reduce by half the proportion of people living without sustainable access to safe drinking water and basic sanitation. WHO, UNICEF and UN-Water,

among many other governmental, nongovernmental, and charitable agencies, have collaborated to address these issues.

Since 2000, 116 countries have met the MDG target for access to clean water and almost 2 billion people gained access to improved sanitation, with 77 countries meeting the MDG target, according to UNICEF's "Progress on Water and Sanitation 2014" report. Nearly 4 billion people have a piped water connection, which is the highest level of water access. Researchers with UN-Water, a subcommittee of the United Nations, also note in their 2014 *Global Analysis and Assessment of Sanitation and Drinking-Water* (GLAAS) report, that between 1990 and 2012 the number of children dying from diarrheal diseases fell from 1.5 million to just over 600,000.

However, about 748 million people still lack easy access to clean drinking water, with the majority living in sub-Saharan Africa. More than 2.5 billion people do not use proper sanitation facilities, according to the UNICEF report, and almost half, about 1 billion, still practice open defecation.

In some of the most affected areas, the WHO and other agencies regularly host campaigns and programs designed to educate people on proper hygiene and safe food handling practices. As part of its "Water Quality and Health Strategy 2013–2020" report, the WHO notes that there is a need to shift from basic responsiveness to "a comprehensive, multidisciplinary approach that works with communities" to improve access to safe drinking water and sanitation while also encouraging behavioral change.

Increased surveillance of vulnerable populations and hot spots for these diseases is also critical. This method allows healthcare workers to get to victims in a timely way, not only to catch and treat these illnesses and control outbreaks as quickly as possible, but also to prevent them.

Vaccinations continue to have a substantial effect in areas where these diseases are endemic. For example, oral cholera vaccines are now part of the cholera control package; they have been shown to provide sustained protection against cholera among all age groups in more than 50 percent of cases, according to the WHO. Two typhoid vaccines are available internationally, and both are considered safe and effective. These vaccines are used to control endemic disease through programs carried out in conjunction with health education, water-quality and sanitation improvements, and training of health professionals in diagnosis and treatment.

Several factors slow the achievement of universal clean water and sanitation. These include rapid urbanization, expanding industrialization, growth in irrigated agriculture, the globalization of corporations, global warming, and a global population expected to reach 8 billion by 2030, according to researchers from Georgia

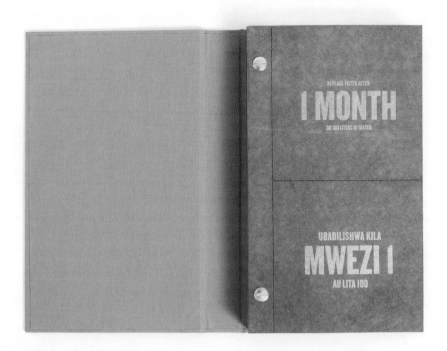

The pages of this book could save thousands of lives because its pages are made of filter paper that stops waterborne diseases like cholera and typhoid. The Drinkable Book's perforated filter sheets are ready to be torn out and used in a custom filter box. Each sheet can reduce bacteria count by 99.99 percent. The project was designed by 26-year-old graphic designer Brian Gartside and developed by scientists and engineers from the University of Virginia and Carnegie Mellon University. Each page is imprinted with bilingual messages designed to educate users on water hygiene and sanitation; one message is in English and the other in the locally spoken language of the area for which the book is headed. The pages use food-based ink, and underneath the words lie silver nanoparticles containing ions capable of killing off the most deadly waterborne diseases. They make the filtered water so pure it is comparable to tap water from the United States and costs just pennies to produce. © *Solent News/REX Features/AP Images.*

Tech Research Institute in their presentation at the 2009 Institute of Medicine (US) Forum on Microbial Threats.

Water scarcity will also increasingly become an issue. The Georgia Tech researchers point out that, "By 2025, more than half the nations in the world will face freshwater stress or shortages, and by 2050 up to 75 percent of an estimated 9.1 billion people could face freshwater scarcity. The future health, prosperity, and security of the human race will be strongly influenced by our ability to access clean water."

The GLAAS report lists other impediments to achieving the goal of universal coverage in water, sanitation, and hygiene. These include lack of resources available to national governments; lack of financing and political wherewithal to implement large-scale water and sewage infrastructure projects; lack of local funding to maintain operation of infrastructure; gaps in monitoring and gathering of data; neglect of water, sanitation, and hygiene in schools and healthcare facilities; and lack of community-wide promotion of hygiene. The GLAAS report also notes that the "vast majority of those without improved sanitation are poorer people living in rural areas. Progress on rural sanitation—where it has occurred—has primarily benefitted the non-poor, resulting in inequalities." Several countries reported efforts to reduce inequalities by making services more affordable to the poor, according to the report, but only half the countries report that these programs are widespread.

SEE ALSO *Bacterial Diseases; Cholera and Dysentery; Epidemiology: Surveillance for Emerging Infectious Diseases; Global Health Initiatives; Health as a Human Right and Health-Care Access; Health-Related Education and Information Access; Neglected Tropical Diseases; Parasitic Diseases; Sanitation and Hygiene; Vaccine-Preventable Diseases; Viral Diseases; Vulnerable Populations; Water Supplies and Access to Clean Water*

BIBLIOGRAPHY

Books

African Conference on Sanitation and Hygiene, and African Ministers' Council on Water. *Meeting Report, AMCOW: Sanitation and Hygiene Task Force.* Kigali, Rwanda: Third Africa Conference on Sanitation and Hygiene, 2011.

Ayisi, R. A. *The Water, Sanitation and Hygiene Promotion (WASH) Programme, Malawi.* Lilongwe, Malawi: UNICEF Unite for Children, 2010.

Burlage, Robert S. *Principles of Public Health Microbiology.* Sudbury, MA: Jones and Bartlett Learning, 2012.

Clark, Robert M. *Modeling Water Quality in Distribution Systems,* 2nd ed. Denver, CO: American Water Works Association, 2011.

Dworkin, Mark S., ed. *Outbreak Investigations around the World: Case Studies in Infectious Disease Field Epidemiology.* Sudbury, MA: Jones and Bartlett, 2010.

Fewtrell, Lorna, and Jamie Bartram, eds. *Water Quality: Guidelines, Standards and Health; Assessment of Risk and Risk Management for Water-Related Infectious Disease.* Geneva: World Health Organization, 2001.

Koch, Tom. *Disease Maps: Epidemics on the Ground.* Chicago: University of Chicago Press, 2011.

Percival, Steven L. *Microbiology of Waterborne Diseases: Microbiological Aspects and Risks,* 2nd ed. Amsterdam: Elsevier Academic Press, 2014.

Thematic Working Group on Water, Hygiene and Sanitation, World Health Organization, and East Asia Ministerial Conference on Sanitation and Hygiene. *Sanitation and Hygiene in East Asia.* Manila: World Health Organization, Regional Office for the Western Pacific, 2010.

World Health Organization. *UN-Water Global Analysis and Assessment of Sanitation and Drinking-Water (GLAAS) 2014 Report: Investing in Water and Sanitation: Increasing Access, Reducing Inequalities.* Geneva: World Health Organization, 2014. Available online at http://www.who.int/water_sanitation_health/glaas/en/ (accessed March 9, 2015).

Websites

"Microbial Agents Associated with Waterborne Diseases." *U.S. National Institutes of Health (NIH).* http://www.ncbi.nlm.nih.gov/pubmed/12546197 (accessed February 13, 2015).

"Waterborne Disease Prevention Branch." *U.S. Centers for Disease Control and Prevention (CDC).* http://www.cdc.gov/ncezid/dfwed/waterborne/ (accessed February 13, 2015).

"Waterborne Diseases and Climate Change." *U.S. National Institutes of Health (NIH).* http://www.niehs.nih.gov/research/programs/geh/climate change/health_impacts/waterborne_diseases/ (accessed February 13, 2015).

"Water-Related Diseases" *World Health Organization (WHO).* http://www.who.int/water_sanitation_health/diseases/en/ (accessed February 13, 2015).

Melanie R. Plenda

Workplace Health and Safety

⊕ Introduction

Workplace health and safety, also known as occupational health, has been defined by the International Labour Organization (ILO) and the World Health Organization (WHO) as "the promotion and maintenance of the highest degree of physical, mental and social well-being of workers in all occupations by preventing departures from health, controlling risks and the adaptation of work to people, and people to their jobs." About half of the world's population is part of the workforce in the formal economy, employed by a company, industry, government, or organization. Their labor is essential to global economic and social development. A healthy workforce, operating at optimum productivity, makes a huge contribution to a nation's economy.

However, workplace health and safety remains a relatively underdeveloped branch of global health, with only a minority of workers currently having access to occupational health services. The ILO has many conventions on working conditions over the years, and seeks to get more countries to adopt and enforce these. Meanwhile, the WHO has put into place a Global Plan of Action on Workers' Health 2008–2017, which covers all aspects of workplace health and safety. The plan includes prevention of hazards at work, a call for better working conditions, and a better response of health systems to issues related to patients' employment. There is an urgent need to reduce inequalities in workplace health seen between countries and within countries and also between different employment sectors. Occupational health for the 21st century, as envisioned by the ILO and the WHO, goes far beyond basic protection from work hazards. It should also encompass health promotion, helping workers reduce the risk of long-term and chronic health conditions, as well as looking after their mental health through stress management and tackling bullying in the workplace.

Employment can involve mechanical, physical, chemical, biological, and psychological risks. Some industries, such as mining, agriculture, construction, chemicals and healthcare, pose more obvious risks than others. For instance, the risks of exposure to pesticides and asbestos are now well known, although many in developing nations are still not protected from these hazards. There are also new threats to workers' health emerging as the global economy develops. These include working for long hours at a computer screen and the trend toward subcontracting and informal labor arrangements, which bring financial insecurity and stress. Women, children, and migrant workers are most at risk of workplace health risks. For many, rising global prosperity has not been paralleled by an improvement in working conditions.

However, the adoption of newer and safer technologies can eliminate or reduce some workplace risks. For instance, there is a move toward eliminating the use of mercury in dentistry and to the use of water-based solvents in the chemical industry. Where processes that do involve an element of risk must still be used, then workers ought to be provided with protective equipment. Another key element of workplace health and safety is ensuring workers know of any risk that they may be exposed to and are fully trained to protect themselves from harm. Successful occupational health policies always begin with a thorough risk assessment. Workplace surveillance and monitoring is important to ensure that safety measures are actually being carried out and are working effectively.

Health and safety regulation is strong in some countries, such as the United States and the European nations, where a culture of risk assessment has grown up since the 1960s. However, only around 10 percent of the global working population currently has access to this kind of protection under occupational health law. The majority are exposed to poor and often insecure working conditions. When things go wrong, there are often no medical facilities to help, owing to the weakness of the health-care infrastructure in many countries. The global weakness of occupational health legislation was highlighted during the 2014 outbreak of the Ebola virus in Sierra Leone, where more than 100 health-care workers became infected. More than half of these died, including one of the country's leading doctors, Sheik Umar Khan, who had led the fight against the disease.

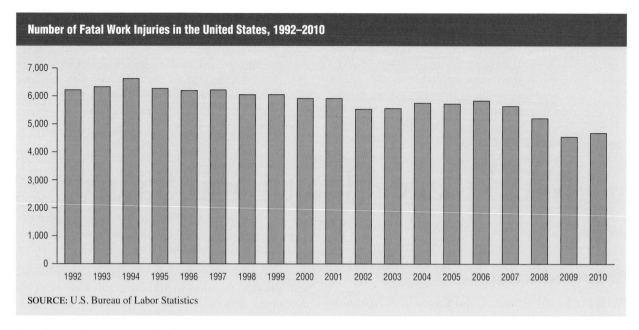

Number of Fatal Work Injuries in the United States, 1992–2010

SOURCE: U.S. Bureau of Labor Statistics

According to the U.S. Bureau of Labor Statistics, the number of workplace fatalities from 1992 to 2010 decreased slightly but overall has remained constant at approximately 5,000 deaths annually.

Both the ILO and the WHO have worked to improve occupational health globally for many years. In 2007, the 60th World Health Assembly launched the WHO's Workers' Health Global Plan of Action, which aims to move workplace health and safety higher up the global health agenda. The plan urges WHO member states to put national plans and policies in place to protect all workers. The WHO itself has a network of collaborating centers whose mission is to support the implementation of the plan. The WHO also aims to strengthen its collaboration with the ILO and other related international organizations.

⊕ Historical Background

In the 19th century, increasing industrialization brought many accidents and deaths as heavy machinery was introduced into industries like mining, railways, manufacturing, and construction. Employees had no legal protections, and their only recourse was to try to sue their employer, if they could even afford a lawyer. Once in court, many cases were won by the employers, which meant workplace accidents and fatalities did not have economic consequences that would create disincentives for unsafe working conditions.

The Beginnings of Health and Safety Legislation

Early attempts were made to regulate mining and manufacturing in the United States and Europe in the mid-19th century. Government inspectors were appointed to oversee safety in the railways, in factories, and in mining. Often, employers saw this as government interference and

declared that voluntary guidelines on workplace health and safety were all that was required. With the growth of the trade union movement, and public concern over the number of accidents, efforts for reform and improvement began to gather pace in the early years of the 20th century.

A landmark incident was a fire at New York City's Triangle Waist Company in 1911 where 146 of 500 employees died. Most of the victims of the tragedy, called the Triangle Shirtwaist Factory fire, were teenaged girls. Managers had locked doors to the stairwell to prevent theft and unauthorized breaks and had not implemented safety measures in case of fire. Many of the trapped workers jumped from the top floors of the 10-story building to their deaths rather than burn. Campaigners on workers' rights used this terrible incident to press their case. New York had already passed a workers' compensation law in 1910, however the Triangle incident spurred further action in New York and around the country. Within a few years, the majority of states had passed new legislation regarding fire safety and addressing labor conditions in the workplace. Companies then had a strong incentive to introduce safer working practices and a healthier environment.

Meanwhile, research into exposures to hazardous chemicals and ergonomic issues formed the basis for more comprehensive legislation. The U.S. Congress passed the Occupational Safety and Health Act in 1970. This led to the creation of the Occupational Safety and Health Administration (OSHA) within the Department of Labor. OSHA sets safety standards, researches workplace hazards, and informs workers of their rights under the law. In the United Kingdom, the Health and Safety at Work Act, which is administered by the Health and Safety Executive, came into being in 1974, and performs broadly similar functions.

⊕ Impacts and Issues

According to figures gathered by the ILO, in 2000 some 2 million people died, at least 271 million were injured, and at least 160 million became ill as a result of occupational hazards. This is only a partial picture, because many countries simply do not have data on the burden of occupational ill health. Nor is there much global data on the ill mental health that can be caused by work. Working conditions for the majority of the world's workers do not even meet minimum standards and guidelines set out by the ILO and the WHO. According to the ILO, as of early 2015, only 24 countries had ratified the ILO Employment Injury Benefits Convention adopted in 1964, which lists the occupational diseases for which compensation should be paid. Only 31 countries had ratified the Convention on Occupational Health Services as of early 2015. These two conventions are the basis of setting up a credible and effective occupational health system.

The developing global economy is leading to new hazards, particularly as workplace health and safety is seen as something that can be adopted at a later stage of development. Thus the electronics industry has led to the creation of large amounts of waste. This has been dumped in vast mountains in China, Ghana, and other developing countries, putting people who scavenge off them at risk. The industry also requires mining for raw materials in Africa, often using child labor under difficult and dangerous conditions. Another sector where companies have been accused of exploiting women and children is the garment industry. The trend toward "fast fashion" and very cheap clothes means that garment workers in countries like China, Vietnam, and Bangladesh may be working in conditions not dissimilar to those prevailing in England before the Industrial Revolution. However, electronics and clothing companies often deny these accusations and claim to operate to high ethical standards. Several garment factory building collapses in the early 21st century have stirred much debate about safety.

Certain other groups of workers are exposed to particularly high risk. For example, agricultural workers in developing countries are often exposed to high levels of pesticides; miners to heavy metals, dust, and explosion risk; construction workers to physical hazards, asbestos, and heavy lifting. Health-care workers may be at risk of needlestick injury. Often, those in the most hazardous

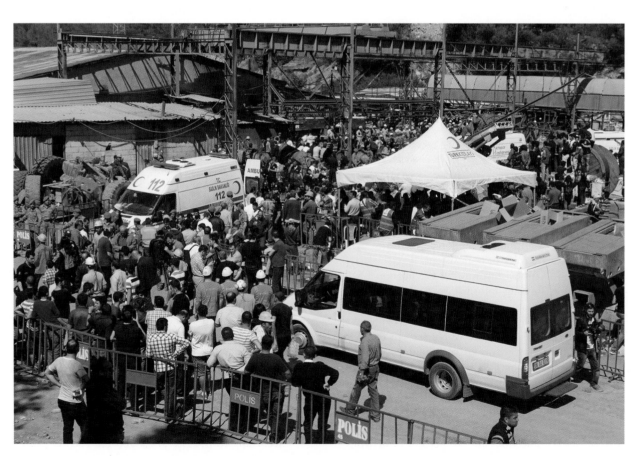

Emergency vehicles and health-care workers arrive after a coal mine explosion and fire in Soma, Turkey, on May 13, 2014. It was one of the the country's worst industrial disasters, killing more than 300 workers. Several executives of the mining company were arrested on charges of negligence following the disaster. Mining is still one of the most dangerous occupations, with safety often giving way to profits.   © *fpolat69 / Shutterstock.com.*

THE BHOPAL DISASTER

On December 3, 1984, a pesticide plant in Bhopal, India, was subject to a leak of methyl isocyanate gas, which immediately killed 3,800 people after being converted by heat to deadly hydrogen cyanide. Thousands more died or became ill over the course of time. The Indian government estimates that around 15,000 people have died as a result of the disaster. It is the worst industrial accident ever to occur as of 2014. A long and bitter legal battle followed between the workers and the parent company, U.S.-based Union Carbide Corporation (now owned by the Dow Chemical Company), which initially disclaimed responsibility. The factory site remained contaminated in 2015, putting people's health at risk.

The Bhopal disaster shows what can happen if rapid industrialization is not accompanied by equally rapidly evolving safety regulation. Though the plant was built to serve a growing Indian economy and expected increase in the need for pesticides, the demand was almost nonexistent. As a result, the plant was scheduled to be closed in the early 1980s. Although the toxic chemicals remained, Union Carbide allowed the safety system to fall into disrepair, even as employees warned of the dangers. An analysis of the Bhopal incident suggests multinational corporations may accept lower safety standards for plants in less developed nations. The surrounding public health infrastructure in Bhopal was very weak in 1984. The site of the factory was in a zone designated for light industrial and commercial use, not for hazardous operations. These factors combined to exacerbate the scale of the disaster. There are signs that the lessons of Bhopal have not been fully taken on board. The Indian economy is growing quickly, but there have not been corresponding improvements in workplace safety. For instance, mining, production, and use of asbestos in India is poorly controlled. Large and small companies throughout the country continue to pollute and put the population at risk.

industries are found in the poorest countries where health services are weak or nonexistent.

The U.S. National Institute for Occupational Safety and Health is funding information tools for reducing needlestick injuries among healthcare workers in Vietnam, South Africa, and Tanzania. The tools are being tested with the International Council of Nurses and the WHO regional offices. Reduction of such injuries is of vital importance in developing countries. Since the number of healthcare workers in such places is relatively small, loss of even one to illness or death from a needlestick injury means loss of a previous resource to the local population. Globally, needlestick injuries account for more than 2.5 percent of HIV infections and 40 percent of hepatitis B and C infections among healthcare professionals. Drug-resistant tuberculosis is another significant biological hazard that affects health workers in many parts of the world and is a particular problem in South Africa.

Global Trade

Increasing mobility of workers across borders brings its own health and safety issues. Many of these workers may be poorly educated with a low level of literacy and may therefore be unaware of hazards associated with their work. Poorly trained workers and supervisors may perpetuate unsafe practices and behaviors across borders when they migrate. This is particularly likely in the construction, agriculture, cleaning, and restaurant industries. In developed countries, this is a relatively new occupational health issue that has arisen through the presence of increasing numbers of migrant workers who may work under very poor conditions, particularly if their paperwork is not in order.

Global economic development has meant that the richer countries rely for their wealth on the labor and resources of poorer countries where wages are low. While outsourcing and trade may provide employment and prosperity to developing nations, occupational health is not given high priority in these countries. People are therefore often working under poor conditions. There has thus been pressure on the multinational companies involved to take the lead in eliminating these "sweatshop" conditions for their workers in such locations.

A significant part of the textile market manufacturing is in countries like Bangladesh, where there is a high incidence of workplace fires. Meanwhile, sandblasted blue jeans are produced in countries where the process causes exposure to crystalline silica, a carcinogen. Breathing in crystallized silica dust also can lead to silicosis, a scarring of the lungs that can be fatal. There are many other examples where the global economy transfers production to sites where occupational health standards are poor or nonexistent.

Child Labor

Many of the worst worker abuses seen in the global economy are among children forced to work under poor and dangerous conditions. The ILO states that children under the age of 15 should not be employed. Child labor robs children of their education, normal childhood, and health. This is particularly so for the worst forms of child labor, namely prostitution, pornography, soldiering, drug trafficking, and slavery. The United Nations Children's Fund (UNICEF), the ILO, and the World Bank estimate that there are 168 million children between the ages of 5 and 17 engaged in child labor, of whom 150 million are under the age of 14. There has, however, been a decline in child labor since 2000, according to an ILO report published in 2012. Child labor among girls fell by 40 percent and among boys by 25 percent from 2000 to 2012. However, at current rates of decline there will still be 100 million children forced into work by 2020.

According to the ILO, Asia and the Pacific regions still have the largest numbers of child laborers, with an estimated 78 million, or 9.3 percent of the children in the region. However, sub-Saharan Africa continues as the region with the highest incidence of child labor, at

21 percent (59 million child laborers). In Latin America and the Caribbean, there are 13 million children (8.8 percent of all children) in work, and in the Middle East and North Africa there are 9.2 million (8.4 percent). More than half of child labor occurs in agriculture, but there are also 54 million child laborers in the service industry and another 12 million in other industry. Child workers are found in many industrial sectors, including mining and quarrying, agriculture, manufacturing, and domestic service. Often, their work is hidden from view. For instance, there are around 15.1 million child domestic workers, most of them female. Child labor occurs as a result of poverty and lack of employment opportunities for adult family members. Too often local social norms permit child labor. This is a short-sighted view, for child labor is a barrier to economic development when children are forced to drop out of school.

Child labor is preventable if the right support systems are put in place. UNICEF, the ILO, and others are working on a plan set out in 2010, which aims to eliminate the worst forms of child labor by 2016. This will involve persuading communities to change their cultural acceptance of child labor and to find alternative sources of income

for a family. There is also a need to work with government on child labor, promoting a path from education to work for young people. Where child labor does still exist, then the workers should be better supported. So far, UNICEF has been able to report promising results from these efforts. For instance, in Burkina Faso, more than 15,000 children have left work in gold mines. This has been achieved by providing support for schooling, vocational training, and literacy, while mothers were given opportunities to develop income-generating activities. In Nepal, over 9,000 child workers have been provided with resources for their rehabilitation, education, and training. Families have been offered financial aid to prevent their children returning to work. Finally, a project in Bolivia has resulted in government establishing a minimum age for employment and protection for adolescent workers.

The Role of the ILO and the WHO

The WHO and the ILO have developed a number of initiatives for the development of workplace health and safety. The ILO has conventions on labor inspection, occupational safety and health, occupational health services, and chemical safety and prevention of major

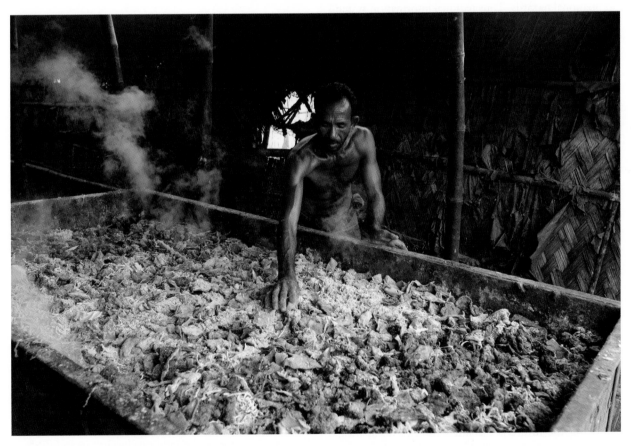

A Bangladeshi man sorts tannery waste for poultry and fish feed on the banks of the Buriganga River in Dhaka, Bangladesh. In a report released in 2012, New York-based Human Rights Watch said tannery workers in Bangladesh's capital are being exposed to serious health risks because of hazardous chemicals and are in danger of accidents due to tannery machinery. Bangladesh annually exports millions of dollars of leather goods to some 70 countries, including the United States and Japan. © *A.M. Ahad/AP Images.*

industrial accidents. There are also ILO conventions on freedom of association, child labor, forced labor, and discrimination issues. Unfortunately, progress on ratifying and implementing these has been very slow, mainly due to lack of funding and political motivation. There has also been some criticism that ILO has moved away from measures that are specific, with high levels of accountability, toward standards that allow more flexibility in application, apparently in line with an individual country's pace of development.

Meanwhile, the WHO is implementing its action plan, supported by its network of Collaborating Centres for Occupational Health by working with a number of stakeholders. These include the ILO and others in the United Nations system, trade unions, and employers' organizations. These groups are "setting standards for protection of workers' health, providing guidelines, promoting and monitoring their use, and contributing to the adoption and implementation of international labour conventions." They also intend to put in place "appropriate scientific and advisory mechanisms to facilitate action on workers' health and safety at global and regional levels." The WHO wants to establish better systems for surveillance of workers' health to better identify and control occupational hazards. Thus national information systems are needed to meet the goal of creating registries of exposure, occupational accidents, and occupational diseases and improved reporting and early detection.

Occupational health often focuses on personal protective equipment. However, more sustainable improvements might be achieved by shifting the emphasis to effective policies on prevention. Furthermore, occupational health needs to be far better integrated within existing systems. The poorest countries need direct support with capacity building and technical assistance. Knowledge of healthcare professionals on the link between health and work should also be improved. Finally, workers' health should be incorporated into economic development, poverty reduction, and international trade strategies. In short, occupational health should be part of national and international plans for sustainable development.

⊕ Future Implications

Thus far, workplace health and safety has not been seen as a priority by many governments, and there is clearly much to be done before the health of employees is seen as an essential part of socioeconomic development. The WHO Global Plan for Action runs to 2017 and sets out an ambitious program of work. What the plan sees as key for the future is the integration of occupational health into national health strategies, particularly where reforms are planned or underway. Occupational health coverage, currently applied to only a minority, needs to be extended. This will require capacity building and

substantial investment. Special efforts will have to be made to extend coverage to those in the informal economy, where short-term contracts are common, and small enterprises and agriculture should be included.

There are deep inequalities in health and safety at work coverage around the world. Remedying these will require a coordinated and multidisciplinary response. Beyond building healthcare infrastructure in developing countries, this will require monitoring of international trade, restructuring trade agreements to include occupational health commitments. Increased government funding should be directed toward the ILO and the WHO so they can put into place occupational health policies, guidance, and training. Regulations to control or ban dangerous products, like the older pesticides, in the workplace are needed. The occupational health community needs to address the issues through advocacy and guidelines by encouraging and supporting occupational health professionals in developing nations. More research and training in occupational health issues will be needed for both healthcare professionals, trade unions, and employers. Finally, consumers have a role to play. They can demand that workers producing goods for the global market are treated fairly.

PRIMARY SOURCE

Occupational Health

SOURCE Occupational Health: A Manual for Primary Health Care Workers. *Cairo: World Health Organization (WHO) Regional Office for the Eastern Mediterranean, 2001, 13. http://www.who.int/occupational_health/ regions/en/oehemhealthcareworkers.pdf?ua=1 (accessed January 25, 2015).*

INTRODUCTION *This primary source is an excerpt from the introduction of a manual prepared by the World Health Organization (WHO) for use by primary healthcare workers. WHO's stated view is that "A healthy workforce is vital for sustainable social and economic development on a global, national, and local level."*

INTRODUCTION

Occupational health: a definition

Occupational health is a multidisciplinary activity aimed at:

- the protection and promotion of the health of workers by preventing and controlling occupational diseases and accidents and by eliminating occupational factors and conditions hazardous to health and safety at work;

- the development and promotion of healthy and safe work, work environments and work organizations;

- the enhancement of the physical, mental and social well-being of workers and support for the development and maintenance of their working capacity, as well as professional and social development at work;

- enabling workers to conduct socially and economically productive lives and to contribute positively to sustainable development.

Occupational health has gradually developed from a mono-disciplinary, risk-oriented activity to a multi-disciplinary and comprehensive approach that considers an individual's physical, mental and social well-being, general health and personal development.

Interaction between work and health

The social and economic importance of work receives considerable attention because a primary function of work in any society is to produce and distribute goods and services. Far less attention is paid to the importance of work to the individual, yet it is clear from recent research that work plays a crucial and perhaps unparalleled psychological role in the formation of self-esteem and a sense of order. Work is a powerful force in shaping a person's sense of identity. It can lend vitality to existence and establishes the cyclical patterns of day, week, month and year. It is believed that work for which there is no economic gain, such as child care, care for the aged and voluntary work, also has its rewards and contributes to personal gratification.

Positive health effects of work

Two-way interaction

There is a continuous two-way interaction between a person and the physical and psychological working environment: the work environment may influence the person's health either positively or negatively and productivity is, in turn, influenced by the workers state of physical and mental well-being. Work, when it is well-adjusted and productive, can be an important factor in health promotion, e.g. partially disabled workers may be rehabilitated by undertaking tasks suited to their physical and mental limitations and, in this way, may substantially increase their working capacity. However, the fact that work can have a positive influence on health has not yet been fully exploited; knowledge of work physiology and ergonomics needs to be further developed and applied to benefit workers health.

Health hazards

When work is associated with health hazards, it may cause occupational disease, be one of the multiple causes of other disease or may aggravate existing ill-health of non-occupational origin. In developing countries, where work is becoming increasingly mechanized, a number of work processes have been developed that treat workers as tools in production, putting their health and lives at risk. The occupational health lessons learned during the Industrial Revolution should be borne in mind in planning for health in developing countries if such problems are to be avoided.

SEE ALSO *Air Pollution: Urban, Industrial, and Transborder; Child Health; Health-Care Worker Safety and Shortages*

BIBLIOGRAPHY

Books

Henmans Freeth LLP. *Health and Safety at Work Essentials*, 8th ed. London: Lawpack, 2014.

Jasanoff, Sheila, ed. *Learning from Disaster: Risk Management after Bhopal*. Philadelphia: University of Pennsylvania Press, 1994.

Smedley, Julia, Finlay Dick, and Steve Sadhra, eds. *Oxford Handbook of Occupational Health*, 2nd ed. Oxford: Oxford University Press, 2013.

Periodicals

Broughton, Edward. "The Bhopal Disaster and Its Aftermath: A Review." *Environmental Health: A Global Access Science Source* 4, no. 1 (May 2005): 1–6. doi:10.1186/1476-069X-4-6. Available online at http://www.ehjournal.net/content/4/1/6 (accessed February 6, 2015).

Lucchini, Roberto, and Leslie London. "Global Occupational Health: Current Challenges and the Need for Urgent Action." *Annals of Global Health* 80 (2014): 251–256.

Macik-Frey, Marilyn, James Quick, and Debra Nelson. "Advances in Occupational Health: From a Stressful Beginning to a Positive Future." *Journal of Management* 33, no. 6 (2007): 809–840.

Websites

"Child Labour." *International Labour Organization*. http://www.ilo.org/global/topics/child-labour/lang--en/index.htm (accessed February 25, 2015).

"Child Protection from Violence, Exploitation and Abuse." *UNICEF.* http://www.unicef.org/protection/ (accessed January 31, 2015).

International Labour Organization. http://www.ilo.org/global/lang--en/index.htm (accessed February 25, 2015).

National Institute for Occupational Safety and Health (NIOSH).http://www.cdc.gov/NIOSH/(accessed January 31, 2015).

"Workers' Health: Global Plan of Action." *World Health Organization (WHO)*. http://www.who.int/occupational_health/publications/global_plan/en/ (accessed January 31, 2015).

Susan Aldridge

World Health Organization: Organization, Funding, and Enforcement Powers

🌐 Introduction

The World Health Organization (WHO) is the agency of the United Nations (UN) that is responsible for public health. Headquartered in Geneva, Switzerland, the WHO has offices around the world and employs over 8,000 people in total, including medical doctors, epidemiologists, and public health experts. The organization is dedicated mainly to advocacy and the sharing of knowledge. The WHO also provides leadership to a number of health campaigns on global health issues, such as malaria, tuberculosis (TB), and HIV/AIDS (human immunodeficiency virus/acquired immune deficiency syndrome).

The stated objective of the WHO is to promote "the attainment by all peoples of the highest possible level of health." It aims to achieve this through a number of activities. These include shaping the global health agenda and setting priorities. It also sets global standards for products such as vaccines and drug therapy for HIV and TB. On the ground, the WHO provides technical assistance to countries on issues including child vaccination and emerging diseases like SARS (severe acute respiratory syndrome). It organizes conferences and forums, and produces many studies and reports. One notable example is the WHO's leading publication, which is its "World Health Report," which highlights a different global health topic each year; the 2013 report focuses on universal health coverage.

The WHO has 194 member states. Any UN country may join the WHO as long as they accept its constitution. Countries that are not UN members can join if the World Health Assembly, the annual meeting of member states, votes them in. The World Health Assembly is the decision-making body of the WHO. It sets policy, approves the budget, and appoints the director-general. Voting is on a "one country, one vote" basis. Thus, smaller countries have equal power with larger ones.

The Geneva headquarters of the WHO houses the director general's office and six teams dedicated to specific health issues. These are: Health Security (including pandemics); HIV, TB, and Malaria; Family, Women's and Children's Health; Non-communicable Diseases and Mental Health; Polio and Emergencies; and Health Systems and Emergencies. The director general of the WHO as of early 2015 was Dr. Margaret Chan, previously director of health in Hong Kong. She was serving a second five-year term in the post, which ends in 2017.

The WHO also has six regional offices. These are: Africa; the Americas; Eastern Mediterranean (which includes parts of North Africa and the Middle East); Europe; Southeast Asia; and Western Pacific. There is also the WHO's Global Service Centre in Malaysia, which handles much of the organization's administration. In addition, the WHO has an office in most of the world's poor countries and in other places where support for health issues is needed. In total, the WHO has a presence in around 150 countries.

The WHO is not a financing agency. Its work is funded by subscriptions from its member states and also from special donations from richer nations. The budget is aligned within the framework of a six-year General Programme of Work. Its 12th program runs from 2014–2019. The budget is set every two years within this framework. The size of the 2014–2015 budget was nearly US$4 billion.

The WHO is governed by the World Health Assembly, which meets in Geneva each May. It tasks an executive board with action on matters where further study or investigation is needed. The board consists of 34 technical experts, each elected for a three-year term, and it reports back to the assembly each year. The board meets each January to set the agenda for the forthcoming World Health Assembly. At this meeting, the board also decides on resolutions to present to the assembly. The board's main function is to carry out decisions and policies of the World Health Assembly, to advise it and generally facilitate the work of the WHO.

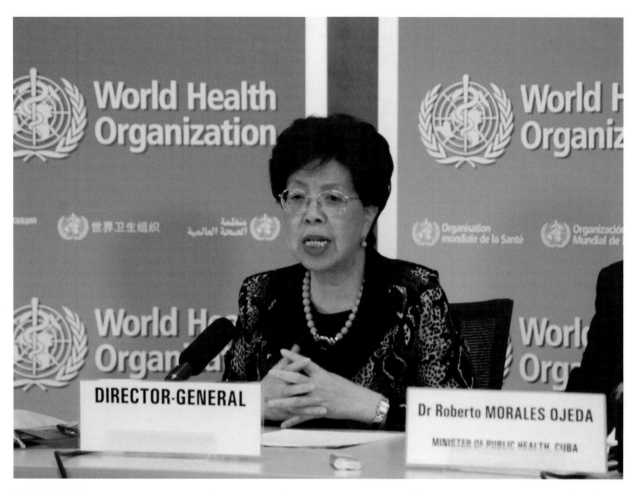

World Health Organization Director-General Dr. Margaret Chan speaks during a press conference on September 12, 2014, in Geneva, Switzerland. © *The Asahi Shimbun via Getty Images.*

⊕ Historical Background

The idea of setting up a global health organization was first discussed when the UN was formed after the World War II (1939–1945) in 1945. Prior to this, work on global health had been conducted by the League of Nations Health Office, set up in 1920 with financial and technical support from the Rockefeller Foundation. The very earliest efforts to develop an international approach to health date back to a conference on cholera in 1851. This was followed by numerous international meetings on health during the second part of the 19th century. The International Commission on Epidemics was created in 1903, followed by the International Office of Public Hygiene.

The WHO Constitution came into force on April 7, 1948, a date which is now celebrated each year as World Health Day. The constitution had previously been signed by all 51 UN members and 10 other nations on July 22, 1946. The early WHO incorporated the International Office of Public Hygiene and League of Nations Health Office. Its first priorities were the control of malaria, TB, and sexually transmitted infections and to improve maternal and child health, all of which are still a major focus of the WHO's work today. The WHO's first major campaign was a drive on mass TB vaccination begun in 1950.

More Than 60 Years of the WHO

Since about the 1950s, the WHO has become a truly global organization. It has expanded in terms of the number of member states, employees, budget, and areas of interest. In the early years, efforts were focused on building capacity for global health campaigns and helping build health-care infrastructure in the many newly independent countries. Another key area was family planning. Here the emphasis has shifted over time from limiting the size of families toward reproductive health and safe motherhood.

The WHO is perhaps best known for its work on infectious disease, and particularly for its various eradication programs. Its campaign to eradicate smallpox began in 1966. The polio eradication program began in 1988. The WHO has also carried out a great deal of work on other communicable diseases that affect mainly the poor, including malaria, leprosy, lymphatic filariasis, and onchocerciasis. Its expanded program on immunization

UN PARTNER AGENCIES

The WHO is one of 15 major agencies of the United Nations (UN). The others include the Food and Agriculture Organization; the United Nations Educational, Scientific and Cultural Organization; the International Labour Organization; and the World Bank. Within these broad categories, there are also many smaller agencies. The UN also has many organizations, like the World Trade Organization, which work closely with its main agencies. The main agencies sharing some of the work of the WHO are the United Nations Children's Fund (UNICEF), the UN Population Fund, and the UN Development Programme.

UNICEF

UNICEF was founded around the same time as the WHO itself, in an effort to help children who were suffering from the aftereffects of World War II. It works to promote the rights of children everywhere in the world, believing this to be a fundamental in human health and progress. As an advocacy organization, UNICEF tackles poverty, disease, and violence in places where it impacts children's lives. It is active, through its programs and campaigns, in more than 190 countries.

UNICEF and the WHO work together on Millennium Development Goal (MDG) 4, which is to reduce the mortality of children under five by two-thirds by 2015. As of a progress check in 2013, this was on track in many parts of the world. However, child mortality remains high in sub-Saharan Africa. To protect children's health, UNICEF and the WHO have many programs on immunization. They also jointly promote breast-feeding and work on maternal health and family planning. UNICEF also has programs in girls' education, which will help build healthier families in the future.

The UN Population Fund

The UN Population Fund (UNFPA) began its work in 1969 and is active in around 150 countries. It works in family planning and maternal health to help ensure that every pregnancy is a wanted one and that every birth is safe. With these aims, it works with partners like the WHO toward MDG 5, improving maternal health. The UNFPA also works to protect young people by mounting campaigns on issues like female genital mutilation and child marriage.

The work of the UNFPA is based on the 1994 Programme of Action of the International Conference on Population and Development. It adopts a human rights approach to its work. Its programs are based upon a knowledge of population dynamics and cultural sensitivities. The UNFPA's progress was reviewed in 2014, which highlighted many achievements but warned of serious coming global inequalities unless the rights, health, and aspirations of women and young people were not given higher priority.

The UN Development Programme

The scope of the UN Development Programme (UNDP) is much broader than that of the WHO or UNICEF. It is dedicated toward the eradication of poverty and reduction of inequalities, working in more than 170 countries and territories. It helps countries to develop leadership, partnerships, better services, and security for its populations. The UNDP's approach aims to be people-centered and sustainable, introducing new systems and innovation from project level up.

The UNDP has been guided by the MDGs, all of which are in some way linked to health and depend upon the reduction of poverty. Its aim is to link together global and national efforts to achieve them. The organization is now focusing upon the post-2015 framework, as the MDGs themselves were scheduled to be completed in 2015. Going forward, it will focus on peace building, climate change, and sustainable development through the UNDP Strategic Plan 2014–2017.

(EPI) began in 1974. The WHO had set up a malaria eradication initiative in the 1970s, but that objective was later dropped as being too ambitious.

Throughout its history, the WHO has articulated a number of visions for global health. One of the most significant was the Alma-Ata declaration of 1978. This called for "health for all" by 2000, through the development of primary care. Looking back, this seems overly optimistic, and some critics say it damaged the credibility of the WHO. One key problem with Alma-Ata is that many countries either could not, or would not, follow through with the primary care strategy. However, the declaration still heralded a new focus upon building primary health care capacity.

In 1986, the WHO responded to the growing threat of HIV/AIDS with a global program that later expanded to become Joint United Nations Programme on HIV/AIDS (UNAIDS) in 1996. Stop TB was formed in 2000, coinciding with the announcement of the UN Millennium Development Goals (MDGs), all of which relate to health. Another key WHO program is Roll Back Malaria, founded with the United Nations Children's Fund (UNICEF) and the World Bank in 1998. Efforts on these three important diseases came together with the formation of the Global Fund to Fight AIDS, Tuberculosis and Malaria, in 2002.

⊕ Impacts and Issues

The WHO is perhaps best known for the eradication of smallpox, a disease that killed an estimated 2 million people annually at the start of the campaign. In fact, the WHO had vowed to beat smallpox in 1959 but it needed the U.S. Centers for Disease Control and Prevention (CDC) to step in with the necessary funding before work could begin on a large scale. Furthermore, mass production and storage of smallpox vaccine without refrigeration was only possible starting in the 1950s.

Thus, like all successful WHO campaigns, smallpox eradication depended upon exploiting technical and scientific advances in partnership with other organizations.

The approach to eradication was not universal vaccination, which would have been impractical. Rather, new cases were sought out and transmission interrupted by vaccinating all of the people around the case. By 1977, the last ever naturally occurring case of smallpox, in Somalia, had been recorded. Smallpox was first eradicated from Latin America in 1971, and from Asia in 1975. The disease was officially declared eradicated worldwide in 1980. The campaign cost an average of $23 million per annum, making it the most cost-effective health intervention ever because of all the lives saved and associated reduction in health-care costs.

The legacy of the smallpox eradication campaign is that many countries were forced to improve their health-care systems. Furthermore, the campaign helped build approaches to mass vaccination, which have been applied to other diseases, like polio. However, there are specific features of smallpox that make it a natural target for eradication. Unlike a disease such as malaria, which has a reservoir in mosquitoes who pass the disease to humans, smallpox is passed directly from person to person. The characteristic rash of smallpox makes it relatively easy to detect new cases, and its severity makes people more likely to take to their beds, where they are less likely to infect others.

Eradicating other diseases is therefore more challenging. The WHO and its partners have made good progress toward eradicating the parasitic disease dracunculiasis, or guinea worm disease, since launching a campaign in 1986. A 2014 report notes that the largest annual decline in the disease since the campaign began occurred from 542 cases in 2012 to 148 in 2013. Similarly, since 1988, when the 41st World Health Assembly adopted a resolution for the worldwide eradication of polio, a total of 125 countries have eliminated polio. It only remained endemic in three countries in 2014: Afghanistan, Nigeria, and Pakistan.

TB, Malaria, and AIDS

The WHO's Stop TB campaign was successful in reducing mortality from TB by 45 percent between 1990 and 2013 and its prevalence by 41 percent over the same period. However, the campaign's 2015 targets to reduce the burden of TB will not be met in the WHO African and Eastern Mediterranean Regions. Thus, TB remains an area where much still needs to be done by the WHO and its partners, particularly with the emerging issues of multidrug-resistant TB and TB and HIV coinfection. A post-2015 plan has been put in place that seeks to "end TB as a global pandemic (an average less than 10 tuberculosis cases per 100,000 population) and to cut the number of deaths from TB by 95% by 2035," according to the Stop TB Partnership.

While the WHO had to abandon its vision of eradicating malaria, much has been achieved by Roll Back Malaria. This program advocates for the control of the disease and for better technologies and approaches. It also helps to spread control and treatment where it is needed. The program has been expanded to various other private and public partners. It has set up the Malaria Medicines and Supplies Service. This helps poorer countries procure the medicines and supplies they need to fight malaria. The global incidence of malaria decreased by 53 percent between 2001 and 2013. Sixty-five countries are now on track to reach the Millennium Development Goal 6, which calls for the incidence of malaria to be halted and reversed by 2015. In 55 of these countries, malaria is down by 75 percent.

Meanwhile, increasing concerns that attempts to address HIV/AIDS were insufficient led to a discussion on global health that broadened to include TB and malaria. This discussion led to the establishment of the Global Fund to Fight AIDS, Tuberculosis and Malaria. The fund is a partnership between WHO, UNAIDS, the World Bank, and a number of other private- and public-sector organizations. It is primarily a funding organization, with a particular interest in ensuring that HIV drugs get to as many of those in need as possible. With experts in over 140 countries, and funding of nearly $4 billion a year, the fund has achieved a great deal. By the end of 2014, it had 7.3 million people on HIV drugs, had 12.3 million tested and treated for TB, and had distributed 450 million insecticide-treated nets to protect against malaria. The WHO collects morbidity and mortality data for all three diseases. However, it is impossible to separate out the impact of WHO-led programs in achieving the overall declines in disease burden from the efforts made by countries themselves and other organizations.

The WHO's Overall Achievements in Global Health

The WHO has undoubtedly made a huge contribution, although it may be difficult to quantify, to improving human life expectancy. In 1999, it predicted that life expectancy would increase to 74 years by 2025 from only 48 years in 1955. According to WHO data, in 2012 global life expectancy at birth was 70 years. Within these global figures there are, however, some marked variations, with ranges from 62 years in low-income countries to 79 years in some high-income countries. TB and AIDS have undermined improvements in sub-Saharan Africa. In Malawi, for instance, HIV/AIDS has reversed gains in life expectancy so that the country is now back to pre–World War II levels (about 59 years).

Child mortality (deaths of children under the age of five), another key indicator of global health, decreased globally from 21 million in 1955 to 11 million in 1995 to 6.3 million in 2013. The WHO's focus on encouraging breast-feeding and its EPI campaign have likely been major factors in this improvement. Child and maternal health continue to be given a strong emphasis in the work of

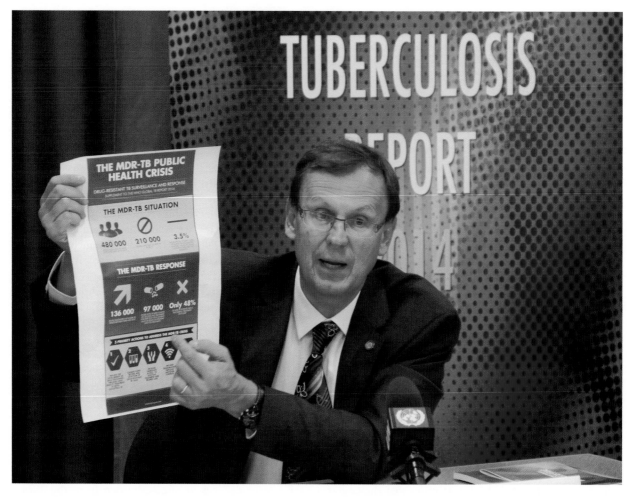

The World Health Organization's director of the Global Tuberculosis Programme, Dr. Mario Raviglione, shows a chart during a press conference about the 2014 global tuberculosis report at the United Nations Office in Geneva, Switzerland, on October 22, 2014. Raviglione mentioned that 1.5 million people died of tuberculosis in the previous year. © *Fatih Erel/Anadolu Agency/Getty Images.*

WHO. The two cannot be separated, because a child that loses its mother runs a strong risk of dying prematurely.

Besides its specific campaigns the WHO has, from the start, sought to inspire member states, health-care workers, and the public through a number of visionary statements. Over time, the emphasis of these statements has changed. The Alma-Ata declaration, mentioned earlier, was thought by many to be overly idealistic and naïve. In 1998, there was the Health for All Declaration, in which the World Health Assembly reaffirmed its commitment to the principle that "the enjoyment of the highest attainable standard of health is one of the fundamental rights of every human being." This was followed, in 1986, by the Ottawa Charter, which many felt was a move toward a more pragmatic approach to global health.

The Ottawa Charter, in short, tried to shift the WHO away from the relatively narrow objectives of fighting specific diseases and reducing child mortality toward a broader program of social, political, and environmental action. Its supporters argued that good health is incompatible with poverty and its attendant conditions such as lack of access to clean water and malnutrition. Therefore, the root causes of ill health should be the focus of global health initiatives. Along with this goes the building of strong health-care structures in countries where these are lacking, which, inevitably, brings great social and political challenges.

Criticisms of the WHO

An organization as large and complex as the WHO, many of whose operations are in the public eye, is sure to attract some criticism. Over the years, the organization has been accused of excessive bureaucracy, secrecy, and lack of accountability and transparency. Lack of leadership and internal feuding are among other observations. There seems to be an overall perception that the WHO could be declining in effectiveness, although it is hard to see how this can be measured.

Given that the WHO derives its power from 194 member states, the accusation of undue political influence and interference is almost inevitable. There have also been suggestions of conflicts of interest. These arose in 2009, when some questioned whether the links between the WHO and drug companies had driven an overreaction to H1N1 flu. Although the WHO declared this new flu to be a pandemic, there were far fewer cases than expected. Overall, however, the WHO is a force for good, although clearly there is room for improvement. Certainly the dedicated work of WHO teams in the field, who work with hard-to-reach populations, often under dangerous conditions, has saved millions of lives over the history of the organization.

⊕ Future Implications

The WHO has to respond to the changing global health scenario. This means monitoring and mobilizing resources to both natural disasters and to disease outbreaks, like that of the Ebola virus outbreak occurring in Africa from 2014 to 2015. In the longer term, attention has to shift away from a narrow focus on infectious disease toward noncommunicable diseases such as diabetes, cancer, heart disease, lung disease, and mental disorders. It is predicted that by 2020, the largest increases in such diseases will be in Africa. Another new, and future, focus is on indoor and outdoor air pollution, which causes 7 million premature deaths each year, according to WHO data.

Noncommunicable diseases are caused to a great extent by increased affluence around the world. In itself, the rise in living standards is a positive factor in health and has certainly helped cut the burden of infectious disease. However, prosperity brings with it risk factors such as decreased physical activity and a higher fat and calorie diet. These have led to an epidemic of obesity. Increased traffic, which also comes with affluence, has had a negative impact on outdoor air quality. Indoor air pollution is more likely in modern homes, while reliance on wood-burning stoves in poorer countries also contributes to poor air quality. Finally, as people in richer countries smoke less, the focus of tobacco companies has moved to lower- and middle-income countries. Increased smoking in these countries has led to an increase in attendant health problems.

The WHO's Response to Future Challenge and Reform

The WHO is tackling the present and future burden of noncommunicable disease by trying to reduce the underlying risk factors. This involves promotion of lifestyle change and healthy living. A major development has been the adoption of the WHO Framework Convention on Tobacco Control, which aims to reduce tobacco use, particularly in developing countries. The focus on behavior change differs somewhat from the more traditional role of the WHO in delivering vaccines and medicines.

The WHO has realized that it needs to reform in order to meet the complex challenges it faces going forward.

Thus, it intends to develop clearer priorities and new work programs. It has also promised to strengthen both its internal governance and its role in global health governance. These changes will be supported by managerial reforms. The process of WHO reform began in 2010, and the hope is that it will make the organization flexible enough to meet the global health needs of the 21st century.

SEE ALSO   *Child Health; Family Planning; Global Health Initiatives; Health as a Human Right and Health-Care Access; Health in the WHO African Region; Health in the WHO Americas Region; Health in the WHO Eastern Mediterranean Region; Health in the WHO European Region; Health in the WHO South-East Asia Region; Health in the WHO Western Pacific Region; Maternal and Infant Health; NGOs and Health Care: Deliverance or Dependence; Pan American Health Organization (PAHO); Pandemic Preparedness*

BIBLIOGRAPHY

Books

Global Health Watch 4: An Alternative World Health Report. London: Zed Books, 2014.

McInnes, Colin, and Kelley Lee. *Global Health and International Relations*. Cambridge, UK: Polity, 2012.

Skolnik, Richard. *Essentials of Global Health*. Boston: Jones and Bartlett, 2008.

Stone, David. *The Growing Global Public Health Crisis and How to Address It*. London: Radcliffe, 2012.

Periodicals

Cavendish, Julius. "The Last Bastions of Guinea-Worm Disease." *Bulletin of the World Health Organization* 92, no. 12 (December 2014): 854–855.

Websites

"About WHO: WHO Reform." *World Health Organization (WHO)*. http://www.who.int/about/who_reform/en/ (accessed March 5, 2015).

"Repaso de la Salud Mundial en 2014." *Organización Mundial de la Salud (OMS)*. http://www.who.int/features/2014/year_review/jan-apr/es/ (accessed March 5, 2015).

Sengupta, Somini. "Effort on Ebola Hurt W.H.O. Chief." *New York Times*, January 6, 2015. http://www.nytimes.com/2015/01/07/world/leader-of-world-health-organization-defends-ebola-response.html?_r=0 (accessed March 5, 2015).

"World Health Report 2013: Research for Universal Health Coverage." *World Health Organization (WHO)*, August 15, 2013. http://www.who.int/whr/en/ (accessed March 5, 2015).

Susan Aldridge

Zoonotic (Animal-Borne) Diseases

⊕ Introduction

Zoonotic diseases, or zoonoses, are diseases that are transmitted naturally from vertebrate animals to humans. The infective agent of a zoonosis may be a virus, bacterium, or parasite. Zoonoses are an increasing public health problem as habitats change, bringing humans and animals into closer contact. There are over 200 common zoonoses. Some of those that have caused deep concern in recent years include HIV, Ebola, yellow fever, Nipah, Lassa, H5N1 and H1NI influenza, Rift Valley fever, and SARS.

Livestock, wildlife, and pets all play a significant role in the transmission of zoonotic disease. According to the World Health Organization (WHO), of the 1,400 or so species of human pathogens, nearly 60 percent come from animal sources. Of these, around three-quarters come from wildlife. Even more important, around two-thirds of emerging pathogens come from animals. Factors that increase the spread of the zoonoses include international travel, globalization, and human encroachment upon animal ecosystems, with changing land use.

The zoonoses are a diverse group of diseases, which makes them challenging to study. They have a global distribution in tropical and subtropical regions, with a variety of different transmission patterns. A zoonosis can be transmitted via direct contact with an animal, by contact with a contaminated environment, or via food. Rabies is transmitted via a bite from a rabid animal, leptospirosis via water contaminated with the urine of an infected animal, and various forms of food poisoning by uncooked or incompletely cooked meat. Zoonoses can also be transmitted indirectly via insect vectors carried by animals. Ticks infected with *Borrelia burgdorferi*, the bacterium that causes Lyme disease, are carried on the coats of deer. Contact with such animals exposes people to the disease.

Zoonotic diseases also occur in a widely diverse range of habitats and health-care settings. However, it is notable that zoonoses disproportionately affect the poorest people in the world, where resources to deal with them tend to be lacking. Zoonoses range in seriousness from mild and self-limiting, like some cases of food poisoning, to life-threatening, like Ebola fever. Often, however, the disease may cause no obvious illness in its animal host.

Bacteria cause food poisoning, which is a particularly common type of zoonotic disease. The main bacteria involved are *Salmonella* and *Camphylobacter* species. While most people get over the symptoms of diarrhea, vomiting, and malaise within a few days, food poisoning can occasionally be fatal if a particularly virulent strain, such as *Escherichia coli* 0157:H7 is involved. The elderly are particularly at risk of potentially fatal food poisoning.

Leptospirosis is the most common of the bacterial zoonoses. It occurs when *Leptospira* species infect rodents and other animals. Humans become infected by coming into contact with contaminated water, when the bacterium enters the body through broken skin or via the mucous membranes of the nose, mouth, and eyes. Also known as Weil's disease, leptospirosis can be very serious, causing kidney failure and lung hemorrhage. It affects those who work in or near water, such as rice paddy and sugarcane workers. The disease can also affect those enjoying recreational activities, like swimming. In a rainy season, or during flooding, leptospirosis may affect cities and reach epidemic proportions. Other significant bacterial diseases derived from animal sources include plague, Q fever, shigellosis, and tularemia.

It is estimated that 50 million people worldwide suffer from a parasitic zoonosis known as cysticercosis or taeniasis. It is caused by the larval cysts of the pork tapeworm *Taenia solium* and is therefore contracted through contact with pigs. Symptoms include headache and seizures. Other zoonoses caused by parasites include toxoplasmosis, which can be caught by contact with cat feces or by eating undercooked meat. As of 2013, 60 million people in the United States were infected with *Toxoplasma gondii*. However, it rarely causes health problems, except in pregnant women and those with compromised immunity.

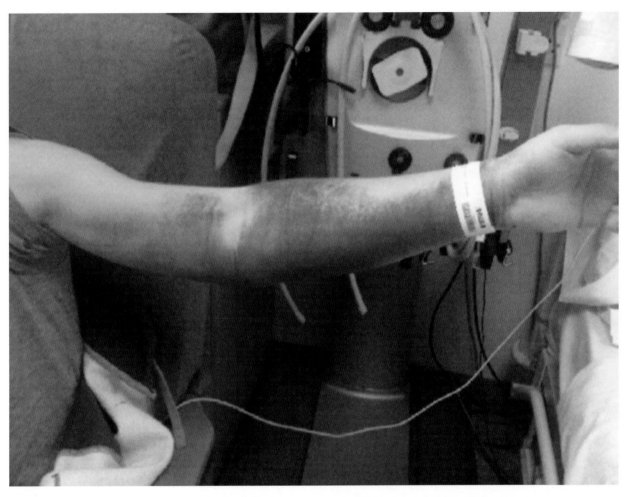

A patient's arm after he contracted Weil's disease (caused by the bacteria *Leptospira*) from rats' urine while kayaking down a river. It is believed the bacteria entered his body through his eyes and nose, as well as grazes on his hands from rock climbing. He was rushed to the hospital after he began vomiting and had an excruciating back ache. If left untreated, leptospirosis attacks the organs and can be fatal. *© Rex Features/AP Images.*

Finally, there are many viral diseases that come from animal sources. One of the most significant is rabies, which is carried by bats and carnivores. If not promptly treated, rabies is nearly always fatal. An estimated 55,000 people, most of them children, die from rabies every year. Bites from dogs infected with rabies are responsible for most of these deaths. Other significant viral zoonoses include Ebola, avian influenza, and Rift Valley fever.

⊕ Historical Background

The zoonoses have a very long history because there has always been close contact between humans, animals, and microbes. However, before the advent of agriculture, when humans existed as small groups of hunter-gatherers, it is likely that outbreaks burned themselves out and never reached epidemic proportions. As populations increased, however, diseases were more likely to jump from animals to humans and become established.

It may be that smallpox, the common cold, and influenza were originally confined to animals but spread to humans over the course of history.

One of the oldest infectious diseases is plague. This disease is caused by the bacterium *Yersinia pestis*, which is carried by fleas living on rodents. Known as the Black Death, plague swept all over Europe between 1347 and 1351, killing more than 25 million people. Plague is still present in parts of Asia, Africa, and the Americas, but it is now treatable by antibiotics.

Viral zoonoses also have a long history. Influenza occurs in both pigs and birds, and mutates to strains that can infect humans. The pandemic of Spanish flu in 1918 claimed an estimated 40 million lives worldwide. There were influenza pandemics in 1957 and 1968, known as Asian flu and Hong Kong flu respectively. The U.S. Centers for Disease Control and Prevention (CDC) warned in 2014 that pandemic flu is likely to strike again within the next 10 years. Another example is hantavirus, which is carried by rodents. It can result in haemorrhagic fever with renal

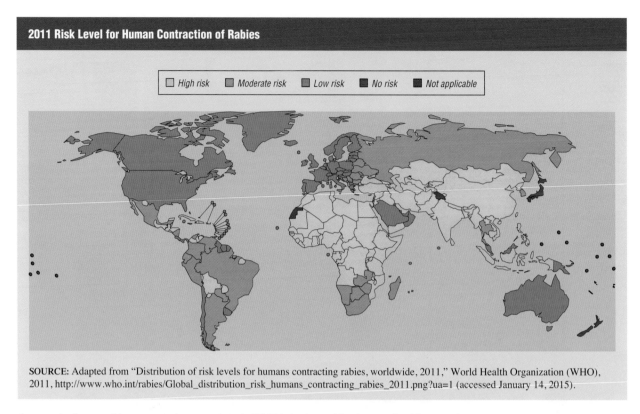

2011 Risk Level for Human Contraction of Rabies

☐ *High risk* ☐ *Moderate risk* ☐ *Low risk* ☐ *No risk* ☐ *Not applicable*

SOURCE: Adapted from "Distribution of risk levels for humans contracting rabies, worldwide, 2011," World Health Organization (WHO), 2011, http://www.who.int/rabies/Global_distribution_risk_humans_contracting_rabies_2011.png?ua=1 (accessed January 14, 2015).

A zoonotic disease, rabies accounts for approximately 55,000 deaths worldwide annually. African and Asian countries are at greatest risk of human rabies cases.

syndrome or hantavirus pulmonary syndrome, both of which can be deadly. This virus has been present for many years in Europe and Asia. It was first identified as being in the United States in 1993, though the CDC now has traced the hantavirus in the United States as far back as 1959.

AIDS and Ebola

In 2000, German American immunologist Beatrice Hahn and her team at the University of Alabama, Birmingham, described AIDS as a zoonosis. They found that HIV-1, which is responsible for the global pandemic of AIDS, spread to humans through contact with chimpanzees, possible as early as the 1920s. HIV-2, a strain confined to Africa, originated in the sooty mangabey, which is another African primate. The group assumes that hunters in the Congo basin came into contact with simian immunodeficiency virus (SIV), which is closely related to HIV. HIV/AIDS remains a global public health threat; although there is now effective treatment for it, there is still no cure or vaccine to prevent it.

In the spring of 1976, hundreds of cases of Ebola, a deadly hemorrhagic disease, were seen in Africa. Researchers observed that the disease first emerged in the dense jungles of Africa. It likely spread to people via contact with monkeys. However, unlike many zoonoses, Ebola usually kills its intermediate monkey hosts. Therefore, for the virus to survive, there must be some other

as yet unconfirmed natural reservoir for the disease. Currently, scientists suspect that fruit bats are the most likely candidates for the natural reservoir of Ebola virus. Clearly there is still much to be learned about this zoonosis that is causing so much current concern, as the largest outbreak of Ebola virus disease in recorded history began in western Africa in 2014 and continued into 2015. As of May 27, 2015, the WHO estimated that there had been more than 27,000 cases and more than 11,100 deaths from the outbreak, occurring in nine countries on three different continents, though the majority of cases and deaths were in Guinea, Liberia, and Sierra Leone.

⊕ Impacts and Issues

There has been a significant increase in zoonotic disease over the 40 years prior to 2014, with 43 new outbreaks since 2004, according to the Institute of Development Studies. There are several reasons for this trend. Increasing populations have meant opening up increasing areas of land for food production and human habitation; therefore, previously inaccessible habitats are being converted into farmland and settlements. This ecosystem change brings both humans and livestock into contact with wildlife, exposing them to previously rare diseases carried by these animals.

Increased urbanization and increased interconnectedness of cities around the globe due to international

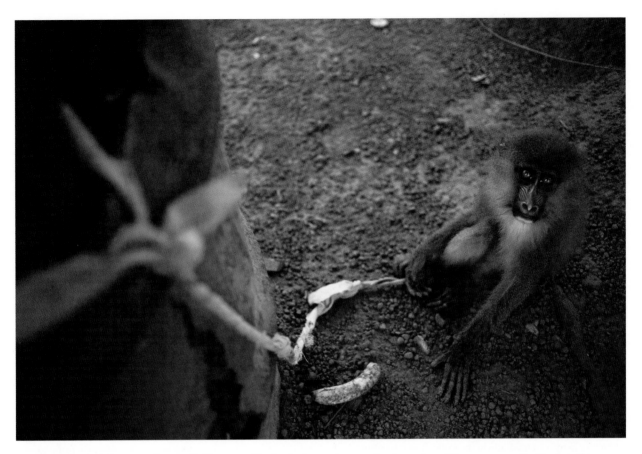

A Drill monkey is tied to a tree in a small village near Ngoilya in the southeastern border region of Cameroon near the Democratic Republic of the Congo. The monkey was for sale, and if not purchased would be butchered for its meat. Researchers have confirmed HIV/ AIDS originated through the hunting and consumption of wild game or bushmeat, particularly nonhuman primate species such as chimps and monkeys such as this one. The virus is theorized to have jumped from a local species of chimpanzee to humans as a result of contact with the animals' blood during hunting and cooking.   © *J Carrier/Getty Images.*

travel spread these diseases more rapidly, as people are more mobile and also crowded together. These diseases may, therefore, appear far from their country of origin, as has happened with West Nile virus, hantavirus, SARS, and Ebola. Finally, the increasing trade in animals and animal products has also contributed to the problem of zoonoses.

The WHO defines emerging zoonosis as one that is either newly recognized, or one that has been observed previously but now shows an increase in its incidence or an expansion in its geographical, host, or vector range. An analysis carried out by researchers at the Zoological Society of London and colleagues in the United States showed that, of 335 events of emerging infections between 1940 and 2004, zoonoses dominated. Over 60 percent of these events had a zoonotic origin. Of these, 71.8 percent originated from wildlife, including Ebola virus and SARS. Moreover, these events have been increasing over time. The researchers concluded that there is a substantial risk of wildlife zoonotic and vector-borne emerging diseases originating at lower latitudes. These are locations where reporting ability happens to be low, which makes a rapid response challenging.

The Burden of Zoonotic Disease

Zoonoses such as avian influenza and Ebola have threatened pandemics in the early 21st century, with frequent international travel being a significant risk factor in their spread. Climate change is also likely to play a role in causing such pandemics in the future by altering habitats and changing human-animal interactions. Thus, developed countries may see more cases of zoonoses like West Nile virus. However, the developed countries are able to call on considerable resources, such as surveillance and monitoring capacity and stockpiled vaccines and drugs, when a pandemic threat is announced or where emerging zoonoses appear on a smaller scale.

In contrast, the problem of zoonoses in poorer countries is chronic and insidious. Communities live closely with livestock and are dependent upon them for their survival. This applies to around 10 percent of the world's population, around 600 million to 1 billion people. Three-quarters of the rural poor and one-third of the urban poor depend upon livestock for food and income. In some parts of the tropics, as much as 70 percent of the population relies upon livestock for their livelihood.

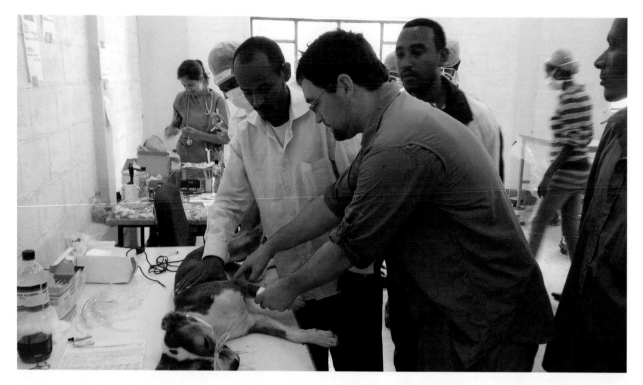

U.S. Centers for Disease Control and Prevention (CDC) Veterinary Medical Officer Ryan M. Wallace trains Ethiopian veterinarians at a spay/neuter clinic in Ethiopia. In many parts of the world, standard veterinary services, an integral component of rabies control, are not present. The CDC is collaborating with the Ethiopian government, the University of Gondar, and Ohio State University to help improve veterinary infrastructure to keep animals healthier and prevent rabies. According to the CDC, Ethiopia has reported some of the highest rates of human rabies deaths in the world. The transmission to humans of the rabies virus from dogs is a major problem in many areas around the world. *Ally Sterman/U.S. Centers for Disease Control and Prevention.*

Furthermore, zoonoses tend to be more common in places that have been affected by natural disasters such as earthquakes, or in conflict or war zones.

An analysis by scientists in Kenya and elsewhere found that the 13 leading zoonoses kill 2.2 million people each year. In poor countries, zoonoses can account for 20 percent of illness and death. The countries most affected were Ethiopia, Nigeria, Tanzania, and India. The 13 diseases were, in descending order: zoonotic gastrointestinal disease; leptospirosis; cysticercosis; zoonotic tuberculosis (TB); rabies; leishmaniasis (caused by a bite from certain sand flies); brucellosis (a bacterial disease that mainly infects livestock); echinococcosis; toxoplasmosis; Q fever; zoonotic *trypanosomiasis* (sleeping sickness); hepatitis E; and anthrax. Moreover, hot spots for emerging zoonotic diseases are Western Europe, particularly the United Kingdom; the northeastern United States; Brazil; and certain areas of southeastern Asia. The analysis also showed high rates of infection among livestock. For instance, 25 percent had signs of current or past infection with Q fever and 26 percent with leptospirosis.

Overall, there is limited information on the global burden of zoonotic disease, because so much of it occurs in remote communities, where surveillance and reporting systems have not been set up. Similarly, there is a lack of diagnostic and treatment facilities in the places most affected. There is also little hard information on the socioeconomic impact of these diseases; they do affect the productivity of livestock, which in turn contributes to poverty and malnutrition.

Zoonoses and the Millennium Development Goals

Millennium Development Goal (MDG) 6 is to combat HIV/AIDS, malaria, and other diseases. The target that would appear to relate to the zoonoses, though they are not specifically mentioned, is to "have halted by 2015 and begun to reverse the incidence of malaria and other major diseases." The gains, in terms of improving the health of those in traditional communities dependent on livestock, would be huge.

However, global health policy has tended to address one disease at a time. It tends to be influenced by donor priorities and the strength of advocates' voices. Thus much effort and investment has been dedicated to the cause of AIDS, tuberculosis, and malaria, as evidenced by the establishment of the Global Fund to Fight AIDS, Tuberculosis and Malaria in 2002. However, a paper from David Molyneux of the Liverpool School of Tropical Medicine has argued that the disease burden of zoonoses is actually higher than that of TB or malaria.

WEST NILE VIRUS

West Nile virus (WNV) can cause a potentially fatal neurological disease in humans, although most of those infected will not show symptoms. Cases of WNV have been on the increase in many countries, including the United States, in recent years. Birds are the hosts for WNV and its vector is the mosquito. There is currently no vaccine for WNV and no treatment other than for symptoms. It is one of the diseases that scientific modeling has predicted to increase with climate change. Both the number of cases and the geographical range of WNV are set to increase as temperatures and rainfall increase.

WNV was first identified in a woman in the West Nile area of Uganda in 1937. In 1953, it was identified in birds of the Nile delta. Human cases of WNV were reported in many countries over the following 50 years. In 1999, WNV infection was imported to New York City from Israel and Tunisia. Since then, there have been around 40,000 reported WNV infections in the United States, according to the Centers for Disease Control and Prevention (CDC). Of these, 17,000 people became seriously ill and more than 1,600 died. The CDC believes there may have been many more WNV cases that were not reported.

Besides the United States, the largest outbreaks of WNV have occurred in Greece, Israel, Romania, and Russia. Outbreak sites are on the migration routes of birds, which helps explain the spread of the disease. Originally, WNV was prevalent in Africa, parts of Europe, the Middle East, West Asia, and Australia. It has now been established in the Americas from Venezuela to Canada.

A variety of birds, including crows, jays, hawks, and owls, can become infected by WNV. The infection occurs when the bird is bitten by an infected mosquito, which has, in turn, been infected by feeding on an already infected bird. Mosquitoes of the *Culex* genus, and especially *C.pipiens*, are the main vectors of WNV. The virus is transmitted within mosquito populations from adults to eggs. Thus the connection between birds and mosquitoes is key to transmission. The bird may get sick and die. The identification of WNV in a dead bird is an important surveillance tool for detecting the presence of the disease in a particular place. Predators, like owls, or scavengers, like crows, can become infected by eating dead birds that had the disease.

Most human WNV infections have occurred through mosquito bites. There have been a few cases where people have contracted WNV via organ transplants, blood transfusion, and breast milk. No case of transmission by casual human-to-human contact has ever been reported, nor have healthcare workers become infected when using standard infection-control procedures. However, the disease has, on occasion, been transmitted to laboratory workers.

People living where WNV is endemic need to be aware of risks. Prevention of mosquito bites via protective clothing, mosquito nets, and insect repellent is vital. Sick and dead birds should never be handled without gloves and their presence should always be reported. When there is an outbreak of WNV, blood and organ donations may have to be restricted and laboratory testing of donations put in place.

Beyond personal protection, it is critical that comprehensive mosquito surveillance and control programs be put in place wherever WNV is found. The mosquito species that forms the important bridge between birds and humans should be identified by research and targeted for strict control measures. An integrated approach to vector control, involving source reduction, water management, and chemical and biological control tools, is required. The World Health Organization in Europe and the Americas is providing intensive support for WNV surveillance and outbreak responsive activities with country offices and international partners.

Action on Zoonoses

The control of zoonoses must be a multidisciplinary effort, involving coordination between the human and veterinary health, agricultural, environmental, and water supply sectors. However, this is hardest to achieve in just those countries where the impact of the zoonoses is highest. This is where global agencies such as the WHO have an important part to play.

The WHO has recognized the need for a multidisciplinary approach to the global control of zoonoses and has put together a number of initiatives. One of these is the Global Early Warning System for Major Animal Diseases, including Zoonoses (GLEWS). Effective containment and control of zoonotic disease depends upon early warning of outbreaks among animals and the ability to predict whether these are likely to spread to humans. Such systems have often been lacking in the places most affected, which contributes to the spread of disease.

GLEWS is a partnership between the WHO, the United Nations Food and Agriculture Organization (FAO), and the World Organisation for Animal Health. They share information and carry out a thorough risk assessment on any significant outbreak threats. Currently, GLEWS has 18 zoonoses on its priority list, including Ebola, Rift Valley fever, West Nile virus, and highly pathogenic avian influenza.

The work of GLEWS is complemented by that of the WHO's Global Outbreak Alert & Response Network (GOARN). This organization has the aim of dealing with the global spread of zoonotic disease by providing assistance to the places affected, which involves both control of the animal vector and management of the human cases of disease. Early and rapid response will mean more effective damage control. As of early 2015, GOARN has dealt with 50 significant outbreaks of disease. The long-term aim of GOARN is to work toward epidemic preparedness and capacity building.

Meanwhile, much more research into zoonoses is needed. It is only by recognizing and understanding human-animal interactions that lead to disease that they can be better controlled. Improved predictive models will also help to identify hot spots throughout the world where zoonoses are likely to emerge from the human-animal interface. Finally, to really make a difference in combating the burden of zoonotic diseases, research findings must be linked strongly to control policies and building stronger health-care infrastructures in the places most affected.

⊕ Future Implications

The public health challenge posed by zoonotic disease will only intensify in the future, because factors driving the increased incidence of zoonosis have an upward trend. For instance, urbanization will continue, with 5 billion of the world's estimated 8.1 billion population living in cities by 2025. Also, by 2020, a growing population is likely to increase demand for animal-based protein by 50 percent, which will increase the number of cases of zoonotic disease. Climate change is another risk factor that is likely to change the pattern of zoonotic disease, as vectors and hosts change their geographical range.

Global response to the future threat from zoonotic disease should be to move this comparatively neglected area higher on the agenda. Response needs to be fully integrated, with a strong focus on preparedness and surveillance. Underlying science needs higher priority and funding. Research should be directed toward improved modeling, so the emergence of zoonotic hot spots can be better predicted. Development of drugs and vaccines for diseases like Ebola and West Nile virus must also be a priority.

SEE ALSO *Avian (Bird) and Swine Influenzas; Bacterial Diseases; Cholera and Dysentery; Ebola Virus Disease; HIV/AIDS; Insect-Borne Diseases; Neglected Tropical Diseases; Parasitic Diseases; Viral Diseases; Waterborne Diseases*

BIBLIOGRAPHY

Books

Armon, Robert, and Uta Cheruti. *Environmental Aspects of Zoonotic Diseases.* London: IWA, 2012.

Choffnes, Eileen R., and David A. Relman. *The Causes and Impacts of Neglected Tropical and Zoonotic Diseases: Opportunities for Integrated Intervention Strategies: Workshop Summary.* Washington, DC: National Academies Press, 2011.

Howard, Colin R. *Lecture Notes on Emerging Viruses and Human Health: A Guide to Zoonotic Viruses and Their Impact.* Singapore: World Scientific, 2012.

Krause, Denis O., and Stephen Hendrick. *Zoonotic Pathogens in the Food Chain.* Wallingford, UK: CABI, 2010.

Mackenzie, John S., Martyn Jeggo, Peter Daszak, and Juergen A. Richt, eds. *One Health: The Human-Animal-Environment Interfaces in Emerging Infectious Diseases: Food Safety and Security, and National Plans for Implementation of One Health Activities.* Berlin: Springer, 2013.

M'ikanatha, Nkuchia M., and John K. Iskander, eds. *Concepts and Methods in Infectious Disease Surveillance.* Hoboken, NJ: Wiley, 2015.

Shakespeare, Martin. *Zoonoses*, 2nd ed. London: Pharmaceutical Press, 2009.

Periodicals

Hallaj, Zuhair. "Global Trends in Emerging Zoonoses." *International Journal of Antimicrobial Agents* 36, no. 1, supp. 1 (November 2010): S1–S2.

Jones, Kate, et al. "Global Trends in Emerging Infectious Diseases." *Nature* 451, no. 7181 (February 2008): 990–993.

Molyneux, David. "Combating the 'Other Diseases' of MDG 6: Changing the Paradigm to Achieve Equity and Poverty Reduction." *Transactions of the Royal Society of Tropical Medicine and Hygiene* 102, no. 6 (June 2008): 509–519.

Websites

"About Zoonoses." *National Consortium for Zoonosis Research Hosted by the University of Liverpool.* http://www.zoonosis.ac.uk/about-zoonoses/ (accessed February 20, 2015).

"Four-Way Linking Project for Assessing Health Risks at the Human-Animal Interface." *World Health Organization (WHO).* http://www.who.int/influenza/human_animal_interface/EN_GIP_FourWay_HAI_2013.pdf (accessed January 17, 2015).

"Research Priorities for Zoonoses and Marginalized Infections." *World Health Organization (WHO).* http://apps.who.int/iris/bitstream/10665/75350/1/WHO_TRS_971_eng.pdf (accessed January 16, 2015).

"Zoonoses—from Panic to Planning." *Institute of Development Studies.* https://www.ids.ac.uk/publications/zoonoses-from-panic-to-planning (accessed January 17, 2015).

"Zoonosis." *World Health Organization (WHO).* http://www.who.int/topics/zoonoses/es/ (accessed January 17, 2015).

"Zoonotic Disease Addendum." *Colorado Department of Agriculture*, January 2011. https://www.colorado.gov/pacific/sites/default/files/Zoonotic%20Disease%20Addendum.pdf (accessed February 20, 2015).

Susan Aldridge

Selected Organizations and Advocacy Groups

The following is an annotated compilation of organizations and advocacy groups relevant to the topics found in *Worldmark Global Health and Medicine Issues*. Although the list is comprehensive, it is by no means exhaustive and is intended to serve as a starting point for assembling further information. Gale, a part of Cengage Learning, is not responsible for the accuracy of the addresses or the contents of the websites, nor does it endorse any of the organizations listed.

AMERICAN ASSOCIATION FOR THE ADVANCEMENT OF SCIENCE

The American Association for the Advancement of Science (AAAS) is an international, nonprofit, professional organization of scientists. Its mission is to promote science worldwide. AAAS publishes the journal *Science*, as well as scientific reports and informational materials.

> 1200 New York Avenue NW
> Washington, DC 20005
> United States
> Phone: (202) 326-6400
> E-mail: media@aaas.org
> Website: http://www.aaas.org/

AMERICAN SOCIETY OF GENE & CELL THERAPY (ASGCT)

The American Society of Gene & Cell Therapy seeks to expand government, industry, and public support for cell and gene therapies to treat and cure human diseases.

> 555 East Wells Street, Suite 1100
> Milwaukee, WI 53202
> United States
> Phone: (414) 278-1341
> Fax: (414) 276-3349
> E-mail: info@asgct.org
> Website: http://www.asgct.org/

AMERICAN SOCIETY OF HUMAN GENETICS

Founded in 1948, the American Society of Human Genetics, founded in 1948, is the primary U.S.-based professional organization for genetics researchers and medical professionals in genetics-related fields. The Society holds an annual meeting and periodically publishes *The American Journal of Human Genetics*.

> 9650 Rockville Pike
> Bethesda, MD 20814
> United States
> Phone: (301) 634-7300
> Phone: (866) HUM-GENE
> E-mail: society@ashg.org
> Website: http://www.ashg.org/

AMGEN, INC.

Amgen, Inc. is a U.S.-based biotechnology company with numerous biopharmaceutical products based on innovations in recombinant DNA and molecular biology.

> One Amgen Center Drive
> Thousand Oaks, CA 91320-1799
> United States
> Phone: (805) 447-1000
> Fax: (805) 447-1010
> Website: http://www.amgen.com

ASSOCIATION FOR ASSESSMENT AND ACCREDITATION OF LABORATORY ANIMAL CARE INTERNATIONAL

The Association for Assessment and Accreditation of Laboratory Animal Care International is a nonprofit organization that promotes the humane treatment of laboratory and other animals used in science through assessment and accreditation programs.

> 5283 Corporate Drive, Suite 203
> Frederick, MD 21703-2879

> United States
> Phone: (301) 696-9626
> E-mail: accredit@aaalac.org
> Website: http://www.aaalac.org

THE BILL & MELINDA GATES FOUNDATION

The Bill & Melinda Gates Foundation is the largest private foundation in the world. In the area of global public health, the foundation's goals center on enhanced health care, reduced poverty, and expanded educational opportunities. Among many other activities, the Gates Foundation funds vaccine programs, disease eradication initiatives, and medical research.

> 500 Fifth Avenue North
> Seattle, Washington 98109
> United States
> Phone: (206) 709-3100
> E-mail: info@gatesfoundation.org
> Website: http://www.gatesfoundation.org

BIOINDUSTRY ASSOCIATION

The BioIndustry Association is a bio-science trade association and lobbying group based in the United Kingdom. It promotes industry interests in government policy formation and supports initiatives to make the UK a global hub for biotechnology.

> 7th Floor, Southside, 105 Victoria Street
> London, SW1E 6QT
> United Kingdom
> Phone: 44 (0)20 7630 2180
> Website: http://www.bioindustry.org

BIOMEDICAL ENGINEERING SOCIETY

Founded in 1968, the Biomedical Engineering Society is an organization of biomedical engineers devoted to advancing human health and well-being through biomedical engineering.

8201 Corporate Drive, Suite 1125
Landover, MD 20785-2224
United States
Phone: (301) 459-1999
Phone: (877) 871-BMES
Fax: (301) 459-2444
E-mail: info@bmes.org
Website: http://www.bmes.org

BIOTECHNOLOGY AND BIOLOGICAL SCIENCES RESEARCH COUNCIL

Biotechnology and Biological Sciences Research Council (BBSRC) directly supports and funds scientific research in the United Kingdom. BBSRC is one of seven government-funded Research Councils.

Polaris House
North Star Avenue
Swindon, Wiltshire SN2 1UH
United Kingdom
Phone: 44 (0)17 9341 3200
Fax: 44 (0)1793 413201
E-mail: press.office@bbsrc.ac.uk
Website: http://www.bbsrc.ac.uk/

BIOTECHNOLOGY INSTITUTE

The Biotechnology Institute is a think-tank and education advocacy group dedicated to educating the public about biotechnology and encouraging young people to pursue studies and careers in biotech fields.

1201 Maryland Avenue SW, Suite 900
Washington, DC 20024
United States
Phone: (202) 312-9269
Fax: (202) 488-6301
E-mail: info@biotechinstitute.org
Website: http://www.biotechinstitute.org/

CALIFORNIA LIFE SCIENCES ASSOCIATION

California Life Sciences Association is the merger of BayBio (originally the Bay Area Bioscience Center) and California Healthcare Institute, a regional bioscience and advocacy organization composed of industry members in California, one of the United States' largest centers for biotech development.

250 E. Grand Ave., Suite 26
South San Francisco, CA 94080
United States
Phone: (650) 871-3250
E-mail: info@califesciences.org
Website: http://califesciences.org/

CANADIAN BIOETHICS SOCIETY

Canadian Bioethics Society, in partnership with the W. Maurice Young Centre for Applied Ethics at the University of British Columbia, is a nonprofit organization that acts as a forum for professionals to discuss bioethics and address potential bioethical problems. The Society advocates teaching of bioethics in all university and graduate-level science course programs.

P.O. Box 33
Hubbards, Nova Scotia B0J 1T0
Canada
Phone: (403) 208-8027
E-mail: amy.middleton@bioethics.ca
Website: https://www.bioethics.ca/

CARE

CARE is a nonprofit organization that works in more than 80 countries around the world, including Syria, India, Mali, and the region of Darfur in Sudan. It is often on the frontline of treating people in areas challenged by conflict and violence.

151 Ellis Street NE
Atlanta, GA 30303
United States
Phone: (800) 422-7385
E-mail: info@care.org
Website: http://www.care.org

CARTER CENTER

The nonprofit Carter Center strives to relieve the suffering caused by war, disease, famine, and poverty by advancing peace and health in neighborhoods and nations around the world. The Center, in partnership with Emory University, is committed to promoting human rights, waging peace by bringing warring parties to the negotiating table, monitoring elections, safeguarding human rights, and building strong democracies through economic development.

One Copenhill
453 Freedom Parkway
Atlanta, GA 30307
United States
Phone: (404) 420-5100
Website: http://www.cartercenter.org/

CENTER FOR BIOLOGICAL DIVERSITY

The Center for Biological Diversity is a U.S. nonprofit organization dedicated to protecting endangered species using scientific information and legal action.

P.O. Box 710
Tucson, AZ 85702-0710
United States
Phone: (866) 357-3349
Fax: (520) 623-9797
E-mail: center@biologicaldiversity.org
Website: http://www.biologicaldiversity.org

CENTER FOR BIOTECHNOLOGY

The mission of the Center for Biotechnology is to support biotechnological and biomedical research and promote the growth of the biotechnology industry in New York State.

Bioengineering Building, 2nd Floor
Stony Brook University
Stony Brook, NY 11794-5280
United States
Phone: (631) 632-8521
Fax: (631) 632-8577
E-mail: center_for_biotechnology@
stonybrook.edu
Website: http://centerforbiotechnology.org/

CENTER FOR SCIENCE IN THE PUBLIC INTEREST

The Center for Science in the Public Interest seeks to educate the public and policy makers in the United States and Canada by providing science-based information on food and nutrition issues. Their newsletter, *Nutrition Action Healthletter*, is the most circulated health newsletter in North America, with over 900,000 subscribers.

1220 L Street NW, Suite 300
Washington, DC 20005
United States
Phone: (202) 332-9110
Fax: (202) 265-4954
E-mail: cpsinews@cpsinet.org
Website: http://www.cspinet.org/

CENTERS FOR DISEASE CONTROL AND PREVENTION (CDC)

The Centers for Disease Control and Prevention (CDC) is a U.S. government agency organized under the United States Department of Health and Human Services. The CDC promotes public health and quality of life initiatives by working with health partners to detect and investigate health problems, conduct research on disease, implement disease prevention strategies, develop public health policies, and promote healthy lifestyles.

1600 Clifton Road
Atlanta, GA 30329-4027
United States
Phone: (404) 639-3534
Phone: (800) 232-4636
E-mail: cdcinfo@cdc.gov
Website: http://www.cdc.gov

CONVENTION ON BIOLOGICAL DIVERSITY SECRETARIAT

The Convention on Biological Diversity (CBD) Secretariat coordinates activities that support the goals of the CBD, an international agreement to conserve biodiversity and promote sustainable development. The CBD Secretariat also coordinates activities related to the Cartagena Protocol on Biosafety, which regulates the transport and trade of living modified organisms.

> 413 Saint Jacques Street, Suite 800
> Montreal H2Y 1N9
> Canada
> Phone: (514) 288-2220
> Fax: (514) 288-6588
> E-mail: secretariat@cbd.int
> Website: http://www.cbd.int

DEFENSE ADVANCED RESEARCH PROJECTS AGENCY BIOLOGICAL TECHNOLOGIES OFFICE

The Biological Technologies Office (BTO) is part of the Defense Advanced Research Projects Agency, the science and technology research arm of the U.S. Department of Defense. The BTO's active programs include battlefield medicine, fighting pathogens, and creating fully-functioning prosthetic limbs that are controlled naturally by the recipient's nervous and muscular systems and have full sensory and motor capabilities.

> 675 North Randolph Street
> Arlington, VA 22203-2114
> United States
> Phone: (703) 526-6630
> E-mail: darpapublicaffairsoffice@darpa.mil
> Website: http://www.darpa.mil/our_work/
> BTO/Programs/index.html

ELECTRONIC PRIVACY INFORMATION CENTER

The Electronic Privacy Information Center (EPIC) is a public interest research center that focuses on electronic privacy and civil liberties issues, including biometric and DNA databases.

> 1718 Connecticut Avenue NW, Suite 200
> Washington, DC 20009
> United States
> Phone: (202) 483-1140
> Fax: (202) 483-1248
> E-mail: info@epic.org
> Website: http://epic.org

EUROPEAN ASSOCIATION OF PHARMA BIOTECHNOLOGY (EAPB)

European Association of Pharma Biotechnology (EAPB) is a nonprofit organization linking academia, industry, and government and trade regulatory agencies to promote and facilitate pharmaceutical biotechnology research throughout Europe.

> Theodor Heuss Allee 25
> 60486 Frankfurt
> Germany
> Phone: 49 69 7564 341
> E-mail: managing.director@eapb.org
> Website: http://www.eapb.org

EUROPEAN CENTRE FOR DISEASE PREVENTION AND CONTROL (ECDC)

The European Centre for Disease Prevention and Control (ECDC) is a European Union agency based in Stockholm, Sweden, that was created in 2005 to fight infectious diseases in the countries of the EU. It works with various national governments, health experts, and scientists across the EU.

> Granits väg 8
> 171 65 Solna
> Sweden
> Phone: 46 (0)8 586 010 00
> Fax: 46 (0)8 586 010 01
> E-mail: info@ecdc.europa.eu
> Website: http://ecdc.europa.eu/en/Pages/
> home.aspx

EUROPEAN PATENT OFFICE

The European Patent Office is the main intergovernmental body that reviews patent applications and grants multinational European patents.

> EPO Post
> 80298 Munich
> Germany
> Phone: 49 (0)89 2399-0
> Website: http://www.epo.org

EUROPEAN SOCIETY OF HUMAN GENETICS

The European Society of Human Genetics is a professional society founded in 1967 that promotes research and the sharing of data among scientists in various applied genetics and medical genetics fields. The Society publishes the *European Journal of Human Genetics* and hosts several conferences for members.

> ESHG c/o Vienna Medical Academy
> Alserstrasse 4
> 1090 Vienna
> Austria
> Phone: 43 (1) 405 13 83 20
> Fax: 43 (1) 407 82 74
> E-mail: office@eshg.org
> Website: https://www.eshg.org/
> home.0.html

FEDERATION OF AMERICAN SCIENTISTS

The Federation of American Scientists is a nonprofit organization that provides policy recommendations on national and international security issues based on an objective analysis of available scientific data.

> 1725 DeSales Street NW, Suite 600
> Washington, DC 20036
> United States
> Phone: (202) 546-3300
> E-mail: fas@fas.org
> Website: http://www.fas.org

FOOD ADDITIVES AND INGREDIENTS ASSOCIATION

Founded in 1977, the Food Additives and Ingredients Association is a trade association that represents the interests of food additive manufacturers in the United Kingdom.

> 16 Smith Square
> London SW1P 3HQ
> United Kingdom
> E-mail: info@faia.org.uk
> Website: http://www.faia.org.uk

FOOD SAFETY CONSORTIUM

The Food Safety Consortium brings together researchers from United States universities to investigate all aspects of meat and poultry production.

> University of Arkansas
> 110 Agriculture Bldg.
> Fayetteville, AR 72701
> United States
> Phone: (479) 575-5647
> Fax: (479) 575-7531
> E-mail: dedmark@uark.edu
> Website: http://www.uark.edu/depts/fsc

GENENTECH, INC.

Genentech, Inc. is a U.S.-based biotechnology corporation that is a wholly owned subsidiary of the Roche Group, a Swiss pharmaceutical company.

> One DNA Way
> South San Francisco, CA 94080
> United States
> Phone: (650) 225-1000
> Fax: (650) 225-6000
> Website: http://www.gene.com

THE GENETICS SOCIETY

The UK-based Genetics Society describes itself as a "learned society" of professionals, educators, and students working in various fields of genetics. The Society publishes the journals *Heredity* and *Genes and Society* and holds an annual conference.

> c/o Portland Customer Services
> Charles Darwin House
> 12 Roger Street
> London WC1N 2JU
> United Kingdom
> Phone: 44 (0) 207 685 2444
> E-mail: theteam@genetics.org.uk
> Website: http://www.genetics.org.uk/

GILEAD SCIENCES

Gilead Sciences is a U.S.-based biopharmaceutical company with an emphasis on liver, cardiovascular, metabolic, and respiratory diseases, and HIV/AIDS.

333 Lakeside Drive
Foster City, CA 94404
United States
Phone: (650) 574-3000
Phone: (800) 445-3235
Fax: (650) 578-9264
E-mail: public_affairs@gilead.com
Website: http://www.gilead.com

GLAXOSMITHKLINE

GlaxoSmithKline is a pharmaceutical, biotechnology, and consumer healthcare company headquartered in the United Kingdom.

980 Great West Road
Brentford, Middlesex TW8 9GS
United Kingdom
Phone: 44 (0)20 8047 5000
Website: http://www.gsk.com

THE INSTITUTE FOR FOOD SAFETY AND HEALTH (IFSH)

The Institute for Food Safety and Health, based at the Illinois Institute of Technology, fosters the exchange of scientific research, industry practices, and regulatory policy on food safety. The Institute aims to brings together disparate voices in the food production, research, and regulation sectors.

Illinois Institute of Technology
Moffett Campus
6502 South Archer Rd.
Bedford Park, IL 60501-1957
United States
Phone: (708) 563-1576
Website: http://www.iit.edu/ifsh/

INTERGOVERNMENTAL PANEL ON CLIMATE CHANGE (IPCC)

The Intergovernmental Panel on Climate Change (IPCC) is an intergovernmental organization that analyzes scientific data on global climate change and assesses its impacts and potential mitigation and adaptation strategies.

c/o World Meteorological Organization
7bis Avenue de la Paix
C.P. 2300
CH-1211 Geneva 2
Switzerland
Phone: 41 (22) 730 82 08
Fax: 41 (22) 730 80 25
E-mail: IPCC-Sec@WMO.int
Website: http://www.ipcc.ch

INTERNATIONAL CENTRE FOR GENETIC ENGINEERING AND BIOTECHNOLOGY

The International Centre for Genetic Engineering and Biotechnology—part of the United Nations system—conducts life sciences research in the fields of agricultural biotechnology, biomedicine, biopesticides, and environmental science for the benefit of developing countries to help strengthen global research capability. It has facilities in Trieste, Italy; New Delhi, India; and Cape Town, South Africa.

AREA Science Park
Padriciano 99
34149 Trieste
Italy
Phone: 39 040-37571
Fax: 39 040-226555
E-mail: icgeb@icgeb.org
Website: http://www.icgeb.trieste.it/
home.html

INTERNATIONAL COMMITTEE OF THE RED CROSS (ICRC)

The International Committee of the Red Cross (ICRC) is an organization dedicated to helping victims of disasters, violence, and war. The ICRC is noted for going into places of conflict and disaster and providing food, shelter, and health care, as well as monitoring adherence to the Geneva Conventions for prisoners of war.

19 Avenue de la Paix
CH 1202 Geneva
Switzerland
Phone: 41 22 734 60 01
Fax: 41 22 733 20 57
Website: http://www.icrc.org/eng/

INTERNATIONAL LABOUR ORGANIZATION (ILO)

The International Labour Organization (ILO) is an agency of the United Nations established in 1919 to encourage dialogue between workers, employers, and governments and ensure safe and humane working conditions around the world.

4 route des Morillons
CH-1211 Genèva 22
Switzerland
Phone: 41 (0) 22 799 6111
Fax: 41 (0) 22 798 8685
Email: ilo@ilo.org
Website: http://www.ilo.org

INTERNATIONAL LIFE SCIENCES INSTITUTE

Founded in 1978, the International Life Sciences Institute is a nonprofit global organization dedicated to fostering public health by collaborating with scientific, industry, and policy experts to provide science-based information, research, commentary, and policy analysis.

1156 15th Street NW
Washington, DC 20005
United States
Phone: (202) 659-0074
Fax: (202) 659-3859
E-mail: info@ilsi.org
Website: http://www.ilsi.org

INTERNATIONAL PLANNED PARENTHOOD FEDERATION

The International Planned Parenthood Federation works in 170 countries to provide information, education, and health care services for family planning, maternal and child health, and prevention and treatment of sexually transmitted diseases, including HIV/AIDS.

4 Newhams Row
London
SE1 3UZ
United Kingdom
Phone: 44(0)20 7939 8200
Fax: 44(0)20 7939 8300
E-mail: info@ippf.org
Website: http://www.ippf.org/

INTERNATIONAL RESCUE COMMITTEE (IRC)

The International Rescue Committee (IRC) is a humanitarian aid organization that responds to emergencies and provides relief and development assistance to refugees and people affected by conflict, persecution, or disasters. The IRC was founded in New York in 1933 at the request of physicist Albert Einstein to aid people affected by crisis in Nazi Germany. It now assists people in more than 40 countries worldwide and 22 cities in the United States.

122 East 42nd Street
New York, NY 10168
United States
Phone: (212) 551 3000
Fax: (212) 551 3179
Website: http://www.rescue.org

INTERNATIONAL SOCIETY FOR IN VITRO FERTILIZATION

The International Society for In Vitro Fertilization is an organization that promotes in vitro fertilization (IVF) research and ethical practice within the IVF field.

2155 Guy Street, 14th Floor, Room 1471
Montreal H3H 2R9
Canada
Phone: (514) 241-2537
E-mail: barcap@sympatico.ca
Website: http://www.isivf.com

INTERNATIONAL SOCIETY FOR PHARMACEUTICAL ENGINEERING

The International Society for Pharmaceutical Engineering is an individual membership society for pharmaceutical manufacturing professionals with 22,000 members in 90 countries worldwide.

600 N. Westshore Blvd., Suite 900
Tampa, FL 33609
United States
Phone: (813) 960-2105
Fax: (813) 264-2816
E-mail: ASK@ispe.org
Website: http://www.ispe.org/

MARIE STOPES INTERNATIONAL

Marie Stopes International works around the world to assist with family planning and reproductive health for impoverished women. They also assist with education programs to improve maternal and child health and combat sexually transmitted diseases, including HIV/AIDS.

1 Conway Street
Fitzroy Square
London W1T 6LP
United Kingdom
Phone: 44 (0)20 7636 6200
Fax: 44 (0)20 7034 2369
E-mail: info@mariestopes.org
Website: http://mariestopes.org/contact-us

MÉDECINS SANS FRONTIÈRES (DOCTORS WITHOUT BORDERS)

Médecins Sans Frontières, also known by its English name, Doctors Without Borders, is dedicated to providing medical aid to those who most need it regardless of race, religion, or political affiliation. They frequently serve in conflict zones.

333 7th Avenue, 2nd Floor
New York, NY 10001-5004
United States
Phone: (212) 679-6800
Fax: (212) 679-7016
Website: http://www
.doctorswithoutborders.org

MERCK & CO., INC.

Merck & Co., Inc. is a U.S. pharmaceutical research and manufacturing company and ranks as one of the largest pharmaceutical companies in the world. Merck & Co. was established as a U.S. subsidiary of Merck KGaA, a German pharmaceutical company, in 1891 but was confiscated during World War I (1914–1918) and re-established as an independent company in 1917.

2000 Galloping Hill Road
Kenilworth, NJ 07033
United States
Phone: (908) 740-4000
Website: http://www.merck.com

NATIONAL ACADEMY OF SCIENCES

The National Academy of Sciences is a nonprofit organization comprised of scientists and engineers that advises the U.S. government on scientific and technological affairs.

Keck Center of the National Academy of Sciences
500 Fifth Street NW
Washington, DC 20001
United States
Phone: (202) 334-2000
Website: http://www.nasonline.org

NATIONAL CENTER FOR BIOTECHNOLOGY INFORMATION

The National Center for Biotechnology Information is a division of the U.S. National Library of Medicine. Its online portal facilitates research by sharing and providing up-to-date information on biomedicine and genomics.

National Library of Medicine
Building 38A
Bethesda, MD 20894
United States
Phone: (888) 346-3656
E-mail: info@ncbi.nlm.nih.gov
Website: http://www.ncbi.nlm.nih.gov/

NATIONAL HUMAN GENOME RESEARCH INSTITUTE

Originally established in 1989 as the U.S. National Institutes of Health liaison to the Human Genome Project, the National Human Genome Research Institute has expanded its role to facilitate and fund research on the applications of genome technologies to specific diseases and the genetics of human disorders.

National Institutes of Health
31 Center Drive, MSC 2152
9000 Rockville Pike
Bethesda, MD 20892-2152
United States
Phone: (301) 402-0911
Fax: (301) 402-2218
Website: http://www.genome.gov/

NATIONAL INSTITUTE OF BIOMEDICAL IMAGING AND BIOENGINEERING

The U.S. National Institute of Biomedical Imaging and Bioengineering, one of the U.S. National Institutes of Health, fosters the development of new medical technologies that can identify, image, diagnose, and treat human diseases.

6707 Democracy Blvd., Suite 202
Bethesda, MD 20892-5469
United States
Phone: (301) 496-8859
E-mail: info@nibib.nih.gov
Website: http://www.nibib.nih.gov/

NOBEL PRIZE FOUNDATION

The Nobel Prize Foundation, founded in 1900, presents awards annually for groundbreaking work in the sciences and arts, as well as in diplomatic or humanitarian efforts in the form of the Nobel Peace Prize.

Sturegatan 14, Box 5232
SE-102 45 Stockholm
Sweden
Phone: 46 8 663 17 22
Fax: 46 8 663 27 69
E-mail: info@nobelmedia.se
Website: http://www.nobelprize.org/

OFFICE OF BIOTECHNOLOGY ACTIVITIES

The Office of Biotechnology Activities (OBA), part of the Office of Science Policy at the U.S. National Institutes of Health (NIH), works to anticipate future developments in human genetics research while considering their possible legal, social, and ethical implications on U.S. and international science policy. OBA manages the NIH Recombinant DNA Advisory Committee and the Department of Health and Human Services Secretary's Advisory Committee on Genetics, Health, and Society, as well as works with international, state, and local regulatory agencies including oversight of Institutional Biosafety Committees.

Rockledge 1, Suite 750
6705 Rockledge Drive
Bethesda, MD 20817
United States
Phone: (301) 496-9838
Fax: (301) 496-9839
E-mail: OBA-OSP@od.nih.gov
Website: http://oba.od.nih.gov/oba/

OFFICE OF SCIENCE POLICY

The Office of Science Policy at the U.S. National Institutes of Health provides lawmakers with science-based information and analysis on policies affecting the medical research and research science industries.

Rockledge 1, Suite 750
6705 Rockledge Drive
Bethesda, MD 20817
United States
Phone: (301) 496-9838
Fax: (301) 496-9839
E-mail: SciencePolicy@od.nih.gov
Website: http://osp.od.nih.gov/

ORGANISATION FOR ECONOMIC CO-OPERATION AND DEVELOPMENT (OECD)

The Organisation for Economic Co-operation and Development (OECD) is a forum for governments to work cooperatively to adopt policies that will aid development, share technology, address global challenges, and improve the economic and social well-being of all global citizens. The OECD periodically publishes *Biotechnology Update* to keep delegates up-to-date on conference proceedings, international initiatives, or regulatory changes specific to biotechnology fields.

2, rue André Pascal
75775 Paris Cedex 16
France
Phone: 33 1 45 24 82 00
Fax: 33 1 45 24 85 00
E-mail: news.contact@oecd.org
Website: http://www.oecd.org

OXFAM INTERNATIONAL

Oxfam deploys a team of public health specialists and water engineers in humanitarian emergencies to deliver water supplies and sanitation facilities.

Suite 20
266 Banbury Road
Oxford, OX2 7DL
United Kingdom
Phone: 44 1865 339 100
Fax: 44 1865 339 101
E-mail: information@oxfaminternational.org
Website: https://www.oxfam.org/en

PAN AMERICAN HEALTH ORGANIZATION (PAHO)

The Pan American Health Organization (PAHO), founded in 1902, is the Regional Office for the Americas of the World Health Organization (WHO), as well as the health agency of the Inter-American System; it is part of the United Nations system.

525 Twenty-third Street, NW
Washington, DC 20037
United States
Phone: (202) 974-3000
Fax: (202) 974-3663
Website: http://www.paho.org/hq/

PHYSICIANS FOR SOCIAL RESPONSIBILITY

Physicians for Social Responsibility is a U.S. nonprofit organization of physicians that works to raise public awareness and set public policy on nuclear non-proliferation and environmental health issues.

1111 14th St, NW, Suite 700
Washington, DC 20005

United States
Phone: (202) 667-4260
Fax: (202) 667-4201
E-mail: psrnatl@psr.org
Website: http://www.psr.org

PROJECT HOPE

Project HOPE "delivers essential medicines and supplies, health expertise, and medical training to respond to disaster, prevent disease, promote wellness, and save lives around the globe."

255 Carter Hall Lane, P.O. Box 250
Millwood, VA 22646
United States
Phone: (540) 837-2100
Website: http://www.projecthope.org

THE ROCKEFELLER FOUNDATION

The Rockefeller Foundation's stated mission, unchanged since 1913, is to improve the well-being of humanity around the world. The foundation states its focus is on the following four goals: to revalue ecosystems, secure livelihoods, transform cities, and advance health.

420 Fifth Avenue
New York, NY 10018
United States
Phone: (212) 869-8500
Fax: (212) 764-3468
Website: http://www.rockefellerfoundation.org

UNITED NATIONS (UN)

The United Nations, founded following World War II (1939–1945), is dedicated to maintaining peace and security and developing peaceful resolution to conflict worldwide. It also protects human rights and promotes better living standards.

777 44th Street
New York, NY 10017
United States
Phone: (212) 963-4440
E-mail: unitg@un.org
Website: http://www.un.org/en/

UNITED NATIONS CHILDREN'S FUND (UNICEF)

The United Nations Children's Fund works worldwide to help children by providing health care, food, education, and emergency relief.

125 Maiden Lane, 11th Floor
New York, NY 10038
United States
Phone: (212) 686-5522
Fax: (212) 779-1679
Website: http://www.unicef.org/

UNITED NATIONS DEVELOPMENT PROGRAMME (UNDP)

The United Nations Development Programme is part of the United Nations dedicated to global development and capacity building.

One United Nations Plaza
New York, NY 10017
United States
Phone: (212) 906-5000
Fax: (212) 906-5001
E-mail: publications.queries@undp.org
Website: http://www.undp.org

UNITED NATIONS DIVISION FOR SUSTAINABLE DEVELOPMENT

The United Nations (UN) Division for Sustainable Development, a division of the UN Department of Economic and Social Affairs, promotes sustainable development through capacity building and technical cooperation at international, regional, and national levels.

United Nations Secretariat Building
405 East 42nd Street
New York, NY 10017
United States
Phone: (212) 963-3170
Fax: (212) 963-4260
Website: http://www.un.org/esa/dsd/

UNITED NATIONS ENVIRONMENT PROGRAMME (UNEP)

The United Nations Environment Programme is the agency responsible for developing and implementing the United Nations' environmental activities.

United Nations Avenue, Gigiri
P.O. Box 30552, 00100
Nairobi
Kenya
Phone: (254-20) 7621234
Fax: (254-20) 7624489
E-mail: unepinfo@unep.org
Website: http://www.unep.org

UNITED NATIONS FOOD AND AGRICULTURE ORGANIZATION (FAO)

The Food and Agriculture Organization is a part of the United Nations that promotes food security and adequate nutrition for all and the development of sustainable agriculture.

Viale delle Terme di Caracalla
00153 Rome
Italy
Phone: (39) 06 57051
E-mail: FAO-HQ@fao.org
Website: http://www.fao.org/home/en/

THE UNITED NATIONS HIGH COMMISSIONER FOR REFUGEES (UNHCR)

The United Nations High Commissioner for Refugees was established to coordinate and resolve refugee problems worldwide and to protect the rights of refugees. Refugee crises can be found throughout the world, but are frequently located in places of violence or in regions hit by environmental catastrophes, such as earthquakes and typhoons.

Case Postale 2500
CH-1211 Genève 2 Dépôt
Suisse
Phone: 41 22 739 8111
Fax: 41 22 739 7377
Website: http://www.unhcr.org/cgi-bin/texis/
vtx/home

UNITED NATIONS WORLD FOOD PROGRAMME (WFP)

The World Food Programme was established by the United Nations to provide food relief during times of crisis in areas of conflict and natural disasters. It serves an estimated 80 million people annually.

Via Cesare Giulio Viola 68
Parco dei Medici
00148 Rome
Italy
Phone: 39-06-65131
Fax: 39-06-6590632
Website: http://www.wfp.org/

U.S. AGENCY FOR INTERNATIONAL DEVELOPMENT (USAID)

The U.S. Agency for International Development (USAID) is the U.S. agency responsible for administering and distributing all non-military foreign aid for the United States. USAID also undertakes agricultural technology and infrastructure development programs to meet longer-term community needs.

Ronald Reagan Bldg., 1300 Pennsylvania
Avenue NW
Washington, DC 20523-1000
United States
Phone: (202) 712-0000
Fax: (202) 216-3524
Website: http://www.usaid.gov

U.S. DEPARTMENT OF AGRICULTURE (USDA)

The U.S. Department of Agriculture is a cabinet-level agency of the U.S. government and is responsible for developing, implementing, and administering U.S. agricultural, farming, and food policies.

1400 Independence Avenue SW
Washington, DC 20250
United States
Phone: (202) 720-2791
Website: http://www.usda.gov

U.S. ENVIRONMENTAL PROTECTION AGENCY (EPA)

The U.S. Environmental Protection Agency (EPA) is a U.S.-government agency dedicated to protecting the environment and human health. The EPA devises and enforces environmental regulations based on U.S. environmental laws.

1200 Pennsylvania Avenue NW
Washington, DC 20460
United States
Phone: (202) 272-0167
Website: http://www.epa.gov

U.S. FOOD AND DRUG ADMINISTRATION (FDA)

The U.S. Food and Drug Administration (FDA) is an agency within the U.S. Department of Health and Human Services that is responsible for regulating the safety of food, drugs, and cosmetics. The FDA must approve the safety and efficacy of drugs, vaccines, medical devices, and biotechnology drugs and treatments before they enter the stream of commerce.

10903 New Hampshire Avenue
Silver Spring, MD 20993-0002
United States
Phone: (888) 463-6332
Website: http://www.fda.gov

U.S. PATENT OFFICE

The U.S. Patent Office is the governmental body that reviews applications and grants patents and trademarks in the United States. The Patent Office also maintains searchable databases of patent applications and numbers to facilitate licensing.

USPTO Madison Building
600 Dulany Street
Alexandria, VA 22314
United States
Phone: (571) 272-1000
Phone: (800) 786-9199
E-mail: usptoinfo@uspto.gov
Website: http://www.uspto.gov/

WORLD BANK

The World Bank, part of the UN system, describes itself as an organization that offers "financing, state-of-the-art analysis, and policy advice to help countries expand access to quality, affordable health care; protects people from falling into poverty or worsening poverty due to illness; and promotes investments in all sectors that form the foundation of healthy societies."

1818 H Street NW
Washington, DC 20433
United States
Phone: (202) 473-1000
Fax: (202) 477-6391
Website: http://www.worldbank.org

WORLD HEALTH ORGANIZATION (WHO)

The World Health Organization is charged with leading the world on global health matters, especially those impacting public health. In addition to other activities, WHO monitors the outbreak of diseases and epidemics and develops programs to address the spread of disease.

Avenue Appia 20
1211 Geneva 27
Switzerland
Phone: 41 (0)22 791 21 11
Website: http://www.who.int/en/

WORLD HEALTH ORGANIZATION REGIONAL OFFICE FOR AFRICA (AFRO)

The World Health Organization is divided into six regions. The Regional Office for Africa, based in Brazzaville, Republic of the Congo, monitors the outbreak of diseases and epidemics and develops programs to address the spread of disease in the countries in its 47 member states.

Cité du Djoué, P.O. Box 06
Brazzaville
Republic of the Congo
Phone: (47 241) 39100
E-mail: regafro@afro.who.int
Website: http://www.afro.who.int/

WORLD HEALTH ORGANIZATION REGIONAL OFFICE FOR THE EASTERN MEDITERRANEAN (EMRO)

The World Health Organization is divided into six regions. The Regional Office for the Eastern Mediterranean, based in Cairo, Egypt, monitors the outbreak of diseases and epidemics and develops programs to address the spread of disease in the countries in its 21 member states and the Palestinian territories.

Monazamet El Seha El Alamia Str
Extension of Abdel Razak El Sanhouri Street
P.O. Box 7608, Nasr City
Cairo 11371
Egypt
Phone: (20) 2 22765000
Fax: (20) 2 23492092
Website: http://www.emro.who.int/

WORLD HEALTH ORGANIZATION REGIONAL OFFICE FOR EUROPE (EURO)

The World Health Organization is divided into six regions. The Regional Office for Europe, based in Copenhagen, Denmark, monitors the outbreak of diseases and epidemics and develops programs to address the spread of disease in the countries in its 53 member states, which range from the Atlantic to the Pacific Ocean.

UN City
Marmorvej 51
DK-2100 Copenhagen Ø
Denmark
Phone: 45 45 33 70 00
Fax: 45 45 33 70 01
Website: http://www.euro.who.int/en/home

WORLD HEALTH ORGANIZATION REGIONAL OFFICE FOR SOUTH-EAST ASIA (SEARO)

The World Health Organization is divided into six regions. The Regional Office for South-East Asia, based in New Delhi, India, monitors the outbreak of diseases and epidemics and develops programs to address the spread of disease in the countries in its 11 member states.

World Health House
Indraprastha Estate

Mahatma Gandhi Marg
New Delhi 110 002
India
Phone: 91-11-23370804
E-mail: registry@searo.who.int
Website: http://www.searo.who.int/en/

WORLD HEALTH ORGANIZATION REGIONAL OFFICE FOR THE WESTERN PACIFIC (WPRO)

The World Health Organization is divided into six regions. The Regional Office for the Western Pacific, based in Manila, Philippines, monitors the outbreak of diseases and epidemics and develops programs to address the spread of disease in the countries in its 37 member states.

P.O. Box 2932
Manila

Philippines
Phone: 63 2 528 8001
Fax: 63 2 521 1036
E-mail: pio@wpro.who.int
Website: http://www.wpro.who.int/en/

WORLD TRADE ORGANIZATION

The World Trade Organization is an international body that helps formulate and regulate trade agreements among its participating nations.

Centre William Rappard
Rue de Lausanne 154
CH-1211 Geneva 21
Switzerland
Phone: 41 (0)22 739 51 11
Fax: 41 (0)22 731 42 06
E-mail: enquiries@wto.org
Website: https://www.wto.org

General Resources

BOOKS

Abramson, Jon Stuart. *Inside the 2009 Influenza Pandemic.* Singapore: World Scientific, 2011.

Abu-Sada, Caroline. *Dilemmas, Challenges, and Ethics of Humanitarian Action: Reflections on Médecins Sans Frontières' Perception Project.* Montreal: McGill-Queen's University Press, 2012.

Acton, Q. Ashton. *Ebola Virus: New Insights for the Healthcare Professional.* Atlanta: Scholarly Editions, 2012.

Adams, Jonathan, Karen Gurney, and David Pendlebury. *Neglected Tropical Diseases.* Leeds: Evidence, 2012.

Aday, Lu Ann. *At Risk in America: The Health and Health Care Needs of Vulnerable Populations in the United States,* 2d ed. San Francisco, CA: Jossey-Bass, 2001.

Agras, W. Stewart. *The Oxford Handbook of Eating Disorders.* Oxford: Oxford University Press, 2010.

Altman, Stuart H., and David Shactman. *Power, Politics, and Universal Health Care: The Inside Story of a Century-Long Battle.* Amherst, NY: Prometheus Books, 2011.

American Psychiatric Association DSM-5 Task Force. *Diagnostic and Statistical Manual of Mental Disorders,* 5th ed. Washington, DC: American Psychiatric Association, 2013.

Arita, Isao, Alan Schnur, and Masanobu Sugimoto. *The Smallpox Eradication Saga: An Insider's View.* New Delhi: Orient Blackswan, 2010.

Atkinson, William, et al., eds. *Epidemiology and Prevention of Vaccine-Preventable Diseases (The Pink Book),* 13th ed. Washington, DC: The Public Health Foundation, 2014.

Awotona, Adenrele A. *Rebuilding Sustainable Communities with Vulnerable Populations after the Cameras Have Gone: A Worldwide Study.* Newcastle, UK: Cambridge Scholars, 2012.

Ayisi, Ruth Ansah. *The Water, Sanitation and Hygiene Promotion (WASH) Programme, Malawi.* Lilongwe, Malawi: UNICEF Unite for Children, 2010.

Baciu, Alina, Kathleen P. Stratton, and Sheila Burke. *The Future of Drug Safety: Promoting and Protecting the Health of the Public.* Washington, DC: National Academies Press, 2007.

Balch, Phyllis, and Stacey J. Bell. *Prescription for Herbal Healing,* 2nd ed. New York: Avery, 2012.

Balenovic, Damijan, and Emilije Stimac. *Radiation Exposure Sources, Impacts, and Reduction Strategies.* New York: Nova Science, 2012.

Ban Ki-moon. *Global Strategy for Women's and Children's Health.* New York: United Nations, 2010. Available online at http://www.who.int/pmnch/activities/advocacy/fulldocument_globalstrategy/en/ (accessed February 11, 2015).

Barrett, Ron, and George J. Armelagos. *An Unnatural History of Emerging Infections.* Oxford: Oxford University Press, 2013.

Barry, John M. *The Great Influenza: The Epic Story of the Deadliest Plague in History.* New York: Viking, 2004.

Basedow, Jurgen, and Ulrich Magnus. *Pollution of the Sea: Prevention and Compensation.* New York: Springer Science & Business Media, 2007.

Benatar, S. R., and Gillian Brock, eds. *Global Health and Global Health Ethics.* Cambridge, UK: Cambridge University Press, 2011.

Biehl, J. Guilherme, and Adriana Petryna. *When People Come First: Critical Studies in Global Health.* Princeton: Princeton University Press, 2013.

Bray, R. S. *Armies of Pestilence: The Impact of Disease on History.* New York: Barnes & Noble, 2000.

Bristol, N. *Global Action Toward Universal Health Coverage: A Report of the CSIS Global Health Policy Center*. Washington, DC: Center for Strategic and International Studies, 2014.

Bristow, Nancy K. *American Pandemic: The Lost Worlds of the 1918 Influenza Epidemic*. Oxford: Oxford University Press, 2012.

Butler, Colin. *Climate Change and Global Health*. Wallingford, CT: CABI International, 2014.

Chen, Sue, Nicole R. Wyre, and Agnes E. Rupley. *New and Emerging Diseases*. Philadelphia: Elsevier, 2013.

Cliff, A. D., and Matthew Smallman-Raynor. *Oxford Textbook of Infectious Disease Control: A Geographical Analysis from Medieval Quarantine to Global Eradication*. Oxford, UK: Oxford University Press, 2013.

Coates, Anthony R. M. *Antibiotic Resistance: Handbook of Experimental Pharmacology*. Heidelberg: Springer, 2012.

Cox, Chad M., and Ruth Link-Gelles. *Manual for the Surveillance of Vaccine-Preventable Diseases*. Atlanta, GA: U.S. Centers For Disease Control and Prevention, 2012.

Crisp, Nigel. *Turning the World Upside Down: The Search for Global Health in the Twenty-First Century*. London: Royal Society of Medicine Press, 2010.

Cueto, Marcos. *The Value of Health: A History of the Pan American Health Organization*, Washington, DC: Pan American Health Organization, 2007.

Davidson, Ronald J. *Neglected Tropical Diseases: Background, Identification, and Prevention*. New York: Nova Science Publishers, 2011.

De Maio, Fernando.*Global Health Inequities: A Sociological Perspective*. Houndmills, Basingstoke, Hampshire: Palgrave Macmillan 2014.

Dehner, George. *Global Flu and You: A History of Influenza*. London: Reaktion Books, 2012.

Donohoe, Martin. *Public Health and Social Justice*. San Francisco, CA: Jossey-Bass, 2013.

Drlica, Karl, and David Perlin. *Antibiotic Resistance: Understanding and Responding to an Emerging Crisis*. Upper Saddle River, NJ: FT Press, 2011.

Dworkin, Mark S. *Outbreak Investigations Around the World: Case Studies in Infectious Disease Field Epidemiology*. Sudbury, MA: Jones and Bartlett Publishers, 2010.

Elliott, Richard L., and K. Arora. *Third World Diseases*. Berlin: Springer, 2011.

Evans, Timothy, et al., eds. *Challenging Inequities in Health: From Ethics to Action*. New York: Oxford University Press, 2001.

Falola, Toyin, and Matthew M. Heaton, eds. *HIV/AIDS, Illness, and African Well-Being*. Rochester, NY: University of Rochester Press, 2007.

Fagan, Brian. *Elixir: A History of Water and Humankind*. New York: Bloomsbury Press, 2011.

Fairman, David, et al. *Negotiating Public Health in a Globalized World: Global Health Diplomacy in Action*. New York: Springer, 2012.

Farmer, Paul, Jim Yong Kim, Arthur Kleinman, and Matthew Basilico. *Reimagining Global Health*. Berkeley: University of California Press, 2013.

Flynn, James, Paul Slovic, and Howard Kunreuther, eds. *Risk, Media, and Stigma: Understanding Public Challenges to Modern Science and Technology*. London: Earthscan, 2004.

Foa, Edna B., and Terence Keane, eds. *Effective Treatments for PTSD: Practice and Guidelines from the International Society for Traumatic Stress*, 2nd ed. New York: Guilford Press, 2008.

Fong, I. W., and Kenneth Alibek, eds. *Bioterrorism and Infectious Agents: A New Dilemma for the 21st Century*. New York: Springer, 2005.

Fox, Renée C. *Doctors Without Borders: Humanitarian Quests, Impossible Dreams of Médicins Sans Frontières*. Baltimore: Johns Hopkins University Press, 2014.

Henderson, Donald A. *Smallpox: The Death of a Disease*. Amherst, NY: Prometheus Books, 2014.

Holtz, Carol, ed. *Global Health Care: Issues and Policies*, 2nd ed. Burlington, MA: Jones & Bartlett Learning, 2012.

Intergovernmental Panel on Climate Change. *Climate Change 2013: The Physical Science Basis*. New York: Cambridge University Press, 2013.

International Diabetes Federation (IDF). *IDF Diabetes Atlas*, 6th Ed. Brussels, Belgium: International Diabetes Federation, 2013.

Kaslow, Richard A., Lawrence R. Stanberry, and J. W. LeDuc. *Viral Infections of Humans: Epidemiology and Control*. New York: Springer, 2014.

Kestenbaum, Bryan, Kathryn L. Adeney, and Noel S. Weiss, eds. *Epidemiology and Biostatistics: An Introduction to Clinical Research*. New York: Springer, 2009.

Koch, T. *Disease Maps: Epidemics on the Ground*. Chicago, IL: University of Chicago Press, 2011.

Langwith, Jacqueline. *Population, Resources, and Conflict*. Detroit: Greenhaven Press, 2011.

Latzer, Yael, Joav Merrick, and Daniel Stein. *Understanding Eating Disorders: Integrating Culture, Psychology and Biology.* New York: Nova Science, 2011.

Lawman, Michael J. P., and Patricia D. Lawman. *Cancer Vaccines: Methods and Protocols.* New York: Springer, 2014.

McGuire, Robert A., and Philip R. P. Coelho. *Parasites, Pathogens, and Progress: Diseases and Economic Development.* Cambridge, MA: MIT Press, 2011.

McInnes, Colin, and Kelley Lee. *Global Health and International Relations.* Malden, MA: Polity, 2012.

McVeigh, Enda, Roy Homburg, and John Guillebaud. *Oxford Handbook of Reproductive Medicine and Family Planning,* 2nd ed. Oxford, UK: Oxford University Press, 2013.

Nellemann, C., et al., eds. *The Environmental Food Crisis: The Environment's Role in Averting Future Food Crises.* Arendal, Norway: UNEP, 2009. Available online at http://www.grida.no/files/publications/FoodCrisis_lores.pdf (accessed June 12, 2015).

Nutt, David J., and Liam Nestor. *Substance Abuse.* Oxford, UK: Oxford University Press, 2013.

Okpaku, Samuel O. *Essentials of Global Mental Health.* Cambridge: Cambridge University Press, 2014.

Plotkin, Stanley A. *History of Vaccine Development.* New York: Springer, 2011.

Plotkin, Stanley A., Walter Orenstein, and Paul Offit, *Vaccines,* 6th ed. Philadelphia, PA: Elsevier Saunders, 2013.

Power, Chris, and Richard T. Johnson. *Emerging Neurological Infections.* Hoboken, NJ: Taylor and Francis, 2013.

Sen, Amartya. *Poverty and Famines: An Essay on Entitlement.* Oxford, UK: Oxford University Press, 1981.

Sen, Gita, and Piroska Östlin. *Gender Equity in Health: The Shifting Frontiers of Evidence and Action.* New York: Routledge, 2010.

United Nations. *Global Strategy for Women's and Children's Health.* New York: UNICEF, 2010. Available online at http://www.who.int/pmnch/activities/advocacy/fulldocument_globalstrategy/en/ (accessed June 12, 2015).

Walraven, Gijsbertus Engelinus Laurentius. *Health and Poverty: Global Health Problems and Solutions.* London: Earthscan, 2011.

World Health Organization (WHO) and Food and Agriculture Organization (FAO) of the United Nations. *Diet, Nutrition and the Prevention of Chronic Diseases: Report of a Joint WHO/FAO Expert Consultation.* Geneva: World Health Organization, 2003.

World Health Organization. *UN-Water Global Analysis and Assessment of Sanitation and Drinking-Water (GLAAS) 2014 Report: Investing in Water and Sanitation: Increasing Access, Reducing Inequalities.* Geneva: World Health Organization, 2014. Available online at http://www.who.int/water_sanitation_health/publications/glaas_report_2014/en/ (accessed June 14, 2015).

Youde, Jeremy. *Global Health Governance.* Cambridge, MA: Polity, 2012.

PERIODICALS

Andrade, L. H., et al. "Barriers to Mental Health Treatment: Results from the WHO World Mental Health Surveys." *Psychological Medicine* 44, no. 6 (April 2014): 1303–1317.

Arvanitakis, Constantine, and Nurdan Tozun. "Mediterranean Diet: Health and Culture." *International Journal of Anthropology* 28, no. 4 (2013): 207–235.

Baker, Michael, and Fidler, David. "Global Public Health Surveillance under New International Health Regulations." *Emerging Infectious Diseases* 12, no. 7 (July 2006): 1058–1065.

Baker, Peter A., et al. "The Men's Health Gap: Men Must Be Included in the Global Health Agenda." *Bulletin of the World Health Organization* 92, no. 8 (August 1, 2014): 618–620.

Bakhshi, Savita. "Women's Body Image and the Role of Culture: A Review of Literature." *Europe's Journal of Psychology* 7, no. 2 (December 2010): 374–394. Available online at http://ejop.psychopen.eu/article/download/135/pdf (accessed April 7, 2015).

Banks, Nicola, and David Hulme. "The Role of NGOs and Civil Society in Development and Poverty Reduction." *Brooks World Poverty Institute Working Paper* 171 (June 1, 2012) Available online at http://www.slideshare.net/purbitaditecha/bwpiwp17112 (accessed April 13, 2015).

Bhutta, Zulfiqar A., and Robert E. Black. "Global Maternal, Newborn and Child Health—So Near and Yet So Far." *New England Journal of Medicine* 369, no. 23 (December 5, 2013): 2226–2235.

Brockwell-Staats, Christy, Robert G. Webster, and Richard J. Webby. "Diversity of Influenza Viruses in Swine and the Emergence of a Novel Human Pandemic Influenza A (H1N1)." *Influenza and Other Respiratory Viruses* 3, no. 5 (2009): 207–213.

Cabral, S. A., A. T. Soares de Moura, and J. E. Berkelhamer. "Overview of the Global Health Issues Facing Children." *Pediatrics* 129, no. 1 (January 2012): 1–3. doi:10.1542/peds.2011-2665.

Cerón, Alejandro. "Review of *Life in Crisis: The Ethical Journey of Doctors Without Borders.*" *Global Public Health* 8, no. 10 (2013): 1180–1181.

Chen, K. "Review of *Doctors Without Borders.*" *Science* 346, no. 6215 (2014): 1304.

Cooley, Alexander, and James Ron. "The NGO Scramble: Organizational Insecurity and the Political Economy of Transnational Action." *International Security* 27, no. 1 (Summer 2002): 5–39.

Costello, Anthony, et al. "Managing the Health Effects of Climate Change." *The Lancet* 373, no. 9676 (May 16, 2009): 1693–1733.

Deer, Brian. "How the Case against the MMR Vaccine Was Fixed." *British Medical Journal* 342, no. 7788 (January 8, 2011): 77–82.

Drazen, Jeffrey M., et al. "Ebola and Quarantine." *New England Journal of Medicine* 371, no. 21 (2014): 2029–2030.

Ernst, Edzard. "The Public's Enthusiasm for Complementary and Alternative Medicine Amounts to a Critique of Mainstream Medicine." *International Journal of Clinical Practice* 64, no. 11 (October 2010): 1472–1474.

Estrin, D. "Small Data, Where n = me." *Communications of the ACM* 57, no. 4 (April 2014): 32–34.

Fidler, David. "From International Sanitary Conventions to Global Health Security: The New International Health Regulations." *Chinese Journal of International Law* 4, no. 2 (September 2005): 325–392.

Fidler, David, and Lawrence Gostin. "The New International Health Regulations: An Historic Development for International Law and Public Health." *Journal of Law, Medicine and Ethics* 34, no. 1 (February 2006): 84–95.

Fineberg, Harvey V. "Pandemic Preparedness and Response—Lessons from the H1N1 Influenza of 2009." *New England Journal of Medicine* 370, no. 14 (April 2014): 1335–1342. Available online at http://www.nejm.org/doi/full/10.1056/NEJMra1208802 (accessed January 23, 2015).

Friedrich, M. J. "Neglected Tropical Diseases." *JAMA* 304, no. 19 (2010): 2116.

Hoang, Van Mingh, and Hung Nguyen-Viet. "Economic Aspects of Sanitation in Developing Countries." *Environmental Health Insights* 5 (2011): 63–70.

Jones, Kate, et al. "Global Trends in Emerging Infectious Diseases." *Nature* 451, no. 7181 (February 2008): 990–993.

Lachat, C., et al. "Diet and Physical Activity for the Prevention of Noncommunicable Diseases in Low- and Middle-income Countries: A Systematic Policy Review." *PLOS Medicine* 10, no. 6 (2013): e1001465.

Lucchini, Roberto, and Leslie London. "Global Occupational Health: Current Challenges and the Need for Urgent Action." *Annals of Global Health* 80 (2014): 251–256.

Martelli, P. "Working Together for Public Health." *Transcultural Psychiatry* 46, no. 2 (2009): 316–327.

Mombouli, J. V., and S. M. Ostroff. "The Remaining Smallpox Stocks: the Healthiest Outcome." *The Lancet* 379, no. 9810 (January 7, 2012): 10–12.

Morens, David M., Gregory K. Folkers, and Anthony S. Fauci. "What Is a Pandemic?" *Journal of Infectious Diseases* 200, no. 7 (August 2009): 1018–1021.

New York Times Editorial Board. "The Race to Improve Global Health." *New York Times* (September 11, 2013): A26. Available online at http://www.nytimes.com/2013/09/11/opinion/the-race-to-improve-global-health.html?_r=0 (accessed February 4, 2015).

Perry, Phil, and Fred Donini-Lenhoff. "Stigmatization Complicates Infectious Disease Management." *AMA Journal of Ethics* 12, no. 3 (March 2010): 225–230. Available online at http://journalofethics.ama-assn.org/2010/03/mhst1-1003.html (accessed June 14, 2015).

Qaim, Matin, and Shahzad Kouser. "Genetically Modified Crops and Food Security." *PLOS ONE* 8, no. 6 (June 2013): e64879.

Ross, Catherine E., Ryan K. Masters, and Robert A. Hummer. "Education and the Gender Gaps in Health and Mortality." *Demography* 49, no. 4 (November 2012): 1157–1183.

Sartorius, Norman. "Stigmatized Illnesses and Health Care." *Croatian Medical Journal* 48, no. 3 (June 2007): 396–397. Available online at http://www.ncbi.nlm.nih.gov/pmc/articles/PMC2080544/ (accessed June 14, 2015).

Scambler, Graham. "Stigma and Disease: Changing Paradigms." *The Lancet* 352, no. 9133 (September 26, 1998): 1054–1055. Available online at http://www.thelancet.com/pdfs/journals/lancet/PIIS0140-6736(98)08068-4.pdf (accessed June 14, 2015).

Stenberg, Karin, et al. "Advancing Social and Economic Development by Investing in Women's and Children's Health: A New Global Investment Framework." *The Lancet* 383, no. 9925 (April 12, 2014): 1333–1354.

Swinburn, B. A., et al. "The Global Obesity Pandemic: Shaped by Global Drivers and Local Environments." *The Lancet* 378, no. 9793 (August 2011): 804–814.

Tognotti, Eugenia. "Lessons from the History of Quarantine, from Plague to Influenza A." *Emerging Infectious Diseases* 19, no. 2 (February 2013): 254–259.

Wickett, J., and P. Carrasco. "Logistics in Smallpox: The Legacy." *Vaccine* 29 (December 30, 2011): D131–134.

Zaidi, S. Akbar. "NGO Failure and the Need to Bring Back the State." *Journal of International Development* 11, no. 2 (March–April 1999): 259–271.

Zhang, Qiucen, et al. "You Cannot Tell a Book by Looking at the Cover: Cryptic Complexity in Bacterial Evolution." *Biomicrofluidics* 8, no. 5 (September 9, 2014): 052004.

Zhou, Xiao-Nong, et al. "Potential Impact of Climate Change on Schistosomiasis Transmission in China." *American Journal of Tropical Medicine and Hygiene* 78, no. 2 (February 2008): 188–194.

Zumla, Alimuddin, Payam Nahid, and Stewart T. Cole. "Advances in the Development of New Tuberculosis Drugs and Treatment Regimens." *Nature Reviews Drug Discovery* 12, no. 5 (May 2013): 388–404.

WEBSITES

"About Pandemics." *Flu.gov.* http://www.flu.gov/pandemic/about/ (accessed June 14, 2015).

"About Us: MyPlate." *United States Department of Agriculture (USDA).* http://www.choosemyplate.gov/about.html (accessed June 14, 2015).

"About WHO: WHO Reform." *World Health Organization (WHO).* http://www.who.int/about/who_reform/en/ (accessed June 14, 2015).

"About Zoonoses." *National Consortium for Zoonosis Research Hosted by the University of Liverpool.* http://www.zoonosis.ac.uk/about-zoonoses/ (accessed June 14, 2015).

"Acting on the Call: Ending Preventable Child and Maternal Death." *United States Agency for International Development.* http://www.usaid.gov/ActingOnTheCall (accessed June 14, 2015).

"Burden of Disease from Air Pollution for 2012." *World Health Organization (WHO).* http://www.who.int/phe/health_topics/outdoorair/databases/FINAL_HAP_AAP_BoD_24March2014.pdf? (accessed February 10, 2015).

"CDC Learns from Katrina, Plans for Pandemic." *U.S. Centers for Disease Control and Prevention (CDC).* http://www.cdc.gov/news/2006_11/katrina.htm (accessed January 27, 2015).

"CDC: Saving Lives. Protecting People." *U.S. Centers for Disease Control and Prevention (CDC),* August 2014. http://www.cdc.gov/about/report/2013/docs/cdcreport_2013.pdf (accessed June 14, 2015).

"Celebrating 110 Years of Health." *Pan American Health Organization (PAHO).* http://issuu.com/paho2012/docs/paho110_album3_screen/1?e=6477936/5775595 (accessed June 14, 2015).

"Celebrating 25 years of the Convention on the Rights of the Child." *World Health Organization (WHO).* http://www.who.int/maternal_child_adolescent/topics/child/en/ (accessed June 14, 2015).

"Child Health." *World Health Organization (WHO).* http://www.who.int/topics/child_health/en/ (accessed June 14, 2015).

"Climate Change and Human Health—Risks and Responses." *World Health Organization (WHO).* http://www.who.int/globalchange/summary/en/index5.html (accessed June 14, 2015).

"Combating Antibiotic Resistance." *U.S. Food and Drug Administration (FDA).* http://www.fda.gov/ForConsumers/ConsumerUpdates/ucm092810.htm (accessed June 14, 2015).

"Comparative Analysis of National Pandemic Influenza Preparedness Plans." *World Health Organization (WHO),* January 2011. http://www.who.int/influenza/resources/documents/comparative_analysis_php_2011_en.pdf (accessed March 20, 2015).

"Complementary, Alternative, or Integrative Health: What's in a Name?" *National Center for Complementary and Integrative Health (NCCIH).* https://nccih.nih.gov/health/integrative-health (accessed June 14, 2015).

"Disasters and Conflicts." *United Nations Environment Programme (UNEP).* http://www.unep.org/disastersandconflicts/ (accessed June 14, 2015).

"E-Cigarette Use Triples among Middle and High School Students in Just One Year." *U.S. Centers for Disease Control and Prevention (CDC),* April 16, 2015. http://www.cdc.gov/media/releases/2015/p0416-e-cigarette-use.html (accessed June 14, 2015).

Gavi: The Vaccine Alliance. http://www.gavi.org (accessed June 14, 2015).

"Global Food Security." *United Nations (UN).* http://www.un-foodsecurity.org/ (accessed June 14, 2015).

"Global Health Initiatives" *World Health Organization (WHO).* http://www.who.int/trade/glossary/story040/en# (accessed June 14, 2015).

Global Polio Eradication Initiative. http://www.polioeradication.org/ (accessed June 14, 2015).

"Global Status Report on Noncommunicable Diseases 2014." *World Health Organization (WHO),* 2014. http://www.who.int/nmh/publications/ncd-status-report-2014/en/ (accessed June 14, 2015).

"Humanitarian Pandemic Preparedness Programme." *International Federation of Red Cross and Red Crescent Societies.* http://www.ifrc.org/en/what-we-do/health/diseases/pandemic-influenza/humanitarian-pandemic-preparedness-programme/ (accessed June 14, 2015).

"Hunger." *World Food Programme.* http://www.wfp.org/hunger (accessed June 14, 2015).

"IHR Review Committee on Second Extensions for Establishing National Public Health Capacities and on IHR Implementation." *World Health Organization (WHO).* http://www.who.int/ihr/qa-ihr-rc-11nov.pdf (accessed June 14, 2015).

"Immunizations, Vaccines, and Biologicals." *World Health Organization (WHO).* http://www.who.int/immunization/en/ (accessed June 14, 2015).

"The Impacts of Climate Change on Health." *Climate and Health Council.* http://www.climateandhealth.org/health_impacts.html (accessed June 14, 2015).

"Influenza." *World Health Organization (WHO).* http://www.who.int/topics/influenza/en/ (accessed June 14, 2015).

International Committee of the Red Cross. https://www.icrc.org/en (accessed June 14, 2015).

International Federation of Red Cross and Red Crescent Societies. http://www.ifrc.org/ (accessed June 14, 2015).

"International Health Regulations (2005)," 2nd ed. *World Health Organization (WHO),* 2005. http://whqlibdoc.who.int/publications/2008/9789241580410_eng.pdf?q=international (accessed June 14, 2015).

"LGBT Health and Well-Being." *U.S. Department of Health and Human Services.* http://www.hhs.gov/lgbt/ (accessed June 14, 2015).

Malaria No More. http://www.malarianomore.org (accessed June 14, 2015).

"Malnutrition." *Médecins Sans Frontières/Doctors Without Borders.* http://www.doctorswithoutborders.org/our-work/medical-issues/malnutrition (accessed June 14, 2015).

"Managing Vulnerable Populations." *World Health Organization (WHO).* http://www.who.int/substance_abuse/publications/vulnerable_pop/en/ (accessed June 14, 2015).

"Marine Toxins." *U.S. Centers for Disease Control and Prevention (CDC).* http://www.cdc.gov/ncidod/dbmd/diseaseinfo/marinetoxins_g.htm (accessed June 14, 2014).

Médecins Sans Frontières/Doctors Without Borders. http://www.doctorswithoutborders.org (accessed June 14, 2015).

"The Millennium Development Goals Report 2014." *United Nations (UN).* http://www.un.org/millenniumgoals/2014%20MDG%20report/MDG%202014%20English%20web.pdf (accessed June 14, 2015).

"Nongovernmental Organizations (NGOs)." *Fogarty International Center, National Institutes of Health (U.S.).* http://www.fic.nih.gov/Global/Pages/NGOs.aspx (accessed June 14, 2015).

Pan American Health Organization (PAHO). http://www.paho.org/hq/ (accessed June 14, 2015).

"Pandemic Flu History." *Flu.gov.* http://www.flu.gov/pandemic/history/index.html (accessed June 14, 2015).

"Preventing Unsafe Abortion." Fact Sheet No. 388. *World Health Organization (WHO),* March 2014. http://www.who.int/mediacentre/factsheets/fs388/en/ (accessed June 14, 2015).

"PTSD: National Center for PTSD." *U.S. Department of Veterans Affairs.* http://www.ptsd.va.gov (accessed June 14, 2015).

"Quarantine and Isolation." *U.S. Centers for Disease Control and Prevention (CDC).* http://www.cdc.gov/quarantine/ (accessed June 14, 2015).

"Quick Guide to Health Literacy." *U.S. Department of Health and Human Services.* http://www.health.gov/communication/literacy/quickguide/ (accessed June 14, 2015).

"Radiation Emergencies." *U.S. Centers for Disease Control and Prevention (CDC).* http://emergency.cdc.gov/radiation/ (accessed June 14, 2015).

"Stigma and Illness." *U.S. Centers for Disease Control and Prevention (CDC).* http://www.cdc.gov/mentalhealth/about_us/stigma-illness.htm (accessed June 14, 2015).

"Strategic National Stockpile (SNS)." *U.S. Centers for Disease Control and Prevention, Office of Public*

Health Preparedness and Response. http://www .cdc.gov/phpr/stockpile/stockpile.htm (accessed June 14, 2015).

Sun, Lena H. "CIA: No More Vaccination Campaigns in Spy Operations." *Washington Post*, May 19, 2014. http://www.washingtonpost.com/ world/national-security/cia-no-more-vaccination-campaigns-in-spy-operations/2014/05/19/406 c4f3e-df88–11e3-8dcc-d6b7fede081a_story.html (accessed June 14, 2015).

"Tobacco." *World Health Organization (WHO)*. http://www.who.int/topics/tobacco/en/ (accessed June 14, 2014).

"Vaccine Safety: Smallpox." *U.S. Centers for Disease Control and Prevention (CDC)*. http://www .cdc.gov/vaccinesafety/emergency/smallpox .htm (accessed June 14, 2015).

"Vaccines and Diseases." *World Health Organization (WHO)*. http://www.who.int/immunization/ diseases/en/ (accessed June 14, 2015).

"Viral Hemorrhagic Fevers." *U.S. Centers for Disease Control and Prevention (CDC)*. http://www.cdc .gov/ncidod/dvrd/spb/mnpages/dispages/vhf .htm (accessed June 14, 2015).

"Vulnerable Populations." *U.S. Department of Health and Human Services.* http://www.hhs.gov/ohrp/ policy/populations/ (accessed June 14, 2015).

"Water & Sanitation Specialists." *Médicins Sans Frontières/Doctors Without Borders.* (accessed June 14, 2015).

"Water Projects & Programs." *The World Bank.* http://www.worldbank.org/en/topic/water/ projects (accessed June 14, 2015).

"WHO PMTCT Guidelines." *AVERT: AVERTing HIV and AIDS.* http://www.avert.org/world-health-organisation-who-pmtct-guidelines.htm (accessed June 14, 2015).

"WHO Raises the Alarm over Nutrition Problems." *World Health Organization (WHO), Regional Office for South-East Asia,* 2011. http://origin .searo.who.int/mediacentre/releases/2011/ pr1528/en/ (accessed June 14, 2015).

"The World Factbook." *U.S. Central Intelligence Agency (CIA).* https://www.cia.gov/library/ publications/resources/the-world-factbook/ (accessed June 14, 2015).

"Workers' Health: Global Plan of Action." *World Health Organization (WHO),* 2007. http://www .who.int/occupational_health/publications/ global_plan/en/ (accessed June 14, 2015).

World Health Organization Regional Office for Africa (AFRO). http://www.afro.who.int/ (accessed June 14, 2015).

World Health Organization Regional Office for Europe (EURO). http://www.euro.who.int/ (accessed June 14, 2015).

World Health Organization Regional Office for the Eastern Mediterranean (EMRO). http://www .emro.who.int/index.html (accessed June 14, 2015).

World Health Organization Regional Office for South-East Asia (SEARO). http://www.searo.who.int/ en/ (accessed June 14, 2015).

World Health Organization Regional Office for the Western Pacific (WPRO). http://www.wpro .who.int/en/ (accessed June 14, 2015).

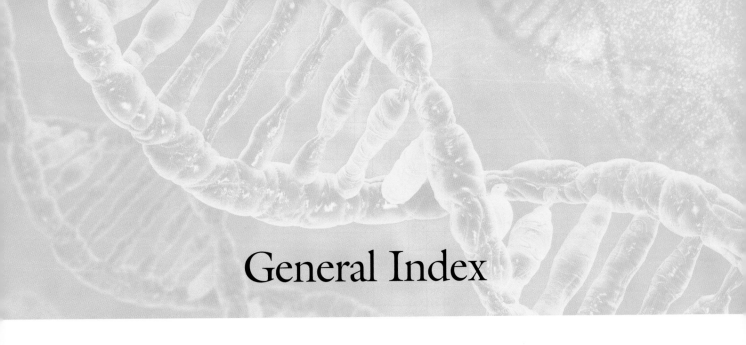

General Index

"Flesh-eating disease." *See* Necrotizing fasciitis

Flexner, Simon, 2:535

Flooding, 1:96–97

Florey, Howard, 1:33

Flu. *See* Influenza

Flucytosine, 1:200

Fluoroquinolones, 1:18–19

Foley, Jonathan A., 1:189

"Folk Remedy–Associated Lead Poisoning in Hmong Children—Minnesota" (CDC), 1:*123*

Food aid, 1:80, 377–380

Food and Agriculture Organization, UN
  Codex Alimentarius, 1:*193–194*
  food assistance, 1:377
  food safety, 1:178–179
  food security and hunger, 1:119, 187
  prevention of food-borne illnesses, 1:183
  zoonotic diseases, 2:709

Food and Drug Administration, U.S.
  cultural and traditional medical products, 1:122
  direct-to-consumer genetic test kits, 1:214
  Exserohilum rostratum outbreak, 1:199–200
  influenza vaccines, 1:330
  pandemic preparedness, 2:501–502
  pharmaceutical research, testing, and access, 2:520–521
  smallpox research stocks, 2:597
  weight-loss drugs, 2:466–467

Food and Drug Administration Modernization Act (U.S.), 2:521

Food fortification, 1:395

Food poisoning, 1:37, 101

Food production. *See* Agriculture and food production

Food safety and food preparation, 1:**178–186,** *179, 181*
  bacterial diseases, 1:37
  Centers for Disease Control and Prevention, 1:68
  common food-borne illnesses, 1:179, *180,* 180–182
  future implications, 1:183–184
  health promotion and social media, 1:300
  historical background, 1:178–179
  listeriosis, 1:184–185
  marine toxins and pollution, 1:383–389
  prevention of food-borne illnesses, 1:182–183

  safe minimum cooking temperatures, 1:*183*
  technology, 1:*184*
  viral hepatitis, 2:662, 663

Food security and hunger, 1:**187–195,** *188, 190, 191*
  children, 1:79–80
  climate change, impact of, 1:190–191
  Codex Alimentarius (FAO), 1:*193–194*
  genetically modified crops, 1:191–192
  Global Day of Action against Hunger, 2:*458*
  historical background, 1:188–189
  malnutrition, 1:374–376, 377–382
  Millennium Development Goals, 1:187
  nutrition, 2:459
  policies, 1:189–190
  population growth, 1:192, 2:543, 544
  The State of Food Insecurity in the World (UN Food and Agriculture Organization), 1:*381–382*
  World Food Summit, 1:187

Food waste reduction, 1:189

Foot binding, 1:44

Ford, Gerald R., 1:25

Former Soviet Union, 1:268

Fort Reilly (Kansas), 1:111

Fossil fuels, 1:1, 95

Foucault, Michel, 2:599

Fouchier, Ron, 1:29

Four humors, 1:47–48

Framework Convention on Tobacco Control (WHO), 2:615, 618, 703

France, 1:214, 409–410

Fraud, research, 2:638

French Guyana, 1:97–98

Freud, Sigmund, 1:145, 410

Frieden, Thomas, 1:69, *69,* 71, 155, 2:539, 540

Friedlander, Carl, 2:528

Frontal lobotomy, 1:410

Fujifilm, 2:*524*

Fukuda, Keiji, 1:*349*

Fukushima Daiichi nuclear power plant, 2:572–573, *573*

Funding
  Centers for Disease Control and Prevention, 1:*67*
  cholera crisis in Haiti, 1:88
  complementary and alternative medicine research, 1:107
  European Centre for Disease Prevention and Control, 1:68

  gender disparities in research, 1:208
  leprosy treatment, 1:35
  malnutrition problems, 1:380
  mobile health technologies, 1:422
  National Center for Complementary and Integrative Health, 1:119
  nongovernmental organizations, 2:444
  President's Emergency Plan for AIDS Relief, 1:231, *232*
  sanitation and hygiene initiatives, 2:579
  universal health coverage, 2:629–630
  vaccines, 2:638–639
  World Health Organization, 2:698

Fungal diseases, 1:19, 20, **196–202,** *197, 201,* 2:526

Funk, Casimir, 2:456

G

Gajdusek, D. Carleton, 2:564, 567

Galen, 1:47–48, 57

Galli, Costanza, 2:566

Gallup, Inc., 2:479

Garment industry, 2:692, 693

Garrastazu Médici, Emilio, 2:492

Gastrointestinal diseases. *See* Diarrhea and diarrheal diseases

Gates, Bill, 2:*441*

Gates Foundation. *See* Bill and Melinda Gates Foundation

Gauhati, India, 1:*275*

Gaupp, Robert, 2:550

Gavi, the Vaccine Alliance 1:78, 234

Gaza Strip, 1:*413*

Gender, 1:**203–209,** *207*
  alcohol use and abuse, 1:13
  body image and eating disorders, 1:40, 41
  cancer, 1:48, 2:449
  cardiovascular diseases, 1:59, 63–64
  drug abuse, 1:149
  obesity, 2:463
  organ donation, 2:480

Gender and Women's Health Program, WHO, 1:209

Gender reassignment, 1:218

General Chiropractic Council, 1:107

Genetic Information Nondiscrimination Act, 1:215

Genetic modification
  crops, 1:191–194, 380
  mosquitoes, 1:131, 340

Genetic testing, 1:**211–217,** *213*

SARS, 2:**584–591**, *586*
 epidemiology, 1:167
 International Health Regulations,
  1:346
 isolation and quarantine, 1:357
 research stocks, 2:596
"SARS and Carlo Urbani" (*New
 England Journal of Medicine*),
 2:*590–591*
Satin, Morton, 1:178
Sato, Hiroko, 2:646
Sato, Yuji, 2:646
Saudi Arabia, 2:*588*
Saxitoxin, 1:384
Scheper-Hughes, Nancy, 2:475
Schistosomiasis, 1:97, 2:434–435,
 437, 687–688
Schmiedeberg, Oswald, 2:520
Schubert, Franz, 1:178
Schuchat, Anne, 1:*314*
Science-Based Medicine (organiza-
 tion), 1:106
Scombroid fish poisoning, 1:386
Scotland, 1:10
Scott, Walter, 2:535
Screening. *See* Testing and screening
Scrimshaw, Nevin, 1:376
Scurvy, 2:455–456, 518
S.E. Massengill Company, 2:520
Sea levels, 1:94, 96, *96*
Sea lions, 1:*385*
Seaman, John, 2:442
Sebelius, Kathleen, 2:477
Secondhand smoke, 2:615
Security, data, 1:426
Sedgh, Gilda, 2:558
Selective serotonin reuptake inhibi-
 tors, 2:553
Self-care, 1:279
Sen, Amartya, 1:379–380
Senegal, 1:225
Septic tanks, 2:676
Sertürner, Friedrich W. A., 1:145
Severe acute malnutrition, 1:73, 74,
 79–80
Severe acute respiratory syndrome.
 See SARS
Sewage. *See* Sanitation and hygiene;
 Water supplies and access to clean
 water
Sex education, 1:302
Sex ratio, 2:*557*
Sexual abuse, 1:74, 205–206
Sexually transmitted diseases
 gender, 1:208
 Pan-American Interoceanic High-
  way, 2:494

stigma, 2:607
 wars, 1:110
Shaikh, Babar T., 2:442
Sharps accidents, 1:291
Shellfish poisoning. *See* Marine toxins
 and pollution
Shiga, Kiyoshi, 1:86
Shigella. See Cholera and dysentery
Shigellosis, 2:686
Shingles, 2:651
Shortages, health-care worker. *See*
 Health-care worker safety and
 shortages
Shumway, Norman, 2:473
Sickle cell gene, 1:369
Sickles, Grace, 2:650
Sickness Insurance Law, 1:237
Sidibé, Michel, 1:*231, 324*, 2:654
Sierra Leone, 1:152, 154
Simian immunodeficiency virus,
 1:319, 320
Singapore, 2:617
Single-payer health insurance model,
 1:239–240
Sirleaf, Ellen Johnson, 1:*303*, 358
Sleep medications, 2:553
Smallpox, 1:166, 2:**592–597**, *593,
 594*, 700–701
Smartphones, 1:422–425, *425*
Smith, Theobald, 2:643
Smog, 1:2, 3, 5
Smoking. *See* Tobacco use
Snider, Dixie E., 1:66
Snow, John, 1:85, 164, 169–170,
 2:575, 684
Sobel, Jeremy, 1:384
Social distancing, 1:333, 356
Social issues
 alcohol use and abuse, 1:9–10, *12*
 behavior change, 1:83
 global health initiatives, 1:230
 obstetric fistula, 1:399
 social determinants of health,
  1:233, 258, 2:666, 672
 stigma, 2:605–611
 viral hepatitis, 2:662
 WHO Americas region, 1:258
Social media, 1:300
Social mobilization campaigns, 1:158
Social networking, 1:424
Social theory, 2:**599–604**
Socioeconomic issues, 1:230,
 285–286, 313
Soil-transmitted helminth infections,
 2:435, 507, 508, 509
Solid fuel stoves, 1:4, 5, 6
Soma, Turkey, 2:*693*

Somali refugees, 1:*191*, 2:*669, 678*
Somalia, 1:225, *235, 375*
Sommer, Hermann, 1:383
Sonograms, 1:*61*
Soper, Fred, 2:483
Soto, Claudio, 2:566
South Africa
 health education and information
  access, 1:300, 301
 health care, 1:239
 mobile health technologies, 1:424
South America. *See* Latin America
South Asia
 child mortality, 1:74
 cholera, 1:85
 diarrheal diseases, 1:90
 food security and hunger, 1:191
 malaria, 1:76
 noma, 1:79
 nongovernmental organizations,
  2:440
South Korea, 1:26, 363
South Sudan, 1:*91*, 2:*507, 636*
South-central Asia, 1:175
Southeast Asia
 dengue, 1:127
 diarrhea, 2:684
 family planning, 1:175
 See also WHO South-East Asia
  region
Southern Asia, 1:398
Soviet Union, 1:12
Soviet Union, former, 2:573
Spain, 1:154, 363
Spay/neuter clinics, 2:*708*
Sporotrichosis, 1:199
Sports facilities, 1:419
Sri Lanka, 1:10, 370
Srinagar, India, 1:*34*
Staging, cancer, 1:53–55
Stanger-Hall, Kathrin F., 1:302
State governments and nongovern-
 mental organizations, 2:440
State health departments, U.S., 1:69
*The State of Food Insecurity in the
 World* (UN Food and Agriculture
 Organization, International Fund
 for Agricultural Development,
 and World Food Programme),
 1:*381–382*
Statistics
 epidemiological concepts,
  1:165–166
 mobile health technologies, 1:426
Stent angioplasty, 1:60, *60*
Sterilization (contraception method),
 1:173
Steroid hormones, 2:512, 515–516